# Practical
# Pediatrics

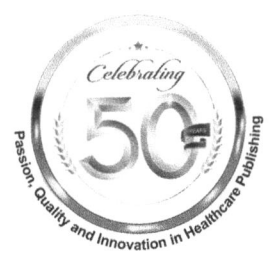

# Practical Pediatrics

**Aruchamy Lakshmanaswamy**
MBBS MD (Pediatrics) DCH
Associate Professor
Department of Pediatrics
Coimbatore Medical College
Coimbatore, Tamil Nadu, India

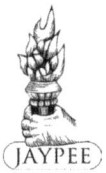

**JAYPEE BROTHERS MEDICAL PUBLISHERS**
*The Health Sciences Publisher*
New Delhi | London

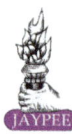 **Jaypee Brothers Medical Publishers (P) Ltd**

**Headquarters**
Jaypee Brothers Medical Publishers (P) Ltd
4838/24, Ansari Road, Daryaganj
New Delhi 110 002, India
Phone: +91-11-43574357
Fax: +91-11-43574314
Email: jaypee@jaypeebrothers.com

**Overseas Offices**
J.P. Medical Ltd
83 Victoria Street, London
SW1H 0HW (UK)
Phone: +44 20 3170 8910
Fax: +44 (0)20 3008 6180
Email: info@jpmedpub.com

Jaypee Brothers Medical Publishers (P) Ltd
Bhotahity, Kathmandu
Nepal
Phone: +977-9741283608
Email: kathmandu@jaypeebrothers.com

Website: www.jaypeebrothers.com
Website: www.jaypeedigital.com

© 2020, Jaypee Brothers Medical Publishers

The views and opinions expressed in this book are solely those of the original contributor(s)/author(s) and do not necessarily represent those of editor(s) of the book.

All rights reserved. No part of this publication may be reproduced, stored or transmitted in any form or by any means, electronic, mechanical, photocopying, recording or otherwise, without the prior permission in writing of the publishers.

All brand names and product names used in this book are trade names, service marks, trademarks or registered trademarks of their respective owners. The publisher is not associated with any product or vendor mentioned in this book.

Medical knowledge and practice change constantly. This book is designed to provide accurate, authoritative information about the subject matter in question. However, readers are advised to check the most current information available on procedures included and check information from the manufacturer of each product to be administered, to verify the recommended dose, formula, method and duration of administration, adverse effects and contraindications. It is the responsibility of the practitioner to take all appropriate safety precautions. Neither the publisher nor the author(s)/editor(s) assume any liability for any injury and/or damage to persons or property arising from or related to use of material in this book.

This book is sold on the understanding that the publisher is not engaged in providing professional medical services. If such advice or services are required, the services of a competent medical professional should be sought.

Every effort has been made where necessary to contact holders of copyright to obtain permission to reproduce copyright material. If any have been inadvertently overlooked, the publisher will be pleased to make the necessary arrangements at the first opportunity. The **CD/DVD-ROM** (if any) provided in the sealed envelope with this book is complimentary and free of cost. **Not meant for sale.**

**Inquiries for bulk sales may be solicited at:** jaypee@jaypeebrothers.com

*Practical Pediatrics*

*First Edition:* **2020**

ISBN: 978-93-89587-07-4

# Preface

Until the last decade the communicable infectious diseases were the most common causes of morbidity and mortality in humans. But today noncommunicable diseases (NCDs) such as autism, bronchial asthma, congenital defects, diabetes, epilepsy, etc. are more common. The problem is that these conditions may become life long problem for the patient, family and the country. Both the patients and the family members have to suffer life long. The resources of the country will be depleted by spending for the care of these patients thereby making the resources unavailable for the development of the country. It is evident that many medicines, wrong dietary habits and nutritional factors are causing most of these noncommunicable disorders. All medicines are associated with one or other adverse effects. So, it is advised not to take medicines unnecessarily. If any new adverse effect occurs following a drug or vaccine administration it should be intimated to appropriate authorities so that steps can be taken to avoid administration of those drugs or vaccines to others. The adverse effects can be prevented in millions of humans.

The important aspects of nutrition, drugs and vaccines are explained in a simple manner so that it will be easily understood. Combination of drugs can be dangerous and should be avoided as far as possible. The indications, contraindications, adverse effects of various medicines and vaccines are discussed in detail which will be helpful for the monitoring of patients.

Almost all the medicines or injections will have one or other side effects ranging from mild side effects like fever, headache to severe side effects like autism, brain damage, convulsions, etc. Many adverse effects are irreversible and one has to regret if any such adverse effect occurs to one of the family member. Before administering any drug or medicine both the medical professionals and the parents/caretakers should be aware of the complications of the medicines they are going to provide to their patients. The adverse effects and the risks should be explained to the parents or caretakers so that they can decide whether to take the risk or not. The benefits and the risks should be known and analyzed before taking a decision to administer the medicine. If any adverse effect like autism, permanent damage to brain occurs, then the child/person is going to suffer life long. The parents or caretakers will also have the guilty feeling for their entire life. As long as the parents are alive they will take care of the child, after that the future of the child will be bleak.

I have provided many medical facts in the form of mnemonics. As the medical field is rapidly advancing it will be easy to remember many facts by having mnemonics. Most of the points are given in the form of mnemonics like A, B, C, D… so that it will be easy to remember and the important points will not be missed.

Basics of X-rays, radiological features of various conditions are discussed in detail.

**Aruchamy Lakshmanaswamy**

*Less the medications, less the complications*
*More the medications, more the complications.*

**Aruchamy Lakshmanaswamy**

# Acknowledgments

I would like to thank my parents B Aruchamy and A Rathinambal and my brothers Lawyer A Sundararaj and Dr Aruchamy Ramalingam (MS Ortho, D Ortho) who encouraged me to come up in my profession and gave me all the support in my life and career.

I would like to thank Dr K Subramaniam (MD DCH), who took care of me and guided me and took special interest throughout my career right from the day I entered the medical field and still guiding me in all aspects of my life. I also thank my colleagues who supported and encouraged me in bringing out the this book.

I like to thank Dr VB Arunkumar MD (Radiodiagnosis), Senior Resident, PSG Institute of Medical Sciences and Research for helping in editing the radiology part of this book. I also thank all those who provided nice X-rays for this book and all others who helped me in preparing and editing this book.

I would also like to thank Shri Jitendar P Vij (Group Chairman), Mr Ankit Vij (Managing Director), Mr MS Mani (Group President), Dr Madhu Choudhary (Publishing Head-Education), Dr Astha Sawhney (Development Editor) and team members of M/s Jaypee Brothers Medical Publishers (P) Ltd, New Delhi, India, for all their support and work in this project.

**Aruchamy Lakshmanaswamy**

# Contents

1. **Nutrition** ................................................. **1**
   - Nutritive Values of Food Items ... 11
   - Recommended Daily Allowance ... 39
   - Nutritional Disorders ... 40

2. **Instruments and Procedures** ......... **48**
   - Antropometry ... 48
   - Skinfold Caliper ... 52
   - Instruments to Record Vital Signs ... 53
   - Blood Pressure ... 55
   - Needles ... 56
   - Biopsy Needles ... 67
   - Syringes ... 73
   - Tubes ... 74
   - Catheters ... 87
   - Bags ... 91
   - Infusion Sets ... 92
   - Oxygen Delivery Systems ... 93
   - Pediatric Breathing Circuit ... 96
   - Newborn Resuscitation ... 97
   - Asthma Devices ... 108
   - Airways ... 113
   - Miscellaneous ... 115

3. **Radiology—X-rays** ......................... **119**
   - General Considerations ... 119
   - X-rays Chest ... 125
   - Cardiovascular System ... 138
   - Respiratory System ... 151
   - Abdomen ... 186
   - Endocrine System ... 192
   - Chromosomal Disorders ... 194
   - Genitourinary System ... 196
   - Hematology ... 198

   **Musculoskeletal System** ... **201**
   - General ... 201
   - Skeleton ... 203
   - Skull ... 218
   - Neck ... 219
   - Pelvis ... 219
   - Newborn ... 221

   **Pediatric Surgery** ... **234**
   - Cardiovascular System ... 234
   - Respiratory System ... 237
   - Gastrointestinal System ... 245
   - Miscellaneous ... 275

4. **Drugs** ........................................... **278**
   - Antibiotics ... 279
   - Antivirals ... 308
   - Antifungals ... 312
   - Antiprotozoal ... 315
   - Anthelmintics ... 319
   - Antihistaminics ... 322
   - Cholinergic Drugs ... 324
   - Sympathomimetic/Inotropic Drugs ... 329
   - Antihypertensives ... 339
   - Antiasthmatics ... 349
   - Sedatives Hypnotics ... 358
   - Opioids ... 363
   - Anticonvulsants ... 368
   - Corticosteroids (Glucocorticoids) ... 384
   - Hormones ... 390
   - Diuretics ... 396
   - Cardiac Glycosides ... 401
   - Chelating Agents ... 407
   - H2-receptor Blockers ... 408
   - Miscellaneous ... 411

5. **Vitamins** ..................................... **449**
   - Vitamin A ... 449
   - Vitamin $B_{12}$ (Cyanocobalamin) ... 453
   - Vitamin D ... 455
   - Vitamin E ... 458
   - Vitamin K ... 459

6. **Intravenous Fluids** ...................... **464**
   - Intravenous Fluid Requirements ... 465
   - Crystalloids ... 467
   - Colloids ... 475
   - Blood Products ... 482

7. **Vaccines** .................................... **483**
- Vaccines for General use        485
- Vaccines used on
  Special Occasions              515
- Combination of Vaccines        534
- Duration of Protection
  Offered by Vaccines            537
- Contradictions Precautions
  for Immunization               537
- Vaccination Failure            538
- Vaccine Storage                538
- Adverse Events following
  Vaccination                    545
- National Vaccine Injury
  Compensation Program           552

8. **Supplement on Vaccines—2019** .... **554**
- Immunization Schedule
  of Vaccines                    554
- High-risk Group                560
- Immunization Schedules         560
- Catch-up Vaccination           560
- Vaccine Schedule for an
  Unimmunized Child              560

*Annexure* .................................................. *563*
*Index* ........................................................ *565*

# CHAPTER 1

# Nutrition

## CHAPTER OUTLINE

- Nutritive Values of Food Items
- Recommended Daily Allowance
- Nutritional Disorders

## INTRODUCTION

Nutrition is the important aspect of every life. Many wrong food habits are resulting in many diseases today. It is important to have a knowledge of the food items so that the diseases occurring due to improper food habits can be prevented. The nutritive values of food items, danger behind improper food habits, method of feeding are discussed in this section.

### Carbohydrates

Carbohydrates should be taken in quantities that will supply about 50-60% on daily required calories.

### Effects of Too Much Carbohydrates

High intake of carbohydrates will predispose to diabetes.

### Effects of Too Little Carbohydrates

- ❖ The source of energy for brain is only carbohydrates.
- ❖ If carbohydrates are not enough or then the functions of brain will get slowed down.

## QUESTIONS

**Q1. How carbohydrates are classified?**
Carbohydrates are classified as follows:
- ❑ *Energy yielding:*
  - ➢ Monosaccharides—glucose, fructose.
  - ➢ Disaccharides—lactose, maltose, sucrose
  - ➢ Polysaccharides—starch
  - ➢ Intrinsic sugars—fruits, milk
  - ➢ Extrinsic sugars—cane sugar, beet root.
- ❑ *Non-energy yielding:* Dietary fibers

**Q2. Mention few monosaccharides.**
- ❑ Glucose (dextrose, grape sugar or corn sugar)
- ❑ Fructose (levulose or fruit sugar).

**Q3. Mention few disaccharides**
- ❑ Lactose or milk sugar
- ❑ Sucrose
- ❑ Maltose

**Q4. Mention few polysaccharides.**
- ❑ Starch
- ❑ Dextrins

- Caramel
- Glycogen
- Cellulose
- Pectin
- Agar

**Q5. Name the reducing disaccharides.**
Lactose and maltose

**Q6. Name few reducing sugars.**
Glucose, fructose and mannose.

## Proteins

Proteins should be taken in quantities that will supply about 15% on daily required calories.

### Effects of Too Much Protein

- Proteins will suppress the appetite
- Increase the solute load on the kidneys.

### Effects of Too Little Proteins

Low intake of proteins will predispose to protein calorie malnutrition.

## QUESTIONS

**Q1. How proteins are classified based on physical basis?**
Simple proteins, conjugated proteins, and derived proteins.

**Q2. Name some simple proteins.**
Albumin, globulin, protamine, lectin, scleroprotein.

**Q3. What are conjugated proteins?**
Combination of a protein group with nonprotein group called prosthetic group.

**Q4. Name few scleroproteins.**
Collagen of bone, cartilage and tendon, keratin of hair.

**Q5. Give an example for reference protein?**
Egg is the reference protein.

**Q6. What is reference protein?**
Egg protein is known as reference protein as it used as reference protein in various studies. It is complete and well digested and contains all essential amino acids. Egg is used as reference protein in nutrition studies.

**Q7. What are the functions of proteins?**
- Tissue synthesis, maintenance and growth.
- Regulation of body processes.
- Source of energy–1 gram of protein will provide 4 calories per gram.

**Q8. What are the essential amino acids?**
- Essential amino acids are amino acids required by the body but not produced in the body.
- Nine amino acids that cannot be synthesized by the body in required amounts and have to be supplied by the diet. These are known as essential amino acids. The essential amino acids are:
  - Methionine
  - Threonine
  - Tryptophan
  - Valine
  - Isoleucine
  - Leucine
  - Phenylalanine
  - Lysine
  - Histidine (in children)
  - Histidine is essential for infants
  - Cystine, arginine, taurine (CAT) is essential for low birth babies

**Q9. What are essential amino acids in newborn apart from the ten amino acids?**
Arginine and histidine.

**Q10. Mention the precursors of essential amino acids.**
Precursors of essential amino acids:
- Cysteine: Methionine, serine
- Tyrosine: Phenylalanine
- Arginine: Glutamine, glutamate, aspartate
- Proline: Glutamate
- Glycine: Serine, choline

# Nutrition

**Q11. Which is the best among the food proteins?**
Egg is the best among the food proteins. It is because of high biological value and digestibility.

**Q12. What is class I protein?**
Proteins which contain all the essential amino acids in the required amounts are known as *class I* proteins.

**Q13. What is complete protein? What is biologically complete protein?**
It contains a balanced set of all essential amino acids. It is a protein which contains all essential amino acids as required by the human body, e.g. egg, milk, meat.

**Q14. What is incomplete protein?**
- The protein which does not contain all essential amino acids and, lack in one or two amino acids. Plant proteins deficient in one or more proteins.
- Protein from vegetable sources is usually biologically incomplete as they lack one or more essential amino acids.

**Q15. What is protein complementation?**
Use of vegetables in combination can lead to complementation of each other so that the net intake will be biologically complete. For example, wheat is deficient in lysine which is present in the legumes. Hence, the combination of the above two will complement each other.

**Q16. What are limiting amino acids?**
Food items lack in one or two amino acids. The essential amino acid which is not present in a particular food is known as limiting amino acid.

**Q17. What are limiting amino acids in cereals and pulses?**
- Cereals proteins are deficient in lysine and threonine.
- Pulse proteins are deficient in methionine. These are called as limiting amino acids.

**Q18. What is the limiting amino acid in soyabean?**
Limiting amino acid in soya bean is methionine.

**Q19. What is the limiting amino acid in cereals?**
- Limiting amino acid in cereals is lysine.
- Mixing foods especially pulses will improve the protein quality.

**Q20. What is the limiting amino acid in roasted nuts?**
Limiting amino acid in roasted nuts is lysine, threonine and methionine.

**Q21. What is the limiting amino acid in pulses?**
Methionine or cysteine is the limiting amino acid in pulses. Lysine is abundant in pulses.

**Q22. What is the limiting amino acid in maize (corn) (legumes)?**
Tryptophan.

**Q23. Legumes are rich in which amino acid?**
Legumes have excess of lysine.

**Q24. What is the limiting amino acid in beef?**
Phenylalanine or tyrosine.

**Q25. What is supplementary action of proteins?**
When two or more vegetarian foods are eaten together and their proteins supplement each other to obtain high grade protein at a low cost comparable to animal proteins.

**Q26. Provide an example for supplementary action of proteins?**
Supplementary action of proteins: Rice and dal.

**Q27. What are branched chain amino acids?**
Leucine, isoleucine and valine acid.

**Q28. Mention few acidic amino acids.**
Aspartic acid, tyrosine, glutamic acid.

**Q29. Mention few basic amino acids.**
Arginine, histidine and lysine.

**Q30. What are sulfur containing amino acids?**
Cysteine, methionine, homocysteine.

**Q31. What is nitrogen balance?**
When proteins are ingested, nitrogen is utilized for the body growth. If the excreted nitrogen is less than the ingested nitrogen, as happens in a normally growing child, it is known as positive nitrogen balance. If the loss is more, it is known as negative nitrogen balance ingested. It is important to maintain a positive nitrogen balance for normal growth. Nitrogen balance is determined by the following formula:
Nitrogen balance = Ingested nitrogen– (urinary nitrogen + fecal nitrogen)

**Q32. What is biological value?**
The biological value of a protein is the fraction of the retained nitrogen compared to the absorbed nitrogen. BV is calculated by the following formula:

$$BV = \frac{\text{Retained nitrogen}}{\text{Absorbed nitrogen}} \times 100$$

| Source of protein | Biological value |
|---|---|
| Egg protein | 96–100 |
| Cow's milk | 90 |
| Rice | 77 |
| Fish | 75 |
| Meat | 74 |
| Wheat | 66 |
| Bengal gram | 74 |
| Milk | 75 |
| Rice | 67 |

**Q33. What is the food item with biological value (BV) of 100?**
Egg protein: 100.

**Q34. What is protein efficiency ratio (PER)?**
Protein efficiency ratio is defined as the gain in weight per unit weight of protein consumed for a period of time for which the gain in body weight is measured.

$$PER = \frac{\text{Weight gain in grams}}{\text{Weight of protein consumed in grams over a period of time.}}$$

| Protein efficiency ratio (PER) | |
|---|---|
| Egg | 3.8 |
| Fish | 3.5 |
| Meat | 3.2 |
| Cow's milk | 2.8 |
| Rice | 1.7 |
| Wheat | 1.3 |
| Bengal gram | 1.1 |

**Q35. What is digestibility coefficient?**
- Digestibility coefficient (DC) is the amount of absorbed nitrogen compared to the nitrogen present in the food.
- Digestibility coefficient =

$$\frac{\text{Absorbed nitrogen}}{\text{Food nitrogen}} \times 100$$

**Q36. What is net protein utilization (NPU)?**
- Net protein utilization (NPU) is the amount of retained nitrogen to the nitrogen present in the food item. It is the product value of biological value (BV) and digestibility (D).
- NPU = BV × D
- NPU can be calculated from the following formula:

$$\frac{\text{Retained nitrogen}}{\text{Food nitrogen}} \times 100$$

Average quality proteins have NPU of 65%. High quality proteins have NPU of more than 65%.

| Net protein utilization (NPU) | |
|---|---|
| Egg | 96 |
| Cow's milk | 85 |
| Rice | 77 |
| Meat | 76 |
| Fish | 74 |
| Bengal gram | 61 |
| Wheat | 61 |

**Q37. What is negative nitrogen balance?**
Negative nitrogen balance is seen in conditions like chronic fever.

**Q38. What is positive nitrogen balance?**
Positive nitrogen balance is seen in conditions like young athlete.

**Q39. Mention few limiting amino acids.**
- Lysine is deficient in rice and wheat
- Methionine is deficient in maize and corn.

**Q40. What is the amount of carbohydrates present in fish and egg?**
Fish and egg contain no carbohydrates.

**Q41. Mention the protein content of various food items.**
- Spinach: 3.2 g/100 g
- Peas: 3.4 g/100 g
- Carrot: 1.1 g/100 g
- Cabbage: 1.3 g/100 g
- Cauliflower: 2.7 g/100 g
- Tomato: 1.1 g/100 g
- Onion: 1.5 g/100 g

**Q42. Which amino acid is present in maximum quantity in plasma?**
Glutamine.

**Q43. Which amino acid is antistress amino acid?**
Glutamine.

**Q44. Which amino acid is known as nature's sleeping pill?**
Tryptophan because it is a precursor of serotonin.

## Fats

### Effects of Too Much Fat Intake

❖ Fats should be taken in quantities that will supply about 30–35% on daily required calories. Too much intake of fat will result in complications like atherosclerosis, obesity, coronary heart disease in later life. Obese children are more likely to suffer from coronary heart diseases. Many adults who had undergone cardiac bypass surgery or coronary stents had a history of over feeding, overweight or obesity during their childhood. The parents should have this in mind while taking care of nutrition of their children.

❖ Fats will be stored in the body so that it can be utilized by the body for energy production during famines or starvation or when energy expenditure exceeds intake. This was the reason that our ancestors used to skip one or two meals in a week or climb hills. During this time the fats will be mobilized for energy production.

### Effects of Too Little Fat Intake

Fat is required for many basic functions in our body.

## QUESTIONS

**Q1. How are fats classified?**
- Simple fats—triglycerides
- Compound fats—phospholipids
- Derived lipids—cholesterol.

**Q2. What are the types of dietary fats?**
- Visible and invisible fats
- Visible fat includes oil, ghee, butter
- Invisible fats are present in the food items.

**Q3. What are the functions of fat?**
- Absorption of fat-soluble vitamins acts as a vehicle for absorption for vitamins A, D, E and K.
- Condensed form of energy: 1 g will provide 9 kcal.
- Source of essential fatty acids.
- Insulation—provide warmth.
- Protein sparing effect—when fat and protein are taken in adequate quantities and the amount of protein utilized for calorie production will be reduced.

**Q4. What is the average amount of fat consumed by normal Indian diet?**
25–30% of fat. Maximum permitted is about 45%.

**Q5. What is the classification of fatty acids?**
Saturated and unsaturated fatty acids.

**Q6. What are the types of fatty acids?**
- Saturated fatty acids
- Monounsaturated fatty acids
- Polyunsaturated fatty acids (PUFA).

**Q7. What are saturated fatty acids?**
Saturated fatty acids—the combining power of carbon atom is satisfied. Examples include palmitic and stearic acids.

**Q8. What are the monounsaturated fatty acids?**
Have only one point of unsaturation, e.g. oleic acid.

**Q9. Name few saturated fatty acids.**
Palmitic acid, stearic acid.

**Q10. Name few unsaturated fatty acids.**
Oleic, linoleic, linolenic and arachidonic acids.

**Q11. What are polyunsaturated fatty acids (PUFA)?**
PUFA include omega-3 and omega-6 fats

**Q12. What are the features of deficiency of long chain polyunsaturated (LCP) fats?**
Deficiency of LCP fats will result in dyslexia, dyspraxia, and hyperactivity.

**Q13. Which food item contains good quantity of PUFA?**
Corn oil, soyabean oil, safflower oil, salmon fish, walnuts are good sources og PUFA.

**Q14. Which food item contains very low quantity of PUFA?**
Animal fats.

**Q15. What is the importance of polyunsaturated fatty acids?**
PUFA are required for:
- Normal functioning of brain and nervous system
- Helps to reduce bad cholesterol and thereby the risk for heart disease.

**Q16. How are triglycerides containing medium chain fatty acids digested?**
Triglycerides containing medium chain fatty acids are hydrolyzed in the gastrointestinal tract by epithelial triglyceride lipase.

**Q17. What are essential fatty acids (EFA)?**
- Essential fatty acids (EFA) are PUFA which are needed in the diet as the synthesis is not enough to meet the body needs.
- These are fatty acids that cannot be synthesized by the human body.
- Essential fatty acids include linoleic acid and linolenic acid.

**Q18. Which is the richest source of essential fatty acids?**
Safflower is the richest source of essential fatty acids.

**Q19. What is the daily requirement of essential fatty acids according to Indian Council of Medical Research (ICMR)?**
Daily requirement of essential fatty acids according to ICMR is fixed as 20% of total energy.

**Q20. What are the essential fatty acids?**
- Arachidonic acid
- Linoleic acid
- Linolenic acid.

**Q21. Which is the most important essential fatty acid?**
- Linoleic acid
- Coconut oil is rich in saturated fatty acid
- Odor of rancid fats is due to volatile fatty acids
- Sunflower oil is rich in linoleic acid.

## Nutrition

**Q22. What are short chain fatty acids?**
Contains fewer than 6 that is 2-5 carbon atoms.

**Q23. What are medium chain fatty acids?**
Contains 6-12 carbon atoms.

**Q24. What are long chain fatty acids?**
Contains 13-21 carbon atoms and above.

**Q25. What are very long chain fatty acids?**
Fatty acids with 22 or more carbon atoms.

**Q26. What are visible fats?**
Visible fats are present in the food items that are purchased as fats. It can be seen by naked eyes. Examples include oil, ghee, butter, margarine, etc.

**Q27. What are invisible fats?**
Invisible fats are present in seeds, wheat, spices, etc.

**Q28. What are essential fatty acids (EFA)?**
- Essential fatty acids are PUFA which are needed in the diet as the synthesis is not enough to meet the body needs. These include linoleic acid and linolenic acid.
- Fatty acids that cannot be synthesized by the body and has to be supplied by the diet.
- Essential fatty acids are linoleic, leinolenic acid and arachidonic acid.
- Most important fatty acid linoleic acid.

**Q29. What are saturated fatty acids?**
Saturated fatty acids have no double bonds.

**Q30. What are unsaturated fatty acids?**
Unsaturated fatty acids will have one or more double bonds between carbon atoms.

**Q31. What are polyunsaturated fatty acids?**
Have two or more points of unsaturation.

**Q32. What is hydrogenation? What are the advantages and disadvantages?**
- Undue optimum temperature, pressure and the presence of catalyst.
- Liquid oil is converted to semisolid or solid fat.
- Advantages—ghee like consistency, keeping quality is hot and humid conditions.
- Disadvantages—essential fatty acids content is reduced.
- Unusual fatty acids are converted to saturated fatty acids.

**Q33. What is saponification?**
Hydrolysis of fat by alkali is called as saponification.

**Q34. What is bad cholesterol?**
Low-density lipoprotein (LDL) cholesterol is known as bad cholesterol it transports cholesterol from liver to peripheral tissues where it gets deposited predisposing to atherosclerosis.

**Q35. What is good cholesterol?**
High-density lipoprotein (HDL) cholesterol is known as good cholesterol because it transports cholesterol from liver to peripheral tissues thereby facilitates excretion of fats. Hence, it is also known as antiatherogenic.

**Q36. What is the ideal fat for good health?**
An ideal fat should contain polyunsaturated fatty acid (PUFA) or saturated fatty acids in a ratio of 0.8/1.0 and linoleic/$\alpha$-linolenic of 5-10 in the diet.

**Q37. How will you balance the fatty acids in cereal based diets?**
Mix two or more oils of different composition. PUFA rich safflower oil and monounsaturated fatty acid (MUFA) rich coconut oil can be mixed.

## Mineral—Zinc

It is a powerful antioxidant.

### Functions of Zinc

They are: Growth, immunity and reproduction, sense perception.

### Uses of Zinc

- Acrodermatitis enteropathica
- Anemia—sickle cell anemia
- Burns
- Bone problems—osteoporosis
- Copper excess—Wilson's disease
- Dermatological problems
- Enteritis or diarrhea
- Foot ulcers in diabetics
- Gestational period
- Hypoguesia (decreased ability to taste)
- Infections—pneumonia.

### Recommended Daily Allowance (RDA)

- RDA for men: 11 mg
- RDA for women: 8 mg/day
- Need more zinc during pregnancy and lactation.

### Dose

- 7 months to 3 years—3 mg/kg
- 4-8 years—5 mg/day
- 9-12 years—8 mg/day
- In diarrhea 10 mg for 4-10 years of age
  - 15 mg/kg of zinc for 14 days
  - 20 mg of zinc for 14 days
- For diarrhea 10-40 mg/day for 7-14 days
- For sickle cell disease 10 mg/day for one year.

### Zinc Rich Foods

**Plant sources:**

- Beans, nuts
- Seeds
- Whole grains

**Animal sources:**

- Red meat
- Shellfish
- Eggs
- Poultry
- Sea food—crab, lobster
- Dairy products.

### Deficiency Symptoms

- Anemia
- Abnormal taste and smell
- Acne
- Acrodermatitis enteropathica
- Appetite loss
- Crohn's disease
- Dermatitis or skin problems-eczema
- Eye lesions
- Gustatory problems—taste problems-impaired taste
- Growth retardation
- Gastrointestinal (GIT)—nausea, vomiting, diarrhea
- Hair loss
- Hypogonadism
- Impaired immune system
- Impotence
- Incomplete or delayed sexual maturity
- Infections—pneumonia
- Wound healing—poor
- Weight loss unexplained
- Wilson's disease.

### Causes of Zinc Deficiency

- Alcohol addiction
- Acrodermatitis enteropathica
- Anemia: Sickle cell disease
- Bowel disorders: Inflammatory bowel disease, ulcerative colitis
- Cancers
- Chronic diarrhea
- Celiac disease
- Decreased intake
- Decreased absorption
- Diabetes
- Diuretics hydrochlorothiazide
- Hepatic disorders
- Hemodialysis
- Kidney disorders: Chronic kidney disease.

## Side Effects

Excess zinc intake can cause following problems:
- Appetite loss
- Brain toxicity
- Cramps
- Copper levels will be low
- Cough
- Diarrhea
- Emesis
- Fever
- Fatigue
- GIT problems: Nausea or vomiting
- Gustatory problems: Metallic taste
- Headache
- Impaired immunity
- Irritability
- Single dose of 10–30 g can be fatal.

Application of zinc on the broke skin may cause:
- Burning
- Itching
- Tingling
- Stinging.

## Interactions

- Zinc will decrease the absorption of Quinolone antibiotics
- Tetracycline—zinc will attach with tetracyclines in the stomach
- Zinc will affect the absorption of penicillamine.

## Pregnancy

The requirement will be more during pregnancy.

## QUESTIONS

**Q1. How will you prevent loss of zinc in the diet?**
- The seeds should be soaked in water before cooking. Soaking in water will reduce the loss of phytates.
- Leavened grain products.

**Q2. What are the problems with excess intake of zinc?**
Too much zinc will cause nausea, vomiting, impaired immune system function.

**Q3. What is the population at high-risk for zinc deficiency?**
- Pregnant women
- Young children
- Old aged more than 65 years of age
- Malnourished
- Starvation
- Legumes and some cereals contain phytic acid which will block absorption of zinc.

## QUESTIONS ON NUTRITION

**Q1. Define nutrition.**
Nutrition is the process by which an organism utilizes food.

**Q2. What are macronutrients?**
Macronutrients are the nutrients that are required in large amounts like carbohydrates, fats and proteins.

**Q3. What are micronutrients?**
- Micronutrients are the nutrients that are required in small quantities. These are divided into minerals and oligo elements and vitamins. They do not provide energy but are essential for life
- Daily requirement should be less than 100 mg/day.

**Q4. How will you classify foods on the basis of origin?**
- Plant origin
- Animal origin.

**Q5. How will you classify foods on the basis of composition?**
- Carbohydrates
- Proteins
- Fats
- Vitamins
- Minerals.

**Q6. How will you classify foods on the basis of functions?**
- Body building foods—milk, meat, fish, eggs, ground nuts, pulses, etc.
- Energy giving foods—cereals, roots, etc.
- Protective foods—vegetables, fruits.

**Q7. What is the respiratory quotient of carbohydrates?**
1

**Q8. What is the respiratory quotient of mixed diet?**
0.82

**Q9. Which food stuff has maximum reactive thermogenesis (specific dynamic action)?**
Proteins.

**Q10. What is the amount of calories generated in carbohydrates, proteins and fats?**
- Calories generated per gram of fat are 9 kcal.
- Calories generated per gram of carbohydrate are 4 kcal.
- Calories generated per gram of protein are 4 kcal.

**Q11. What is poor man's meat?**
Pulses.

**Q12. What is protective food?**
Fruits as it contain more vitamins.

**Q13. Which is the best and complete food?**
- Milk
- Green leafy vegetables.

**Q14. What are the food items that do not swell on cooking?**
Egg, potato.

**Q15. What are isodense feeds?**
100 mL of food will contain 100 calories. 100 mL of milk will give about 70 calories, when sugar is added the calorie content can be increased to 100 kcal/100 mL. This is known as isodense feeds.

**Q16. What are hypodense feeds?**
100 L of milk will give about 70 calories.

**Q17. What are hyperdense feeds?**
100 mL of milk will give about 70 calories, when sugar or oil is added to the milk in large quantities the calorie content will increase to more than 100 kcal/100 mL. This is known as hyperdense feeds.

**Q18. What is the difference between the teeth in calcium and phosphorus deficiency?**
- Pulp defects (phosphate deficiency)
- Enamel defects (in calcium deficiency).

**Q19. What is Pica?**
Pica is ingestion of inedible things like mud or pencil commonly seen in children with iron deficiency anemia, worm infestation or mental retardation.

**Q20. What is the difference between food allergy and food intolerance?**
- *Food allergy:* Food allergy is abnormal response to food. There is exaggerated susceptibility to certain food items. For instance, allergy to sea foods or cow's milk may manifest as asthma, abdominal pain, anaphylaxis, urticaria, angioneurotic edema, etc.
- *Food intolerance:* Intolerance to food items is present when a child is not able to tolerate certain foods and presents with diarrhea or vomiting. For instance, a child may not tolerate breast milk, cow's milk and egg due to protein intolerance.

**Q21. What are food fads?**
Custom or culture that the family follows with respect to nutrition.

**Q22. What are essential fatty acids?**
Fatty acids that cannot be synthesized by the body and has to be supplied by the diet.

**Q23. When is national nutrition week?**
1–7 September.

# NUTRITIVE VALUES OF FOOD ITEMS

## Cereals and Millets

### Cereals

- Cereals like rice, wheat, maize are the staple diet in India.
- Cereals contain 7–11 g% protein and 2–5% fat.
- Wheat, ragi, oats and barley contain gluten.
- Cereals are deficient in lysine, vitamin A and vitamin C.
- Wheat lacks lysine and threonine.

| Cereals (100 g) | Energy (kcal) | Protein (g) | Carbohydrate (g) | Fat (g) |
|---|---|---|---|---|
| Rice | 345 | 6.8 | 78.2 | 0.5 |
| Whole wheat | 341 | 11.8 | 69.4 | 1.7 |
| Maize | 342 | 11.1 | 66 | 3.6 |
| Ragi | | | | |
| Barley | 336 | 11.5 | 69.6 | 1.3 |
| Bajra | 361 | 11.6 | 67.5 | 5.0 |
| Jowar | 331 | 12.3 | 60.9 | 1.9 |
| Kambu | 378 | 11 | 73% | 4 |

## QUESTIONS

**Q1. What are the nutrients deficient in cereals?**
Cereals are poor sources of vitamin A and vitamin C, iron, calcium.

**Q2. How does washing affect the nutritive value of cereals?**
Washing will remove 60% of water soluble vitamins and minerals.

**Q3. How does milling affect the nutritive value of cereals?**
Milling will remove large amount of protein, thiamine and riboflavin from rice.

**Q4. How does soaking affect the nutritive value of cereals?**
Soaking of cereals like rice and pulses like black gram for a short period will increase the vitamin contents, digestibility. It also makes the cooking easier.

**Q5. What is the advantage of parboiling?**
Parboiling will result in retention of vitamins. The vitamins seep into the inner portions of the grain. Even on milling or polishing the vitamins will not be lost parboiled rice will be rich in thiamine. Parboiling will increase the shelf life and ability to resist insects.

**Q6. Mention the nutritive value of whole grains.**
Whole grain contains:
- Carbohydrates: 75%
- Protein: 12%
- Fat: 2%
- Minerals and vitamins: 1%.

**Q7. What are the vitamins not present in cereals?**
Cereals do not contain vitamin A and vitamin C except yellow maize which contains α-carotene.

**Q8. Which cereals contain carotenes?**
Yellow maize.

### Rice

- *Nutritive values:* Each 100 g contains:
  - Calories (kcal): 345
  - Protein (g): 6.8
  - Carbohydrate (g): 78.2
  - Fat (g): 0.5
  - Fiber: 0.2 g
- Rich in thiamine
- Limiting amino acid—lysine
- Deficient in vitamin A and vitamin C
- Of all cereals NPU of rice is more.

### Parts of Rice Grain

- Endosperm
- Outer pericarp
- 1 cup of rice will provide 175 calories.

## QUESTIONS

**Q1. What are the forms in which rice is consumed?**
- Cooked rice
- Uncooked.

**Q2. What is the calorie content of rice?**
- Rice contains 4 calories per gram
- As the rice contains nondigestible parts like fiber and husk, the actual calorie will be lesser than the calculated calories.
- *Protein content:* 6–9%
- *Vitamins:* Rice is a good source of B group vitamins especially thiamine contains fiber.
- 100 g of cooked rice contains 175 kcal and 4 g of protein
- When rice is cooked, it increases the volume by 3 times,
  So, one cup (150 g) of cooked rice will contain 150/3 that is 50 g of rice only.

**Q3. What are the nutrients that are deficient in rice?**
- Rice does not contain vitamin A, vitamin D and vitamin C.
- Poor source of calcium and iron.

**Q4. What is the disadvantage of polished rice?**
Polished rice is devoid of thiamine.

**Q5. What are the limiting amino acids in rice?**
Lysine and threonine.

**Q6. Why rice protein is considered to be best quality?**
Rice protein is considered to be best quality because it is rich in lysine.

**Q7. What are the forms of rice?**
- Cooked rice
- Raw rice
- Milled rice
- Polished rice
- Parboiled rice.

**Q8. What are the parts of rice grain?**
- Germ (embryo)
- Endosperm (inner) contains starch and (outer) pericarp and aleurone layer contains most of the essential nutrients.

**Q9. Is beriberi common in breastfed infants?**
Beriberi will occur in infants, breastfed by thiamine deficient mothers.

**Q10. Why beriberi is common in people eating rice?**
Most people eat polished rice. This will be deficient in thiamine.

**Q11. What are the types of beriberi?**
- Wet beriberi presents with cardiac failure (palpitation, dyspnea, edema and tachycardia).
- Dry beriberi presents with neurological symptoms.

**Q12. What are the three ways infantile beriberi can present?**
1. Cardiovascular type—acute onset with palpitation, dyspnea, edema and tachycardia.
2. Aphonic type—subacute onset with hoarseness of voice.
3. Neurological type—chronic course with vomiting, tremors, nystagmus and convulsions.

**Q13. What is the age of onset of beriberi?**
- 2–3 months.
- Onset of neurological type is by 6–12 months.

## Method of Cooking Cereals

- *Soaking of cereals* will increase vitamins, digestibility and makes cooking easier.
- *Sprouting* improves digestibility by production of amylase. It includes:
  - Increases vitamins, decrease bulk on cooking, decreases phytate levels.
  - Amylase rich foods wheat, bajra, jowar, green grains. Useful in persistent diarrhea, malnutrition.

- *Parboiling,* hot soaking followed by steaming of paddy then milling. It includes:
  - In parboiling, no vitamins will be lost.
  - During steaming, minerals and vitamin from the outer aleurone layer reaches the endosperm.
- *Milling* of cereals removes protein, thiamine and riboflavin from rice. It includes:
  - Milling does not remove nutrients.
  - Milling will reduce the following:
    - 15% of protein
    - 75% of B1
    - 60% riboflavin.
- *Washing and cooking* will limit amino acid lysine and threonine and will remove 60% of water soluble vitamins and minerals.

# QUESTIONS

**Q1. What is parboiling? What are the benefits of parboiling?**
- Parboiling is partial cooking in steam.
- The advantages of parboiling are:
  - This will preserve the nutritive value of rice.
  - Increases the shelf life
  - Will become more resistant to insects
  - Will remove toxic amino acids β-oxalyl-amino-L-alanine acid (BOAA) from kesari dal.

**Q2. What is the disadvantage of parboiling?**
Develops peculiar smell and off flavor.

**Q3. What is hot soaking processes?**
The paddy is soaked in hot water at 65–70°C for 3–4 hours.

**Q4. What happens during steaming process? What is the advantage?**
The greater part of the vitamins and minerals present in the outer aleurone layer will be driven into the inner endosperm. Milling of the rice after steaming process will not result in nutrient loss.

**Q5. What are the benefits of drying?**
- Grains become more resistant to insect invasion
- Rice can be stored for longer time
- Starch gets gelatinized.

**Q6. What is the vitamin that is lost by polishing rice?**
Thiamine will be lost and will result in beriberi.

**Q7. What is the disease is common in rice eating people? Why?**
Beriberi is common due to thiamine deficiency.

**Q8. What are the effects of milling of rice grain?**
The proteins, riboflavin and thiamine will be lost on milling.

**Q9. What are the effects of washing of rice grain?**
Washing will remove about 60% of the water soluble vitamins and minerals.

**Q10. What are the effects of cooking rice grain in large quantities and draining the water?**
- There will be loss of B group vitamins.
- It is better to cook rice in 3 to 4 times water for 1 measure of rice.

## Wheat

- Wheat, the second most commonly used cereals after rice in India.
- Whole grain is rich in B vitamins
- *Nutritive values*-each 100 g contains:
  - Calories (kcal): 341
  - Protein (g): 11.8 (9–16%)
  - Carbohydrate (g): 69.4
  - Fat (g): 1.7

# QUESTIONS

**Q1. What are the forms in which wheat is consumed?**
*Chapati*, bread, upma and atta.

**Q2. What is the limiting amino acid in wheat?**
Wheat is deficient in lysine and threonine.

**Q3. What is the significance of white wheat flour?**
White bread contains less minerals and vitamins.

## Maize

- Maize is rich in fat.
- Yellow maize is rich in carotenoid pigments.
- *Nutritive values:* Each 100 g contains:
  - Calories (kcal): 342
  - Protein (g): 11.1
  - Carbohydrate (g): 66
  - Fat (g): 3.6
- Maize contains excess of leucine.

**Q4. What are the forms in which maize is consumed?**
- Used in cornflakes
- Maize flour
- Used in preparation of custards.

**Q5. What is the limiting amino acid in maize?**
Limiting amino acid in maize is tryptophan and lysine.

**Q6. How will you increase the quality of protein in maize?**
By adding *opaque-2* gene into maize.

## Barley

- *Nutritive values:* Each 100 g contains:
  - Calories (kcal): 336–354
  - Protein (g): 11.5 (9–12%)
  - Carbohydrate (g): 69.6
  - Fat (g): 1.3
  - Dietary fiber (g): 15.6
- Barley is rich in protein, vitamins and minerals.

## Millets

- These can be grown in short period during summer under dry, high temperature conditions.
- Millets are small grains. The millets are ground and consumed without removing the outer layer.

**Types of millets:**
- Millets (Siruthaniyam)
- Barnyard millet (Kuthirai valli, Sanwa, Jhangora, Kavadapullu, Odalu, Oodalu)
- Finger millet (Red millet, Ragi/Kezhvaragu, Panji pullu, Ragulu, Bhav, Nachni, Mandia)
- Fox tail millet (Thinai/Tenai, Kangni, Thina, Korra, Navane, Kang, Rala)
- Kodo millet (Varagu, Kodra, Koovaraghu, Arikelu, Harka, Kodri)
- Little millet (Samai, kutki, chama, Sama, Same, uri, vari), Kang
- Pearl millet (Kambu, Bajra, Kambam. Gantilu/Sajjalu, Sajje, Bajri)
- Sorghum (White millet, Cholam, Jowar/jwaarie, Cholum, Jonnalu, Jola, Juvar/jowar, Jowar, jonhahlaai)
- Proso millet (Panivaragu, Barri, Varigulu, Baragu)

**Q1. What are millets?**
Millets are smaller grain like Jowar, bajra and ragi that are ground and eaten without removing the outer skin.

**Q2. Mention few millets.**
- Jowar, bajra and ragi.
- Little millet samai (kutki).

**Q3. What are the parts of millets?**
- Bran, germ and endosperm.
- Bran protects the millets from sunlight, pests and diseases. It contains antioxidants iron, zinc, copper, magnesium, vitamin B and phytonutrients. It also contains fibers.
- Germ contains vitamin B and vitamin E, antioxidants, phytonutrients, unsaturated fats.
- Endosperm contains starchy carbohydrates, proteins, small amounts of vitamins and minerals.

**Q4. What are minor millets?**
- Panivaragu or proso millet.
- Foxtail millet or Thenai.

# Nutrition

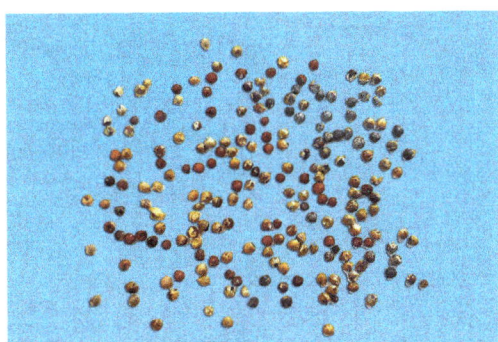

**Fig. 1.1:** Ragi.

**Q1. What is the nutritive value of ragi?**
- Six teaspoon of ragi will give 100 calories and 6 g of protein.
- Calcium 340 mg
- Iron 3.9 mg

**Q2. What is the benefit of sprouted ragi?**
Sprouted ragi is rich in amylase.

**Q3. What are the micronutrients present in ragi?**
Ragi is rich in iron and calcium.

**Q4. What are the advantages of ragi?**
Ragi is the cheapest among millets. It is rich in iron and calcium.
- English: Fox tail millet
- Tamil: Thinai/Tenai
- Hindi: Kangni
- Malayalam: Thina
- Telugu: Korra
- Kannada: Navane
- Gujarathi: Kang
- Marathi: Rala

**Q5. What are little millets?**
Samai.

**Q6. What is the cheapest millet?**
Ragi

**Q7. What are pseudocereals?**
Jowar, bajra, ragi, kodo are minor millets or pseudocereals.
- English: Barnyard millet
- Tamil: Kuthirai valli
- Hindi: Sanwa, Jhangora
- Malayalam: Kavadapullu
- Telugu: Odalu
- Kannada: Oodalu

## *Ragi (Fig. 1.1)*

English: Finger millet (Red millet)
Tamil: Ragi/Kezhvaragu
Hindi: Ragi/Nachani, mundua
Malayalam: Panji pullu
Telugu: Ragulu
Kannada: Ragi
Gujarathi: Bhav
Marathi: Nachni
Oriya: Mandia

- *Nutritive values:* Each 100 g of ragi contains:
  - Calories (kcal): 328
  - Protein (g): 7.3
  - Carbohydrate (g): 72.0
  - Fat (g): 1.3
  - Calcium: 344 mg
  - Iron: 3.9 mg
- Ragi is rich in calcium, iron and iodine.

## *Bajra (Pearl Millet)*

- English: Pearl millet
- Tamil: Kambu
- Hindi: Bajra
- Malayalam: Kambam
- Telugu: Gantilu/Sajjalu
- Kannada: Sajje
- Gujarathi: Bajri

**Q1. What is the nutritive value (protein and calorie content) of bajra?**
- Energy (kcal): 361
- Protein (g): 11.6 (10-14%)
- Carbohydrate (g): 67.5
- Fat (g): 5.0

## *Jowar (Sorghum) (Fig. 1.2)*

English: Sorghum (white millet)
Tamil: Cholam
Hindi: Jowar/jwaarie
Malayalam: Cholam
Telugu: Jonnalu
Kannada: Jola
Gujarathi: Juvar/jowar
Marathi: Jowari/jonhahlaa

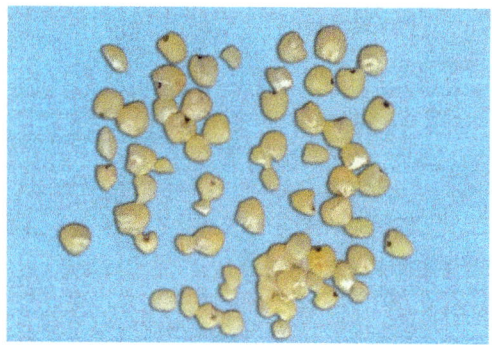

Fig. 1.2: Jowar.

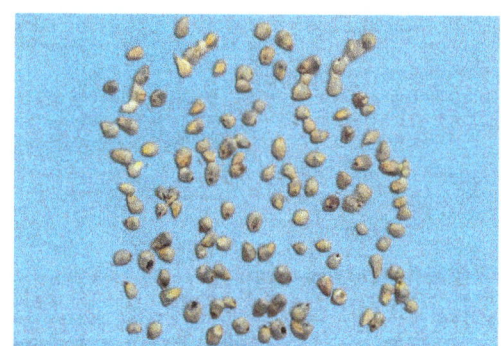

Fig. 1.3: Kambu/Bajra.

**Q1. What is the nutritive value (protein and calorie content) of jowar?**
- ❏ Energy (kcal): 349
- ❏ Protein (g): 10.4 (9–14%)
- ❏ Carbohydrate (g): 72.6
- ❏ Fat (g): 1.9

### Nutritive Value of Ragi

|  | Ragi | Jowar | Bajra |
|---|---|---|---|
| Energy (kcal) | 328 | 349 | 361 |
| Carbohydrate (g) | 72.0 | 72.6 | 67.5 |
| Protein (g) | 7.3 | 10.4 | 11.6 |
| Fat (g) | 1.3 | 1.9 | 5.0 |
| Calcium (mg) | 344 | 25 | 42 |
| Iron (mg) | 3.9 | 8 | 4.1 |

### Bajra

*Nutritive values:* Each 100 g contains:
- ❖ Calories (kcal) 361
- ❖ Protein (g) 11.6
- ❖ Carbohydrate (g) 67.5
- ❖ Fat (g) 5.0

### Jowar

*Nutritive values:* Each 100 g contains:
- ❖ Energy (kcal) 331
- ❖ Protein (g) 12.3
- ❖ Carbohydrate (g) 60.9
- ❖ Fat (g) 1.9

**Q1. What are the limiting amino acids in jowar?**
Lysine and threonine.

### Kambu (Fig. 1.3)

*Nutritive values:* Each 100 g contains:
- ❖ Calories: 360 calories
- ❖ Protein: 12 g
- ❖ Carbohydrate: 67 g
- ❖ Fat: 5 g
- ❖ Minerals:
  - ▪ Calcium: 42 mg
  - ▪ Phosphorus: 242 mg
  - ▪ Iron: 8 mg
- ❖ Fibers: 1 g

### Pulses or Legumes

Pulses are called poor man's meat.

### Pulses

- ❖ Pulses are deficient in methionine, cysteine
- ❖ After germination vitamin B and vitamin C content increases
- ❖ Sprouted pulses will have more nutrients.
- ❖ Pulses are rich in lysine
- ❖ Rich in minerals, B complex vitamins riboflavin, thiamine.

**Q1. Name few pulses.**
- ❏ Bengal gram
- ❏ Black gram (urad dal)
- ❏ Green gram
- ❏ Red gram
- ❏ Soyabeans
- ❏ Peas
- ❏ Horse gram
- ❏ Channa (kondai kadalai).

## Nutrition

**Q2. What is the nutritive value of pulses?**
- Contains 20-25 g% of protein, soya beans contains 40% protein.
- Rich in minerals and B vitamins like riboflavin and thiamine.
- Pulses are rich in lysine.

**Q3. What is the amount of proteins present in the pulses?**
- Pulses are rich sources of protein. Pulses contain 20-25% of proteins. It is two times that is found in wheat and three times found in rice.
- Pulses contain more protein than eggs, fish and flesh foods.

**Q4. Why quality wise pulse proteins are inferior to animal proteins?**
Pulses are deficient in methionine and to a lesser extent cysteine. Pulses lack vitamin A and vitamin C.

**Q5. What is the disadvantage of pulses?**
- Pulses contain phytates and tannins in raw state. These antinutrients will be destroyed by heat.
- Flatulence due to high amount of oligosaccharides.

**Q6. What is the importance of pulses?**
Rich in protein pulses are also rich in minerals and vitamin B.

**Q7. What are the limiting amino acids in pulses?**
Methionine and to a lesser extent cysteine.

**Q8. Which is the amino acid that is rich in pulses?**
Pulses are rich in lysine.

**Q9. What is the amount of vitamin C in the pulses?**
In dry states pulses lack vitamin C. But germinating pulses are rich in vitamin C and vitamin B.

**Q10. What is the advantage of fermentation of pulses?**
Fermentation also modifies the food value of pulses. It enhances the content of riboflavin. Niacin and thiamine pulses will make food palatable.

**Q11. What are the antinutrients factors present in pulses?**
In the raw state it contains anti nutrients like phytates and tannins.

**Q12. What is the disadvantage of oligosaccharides in pulses?**
Oligosaccharides in pulses will cause flatulence.

**Q13. What are the antinutritional factors present in the pulses?**
Phytates and tannins. Most of the antinutritional factors are lost by heat.

**Q14. How will you destroy the antinutrient factors present in pulses?**
- The antinutrient factors present in pulses can be destroyed by heating.

*Pulses: Nutritive values*

| Pulses | Calories (kcal) | Carbohydrate (g) | Proteins | Fat |
|---|---|---|---|---|
| Bengal gram | 360 | 60 | 17 | 5.3 |
| Black gram (Ulunthu) | 347 | 60 | 24 | 1.4 |
| Green gram (Pasi payaryu) | 348 | 57 | 24.5 | 1.2 |
| Horse gram (Kollu, Kulthi) | 321 | 57 | 22 | 0.5 |
| Red gram (Thuvarai) | 335 | 58 | 22.3 | 1.7 |
| Soya bean | 432 | 20 | 43.2 | 19.5 |
| Peas dry (Pattani) | 315 | 14 | 19.7 | 1.1 |
| Chana (kondai kadali) | 340 | 62.0 | 13.0 | 5.0 |
| Beans | 156 | 29.8 | 7.4 | 0.1 |

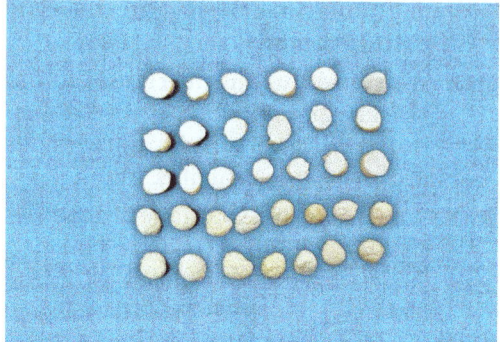

Fig. 1.4: Bengal gram.

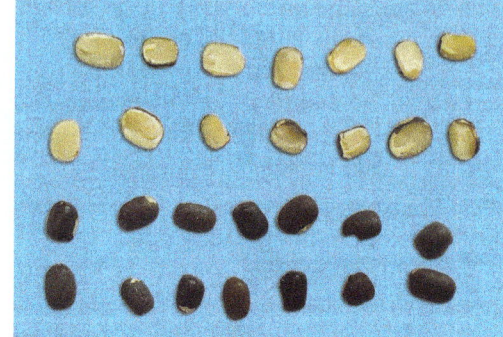

Fig. 1.5: Black gram.

One gram of dal will provide 18 calories:
- **Bengal gram (Fig. 1.4):**
  English: Bengal gram
  Tamil: Kadalai/Kothukadalai
  Hindi: Chana
  Malayalam: Kadala
  Telugu: Sanaga/Sanagalu
  Kannada: Kadale/Chana
  Gujarathi: Chana
  Marathi: Harbara
  Bengali: Chola
  Punjabi: Chole/Channa
  Kashmiri: Chanu
  - *Nutritive values:*
    - Calories (kcal): 360 calories
    - Protein (g): 17 g
    - Carbohydrate: (g) 60
    - Fat (g): 5.3
    - Iron: 4.6 mg
    - Limiting amino acids—methionine and cysteine.
- **Black gram (urad dal) (Fig. 1.5):**
  English: Black gram (Urad Dal)
  Tamil: Ulundhu
  Hindi: Subat Urd/Urid
  Malayalam: Uzhunnu
  Telugu: Minu mullu/Manipa/Uddulu
  Kannada: Uddu
  Gujarathi: Aalad/Udad
  Marathi: Uddachi/Udid
  Bengali: Mashkolir Dal/Kalai
  - *Nutritive values:*
    - Calories (kcal): 347
    - Protein (g): 24

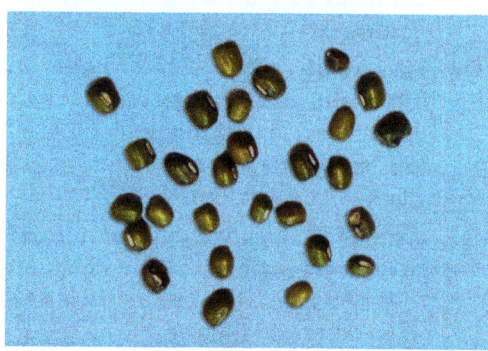

Fig. 1.6: Green gram.

- Carbohydrate (g): 60
- Fat (g): 1.4
- Potassium: 983 mg

- **Green gram (Fig. 1.6):**
  English: Green gram (Moong dhal)
  Tamil: Pachai payiru/Payatham paruppu/Pasipayir
  Hindi: Sabut Mung
  Malayalam: Cherupayaru
  Telugu: Pesaru pappu/Pesalu/pacha-pesalu
  Kannada: Hesare
  Gujarathi: Muga
  Marathi: Mung/Hirave Mug
  Bengali: Mug
  Kongani: Moogu
  Punjabi: Mung/ Moongi
  - *Nutritive values:*
    - Calories (kcal): 348
    - Protein (g): 24
    - Carbohydrate (g): 57
    - Fat (g): 1.2

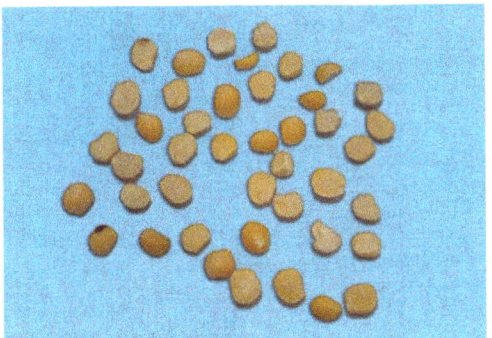

**Fig. 1.7:** Red gram.

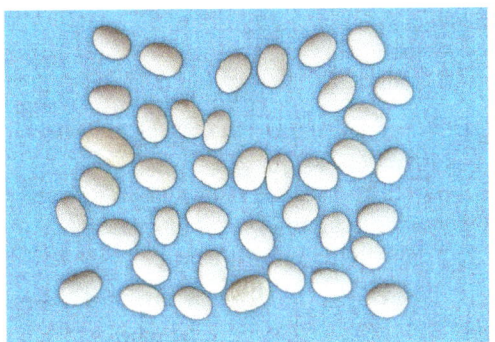

**Fig. 1.9:** Soyabeans.

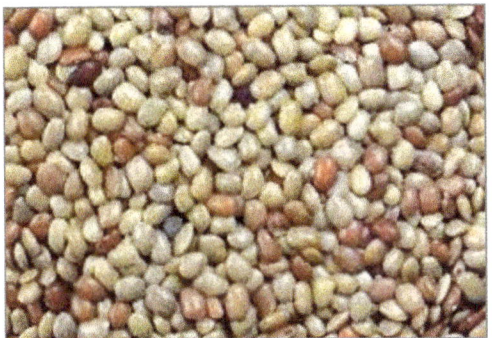

**Fig. 1.8:** Horse gram.

- **Red gram (Fig. 1.7):**
  English: Red gram (Pigeon pea)
  Tamil: Thuvarai/Thuvaram paruppu/Mysore Paruppu
  Hindi: Rahar/Arhar dal
  Malayalam: Thuvara Parippu
  Telugu: Missu Pappu/Kandi Pappu/Kandalu Pappu
  Kannada: Thugari Bele/Masoor Dhal
  Gujarathi: Tuver Dal/Thuvare
  Marathi: Tur Dal
  Bengali: Arhar Dal/Moshoor
  - *Nutritive values:*
    - Calories (kcal): 335
    - Protein (g): 22.3
    - Carbohydrate (g): 57.6
    - Fat (g): 1.7
- **Horse gram (Fig. 1.8):**
  English: Horse gram
  Tamil: Kollu
  Hindi: Kulthi/Hulthi
  Malayalam: Mudhira
  Telugu: Ulavulu
  Kannada: Hurule
  Gujarathi: Kuleeth
  Marathi: Kuleeth
  Bengali: Kulthi-Kalai
  - *Nutritive value:* 100 g contains
    - Calories: 321
    - Protein: 22 g
    - Fat
    - Minerals:
      - Calcium: 287 mg
      - Phosphorus: 311 mg
      - Iron: 7 mg

## *Soyabeans (Fig. 1.9)*

English: Soya beans
Tamil: Soya
Hindi: Bhatma
Malayalam: Soya
Telugu: Soya ginjalu
Kannada: Soyabin
Gujarathi: Soya bina
Marathi: Soya

- Soya beans are rich in protein and fibers.
- It has high nutritive value. It contains 40% protein and 20% fats and 4% minerals.
- It contains 43.2 g of protein and 430 kcal per 100 g.
- Soya bean rich in Fe 10.4 mg.
- *Nutritive values:* Each 100 g contains:
  - Calories (kcal): 432
  - Protein (g): 43.2
  - Carbohydrate (g): 20.9

- Fat (g): 19.5
- Iron: 10.4 mg
- Calcium: 240 mg.

**Q1. What is the importance of proteins in soya beans?**
- Richest source of protein in pulses
- The protein present in the soya beans are of high nutritive value.

**Q2. What is the limiting amino acid in soya beans?**
The limiting amino acid in soya beans is methionine.

**Q3. What are the ways soya beans are consumed?**
- Eaten as dal
- Soya powder can be mixed with atta or making chapatti.
- Soya beans milk and curd
- Used in baby foods
- Richest among the pulses.

### Peas–dry (Pattani)
- Calories (kcal): 315
- Protein (g): 19.7
- Fat (g): 1.1
- Peas are rich in mineral, vitamins and fibers.

### Horse Gram (Kollu, Kulthi, Kulthikalai)
English: Horse gram
Tamil: Kollu
Hindi: Kulthi/Hulthi
Malayalam: Mudhira
Telugu: Ulavulu
Kannada: Hurule
Gujarathi: Kuleeth
Marathi: Kuleeth
Bengali: Kulthi-Kalai
- Calories (kcal): 321
- Protein (g): 22
- Fat (g): 0.5
- Fiber (g): 5
- Calcium: 287 mg
- Phosphorus: 311 mg
- Iron: 7 mg

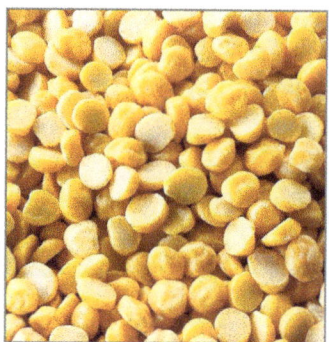

**Fig. 1.10:** Chana dal.

### Chana (Kadalai paruppu) (Fig. 1.10)
- Calories (kcal): 340
- Carbohydrate (g): 62.0
- Protein (g): 13.0
- Fat (g): 5.0
- Dietary fiber: 10.0g
- Does not contain cholesterol.

| Vegetable | Energy (kcal) | Protein (g) | Carbohydrate (g) | Fat (g) |
|---|---|---|---|---|
| Cauliflower | 30 | 2.6 | 4.0 | 0.4 |
| Tomato | 20 | 0.9 | 3.6 | 0.2 |

### Vegetables
Vegetables are the edible parts of plants consumed by humans as food as a part of a meal. This includes stems, leaves, roots, seeds, etc.

**Q1. What are the advantages of vegetables?**
- Vegetables are protective foods.
- Vegetables will provide minerals, vitamins and fibers.
- Vegetables contains high amount of water and low energy.
- Green, yellow, orange and red vegetables are sources of β-carotene.
- Green peas, beans are rich source of proteins.

**Q2. How are vegetables classified?**
Vegetables are classified in to three groups:
- Green leaves, roots and tubers and others:
  - Green leaves—spinach, cabbage

# Nutrition

- ➢ Roots and tubers—potato, tapioca, carrots, radish, colocasia
- ➢ Others—tomatoes, cauliflower.
- ❖ *Green leaves:*
  - Spinach
  - Cabbage
- ❖ *Roots and tuber:*
  - Potato
  - Carrots
  - Radish
  - Colocasia
  - Tapioca
  - Sweet potato
  - Yam
  - Onion
- ❖ *Others:*
  - Tomatoes, cauliflower.
  - Potato and tapioca are good sources of carbohydrates.

## Green leaves:

- ❖ Spinach
- ❖ Cabbage
- ❖ Green leafy vegetables are low in calories.
- ❖ Calcium, iron, vitamin C and vitamin $B_{12}$, folic acid.
- ❖ Green leafy vegetables are rich in calcium, iron, β-carotene, vitamin and B complex.
- ❖ Green leafy vegetables contains chlorophyll which will destroy bacteria from the teeth, intestine. *Green leafy vegetables contain vitamin A (β-carotene), iron, calcium, carotene, riboflavin, folic acid, vitamin C and vitamin K.*
- ❖ These are cheapest protective foods.
- ❖ Chlorophyll contains high quality protein.
- ❖ *Examples of Green leafy vegetables are:*
  - Spinach
  - Amaranth
  - Cabbage
  - Fenugreek
- ❖ Possess low calories 25–50 kcal per 100 g, large bulk.
- ❖ Recommended daily intake is about 40–50 g for an adult.

- ❖ Green leaves are rich in B group proteins except vitamin $B_{12}$
- ❖ Green leaves are rich in carotenes, calcium, iron, and vitamin C.
- ❖ Leaf proteins are good sources of lysine but are deficient in sulfur containing amino acids.
- ❖ The bioavailability of calcium and iron are poor in green leaves because of the presence of high amount of oxalates.
- ❖ Drumstick leaves: GYO (green yellow orange vegetables are rich in β-carotene).
- ❖ Green leafy vegetables good sources of iron:
  - Cauliflower: 40 mg%
  - Gathui, amaranth: 4 mg%
  - Drumstick leave: curry leave, spinach: 1 mg%

*Green leafy vegetables: Nutritive value.*

| Vegetable | Energy (kcal) | Protein (g) | Carbohydrate (g) | Fat (g) |
|---|---|---|---|---|
| Cabbage | 27 | 1.8 | 4.6 | 0.1 |
| Spinach | 26 | 2.0 | 2.9 | 0.7 |

Q1. **What are the conditions in which leafy vegetables should be restricted?**
- ❑ Peptic or duodenal ulcer
- ❑ Diarrhea
- ❑ Kidney stones.

Q2. **What is the daily recommended intake of green leafy vegetables?**
40 g for an adult.

## Spinach (Fig. 1.11)

English: Spinach
Tamil: Pasalai keerai
Hindi: Palak/Poi
Malayalam: Palak Cheera
Telugu: Paalak
Kannada: Paalak/Kemp Baayi Basalae
Gujarathi: Palak
Marathi: Sag/Velbondi
Punjabi: Poi/Palak
Bengali: Palang/Puin/Pui Shaakh

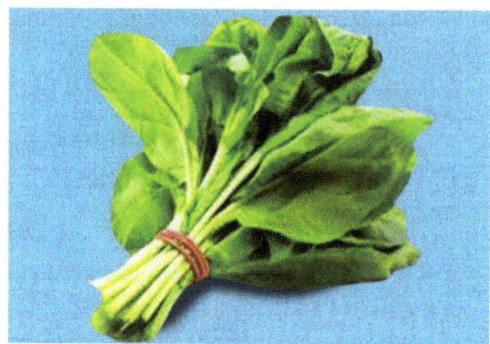

**Fig. 1.11:** Spinach.

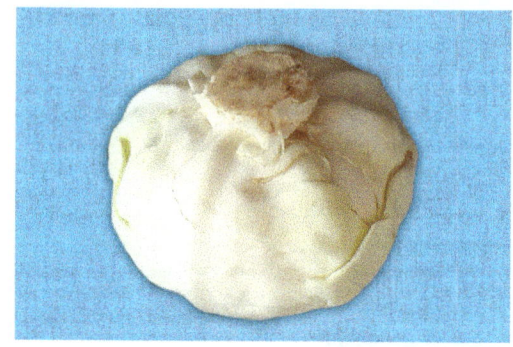

**Fig. 1.12:** Cabbage.

**Q1. What is the nutritive value of spinach?**
- Water: 91.7%
- Protein: 1.9%
- Fat: 0.9%
- Carbohydrates: 4%
- Minerals: 1.5%
  - Calcium: 0.06%
  - Phosphorus: 0.01%
  - Iron: 5 mg/100 g
- Vitamin A: 2,600–3,500 IU/100 g
- Vitamin B: 70 IU/100 g
- Vitamin C: 48 mg/100 g
- It also contains magnesium, sulfur, sodium, silicone, potassium.
- Spinach is rich in iron and is useful in iron deficiency anemia.

**Q2. What is the condition in which spinach should be restricted?**
Spinach contains salts of oxalic acid and may predispose to kidney stones.

## Cabbage (Fig. 1.12)

English: Cabbage
Tamil: Muttaikosu
Hindi: Bandh Gobi/patta Gobi
Malayalam: Muttaikose
Telugu: Gos Koora/Kosu/Gobi
Kannada: Kosu/Ele Kosu
Gujarathi: Kobi
Marathi: Pan Kobi
Punjabi: Gobi
Kashmiri: Band

**Q1. What is the nutritive value of cabbage?**
- Water: 90.2%
- Protein: 1.8%
- Fat: 0.1%
- Carbohydrates: 6.3%
- Minerals: 0.6%
  - Calcium: 0.03%
  - Phosphorus: 0.05%
  - Iron: 0.8 mg/100 g
- Vitamin A: 2,000 IU/100 g
- Vitamin B1: 60 µg/100 g
- Vitamin B2: 30 µg/100 g
- Niacin: 0.4 mg/100 g
- Vitamin C: 124 mg/100 g
- The outer leaves are rich in vitamin A and iron.
- Excessive cooking will decrease the vitamin B and vitamin C.

## Drumstick Leaves (Fig. 1.13)

English: Drumstick leaves
Tamil: Murungai Keerai/Murungai Ilai
Hindi: Saijan Patta
Malayalam: Murungai Ela
Telugu: Mulagu Akulu
Kannada: Nuggekai
Gujarathi: Sarangvani
Marathi: Shevaga Pan
Bengali: Sajna Sag

**Q1. What is the nutritive value of drumstick leaves?**
- Water: 75%
- Protein: 6.7%

Nutrition

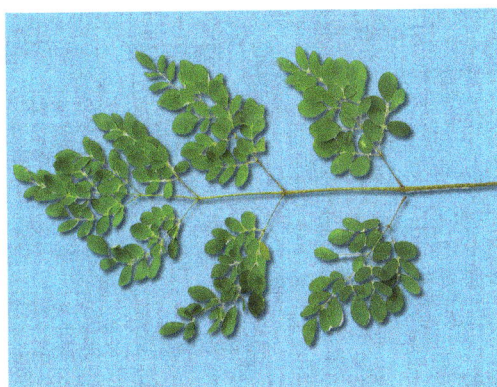

Fig. 1.13: Drumstick leaves.

- Fat: 1.7%
- Carbohydrates: 13.4%
- Minerals: 2.3%
  - Calcium: 0.44%
  - Phosphorus: 0.07%
  - Iron: 7 mg/100 g
- Vitamin A: 11,300 IU/100 g
- Vitamin B: 70 IU/100 g
- Vitamin C: 220 mg/100 g
- High vitamin A content
- Rich in vitamin A, iron.

## Agathi Keerai (Fig. 1.14)

English: Spinach/Agathi keerai
Tamil: Agathi keerai
Hindi: Agasti
Malayalam: Agathi Cheera/Pacha Cheera/
Bombay: Cheera

Telugu: Avisi
Kannada: Agase/Agasthi
Gujarathi: Agathio
Marathi: Agasti/Agasta
Bengali: Bakful/Buko

- Protein 8.4%
- Fat 1.4%
- Carbohydrates 13.4%

Contains minerals, iron, vitamin A and vitamin C.

## Other Vegetables

### Tomato (Fig. 1.15)

Tomato is rich in vitamin A (β-carotene) and vitamin C. Tomato contains β-carotene and antioxidants.

**Q1. What is the nutritive value of tomato?**
- *Per 100 g:*
  - Water: 95%
  - Protein: 0.9%
  - Fat: 0.2 g
  - Carbohydrates: 4%
  - Dietary fibers: 1.2 g
  - Calorie: 18 kcal
  - Rich in potassium
  - Minerals:
    - Calcium
    - Phosphorus
    - Iron
  - Vitamin B1
  - Vitamin B2
  - Vitamin C

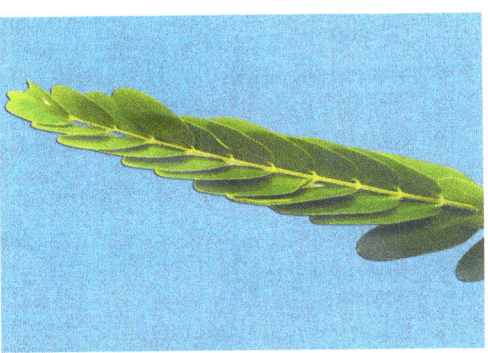

Fig. 1.14: Agathi keerai.

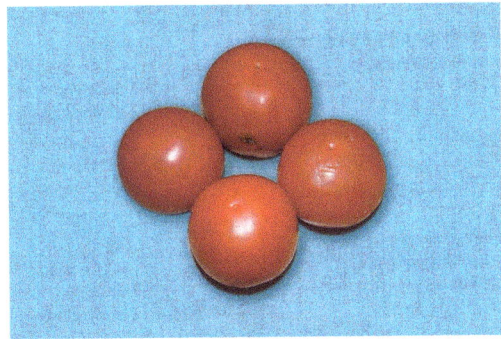

Fig. 1.15: Tomato.

- Excess intake may predispose to renal stone formation.
- About 150 mL of tomato juice will supply about one-third of vitamin C required for the day.
- Vitamin C present in the tomato will not easily destroyed because it is protected by acid.
- Iron in tomato is easily digestible.

**Q2. What is the difference between ripe and unripe tomato?**
- Only ripe tomato contains vitamin B2
- The vitamin C content will increase as the tomato ripens.

**Q3. How tomatoes are used in the diet?**
- Salad
- Tomato juice
- Can be eaten raw
- Used in rasam
- Can be used as soup, by boiling tomatoes in water.

**Q4. Why tomato is good for diabetic patients?**
The carbohydrate content in tomato is very low. Hence it is useful in diabetic patients. For the same reason it is useful for those who want to reduce weight.

**Q5. Why tomato is not good for kidney patients?**
Because it is rich in potassium.

## *Cauliflower (Fig. 1.16)*

- Low in fat
- Nutritive value: per 100 g:
  - Water: 92.0%
  - Protein: 1.9%
  - Fat: 0.3 g
  - Carbohydrates: 5 g
  - Calories: 104 kilocalories
  - Dietary fibers: 2 g
- Rich in vitamins (vitamin B1, vitamin B2, vitamin C) and minerals.
- Minerals:
  - Calcium
  - Phosphorus
  - Iron.

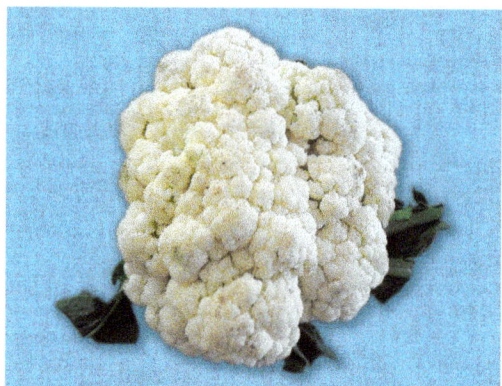

Fig. 1.16: Cauliflower.

- *Nutritive value*:

| Vegetable | Energy (kcal) | Protein (g) | Carbohydrate (g) | Fat (g) |
|---|---|---|---|---|
| Cauliflower | 25 | 1.9 | 5 | 0.3 |

**Roots and tubers:**

**Carrot:**

- *Nutritive values:* each 100 g contains:
  - Calories (kcal): 50
  - Protein: 1 g
  - Carbohydrate (g) 8.8
  - Carbohydrates 10.7%
  - Fats: 0.2%
  - 1 g of protein, 1 g fiber, 1 mg of iron
  - Water 86%
  - Protein 0.9%
  - Fat 0.2%
  - Minerals:
    - Calcium 0.08%
    - Phosphorus 0.53%
    - Iron 1.5 mg/100 g
  - Vitamin A: 2,000–4,300 IU/100 g
  - Vitamin B: 60 IU/100 g
  - Rich in vitamin A: β-carotene
  - Antioxidants
  - Fibers
  - Good source of carotene and calcium. The carotene will be converted to vitamin A by the liver.
  - Carrot contains six times more calcium than potato
  - Rich in vitamin A precursor β-carotene.

## QUESTIONS

**Q1. How β-carotene is absorbed?**
Absorbed through intestinal lymphatics.

**Q2. How will you calculate β-carotene and retinol into retinol equivalents?**
- 1 μg of β-carotene is equal to 0.167 μg of retinol equivalent.
- 1 μg of retinol is equal to 1 μg of retinol equivalent.

**Q3. What are the other plants sources containing β-carotene?**
- GYOR green, yellow, orange, red vegetables.
- Green: Green leafy vegetables (GLV)
- Yellow: Mango, lemon
- Orange
- Red: Red carrot, beet root (Fig. 1.17).

**Q4. What are the disadvantages of roots and tubers?**
Poor sources of protein, minerals and vitamins.

**Q5. What is the recommended intake of roots and tubers by an adult?**
50–60 g per day.

**Potato:**
- Potato is alkaline and will be helpful in maintaining the alkali reserve of the body and preventing acidosis.
- Potatoes are energy dense foods.
- Potatoes do not swell on cooking.

**Q1. What is the protein and calorie content of potato?**
- Energy (kcal): 97
- Protein (g): 1.6
- Water: 74.7%
- Fat: 0.1
- Carbohydrates: 22.9%
- Minerals:
  - Calcium: 0.01%
  - Phosphorus: 0.03%
  - Iron: 0.7 mg/100 g
- Vitamin A: 40 IU/100 g
- Potato also contains vitamin B1, vitamin B2 and vitamin C
- 95% of potatoes are digestible. It will be completely absorbed from the gut in about two and hours after eating it.

## QUESTIONS

**Q1. What is the recommended daily intake?**
Recommended daily intake 50–60 g for an adult.

**Q2. Why potatoes, roots and fibers are not consumed as staple foods?**
These are bulky and low in protein.

**Potato and tapioca:**
- Rich in carbohydrate
- Good source of energy and calcium.
- Poor source of protein, minerals and vitamins
- Potatoes contain vitamin C

### Nuts and Oil Seeds (Fig. 1.18)

Groundnut, cashewnut, coconut, walnut, almonds, pistachio, mustard seeds, sesame seeds, cotton seeds, sunflower seeds, maize germ, pistachio nuts.

### *Nutritive Values*

- Nuts and oil seeds are good sources of good quality protein, vitamins and fat.

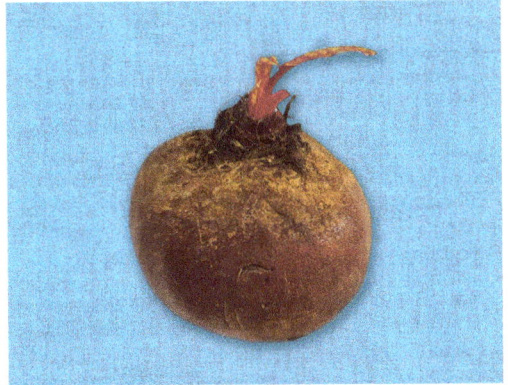

**Fig. 1.17:** Beet root.

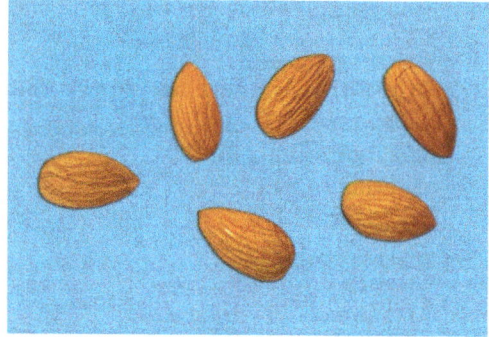
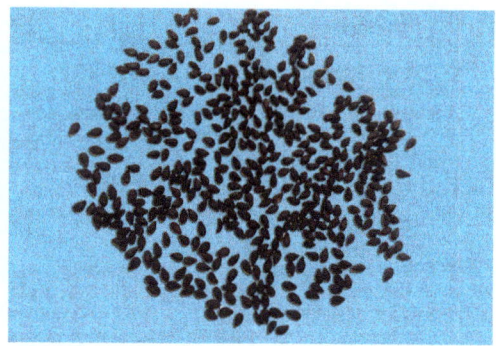

Fig. 1.18: Nuts and oil seeds.

- Nuts are good source of B group vitamins, minerals like calcium, phosphorus and iron.
- Cashewnuts and almonds are rich in iron.

**Q1. Which nut is the richest source of iron?**
- Pistachio is the richest source of iron. It contains 14 mg of iron per 100 g.
- Cashew, almonds, pista are rich in iron.
- Most of the vegetable oils are rich in essential fatty acids.

### Nuts and Oil Seeds Nutritive Value

| Nuts | Energy (kcal) | Protein (g) | Carbohydrate (g) | Fat (g) |
|---|---|---|---|---|
| Groundnut (Peanut) | 567 | 25.3 | 26.1 | 40.1 |
| Groundnut (roasted) | 570 | 26.2 | 26.7 | 39.8 |
| Mustard (seeds) | 541 | 20.0 | 23.8 | 39.7 |
| Coconut (dry) | 662 | 6.8 | 18.4 | 62.3 |
| Almond | 655 | 20.8 | 10.5 | 58.9 |
| Cashewnut | 596 | 21.2 | 22.3 | 46.9 |

### Coconut (Fig. 1.19)
- Coconut oil contains less essential fatty acids.
- Coconut oil contains more medium chain triglycerides (MCT). MCT will be directly absorbed into the portal vein. MCT are C8–C10 fatty acids.
- Monosaturated fatty acid will raise the HDL.

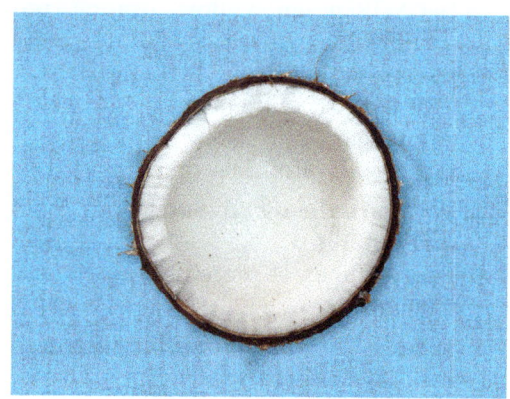

Fig. 1.19: Coconut.

### Groundnut (Fig. 1.20)
- Contains 40% fat and 20% protein
- When peanuts are stored in humid conditions a fungus *Aspergillus flavus* will grow. This fungus will produce aflatoxin.
- *Nutritive values:* 100 g contains:
  - Calories: 550
  - Protein: 25 g
  - Carbohydrate: 25 g
  - Fats: 40 g
  - Calcium: 90 mg
  - Iron: 2.5 mg
  - Carotene: 37 µg

### Fruits
- Amla
- Apple
- Banana

# Nutrition

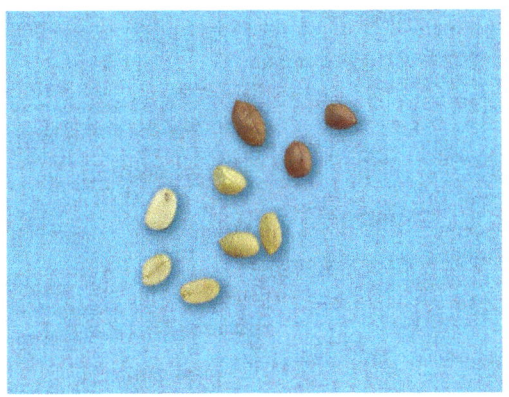

**Fig. 1.20:** Groundnut.

- Citrus fruits–lemon
- Dry fruits
- Gooseberry
- Grapes
- Guava
- Jack fruit
- Mango
- Orange
- Papaya
- Seetapal

*Nutritive Value of Fruits*

- Fruits are protective foods.
- Carbohydrates—many fruits are low in energy but for banana and mango which are rich in carbohydrates.
- Fruits are rich in vitamins, minerals and are easily available.
- Fruits are rich in fibers.
- Can be eaten raw and fresh.
- Pectin is a kind of sugar present in certain fruits like guava. It is helpful in preparation of fruit jellies and fruit sugars.
- More ripe fruit more will be the sugar content.
- Seasonal fruits should be consumed.
- Vitamin C rich fruits are amla, guava and citrus fruits.
- Dried fruits like dates are rich in iron.
- Recommended daily intake fresh fruits for an adult are 85 g or more per day.

❖ *Nutritive value of fruits* per 100 g of edible portion:

| Fruits | Energy (kcal) | Protein (g) | Carbohydrate (g) | Fat (g) |
|---|---|---|---|---|
| Amla | 58 | 0,5 | 13.7 | 0.1 |
| Apple | 59 | 0.2 | 13.4 | 0.5 |
| Banana (ripe) | 104 | 1.2 | 27.2 | 0.3 |
| Grapes | 58 | 0.6 | 13 | 0.4 |
| Guava | 51 | 0.9 | 11.2 | 0.3 |
| Lemon | 57 | 1.0 | 11.1 | 0.9 |
| Mango (ripe) | 74 | 0.6 | 16.9 | 0.4 |
| Orange | 48 | 0.7 | 10.9 | 0.2 |
| Papaya (ripe) | 32 | 0.6 | 7.2 | 0.1 |
| Pine apple | 46 | 0.4 | 10.8 | 0.1 |
| Pomegranate | 65 | 1.6 | 14.1 | 0.1 |
| Tomato | 20 | 0.9 | 3.6 | 0.2 |

❖ Dry fruits:

| Fruits | Energy (kcal) | Protein (g) | Carbohydrate (g) | Fat (g) |
|---|---|---|---|---|
| Dates (dried) | 317 | 2.5 | 75.8 | 0.4 |
| Raisins | 308 | 3.1 | 79 | 0.5 |

## QUESTIONS

**Q1. What are the nutrients present in the fruits?**
- Fruits are rich sources of vitamin, minerals (sodium and potassium) and fiber.
- Fruits are protective foods.

**Q2. What are the fruits rich in vitamin A precursors?**
- GYO (green, yellow and orange) fruits are rich in β-carotene.
- Mango and papaya are rich in carotene (vitamin A).

**Q3. What are the fruits rich in vitamin C?**
Citrus and amla (Indian gooseberry), guava are rich in vitamin C.

**Q4. What are the nutrients in dry fruits?**
- Dried fruits like raisins, apricots and dates are rich in calcium and iron.
- Seetapal*(custard apple) is rich in calcium.

**Q5. What are the fruits rich in energy?**
Banana, jack fruit, mango are good sources of energy.

**Q6. How do fruits help in bowel movements?**
Fruits contain cellulose which assists in normal bowel movements.

**Q7. What is the recommended intake of fruits per day?**
85 g of fruit per day.

**Q8. What are the fruits rich in vitamin C?**
Amla, citrus, guava are rich in vitamin C.

### *Amla (Indian gooseberry) (Fig. 1.21)*
- Water: 81.2%
- Protein: 0.5%
- Fat: 0.1%
- Carbohydrates: 14.1%
- Minerals:
  - Calcium: 0.05% (calcium 50 mg)
  - Phosphorus: 0.02%
  - Iron: 1.2 mg/100 g
- Calories: 58
- Carotene: 9 µg
- Amla contains gallic acid and albumin.
- Vitamin C 600 mg/100 g. When it is dried the vitamin C contents will increase. The dried amla will contain 2,400–2,600 mg of vitamin C per 100 g.

### *Apple (Fig. 1.22)*
- Water: 85.9%
- Protein: 0.3%

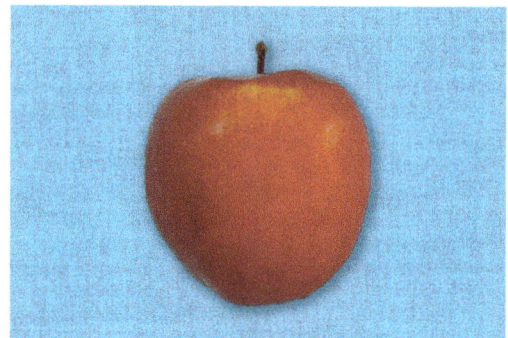

**Fig. 1.22:** Apple.

- Fat: 0.1%
- Carbohydrates: 9.5%
- Minerals: 0.4%
  - Calcium: 0.01%
  - Phosphorus: 0.02%
  - Iron: 1.7 mg/100 g
- Vitamin B: 40 IU/100 g
- Vitamin C trace
- Apple has laxative qualities Pectin in it will control diarrhea.

### *Plantain*
- Rich in carbohydrates.
- Contains 50 calories and 1 g of protein.

### *Banana (Fig. 1.23)*
- *Nutritive values*: 100 g contains:
  - Calories: 111 calories
  - Protein: 1 g
  - Rich in carbohydrates: 27 g carbohydrate

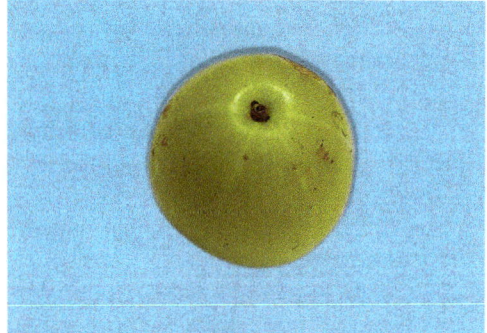

**Fig. 1.21:** Amla.

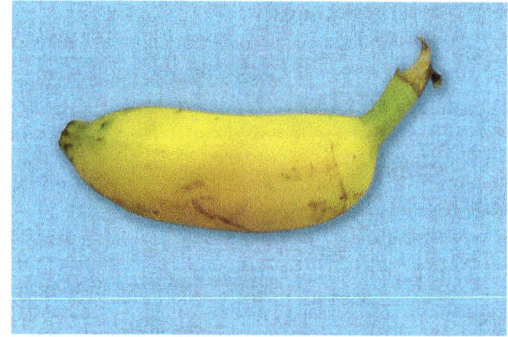

**Fig. 1.23:** Banana.

- Fiber: 0.4 g
- Iron: 0.4 mg
- Rich in vitamin A
- Rich in fibers–helps to relieve constipation
- Calcium: 10 mg
- Iron: 0.5 mg
- Carotene: 124 µg
- Vitamin C: 7 mg

❖ Rich in potassium, magnesium (Mg), dietary fiber, manganese, vitamin B6.
❖ Banana contains potassium, magnesium, dietary fibers, manganese and vitamin B6.
❖ *Banana (ripe and unripe).*

**Q1. What is the difference between ripe and unripe banana?**
Ripe banana contains more of pectin.

## Grapes (Fig. 1.24)
❖ Calories: 71
❖ Calcium: 20 mg
❖ Iron: 1.5 mg
❖ Carotene: 0 µg
❖ Vitamin C: 1 mg

**Q1. What is the difference between raw and ripe grapes?**
Ripe grape contains more sugar.

## Guava (Fig. 1.25)
❖ Calories: 51
❖ Calcium: 10 mg
❖ Iron: 0.27 mg
❖ Vitamin: C 212 mg

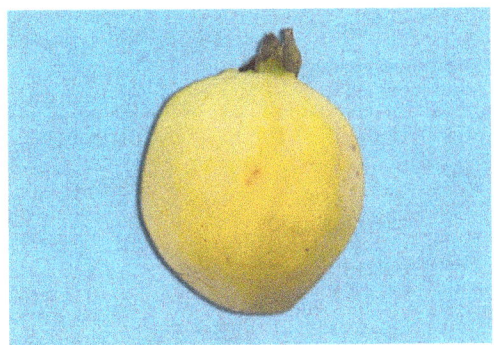

**Fig. 1.25:** Guava.

## Lemon (Fig. 1.26)
❖ It contains more acid and less sugar.
❖ Lemon juice is powerful antibacterial (this was proved by the Nobel Prize winner Professor Fanmuller).
❖ When Vasco da Gama made his voyage to Cape of Good Hope nearly two-third of his crew died of scurvy.
❖ Lemon contains more potassium and vitamin C.
❖ Water: 85%
❖ Protein: 1%
❖ Fat: 0.9%
❖ Carbohydrates: 11.1%
❖ Minerals: Fibers: 1–8%
  - Calcium: 0.07%
  - Phosphorus: 0.03%
  - Iron: 2.3 mg/100 g
❖ Vitamin C 39 mg/1000 g

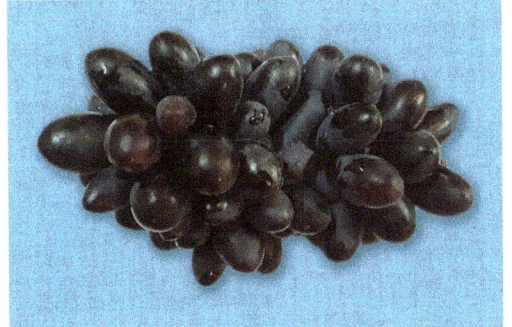

**Fig. 1.24:** Grapes.

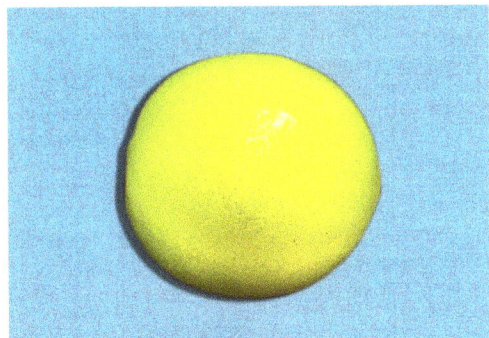

**Fig. 1.26:** Lemon.

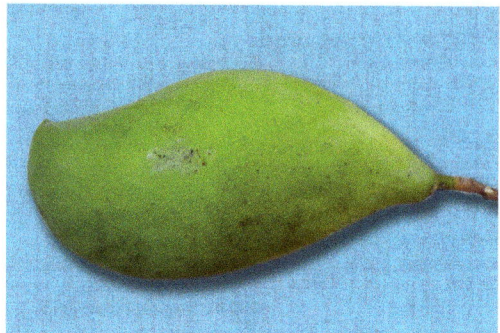

**Fig. 1.27:** Mango.

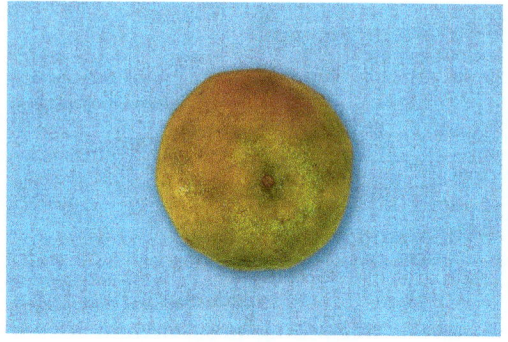

**Fig. 1.28:** Orange.

❖ Contains some vitamin A, niacin and thiamin.

**Q1. Why vitamin C in lemon is more effective?**

Vitamin C in lemon is more effective because it is combined with riboflavinoids.

**Q2. Why lemon juice should be taken diluted in water?**

Pure lemon juice contains acid which will cause injury to the enamel.

### Mango (Fig. 1.27)

Mangoes are rich in vitamin A and vitamin C, B complex.
- ❖ Calories: 74
- ❖ Calcium: 14 mg
- ❖ Iron: 1.3 mg
- ❖ Carotene: 2,210 µg
- ❖ Vitamin C: 16 mg

### Orange (Fig. 1.28)

It is an alkali forming food although acidic in taste.

**Q1. What is the protein and calorie content of orange?**
- ❑ Calories: 47
- ❑ Protein (g): 0.7
- ❑ Carbohydrate (g): 10.9
- ❑ Fat (g): 0.2
- ❑ Water: 87.8%
- ❑ Minerals:
  - ➢ Calcium: 0.05%
  - ➢ Phosphorus: 0.02%
  - ➢ Iron: 0.1 mg/100 g
  - ➢ Sodium: 2.1 mg/100 g
  - ➢ Potassium: 19.7 mg/100 g
  - ➢ Magnesium: 12.9 mg/100 g
  - ➢ Copper: 0.07 mg/100 g
  - ➢ Sulfur: 9.3 mg/100 g
  - ➢ Chlorine: 3.2 mg/100 g

**Vitamins**
- ❑ Vitamin A: 350 IU/100 g
- ❑ Vitamin B: 120 IU/100 g
- ❑ Carotene: 2,240 µg
- ❑ Vitamin C: 68 mg/100 g
- ❑ Orange is a rich source of vitamin A.
- ❑ Orange juice is considered superior to lemon juice because it contains less acid than lemon juice.
- ❑ 125–150 mL of orange juice will provide the daily requirement of vitamin C.
- ❑ Vitamin C content of orange is not easily destroyed because it is protected by citric acid.
- ❑ Vitamin C is blended with calcium which increases the qualities of each other.

### Papaya (Fig. 1.29)

Papaya is rich in fiber, vitamin C, antioxidants, vitamin A. Unripe green papaya fruit and the leaves will contain an enzyme papain. When eaten in larger quantities it can be natural contraceptive and also cause abortion.

**Q1. What is the protein and calorie content of papaya?**
- ❑ Calories energy (kcal): 32
- ❑ Protein (g): 0.6

# Nutrition

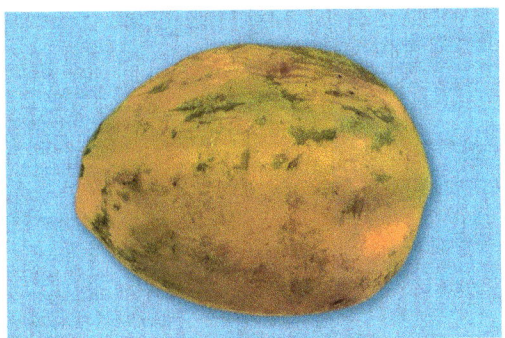

**Fig. 1.29:** Papaya.

- Carbohydrate (g): 7.2
- Water: 89.6%
- Fat: 0.1%
- Minerals: 0.4%
  - Calcium: 0.01%
  - Phosphorus: 0.01%
  - Iron: 0.4 mg/100 g

**Vitamins**
- Vitamin A: 2,020 IU/100 g
- Vitamin C: 46–136 mg/100 g
- Carotene: 2,740 μg
- Vitamin C: 57 mg
- Vitamin B1 and vitamin B2 and niacin
- The sugar and vitamin C contents will be high in papaya during the months of May to October.

**Q2. What are the sugars present in papaya?**
Glucose and fructose (fruit sugar) are present in equal amounts.

**Q3. What are the vitamins present in papaya?**
Vitamin A, vitamin C, vitamin B1, vitamin B2 and niacin.

**Q4. What are the differences between raw papaya and ripe papaya?**
- Raw papaya is green in color. Ripe papaya is yellow in color.
- The content of vitamin C will increase with maturity raw papaya contains 32 mg of vitamin C per 100 g. Ripe papaya contains 68–136 mg of vitamin C per 100 g.

**Q5. What is papain?**
It is a protein digesting enzyme present in the white secretion of raw papaya.

## Seetapal

- Calories: 104
- Calcium: 17 mg
- Iron: 4.31 mg
- Vitamin C: 37 mg

## Fats and Oils

**Q1. What are the differences between fats and oils?**
Fats are solids and oils are liquids at room temperature.

## Oil

- One teaspoon will provide 45 calories. 1 g of fat provides 9 calories.
- This will help to provide more calories without increasing the volume of food taken.
- One teaspoon of oil contains 45 calories.
- Coconut oil is without fatty acids.
- Red palm oil contains vitamin A.
- Animal source of essential fatty acids are sardine oil and cod liver oil.
- Safflower oil is rich in linoleic acid.

| Fats and oils | Energy (kcal) | Protein (g) | Carbohydrate (g) | Fat (g) |
|---|---|---|---|---|
| Butter | 729 | Nil | Nil | 81 |
| Ghee | 900 | Nil | Nil | 100 |
| Vegetable oils (coconut, groundnut, palm, mustard) | 900 | Nil | Nil | 100 |

- Red palm oil is a rich source of β-carotene (about 800 μg/g).
- Total calories from visible fat should not be more than 10–15% with a maximum up to 20%.

**Q2. What are refined oils?**
Refining is done by treatment of oils by alkali, steam, etc. It improves the quality and taste of oils.

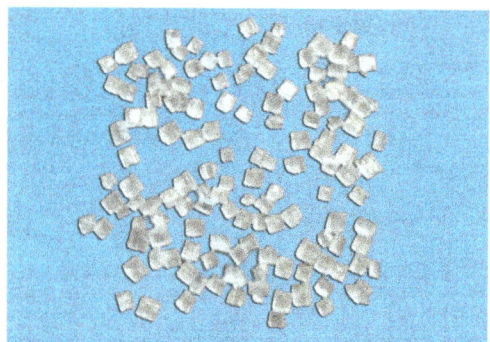

**Fig. 1.30:** Sugar.

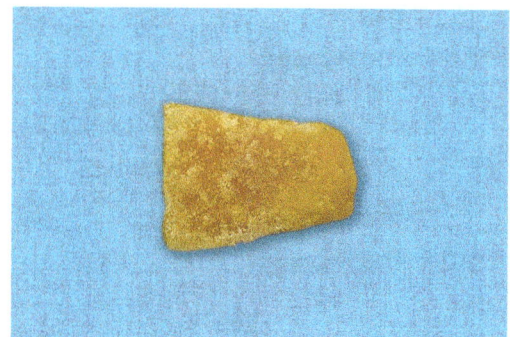

**Fig. 1.31:** Jaggery.

**Q3. Does refining of oils change the unsaturated fatty acid content of oils?**
No refining of oils will not change the unsaturated fatty acid content of oils.

## Sugars
- Sugar
- Jaggery
- Honey

### Sugar (Fig. 1.30)
- Sugars are good energy concentrates. 1 teaspoon of sugar will provide 20 calories. There is no protein or fats. 1 g of carbohydrate will provide 94 calories.
- *Sugar* contains 20 calories per teaspoon and the daily intake from refined sugars should not exceed 10% of total calorie requirement.
- *Nutritive value:*
    - Energy (kcal): 398
    - Protein (g): 0.1
    - Carbohydrate (g): 99.4
    - Fat (g): Nil

## QUESTIONS

**Q1. What is the calorific value of sugar?**
Calorific value: One teaspoon will provide 20 calories.

**Q2. What are refined sugars?**
Pure sucrose with no other nutrients.

**Q3. What is the maximal permissible limit of refined sugars in a balanced diet?**
The amount of the intake of the refined sugars should be restricted, so that it supplies less than 5–10% of the total calorie needs. The total amount of energy derived from refined sugar should not exceed 10% of the total daily requirement.

**Q4. What are the problems associated with intake of refined sugars?**
The ingestion of refined sugars increases the risk of dental caries. It also causes hyperinsulinemia, which predisposes to hyperlipoproteinemia, atherosclerosis. It has been associated with certain tumor growths like breast and colonic carcinoma in the adult life.

**Q5. What are the disadvantages of excessive intake of sugars?**
- There will be wide fluctuations in blood sugar.
- Incidence of caries tooth will be more.

### Jaggery (Fig. 1.31)
- This is an unrefined sugar made from sugar cane juice or palm. It is made by evaporating water from the sugar can juice.
- This is becoming a healthy replacement for sugar.
- Jaggery is rich in iron and carotene.
- *Nutritive value:*
    - Energy (kcal): 383
    - Protein (g): 0.4
    - Carbohydrate (g): 95
    - Fat (g): 0.1

- Sucrose: 65–85 g
- Fructose and glucose: 10–15 g
- Iron: 11 mg
- Potassium: 1,050 mg
❖ Jaggery contains vitamin B, minerals, calcium, phosphorus and copper.

## QUESTIONS

**Q1. What are the health benefits of jaggery?**
- ❏ Agent for cleaning
- ❏ Boosts energy
- ❏ Constipation is relieved
- ❏ Digestion is improved
- ❏ Extra nutritious than sugar.

### *Honey*

❖ Consists of 75% sugar fructose and glucose.
❖ *Nutritive value:*
- Energy (kcal): 319
- Protein (g): 0.3
- Carbohydrate (g): 79.5
- Fat (g): Nil

❖ Botulism is associated with intake of honey.

| Sugars | Energy (kcal) | Protein (g) | Carbohydrate (g) | Fat (g) |
|---|---|---|---|---|
| Sugar | 398 | 0.1 | 99.4 | Nil |
| Jaggery (cane) | 383 | 0.4 | 95.0 | 0.1 |
| Honey | 319 | 0.3 | 79.5 | Nil |

## Condiments or Spices

Condiments or spices are supplemental food items that are added to food to impart or add flavor or enhance flavor:

- ❖ Asafetida
- ❖ Barbecue
- ❖ Cardamom
- ❖ Chilies
- ❖ Cloves
- ❖ Coriander
- ❖ Cumin seeds
- ❖ Dip
- ❖ Epazote
- ❖ Enchilada sauce
- ❖ Frosting
- ❖ Garlic
- ❖ Ginger
- ❖ Honey
- ❖ Idli podi
- ❖ Jalapenos
- ❖ Kadugu
- ❖ Lemon
- ❖ Lecithin
- ❖ Mustard
- ❖ Nutritional yeast
- ❖ Nutmeg
- ❖ Olive oil
- ❖ Onion
- ❖ Pepper
- ❖ Poppy seeds
- ❖ Piccalilli
- ❖ Raisins
- ❖ Salt and pepper
- ❖ Tamarind
- ❖ Turmeric
- ❖ Vanilla
- ❖ Vinegar
- ❖ Yeast

### *Benefits of Condiments or Spices*

- ❖ Increase palatability
- ❖ Give taste to food
- ❖ Supply $\alpha$-carotene, vitamins and minerals
- ❖ Green chilies will supply $\beta$-carotene
- ❖ Garlic is rich source of selenium
- ❖ Turmeric is good source of iron but tannin in it will interfere with iron absorption.
- ❖ Nutritive value is less

## QUESTIONS

**Q1. Which condiment is known as black gold of India?**
Pepper.

**Q2. Which condiment is known as king of spices?**
Pepper.

**Q3. Which condiment is known as queen of spices?**
Cardamom.

## Beverages

- Beverages are liquids intended for human consumption.
- Coffee, tea
- Beverages are used to quench thirst and not consumed for their food value.

### Types of Beverages

- Alcoholic beverages—wine, beer, whisky.
- Nonalcoholic beverages contain no alcohol. They can be soft drinks or hot drinks.
- Soft drinks: Aerated water
- Hot drinks: Coffee, tea

### Soft drinks:

- *Bottled drinks—carbonated:* Carbonated drinks will have carbon dioxide dissolved in it.
    Example–soda.
- *Bottled drinks—noncarbonated:* Comes in various names.

### Fruit juices:

- Orange juice
- Grape fruit juice
- Coconut water
- Vegetable juices
- Sugar cane juice
- Neera
- Milk based beverages: Butter milk, lassi
- Flavored milk: Rose milk, badam milk.

## QUESTIONS

**Q1. What are the advantages of beverages?**
Quenches thirst.

**Q2. What are the disadvantages of beverages?**
- Not useful for treating rehydration
- No nutritive value.

## Animal Foods

- Milk and dairy products
- Egg
- Meat
- Poultry
- Fish
- *Animal foods* are good sources of high quality protein, which contains all amino acids, and good amount of fats, vitamins and minerals.
- *Animal foods* will provide vitamin $B_{12}$.
- Milk and dairy products: Egg.

### Milk and Dairy Products

- Milk is the most complete of all foods.
- Milk is a good source of protein, fats, sugars, calcium, vitamins and minerals. Milk is deficient in iron and vitamin C.
- High phosphate content in cow's milk will interfere with iron and calcium absorption.
- Human milk contains high lactose about 7 g%.
- Buffalo milk will contain high fat about 7 g% which is mostly saturate fat.

Nutritive value of milk and milk products:

| Milk product | Energy (kcal) | Protein (g) | Carbohydrate (g) | Fat (g) |
|---|---|---|---|---|
| Milk (cow) | 67 | 3.2 | 4.4 | 4.1 |
| Milk (Human) | 65 | 1.1 | 7.4 | 3.4 |
| Milk (Buffalo) | 117 | 4.3 | 5.0 | 6.5 |
| Butter milk | 15 | 0.8 | 0.5 | 1.1 |
| Curd | 60 | 3.1 | 3.0 | 4.0 |
| Cheese | 348 | 24.1 | 6.3 | 25.1 |

### Milk:

- 67 calories in 100 mL
- 3 g protein
- Milk is deficient in vitamin C
- Mineral deficient is iron
- Rich in calcium, potassium, sodium, magnesium, cobalt, copper.

**Q1. What are the proteins present in milk?**
Casein, lactalbumin and lactoglobulin.

**Q2. What is the chief protein in cow's milk?**
- Casein
- Milk proteins will contain all essential amino acids.

- Greater amounts of tryptophan. Sulfur containing amino acids especially cysteine.

**Q3. What is the fat content of human milk?**
3.4%

**Q4. What is the fat content of buffalo milk?**
- 8.8%
- Human milk will contain higher percentage of linoleic acid and oleic acid.
- Milk fat is rich source of retinol and vitamin D.
- Milk contains all minerals needed by the body like calcium, phosphorus, sodium, potassium, magnesium, cobalt, copper, iodine.
- Milk is a poor source of iron.
- Milk is poor source of vitamin C, but rich in all other vitamins.

**Milk products:**
Butter, ghee, dried and condensed milk, khoa, ice cream.

**Q1. What is skimmed milk?**
- The milk from which fats are removed resulting in poor source of fat and fat soluble vitamins.
- But it is a good source of milk protein and calcium.

**Q2. What is toned milk?**
It is blend of 1 part of water, 1 part of natural milk and 1.8 part of skim milk powder.

**Q3. What is vegetable milk?**
It is the milk prepared from vegetables, like groundnut, soybeans.

**Egg:**
- *Weight wise composition of egg:*
  - 58-60% of egg will be egg white
  - 30% will be egg yolk
  - 10-12% is the weight of shell.
  - Average egg will provide 66-70 calories of which 80% comes from the yolk.
  - Vitamin C, carbohydrates, fibers are absent-egg is good source of good quality protein, vitamins and fat. But poor source of carbohydrate, fibers, sugars and vitamin C.

**Q1. What is the nutritive value of egg?**
- *Nutritive value per egg* (60 g):
  - Calories: 66-70 kcal
  - Protein: 6 g
  - Fat: 6 g
  - Cholesterol: 250 mg/egg
- Rich in high quality protein and easily digestible
- Contains no carbohydrates or fibers
- Reference protein as it contains all essential amino acids in right proportions
- *Rule of six:* 66 calories and 6 g of protein and 6 g of fat:
  - An average sized egg will be 60 g in weight will contain 6 g of protein and 66 calories
  - Egg does not contain trans fats.
- *Minerals:*
  - Contains other minerals like calcium, phosphorus, zinc, iron. Good source of iron and phosphorus.
  - Iron: 1.5 mg
  - Rich in calcium 30 mg of calcium
- *Vitamins:*
  - Rich in vitamin A and vitamin D.
  - Egg contains all fat soluble and water soluble vitamins except vitamin C.
- *Electrolytes:*
  - Sodium: 65 mg
  - Potassium: 126 mg
  - Biological value (BV) of Egg is 96
  - Net protein utilization (NPU) of egg is 100
  - Protein efficiency ratio (PER) of egg is 3.8
  - Deficient in iron
  - Biotin is present in the egg
  - Avidin in raw duck egg will prevent body from obtaining biotin and cause biotin deficiency.
  - Boiling will destroy avidin.
  - Boiled egg is superior to raw egg.
  - Raw egg will not be assimilated by the gastrointestinal tract so it should be cooked before consumption.

| Part of egg | Composition |
|---|---|
| White | High quality protein<br>Riboflavin<br>Selenium<br>Avidin |
| Yolk | Vitamin A, D, E and K<br>Choline<br>Antioxidants–lutein and zeaxanthin<br>Cholesterol<br>DHA<br>Carotenoids<br>Amino acid (AA)<br>Biotin |

| Constituents | Egg white | Egg yolk |
|---|---|---|
| Protein (g) | 3.6 | 2.7 |
| Fat | 0.05 | 4.5 |
| Calcium (mg) | 2.3 | 21.9 |
| Phosphorus (mg) | 5 | 66.3 |

## QUESTIONS

Q1. **What is the average weight of an egg?**
60–80 g.

Q2. **What is the amount of carbohydrate present in the egg?**
Egg contains no carbohydrates.

Q3. **What is the amount of vitamin C present in the egg?**
Egg contains no vitamin C.

Q4. **What is the amount of fibers present in the egg?**
Egg contains no fibers.

Q5. **What are the minerals present in the egg?**
Egg contains minerals like phosphorus and zinc.

Q6. **What are the features of egg?**
- High density
- Does not swell on boiling
- Weight 60 g.

Q7. **Egg yolk is rich in what nutrient?**
Egg yolk is rich in cholesterol.

Q8. **What is the proportion of egg white and yolk?**
Weight wise 60% of the egg is of white. 30% is egg yolk, 10–12% is shell.

Q9. **What is the nutrient present in egg white and yolk?**
Egg white is rich in salt and egg yolk is rich in cholesterol.

Q10. **What is the amount of calcium present in one egg?**
About 30 mg.

Q11. **What are the forms in which the egg is eaten?**
- Scrambled egg
- Fried egg
- Boiled egg
- Half boiled egg

Q12. **What is the net protein utilization value of egg?**
- Net protein utilization (NPU) for egg is 100 (NPU for milk is 75, NPU for meat is 80).
- Egg contains 30 mg of calcium and 1.5 mg of iron. Egg contains all nine essential amino acids in adequate proportions needed by the human body.

Q13. **What are the minerals present in egg?**
Calcium, phosphorus, iron, zinc, other trace elements.

Q14. **What is the effect of eating raw duck's egg?**
- Raw duck's egg contains avidin which will bind with biotin in the intestines and predispose to biotin deficiency.
- The intestine will not assimilate raw egg white.

Q15. **Why boiled egg is nutritionally superior to raw egg?**
Boiling will destroy avidin which prevents body from obtaining biotin. Hence boiled egg is superior to raw egg.

Q16. **What is the disadvantage of consuming raw egg white?**
The intestine will not assimilate raw egg white.

# Nutrition

**Q17. Will cooking increase the calorific value of egg?**
- Yes, cooking will increase the chance of extracting and preserving nutrients.
- Cooking will increase the digestibility.

**Q18. What is the effect of boiling the egg?**
Boiling the egg will result in loss of vitamin B1.

**Q19. Egg is rich in which mineral?**
Egg is rich in calcium.

**Q20. What are the disadvantages of egg?**
- The intestine will not assimilate egg white.
- Antinutritive factor present in egg is trypsin inhibitor in egg white
- Raw egg interferes with digestion by inhibiting trypsin.

**Q21. What is rule of six for nutritive value of egg?**
Rule of six:
- Weight of egg is 60 g weight
- 66 calories
- 6 g fat
- 6 g protein
- 1.5 mg of iron (6/4 = 1.5)
- 30 mg of calcium (6 × 5 = 30)

**Q22. Why egg is known as reference protein?**
- Reference protein: It contains all essential amino acids, net protein utilization is 100%.
- Egg and breast milk are reference proteins because their AA profile is close to that of our body tissue protein and contains all essential amino acids.

**Q23. What are the positive aspects of egg?**
- Reference protein
- Calories 80 calories
- Easy availability and easy storage.

**Q24. What is the problem of consuming unboiled egg?**
- Avidin is present in the egg white. The avidin will be destroyed by the heat while cooking. Hence consuming unboiled egg will predispose to biotin deficiency.
- Salmonella infection.

**Q25. What is the advantage of choline and lutein in egg?**
Contains choline and lutein which has a positive influence of cognitive development and academic performance.

**Q26. How will you test for good egg?**
- Water density test should be done.
- Fresh egg will sink to the bottom of water and lie on the side.
- Less fresh eggs will sink to bottom and stand at an angle to the bottom.
- Old eggs will float on the water.

**Q27. Why old eggs float in the water?**
All the eggs becomes old the air sacs inside will become larger.

## Meat and Meat Products

**Meat:**
- Contains 15–20% of protein
- Good source of essential amino acids
- Iron 2–4 mg per 100 g.
- Iron is more easily absorbed than from plant sources.
- Fat composed of essential fatty acid
- Minerals zinc and B complex vitamins
- Poor in calcium rich in phosphorus
- Potassium: 421 mg
- Sodium: 57 mg
- Contains no carbohydrates, fibers, sugar.

### Pork

*Nutritive value*: 100 g will provide
- Protein: 18
- Fat: 4.4
- Energy: 114 calories
- Rich in potassium, riboflavin, zinc

### Liver
- Cholesterol: 355 mg
- Carbohydrate: 3.8 g
- Potassium: 150 mg
- Calcium: 10 mg

- Iron: 23 mg
- No fibers

*Poultry*

**Chicken:**

- Energy (kcal): 190
- Protein (g): 28
- Carbohydrate (g): Nil
- Fat (g): 7.4
- Cholesterol (mg): 89
- Contains no carbohydrates, fibers, sugars
- Calories from fat: 69%

Nutritive value per 100 g of animal foods or meat and meat products:

| Meat and meat products (100 g) | Energy (kcal) | Protein (g) | Carbohydrate (g) | Fat (g) | Cholesterol (mg) |
|---|---|---|---|---|---|
| Egg | 173 | 13.3 | Nil | 13.3 | 373 |
| Meat | 194 | 21–26 | Nil | 3.6 | 73 |
| Liver | 134 | 20–26 | 2.5–3.8 | 3.7 | 355 |
| Fish | 100–300 | 19–60 | Nil | 1–12 | 63 |
| Chicken | 190 | 28 | Nil | 7.4 | 89 |

*Fish and Sea Foods*

- Fishes are rich in proteins, vitamin D.
- Fish oil contains unsaturated fats
- Fish is rich in proteins 15–25%
- Rich in unsaturated fatty acids
- Vitamin A and vitamin D
- Poor sources of iron 0.7–3 mg per 100 g.
- Sea fish contains iodine
- Carbohydrates and fibers are absent in fish
- Cholesterol 63 mg
- Potassium 384 mg

**Miscellaneous**

*Tender Coconut*

**Q1. What is the amount of potassium present in tender coconut?**
- Energy: 160–200 kcal/L
- Carbohydrates: 8.9 g
- Sugars: 6.3 g
- Fibers: 2.6 g
- Protein: 1.78 g
- Fat is less than 1 g
- Electrolytes:
  - Coconut water contains sodium and potassium.
  - It should be avoided in renal failure cases as it contains more potassium.
  - Used for rehydration.
  - Contains vitamin C, calcium and iron.
  - Contains less sugar than soft drinks.
  - Does not contain cholesterol, vitamin A.

*Tomato*

Tomato is rich in vitamin A (β-carotene) and vitamin C. Tomato contains β-carotene and antioxidants.

**Q1. What is the nutritive value of tomato?**
- Water: 94.3%
- Protein: 0.9%
- Fat
- Carbohydrates
- Minerals:
  - Calcium
  - Phosphorus
  - Iron
- Vitamin B1
- Vitamin B2
- Vitamin C
- Calories
- Rich in potassium
- Excess intake may predispose to renal stone formation.
- About 150 mL of tomato juice will supply about one-third of vitamin C required for the day.

- Vitamin C present in the tomato will note easily destroyed because it is protected by acid.
- Iron in tomato is easily digestible.

**Q2. What is the difference between ripe and unripe tomato?**
- Only ripe tomato contains vitamin B2
- The vitamin C content will increase as the tomato ripens.

**Q3. How tomatoes are used in the diet?**
- Salad
- Can be eaten raw
- Used in rasam
- Tomato can be used as soup, by boiling tomatoes in water.

**Q4. Why tomato is good for diabetic patients?**
The carbohydrate content in tomato is very low. Hence it is useful in diabetic patients. For the same reason it is useful for those who want to reduce weight.

**Q5. Why tomato is not good for kidney patients?**
Because it is rich in potassium.

# RECOMMENDED DAILY ALLOWANCE

Recommended daily allowance are levels of intake of essential nutrients that on the basis of scientific knowledge are adequate to meet the known nutrient needs of all healthy persons.

## Indian Council of Medical Research (ICMR) Recommendations

- Calories 1 year 1,000 calories
- For every another year add 100 calories/year.

## Minerals

| Minerals | Recommended daily allowance |
|---|---|
| Calcium | 500–1,000 mg/day |
| Magnesium | 200–300 mg/day |
| Phosphorus | 800–1,000 mg/day |

## Trace Elements

| Trace elements | Recommended daily allowance |
|---|---|
| Chromium | 10 µg/day |
| Copper | 1–2 mg/day |
| Fluoride | 1–5 mg/day |
| Iodine | 50–100 µg/day |
| Iron | 10–20 mg/day |
| Manganese | 1–5 mg/day |
| Molybdenum | 200–500 µg/day |
| Selenium | 100 µg/day |
| Zinc | 5–15 mg/day |

## Vitamins

| Vitamins | | Recommended daily allowance |
|---|---|---|
| Vitamin A | | 1,500 IU/day (500 µg/day) |
| Vitamin B | $B_1$-Thiamine | 0.9 mg/day |
| | $B_2$-Riboflavin | 1 µg/day |
| | $B_3$-Niacin | 8–13 mg/day |
| | $B_6$-Pyridoxine | 1.6 mg/day |
| | $B_{11}$-Folic acid | 50 µg/day |
| | $B_{12}$Cyanocobalamine | 0.2–1.0 µg/day |
| Vitamin C | | 40 mg/day |
| Vitamin D | | 400 IU/day (10 µg/day) |
| Vitamin E | | 5–15 IU/day |
| Vitamin K | | 5–15 µg/day |

# QUESTIONS

**Q1. What is recommended daily allowance—RDA?**
- Recommended daily allowance is the nutrient intake considered adequate to meet the known nutrient needs of practically all healthy children in a particular age.
- Energy requirement of a child is defined as the amount of energy needed to balance total energy expenditure.

Q2. What are the amounts of energy expenditure in various conditions?
- Light work: 70 cal/h
- Moderate work: 1,000 cal/h
- Heavy work: 200 cal/h
- Very heavy work: 300 cal/h.

Q3. What is the calories requirement of a 60 kg person doing sedentary work?
The calories requirement of a 60 kg person doing sedentary work is approximately 2,000 kcal.

## NUTRITIONAL DISORDERS

There are many disorders which can be prevented by taking care of nutrition. Some of the disorders where nutritional factors play a role are discussed in this chapter.

### Nutritional Disorders due to Excess Intake of Feeds or Overfeeding or Overnutrition

- Overweight—the weight of the child will be more than the normal for that age.
- Obesity
- Malnutrition—impaired function resulting from prolonged deficiency or excess of total energy or specific nutrient such as protein, essential fatty acids, vitamins, minerals.

### Nutritional Deficiency Disorders

*Acrodermatitis Enteropathica*

Acrodermatitis enteropathica is due to zinc deficiency. There is vesiculation and ulceration around the nose, mouth, anal opening and genitalia. Acral areas like hands and feet are involved.

*Anemia—Iron Deficiency Anemia*

Iron deficiency anemia can occur due to decreased intake of iron. With adequate intake of iron, iron deficiency anemia cannot occur when there is malabsorption. Increased or chronic blood loss also can predispose to iron deficiency anemia.

**Sources of iron:**
- Dates, jaggery, green leafy vegetables
- Animal foods—Liver, kidney
- Treatment—oral or parenteral iron.

**Megaloblastic anemia**
- Due to vitamin $B_{12}$ or folic acid deficiency
- Treatment—vitamin $B_{12}$ or folic acid supplements.

**Hemolytic anemia:** Due to vitamin E deficiency.
Vitamin E is an antioxidant which protected our body cells against damage by antioxidants. In case of deficiency the radicals will cause various cells like blood cells, muscle (myopathy) nerve cell (neuropathy) reproductive cells (infertility).

**Pernicious anemia:** Due to vitamin $B_{12}$ deficiency.

*Beriberi*
- This is due to thiamine deficiency. Thiamine will be lost from rice on polishing.
- There are three types of beriberi dry, wet and infantile beriberi
- Dry beriberi is associated with neurological symptoms
- Wet beriberi is associated with cardiac symptoms like cardiac failure.

**Foods Rich in Thiamine**
- Meat, eggs, whole grains, dried beans
- Treatment is by administration of thiamin.

*Bitot's Spots*

It is seen in vitamin A deficiency. Bitot's spots are small plaque of silver gray color with a foamy surface. It is seen in the lateral half of the bulbar conjunctiva just close to the limbus. The shape is triangular, usually. The spots vary in size from 2 mm to 10 mm. These are usually seen bilaterally.

*Bleeding Problems*
- Perifollicular hemorrhages, easy bruising, petechiae.
- These are seen in scurvy.

## Burning Feet Syndrome (Also Known as Grierson-Gopalan Syndrome)

This condition is associated with the following features:

- Aching of the feet
- Burning—severe burning heat in the soles, ankles and lower legs
- Color change absent over the feet (No redness)
- Diurnal variation-more intense at night becoming better by day
- Excessive sweating due to vasomotor changes
- Eye problems—scotoma, amblyopia
- Foot is involved
- Feeling of pins and needles
- Gait disturbances
- Hot foot
- Hyperesthesia
- Increased sensitivity to pressure
- Burning feet syndrome is seen in pantothenic acid deficiency.

## Cardiomyopathy

The heart will get enlarged and will not contract well enough to pump enough blood to the organs. Selenium deficiency will result in dilated cardiomyopathy. The incidence of cardiomyopathy is rising alarmingly without the cause being found out. The condition may need cardiac transplantation.

## Congestive Cardiac Failure

Wet beriberi is associated with thiamine deficiency, which will present as cardiac failure.

Sources of thiamine—pulses, yeast, oil seeds

## Corneal Xerosis

*Corneal xerosis* seen in vitamin A deficiency.

## Corneal Ulcer

Corneal ulcer seen in vitamin A deficiency.

## Conjunctival Xerosis

Conjunctival xerosis is seen in vitamin A deficiency.

## Conjunctival Ulcer

Conjunctival ulcer seen in vitamin A deficiency.

## Cheilosis

Cheilosis—red, swollen patches at the corners of the mouth is seen in riboflavin deficiency or iron deficiency:

- Bleeding
- Blister
- Cracked
- Crusty
- Itching
- Painful
- Red
- Scaly swollen.

## Dead in Bed Syndrome or Bed's Syndrome

Dead in Bed syndrome or Bed's syndrome—is common in young aged with type 1 diabetics, sudden unexplained deaths. This occurs due to deficiency of biotin.

## Diarrhea

Diarrhea is seen in niacin deficiency.

## Dermatitis

Dermatitis is seen in niacin deficiency.

## Death

**Death** is seen in niacin deficiency.

## Dementia

*Dementia*—is seen in niacin deficiency, vitamin $B_{12}$ deficiency.

## Depression

Depression is seen in vitamin $B_{12}$ deficiency.

## Dermatitis

*Dermatitis*—itchy, erythematous, vesicular crusting patches in the skin. Dermatitis is seen *in protein*, essential fatty acid, niacin, zinc deficiency.

## Seborrheic Dermatitis

*Seborrheic dermatitis* is caused by vitamin B6, biotin and zinc deficiency.

## Scrotal Dermatitis

*Scrotal dermatitis* is caused by riboflavin deficiency:
- Biotin
- Niacin pellagra due to niacin deficiency
- Pyridoxine
- Riboflavin deficiency.

## Dyssebacea

Dyssebacea (also known as seborrheic dermatitis)—plugs of inspissated sebum projects from the orifices of the sebaceous glands. This is seen in pellagra due to niacin deficiency (Considered as fifth D after diarrhea, dermatitis, dementia and death). The areas commonly affected are nasolabial folds, external ears, eyelids, scrotum in the male and labia majora in the females.

## Edema

- Generalized edema will occur in thiamine deficiency.
- *Encephalopathy* diffuse cerebral dysfunction is due to abnormal brain function.
- The function or the structure of the brain will be affected.
- Pellagrous encephalopathy due to niacin deficiency.
- Encephalopathy is associated with the following:
  - Apathy
  - Altered mental state
  - Breathing abnormalities
  - Brisk tendon reflexes
  - Confusion
  - Concentration problems
  - Convulsions
  - Coma
  - Decision making will be difficult
  - Disorientation
  - Depression
  - Dysphagia
  - Dysphasia
  - Eye movements abnormal
  - Fainting or fatigue
  - Focal neurological deficits
  - Gait abnormalities
  - Hypervigilance
  - Hallucinations
  - Impaired memory
  - Inattentiveness
  - Judgment poor
  - Korsakoff psychosis (Wernicke encephalopathy)
  - Lethargy
  - Memory problems
  - Muscle weakness
  - Neurological deficits—spastic quadriplegia
  - Oculocephalic response lost
  - Personality changes.

## Follicular Hyperkeratosis

It is seen in vitamin A deficiency.

## Glossitis

Inflammation of the tongue results in swelling of the tongue with color change. There will be a change in the surface of the tongue due to change in size and shape of the papillae. This will be associated with pain in the tongue. Glossitis is seen in the following nutritional conditions:
- Cobalamin deficiency
- Iron deficiency anemia.

## Goiter

- Enlargement of thyroid glands in the front of the neck occurs in goiter.
- Goiter is due to iodine deficiency.
- Clinical features:
  - Anemia
  - Cretinism
  - Enlarged thyroid gland
  - Growth poor in infancy
  - Intellectual disability
  - Poor school performance.
- Sources of iodine—salt water fish, sea foods, iodine fortified salt.

## Gopalan's Feet

Gopalan's feet are seen in pantothenic acid deficiency. Burning feet syndrome is also known as Gopalan's feet.

## Guttoral Pigmentation

Guttoral pigmentation is seen in vitamin A deficiency.

## Growth Retardation

Growth retardation is seen in malnutrition.

## Hair Loss, Thinning

Hair loss, thinning—due to niacin, biotin deficiency

## Hemolysis

Hemolysis is seen in vitamin E deficiency.

## Intellectual Disability

Intellectual disability (mental retardation) in iron deficiency anemia the mental functions will be affected.

## Jaundice

Jaundice—in nutritional cirrhosis.

## Keratomalacia

Keratomalacia—drying, softening and clouding of cornea due to vitamin A deficiency.

## Keshan Disease

- Allergy—skin rash
- Brittle nails
- Blood clotting problems
- Congestive cardiomyopathy
- Dental problems— mottled teeth
- Extreme fatigue
- Facial flushing
- Gastrointestinal upset—vomiting
- Hair loss or brittle hair
- Irritability
- Intellectual disability
- Joint problems (necrosis of cartilage tissue in joints)
- Kidney problems
- Liver problems
- Male infertility
- Mild nerve damage
- Nail inflammation
- Nausea
- Odor—garlic breath odor.
- It is seen in selenium deficiency.
- Selenium deficiency also can cause features of hypothyroidism like extreme fatigue, mental slowing, goiter, intellectual disability, miscarriages.

*Koilonychia*—spoon shaped nails. It is seen in iron deficiency and protein deficiency especially sulfur-containing amino acids.

*Korasakoff syndrome or Korasakoff psychosis*—psychosis is due to thiamine deficiency. This will be associated with the following:
- Ability to recall recent conversation or event will be affected
- Amnesia
- Behavior changes
- Confusion
- Confabulation
- Defects in memory
- Educational problems-learning difficulties
- Fall in mentation
- Gaps in long-term memory
- Predisposing factors: Thiamine deficiency may cause Wernicke's encephalopathy. If this is not treated it may progress to Korsakoff psychosis.

## Kwashiorkor

- Psychic changes—apathy and misery, lethargy, irritability, state of prostration.
- Hair changes-sparse, flag sign, hypopigmented, easily pluckable.
- Skin changes (hypo or hyperpigmentation, paddy field dermatosis, crazy pavement epithelium, bullous lesions, flexural ulcers, etc).
- Edema.

## Lethargy

It is a state of weariness with diminished energy, mental capacity and motivation.

## Malnutrition

### Marasmus

- Nonedematous malnutrition without edema due to inadequate intake of energy or both protein and calories
- Weight of the child will be less than 60% of the expected for the age
- No edema
- Appetite good
- Old man appearance.

### Marasmic Kwashiorkor

Will be associated with features of marasmus including wasting with edema.

### Nail Changes: Beau's Lines

- These are transverse depressions in the nail plate due to temporary cessation of nail growth. This is seen in zinc deficiency.
- Toenail Brown-grey discoloration will be seen in vitamin $B_{12}$ deficiency.
- White nails are seen in malnutrition.

### Neural Tube Defects

In antenatal mothers with folate deficiency the risk of neural tube defects like meningocele, meningomyelocele will be high.

### Night Blindness (Nyctalopia)

- A child who is playing throughout the day will become quiet by evening. The child will avoid playing in the evening. The movements will be restricted as the vision in the dim light will be poor. There will be defective dark adaptation.
- Cause—vitamin A deficiency.
- Other clinical features of vitamin A deficiency:
  - Bitot's spots
  - Corneal xerosis
  - Conjunctival xerosis
  - Conjunctival ulcer
  - Corneal ulcer
  - Keratomalacia.
- Foods rich in vitamin A—carrots, green leafy vegetables.
- Animal foods—liver, egg, fish.
- Treatment—administrations of oral or parenteral iron.

### Ophthalmoplegia

Internal ophthalmoplegia is involvement of pupillary sphincter and ciliary muscle. External ophthalmoplegia is involvement of extraocular muscles. Complete ophthalmoplegia is involvement of both internal and external ophthalmoplegia.

Ophthalmoplegia is seen in thiamine deficiency.

### Oro-Oculo-Genital Syndrome

It is due to deficiency of vitamin B2 and B6:
- Angular stomatitis
- Atrophic tongue (bright red)
- Blepharoconjunctivitis
- Burning eyes—red
- Cheilosis
- Corneal vascularization
- Dermatitis in pubic area (seborrheic scrotal dermatitis)
- Eczema-like changes in the face, genital region
- Epidermal necrolysis
- Excoriation
- Fissuring of lips
- Fissures (palpebral fissures excoriated)
- Free border of prepuce, vulva and anus involved
- Genital skin
- Glossitis
- Healthy granulation tissue over tender ulcers
- Irritated angle of mouth
- Interspersed lips
- Keratitis
- Photophobia
- Rhagades
- Treatment—oral riboflavin and pyridoxine.

### Osteoporosis

- The bone density will be decreased and the bones will become weaker. The risk

- for fracture will be high especially in the spine, hip and wrists.
- ❖ It may occur due to deficiency of vitamin D or calcium or both.
- ❖ Extra calcium intake along with vitamin D will be helpful in treating osteoporosis.
- ❖ *Sources of calcium*—milk, egg, green leafy vegetables and ragi.

## *Pellagra*

It is due to niacin deficiency. This will be associated with the following features:
- ❖ Dermatitis
- ❖ Diarrhea
- ❖ Dementia
- ❖ Death.

### Foods Containing Niacin

- ❖ Whole grains, peanuts, mushrooms, chicken
- ❖ Treatment—administration of niacin.

## *Peripheral Neuropathy*

- ❖ Will be seen in the following conditions:
  - Cobalamin deficiency
  - Thiamine deficiency
  - Vitamin $B_{12}$ deficiency.
- ❖ Clinical features of peripheral neuropathy:
  - Sensory (skin):
    - ♦ Tingling, stabbing pains, numbness, heavy feeling in the hands and feet
    - ♦ Shocking sensations
    - ♦ Thinning of skin.
  - Motor (muscles): Dropping things from hands.
  - Autonomic (internal organs)
    - ♦ Blood pressure: Fall in blood pressure
    - ♦ Constipation
    - ♦ Diarrhea
    - ♦ Erectile (sexual) dysfunction
    - ♦ Excessive sweating.

## *Petechiae*

These are 1–2 mm red or purple spots due to minor hemorrhage from broken capillary blood vessels. Petechiae are seen in niacin, vitamin C deficiency.

## *Phrynoderma*

It is follicular hyperkeratosis due to nutritional deficiency. Hyperkeratotic papules and plaques will appear on the extensor surfaces of the extremities shoulders and buttocks.

The skin will resemble toad skin.

### Causes of Phrynoderma

- ❖ Vitamin A deficiency
- ❖ Essential fatty acid deficiency.

## *Quadriplegia*

Flaccid quadriplegia will be associated with Wernicke's encephalopathy due to thiamine deficiency.

## *Rickets*

- ❖ Bony deformities—softening of bones due to vitamin D deficiency.
- ❖ Clinical features:
  - Bone deformities
  - Bow legs
  - Craniotabes
  - Caput quadratum
  - Chest deformities-Harrison sulcus
  - Costochondral beading
  - Delayed motor milestones
  - Dwarfism—short stature
  - Enlargement of ends of long bones (Widening of wrist)
  - Eruption of teeth delayed
  - Fontanel closure delayed
  - Genu varum or genu valgum or genu recurvatum
  - Hypotonia.
- ❖ Treatment—oral or parenteral vitamin D.
- ❖ *Foods rich in vitamin D*: Milk.
- ❖ *Predisposing factors:*
  - Poor intake of vitamin D
  - Lack of sun exposure.
- ❖ Prevention
  - Sun exposure
  - Adequate foods rich in vitamin D.

## Scurvy

- It is due to vitamin C deficiency.
- Vitamin C is needed for collagen formation.
- Clinical features:
  - Anemia
  - Arthralgia
  - Bleeding (Fatal bleeding in vital organs)
  - Corkscrew hairs or coiled hairs
  - Delayed healing of wounds
  - Ecchymosis
  - Edema
  - Fatigue
  - Follicular hyperkeratosis
  - Gum diseases: Gingival bleeding, ulceration
  - Hemorrhage: Perifollicular hemorrhages
  - Irritability
  - Infections
  - Jaundice due to hemolysis
  - Pseudoparalysis due to pain in the limbs
  - Weakness
  - Weight loss
  - Woody leg.
- Predisposing factors—diet lacking fresh fruits
- Exclusive milk ingestion can manifest as scurvy.

### Vitamin C Containing Foods

- Fruits—fresh citrus fruits like lemon, oranges, strawberry, guava, kiwi fruit and papaya.
- Vegetables—tomatoes, carrots, potatoes, broccoli, cabbage and spinach.

## Subacute Combined Degeneration of Spinal Cord (SACD)

It is due to vitamin $B_{12}$ deficiency. Both sensory and motor systems are affected. This will be associated with degeneration of posterior and lateral columns of spinal cord. It is associated with sensorimotor disturbances in the lower limbs:

- Ataxia (dosrsal spinocerebellar tract involvement)
- Babinski sign positive
- Bladder or bowel dysfunction
- Bilateral involvement (Progressive symmetrical involvement)
- Corticospinal signs—spasticity (lateral corticospinal tract dysfunction)
- Developmental delay
- Dementia
- Eye problems—vision changes, visual loss due to optic atrophy
- Failure to thrive
- Fatigue
- Gait ataxia
- Glossitis
- Glove and stock pattern of sensory loss
- Hyper-reflexia or hyporeflexia
- Irritability
- Joint position and vibration sense are affected first (posterior column dysfunction)
- Knee reflex brisk
- Loss of ankle reflexes
- Lethargy
- Memory loss
- Numbness
- Optic atrophy
- Paresthesia
- Paresis or weakness of legs, arms and trunk
- Personality changes—dementia, psychosis
- Romberg test will be positive.

Magnetic resonance imaging (MRI) will show dilated ventricles, brain atrophy, thin corpus callosum, delayed myelination.

Classical triad of SACD is absent ankle jerk, brisk knee jerk and extensor plantar reflex.

*Toad skin* is seen in vitamin A deficiency. It is also known as phrynoderma.

## Tongue

- Glossitis (in vitamin riboflavin deficiency)
- Bald tongue (in vitamin $B_{12}$ deficiency).
- Magenta red tongue (in riboflavin deficiency)
- Beefy red tongue (in niacin deficiency)

- Painful tongue (in folate deficiency)
- Raw leaf tongue (in vitamin B1 deficiency).

## Ulcer
Corneal and conjunctival ulcers are seen in vitamin A deficiency.

## Vascularization of Cornea
It occurs in riboflavin deficiency.

## Weakness
It is seen in vitamin C deficiency.

## Wernicke Encephalopathy
It occurs in thiamine deficiency. This will be associated with a triad of eye movement disorders like ophthalmoplegia, cerebellar signs like ataxia and mental changes like confusion.

Polished rice will be deficient in thiamine. The rice with dull color should be preferred.

## Wernicke Korsakoff Syndrome
It occurs in thiamine deficiency associated with a triad-confusion, ataxia, nystagmus

*Woody leg* is seen in scurvy

*Wound healing* poor in vitamin C deficiency.

## Xerosis
The skin, cornea or conjunctiva will be dry. Corneal xerosis and conjunctival xerosis will be seen in zinc and vitamin A deficiency.

## Xerophthalmia
It is abnormal dryness of cornea or conjunctiva seen in vitamin A deficiency. The conjunctiva will become dry and wrinkled.

## QUESTIONS

**Q1. What are the causes of night blindness?**
- Vitamin A deficiency
- High myopia
- Retinitis pigmentosa.

**Q2. What are the changes seen in the tongue in vitamin deficiencies?**
- Glossitis (in vitamin riboflavin deficiency)
- Bald tongue (in vitamin $B_{12}$ deficiency)
- Magenta red tongue (in riboflavin deficiency)
- Beefy red tongue (in niacin deficiency)
- Painful tongue (in folate deficiency).

**Q3. What is the difference between the teeth in calcium and phosphorus deficiency?**
- Pulp defects (phosphate deficiency)
- Enamel defects (in calcium deficiency).

**Q4. What are the skin manifestations of vitamin C deficiency?**
- Poor wound healing
- Petechiae

**Q5. What is potbelly? What are the conditions associated with Pot belly?**
Potbelly is distension of abdomen due to hypotonia of anterior abdominal wall muscles.

The conditions associated with potbelly are:
- Hypocalcemia
- Rickets.

**Q6. What is the cause of woody leg?**
Woody leg is seen in scurvy.

# CHAPTER 2

# Instruments and Procedures

## CHAPTER OUTLINE

- Antropometry
- Skinfold Caliper
- Instruments to Record Vital Signs
- Blood Pressure
- Needles
- Biopsy Needles
- Syringes
- Tubes
- Catheters
- Bags
- Infusion Sets
- Oxygen Delivery Systems
- Pediatric Breathing Circuit
- Newborn Resuscitation
- Asthma Devices
- Airways
- Miscellaneous

## INTRODUCTION

Instruments should be handled carefully to avoid complications. Also one should anticipate all the complications that can occur during various procedures and be ready to prevent or manage them. Insertion of needle or tube for Intercostal drainage can cause pleural shock due to stimulation of vagal nerve and cause sudden death. Administration of atropine can prevent this complication. Lumbar puncture in a patient with increase intracranial tension can cause herniation of brainstem and cause sudden death. Increased intracranial tension should be ruled out by fundal examination before performing lumbar puncture to avoid this complication. The indications, contraindications, complications and other salient features of various instruments are discussed in this chapter.

## ANTROPOMETRY

### Weighing Machine (Fig. 2.1)

Types of weighing machines are as follows:
- ❖ Salter spring weighing machine
- ❖ Beam weighing machine
- ❖ Electronic weighing machine

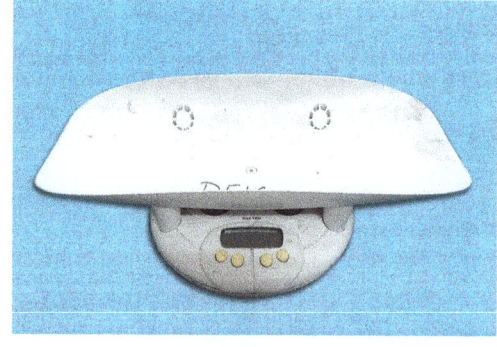

**Fig. 2.1:** Weighing machine.

- Spring weighing machine
- Bathroom scale weighing machine
  - Spring type
  - Interpersonal observation variation is high
- Detecto scale weighing machine.

If the child is not cooperating by standing on the weigh machine, the mother and the child can be asked to stand on the weighing machine. First the mother should stand with the child in her hands, later the mother alone should be weighed. By deducting the mother's weight from the first value, the weight of the child can be known.

The weight should be plotted in the road to health chart and verified if the weight falls in between the normal percentiles.

## Precautions

- The accuracy of the machine should be checked periodically by placing standard weights on the weighing scale.
- Recording of weight at birth and daily in newborn will help to monitor the nutrition and fluid balance of the babies. Also it is important for growth monitoring of children.
- The weighing machine should be placed on a flat, stable surface.
- Before putting the baby on the weighing machine zero marking should be ensured.
- The baby should be kept naked with all equipments detached.
- The baby should be kept on the middle of the scale.
- The weight should be better recorded prior to feeding.

## Significance

Excessive weight gain should be a warning sign for fluid overload, congestive cardiac failure, and renal failure.

## Expected Weight in Relation to Birth Weight

- Birth weight = x
- 5 months = 2×
- 1 year = 3×
- 2 years = 4×
- 3 years = 5×
- 5 years = 6×
- 7 years = 7×
- 10 years = 10×

## Expected Weight using Formula

### Weech's formula

**3–12 months**

$$\text{Expected weight (Kg)} = \frac{\text{Age (months)} + 9}{2}$$

**1–6 years**

Expected weight (Kg) = Age (years) × 2 + 8

**7–12 years**

$$\text{Expected weight (Kg)} = \frac{\text{Age (years)} \times 7 - 5}{2}$$

## Infantometer (Fig. 2.2)

It is used to measure the length of the newborn babies.

### Technical Aspects

- Markings inches and centimeters
- Measuring range 5–80 cm
- Graduations 1 mm
- Head rest fixed with other end adjustable

### Uses

The length of the following children can be measured using an infantometer.

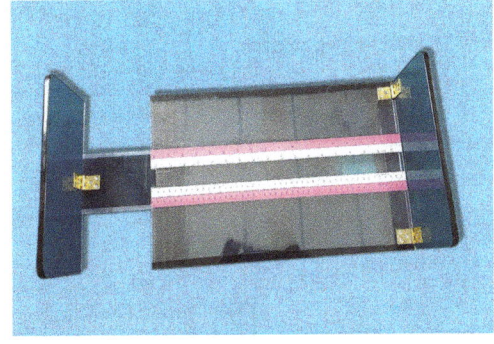

**Fig. 2.2:** Infantometer.

- ❖ Newborn
- ❖ Infants.

### Technique of Measurement of Length

Squaring of the pelvis—the anterior superior iliac spine should be perpendicular to the body.

### Advantages

- ❖ Easy and quick measurement
- ❖ Easily transportable
- ❖ Easily disinfected.

## QUESTIONS

**Q1. What is the length of the normal newborn?**
50 cm.

**Q2. What is the expected length of the infant at 1 year of age?**
75 cm.

**Q3. In normal children up to what age length is measured?**
Up to 2 years of age.

### Stadiometer (Fig. 2.3)

Stadiometer has affixed wooden or aluminum height scale and a sliding platform. The height of the children above 2 years can be measured using stadiometer. The child should be asked to stand on the stadiometer with three points touching the stand. The occiput, shoulders, buttocks back, and heel should touch the stand. The face should look straight in Frankfort plane.

Steps to be followed before measuring the height are as follows:

- ❖ The patient should stand straight and look forward
- ❖ The patient should look straight
- ❖ The patient should stand with both the feet kept closed
- ❖ The patient should be bare footed
- ❖ Arms should hang by the sides
- ❖ *Frankfurt plane*: The external auditory meatus and lower border of the orbits should be parallel to the floor. The line joining the outer canthus and the lower margin of the external auditory canal should be straight.

Expected length/height of the child:
- ❖ Length at birth: 50 cm
- ❖ Length at 1 year: 75 cm
- ❖ Length/height at 2 years: 87 cm
- ❖ Height at 3 years: 93 cm
- ❖ 2–12 years: Add 6 cm per year.

### Tapes

#### Measuring Tape

The tape will have markings in centimeters and inches. The measuring tape or inch tape is used for the measurement of the following:
- ❖ Head circumference
- ❖ Mid-arm circumference (MAC)
- ❖ Chest circumference
- ❖ Arm span
- ❖ Upper segment to lower segment ratio.

**Precautions:**

- ❖ *Head circumference*: The measurement should be taken at the side of the head. Do not manipulate in front of the eyes which will be uncomfortable to the child. Also you may accidentally hit the eyes.
- ❖ *Mid-arm circumference*: Measure at the midpoint in between the acromion and olecranon process with the arm hanging by the side. The MAC will be 13.5–16 cm from 1 year to 4 years of age. This is because the fat in the infant will be replaced by the growing muscle mass.

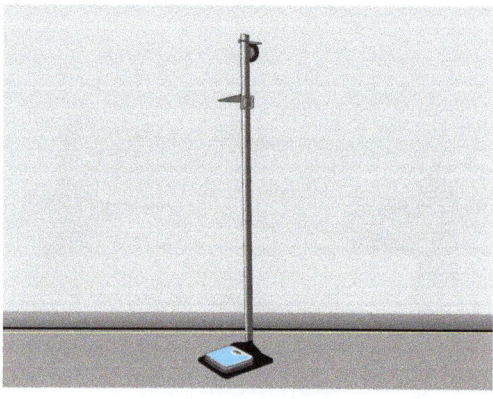

**Fig. 2.3:** Stadiometer.

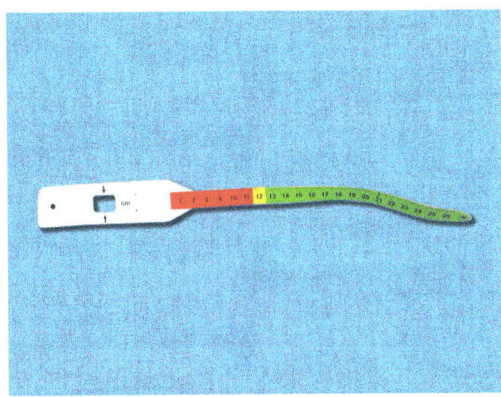

**Fig. 2.4:** Shakir tape.

- *Length*: Squaring of pelvis—the line joining both anterior superior iliac spine should be perpendicular to the vertebral column. If this is not done the length may not be correct.

## Shakir Tape (Fig. 2.4)

Shakirs tape is a simple easy way of assessing MAC. The tape shows color coded cutoff points indicating various levels of malnutrition.

**Shakirs tape (color):**

| MAC | Color |
|---|---|
| 13.5–16 cm | Green |
| 12.5–13.5 cm | Yellow |
| <12.5 cm | Red |

It should be measured at the midpoint between the tip of the shoulder and elbow (between olecranon process and acromion). Measure with the arms hanging down.

## QUESTIONS

**Q1. What are the significances of MAC?**
Mid-arm circumference is a good indicator of muscle wasting. This is also a good predicator of mortality. The mid-upper arm circumference is measured from the age of 6 months to 59 months.

**Q2. What are the methods used for measurement of mid-upper arm circumference?**
Measure MAC using an inch tape, Shakir tape, Quack stick method, Kanawati index, and bangle test using a bangle with an internal diameter of 4 cm.

**Q3. What are the two determinants of MAC?**
Muscle and subcutaneous fat.

**Q4. Why MAC is a better indicator of malnutrition than the other indices like body mass index?**
It is because MAC is less affected by accumulation of fluid like nutritional edema, ascites, etc. MAC less than 11.5 cm indicates severe acute malnutrition. This is an indication for admission and therapeutic feeding program.

**Q5. What are the age-dependent criteria?**
- Weight for age
- Height for age
- Head circumference

**Q6. What are the age-independent criteria?**
The following criteria does not vary with the age. These remain constant irrespective of the age.
- Weight for height
- Mid-arm circumference (1–5 years)
- Rao and Singh's criteria
- Dugdale's index
- Enderberg index
- Kanawati index
- Mid-upper arm/height ratio
- Quetelet index
- Ponderal index
- Body mass index.

**Q7. How will you grade PEM according to MAC in Arnold classification?**

| Grades | Cm |
|---|---|
| Normal | 16 cm |
| Mild protein energy malnutrition (PEM) | Between 13.5 cm and 16 cm |
| Moderate PEM | Between 12.5 cm and 13.5 cm |
| Severe PEM | Less than 12.5 cm |

**Q8. What is Rao and Singh's criteria?**

$$\frac{\text{Weight (Kg)}}{(\text{Height in cm})^2} \times 100$$

Normal 0.15–0.16
PEM less than 0.14

Normal value 0.15–0.16 is constant for growth up to 5 years. Since, it depends on the body mass, any change indicates malnutrition.

**Q9. What is Dugdale's index?**

$$\frac{\text{Weight of the child}}{(\text{Height in cm})^{1.6}} \times 100$$

0.88 is the expected normal value.

**Q10. What is Enderberg index?**
$C = \log(Wt) - 1.6\, Ht$
Normal value of C will be 40. This remains a constant up to 13 years of age.

**Q11. What is Kanawati index?**

$$\frac{\text{Mid-arm circumference}}{\text{Head circumference}}$$

- This ratio remains constant for children between 4 months and 4 years irrespective of sex.
- The normal value is more than 0.32
- The malnutrition can be graded according to the values of the index as follows:

| Classification of PEM according to Kanawati index | |
|---|---|
| Mild PEM | 0.28–0.32 |
| Moderate PEM | 0.25–0.28 |
| Severe PEM | <0.25 |

**Q12. What is mid-arm/height ratio?**
- Less than 0.29 indicates gross malnutrition
- Normal: 0.32–0.33.

**Q13. Describe Quack stick method.**
The Quack stick will have markings of MAC on one side and the height on the other side. The MAC should be measured and the height of the child should be checked. If the height is more than the height for MAC the child is considered as malnourished.

**Q14. Describe bangle test.**
A bangle with an inner diameter of 4 cm should be slipped up arm. If the bangle passes above the elbow the child is considered as malnourished.

## SKINFOLD CALIPER

### Herpenden Caliper (Fig. 2.5)

- This indicates the status of fat deposits in the body.
- Herpenden caliper is used to measure the skinfold thickness. Adequate pressure should be maintained while taking the measurements. This is important as more pressure results in falsely low values, while low pressure will give abnormally high values. Maintain a pressure of 10 g/mm².
- *Measuring pressure*: 10 gm/mm²
- *Accuracy*: 99%
- *Measuring range*: 0–80 mm
- *Graduation*: 0.2 mm.

### Sites in which Skinfold Thickness is Measured

- Triceps
- Subscapular
- Suprailiac
- Abdomen
- Upper thigh

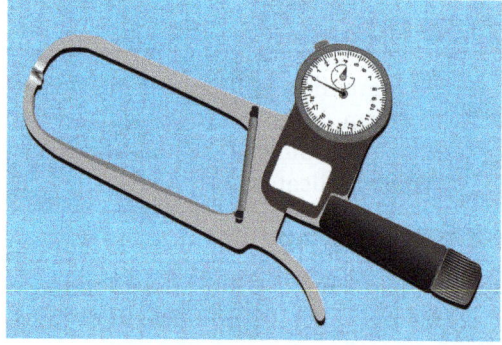

**Fig. 2.5:** Herpenden caliper.

## Normal Skinfold Thickness

- *Children*: 10 mm
- *Adults*:
  - Male: 12.5 mm
  - Female: 16.5 mm

## Significance of Skinfold Thickness

- *Normal*: 90–100% of expected
- *Mild malnutrition*: 80–90%
- *Moderate malnutrition*: 60–80%
- *Severe malnutrition*: Below 60%

# INSTRUMENTS TO RECORD VITAL SIGNS

## Temperature

### Thermometers (Fig. 2.6)

Thermometers are devices that measure the temperature or temperature gradient.

### Temperature Assessment

- *Clinical examination*: Feel the temperature by placing the dorsum of the fingers over the neck of the child. It is not advised to feel the temperature at the periphery, as it will give false values in the presence of abnormal blood flows. For example in shock, the peripheries will be cold in spite of a normal core temperature.
- Temperature can be measured by using clinical thermometers. Core temperature is measured by using a rectal thermometer.

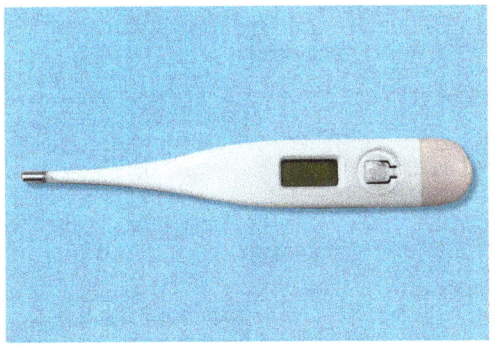

**Fig. 2.6:** Thermometer.

### Sites to Record the Temperature

The temperature can be measured in the sites where the body maintains a stable temperature. These sites are:

- Forehead
- Oral
- Axilla
- Rectum
- Vagina
- Groin (between the abdomen and the flexed thigh).

Rectal temperature is 1°F more than oral temperature and oral temperature is 1°F more than axillary temperature.

### Temperature Range

| Temperature | Centigrade | Fahrenheit |
|---|---|---|
| Normal | 36.6–37.2° | 98–99° |
| Subnormal | <36.6° | <98° |
| Febrile | >37.2° | >99° |
| Hyperpyrexia | >41.6° | >107° |
| Hypothermia | <35° | <95° |

The pulse, respiration, and temperature (PTR).

- For each degree rise in temperature the heart rate increases by 10/min.
- The ratio between the heart rate to respiratory rate is 4:1
- Increase of 1°F produces increase of pulse rate by 10 beats/min and respiratory rate by 4/min.

### Types of Thermometer

Clinical and rectal thermometer.

**Clinical Thermometer:** There will be a constriction which will prevent leakage of mercury and rapid back flow of the mercury during recording of temperature.

**Rectal Thermometer:** The bulb will be short, rounded, and thick. This will decrease the risk of injury to the rectum. As the thermometer is inserted blindly into the rectum, long and thin bulb will cause injury to the rectal mucosa.

## Differences between clinical and rectal thermometer

| Features | Clinical thermometer | Rectal thermometer |
|---|---|---|
| Site | Oral or axilla | Rectum |
| Color coding on the stem | Blue | Red |
| Tip of the bulb | Pointed | Short, rounded and thick (to prevent injury of rectal mucosa) |
| Temperature measured | High reading | Low reading 25–40°C |

## QUESTIONS

**Q1. What is the principle of thermometers?**
Thermal expansion of solids and liquids with temperature.

**Q2. What are the properties of thermometric materials used in thermometers?**
- Heating and cooling should be rapid
- Heating and cooling should be monotonic.

**Q3. What are the types of thermometers?**
Clinical and rectal.

**Q4. What are the units for temperature?**
Centigrade (C) and Fahrenheit (F).

**Q5. What are the substances used in the thermometers for measuring temperature?**
- Mercury
- Alcohol.

**Q6. What are the parts of the body where the temperature is recorded?**
- Oral
- Rectum
- Eardrum
- Skin.

**Q7. How long the thermometer should be placed in oral cavity and axilla for recording temperature?**
- *Oral cavity*: 1 minute
- *Axilla*: 3 minutes.

**Q8. What is low reading thermometer?**
Rectal thermometer is known as low reading thermometer. It measures the temperature from 25°C to 40° C.

**Q9. What is the relation between heart rate, respiration, and pulse?**
For every 1° rise in temperature the pulse will increase by 10 and respiratory rate by 4.

**Q10. What are the precautions to be taken before taking temperature?**
- The thermometer should be shaked so that the mercury returns to the bulb.
- Axilla should be dry.
- Place the bulb of the thermometer at the roof of axilla and hold the arm firmly against the chest wall for 5 minutes.
- It is better to have separate thermometers for each babies, especially newborn babies.
- The thermometer should be kept in a bottle filled with disinfectant 70% isopropyl alcohol plus 1% iodine.

**Q11. What are the conditions in which rectal temperature is measured?**
- Heat stroke
- Drowning
- Malnutrition
- Hypothermia
- Newborn.

**Q12. What is the relation between the rectal, oral, and axillary temperature?**
Rectal > oral > axillary by 0.5°C

### Types of Fever

| | |
|---|---|
| Continuous fever | Fever which does not fluctuate more than 1°C during 24 hours and never touches the normal; e.g. viral fever. |
| Intermittent fever | Fever is present only for few hours in a day; e.g. malarial and filarial fever. |
| Remittent fever | A type of continuous fever where the fluctuation is more than 2°C; e.g. enteric fever. |

| | |
|---|---|
| Step ladder fever | Fever rises like a ladder in enteric fever. |
| Saddle back fever | Fever present for 2–3 days followed by afebrile period for 2–3 days; e.g. dengue fever. |
| Pel-Ebstein fever | Fever present for 3–10 days followed by afebrile period for 3–10 days. |
| Undulant fever | Fever rises and falls like a wave in brucellosis. |
| Fever with rigors | Occurs in malaria, filaria, urinary track infection (UTI), and follicular tonsillitis. |
| Tertian fever | Fever relapses every 3rd day (benign—vivax, malignant—*Plasmodium falciparum*) |
| Quartan fever | Fever relapses every 4th day in malaria (*Plasmodium malariae*) |

## BLOOD PRESSURE

Blood pressure is the pressure of the circulating blood on the walls of the blood vessels. It is indicated by systolic pressure and diastolic pressure. For example 120/80 mm Hg indicates systolic pressure of 20 mm Hg and diastolic pressure of 80 mm Hg. Normal blood pressure will vary according to the age. In hypertension the blood pressure will be increased and in hypotension it will be decreased.

## Blood Pressure Apparatus (Fig. 2.7)

### Sphygmomanometer to Measure Blood Pressure

Sphygmomanometer is a blood pressure meter used to measure the blood pressure.

### Types
- Manual sphygmomanometer
- Digital sphygmomanometer
- Aneroid sphygmomanometer

### Parts of Manual Sphygmomanometer
- Air valve
- Bulb to pump air into the cuff

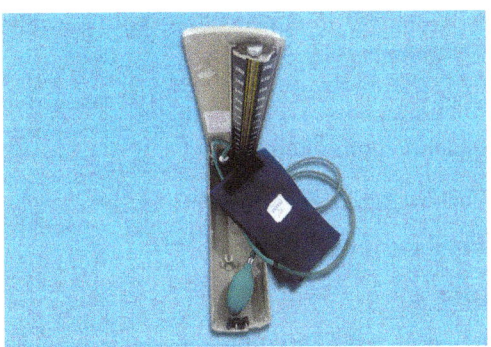

**Fig. 2.7:** Blood pressure apparatus.

- Column of mercury indicating the pressure
- Deflation valve which allows controlled deflation
- External cuff to hold the bladder around the limb
- Glass tube
- Hinges—metal and plastic
- Inflatable bladder to occlude the artery
- Manometer to measure the pressure
- Mercury tank.

### Cuff Size for various Age Groups
- If the size is small the reading will be high
- The cuff should fit to the limb.

| Age group | Cuff width (cm) | Bladder length |
|---|---|---|
| Neonate | 2.5–4 | 5–9 |
| Infant | 4–6 | 10–13 |
| Child | 6–12 | 12–18 |
| Adult | 12–14 | 22–26 |

### Criteria to be followed to Measure the Blood Pressure
- The cuff should be selected so that the bladder width is more than and equal to 40% of the MAC.
- The bladder length is 80-100% of arm circumference.

### Methods used to Measure Blood Pressure
- Conventional method using sphygmomanometer

- ❖ Palpatory method using sphygmomanometer
- ❖ Oscillometry method
- ❖ Flush method
- ❖ Doppler method.

### Normal Blood Pressure in Children

Blood pressure varies with age.

## NEEDLES

Needles are thin, metallic hollow cylindrical objects with sharp point at the end. Needles are used to inject medicines into the body.

### Intramuscular Needle (Fig. 2.8)

Parts of needle:
- ❖ Hub
- ❖ Shaft
- ❖ Needle cap
- ❖ Lumen
- ❖ Bevel

The following points should be noted before giving intramuscular injections.
- ❖ Length
- ❖ Gauge
- ❖ Syringe tip
- ❖ Site of injections.

### Site of Intramuscular Injections

For newborn and children below 18 months the intramuscular injections can be given in the vastus lateralis muscle. This lies at the anterolateral aspect of the thighs. This site is selected because no major vessels or nerves are present in this site.

For children aged less than 18 months the intramuscular injections can be given at the upper and outer quadrant of the gluteal region.

The needle should be long enough to pierce the skin, subcutaneous tissue and the muscle and delivers medicine deep into the muscle.

The needle should be inserted in one prick with the angle between the needle and the site being 80–90°.

### Recommended Tip of the Syringes

- ❖ Luer-Lok type with secure screw type connection. This is most commonly used. This is more safe and secure.
- ❖ Slip tip syringe or push on connection
- ❖ Eccentric tip used for surface veins or artery
- ❖ Longer catheter tip with longer and tapered tip. This will be used for irrigation.

### Method of Intramuscular Injection

Load the syringe and discard the needle used to load the syringe. Use a fresh needle to inject as the needle used to loading may have got blunted.

## QUESTIONS

**Q1.** What is the length of the IM needle used for intramuscular injection?
2.5 cm.

**Q2.** What is the recommended length of the IM needle for gluteal injections?
- ❑ For children weighing 31–40 kg: 2.5 cm
- ❑ For those weighing 40.5–90 kg: 5–7.5 cm.

**Q3.** What is the gauge of the IM needle?
Gauge of the IM needle is the outer diameter of the needle. Smaller gauge number is indicated for larger diameters. The gauge of the needle is selected on the basis of the viscosity of the fluid to be injected.

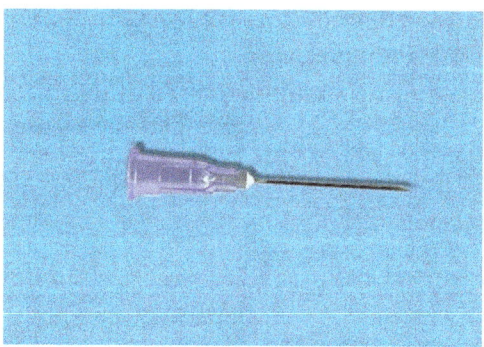

**Fig. 2.8:** IM needle.

**Q4. What is the gauge for an intramuscular injection?**
- 21–23 G.
- For dense solutions like benzathine penicillin 20–21 G can be used
- For thin solutions 24 G can be used.

**Q5. What are the sites used to give intramuscular injections?**
- Deltoid
- Gluteal region—ventrogluteal area (upper and outer quadrant)
- Anterolateral aspect of thigh.

**Q6. Why intramuscular injections should be avoided in infancy?**
The gluteal region will be under developed until the child starts to walk.

**Q7. Why anterolateral aspect of thigh is selected for intramuscular injection?**
This part is not having any major vessels or nerves.

**Q8. What are the steps to be followed while giving intramuscular injection?**
- The needle should be pierced at 45–90°.
- The needle should be aspirated after entering the muscle to rule out entry into a vessel.

**Q9. What does 22 G½ indicates?**
22 indicates the gauge of the needle and ½ indicates the length of the needle that is half an inch.

**Q10. What is the size of the needle recommended for subcutaneous injections?**
28 gauge needles are recommended.

**Q11. What is the size of the needle recommended for intramuscular injections?**
22–23 gauge needles with 1–1.5 cm long are recommended.

**Q12. What is the gauge for an intradermal injection?**
26–27 G.

## Intravenous Needle (Fig. 2.9)

Intravenous (IV) needle is inserted into a vein to administer medications.

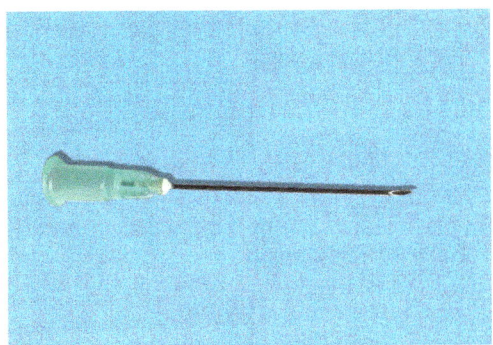

**Fig. 2.9:** IV needle.

Parts of IV needle are:
- Cannula or inner needle is the hollow tube.
- Trocar or external plastic/polyethylene—outer sheath
- Connecting hub is the part of the needle lying outside the skin after insertion of the needle
- Hep lock or saline lock—the cap used to.

### Intravenous Infusion

Intravenous access should be established. The skin should be pricked at the side of the selected vein. After entering the skin the needle should be brought between the skin and the vein, now advance the needle into the vein.

Syringe should be selected with adequate capacity to collect enough blood needed for various tests. All the blood should be collected at the same time.

### Sites for Blood Collection

**Veins in the antecubital fossa:** A prominent vessel may be an artery and one should be careful in selection a vein for blood collection.

Prolonged application of tourniquet, squeezing of the arm, clenching, and unclenching the arm while collecting the blood may give wrong electrolyte values.

### Veins used for Peripheral Vein Transfusion

- *Head*: Scalp veins
- *Neck*: External jugular vein
- *Arms*:
  - Cephalic veins: Antecubital fossa
  - Veins in the wrist: Dorsum of the hand
- *Legs*: Internal saphenous vein, anterior to medial melleolus.

### Risks of Intravenous Cannula

- Infiltration of tissues causing necrosis
- Insertion point is a portal of entry for organisms.

### Complications of Intravenous Needle Insertion/Peripheral Vein Infusion

- Air embolism
- Blowing of vein
- Bleeding
- Cellulitis
- Damage to surrounding tissues: Nerve damage
- Electrolyte imbalance due to administration of too dilute or too concentrated solutions
- Embolism
- Extravasation of medicines or fluid
- Fluid overload predisposing to hypertension, heart failure, and pulmonary edema
- Fragment embolism: Catheter shearing when the beveled edge of the trocar is cutting the catheter and resulting in foreign body embolus
- Gangrene
- Hematoma
- Hypothermia
- Infection: Thrombophlebitis
- Injuries:
  - Injury to the vein
  - Hemorrhage
  - Introduction of infection
  - Infiltration into the surroundings
- Infection: Phlebitis, cellulitis, and sepsis

Frequent use of a vein may result in scarring or narrowing of the vein resulting in difficulty in using it or not usable.

## QUESTIONS

**Q1. How to calculate the amount of fluid to be given?**
Each mL contains 15 macrodrops or 60 microdrops. Suppose you have to give 100 mL in 1 hour:
- *Macrodrops*:
  - 100 × 15 in 60 minutes
  - That is 1,500/60 = 25 drops per minute.
- *Microdrops*:
  - 100 × 60 in 60 minutes
  - That is 6,000/60 = 100 drops per minute

In other words, divide the amount in mL/1 hour to be given by 4 gives the macrodrops per minute. Amount of fluid in ml to be given in 1 hour will be equal to number of microdrops.

**Q2. Why intravenous route is preferred over arterial route for administration of fluids?**
It is because the fluid will pass through the lungs before passing through the body. The lungs will prevent embolisms and air bubbles from entering the systemic circulation.

**Q3. How will you prevent clotting when the intravenous line is not in use?**
This can be done by filling the needle portion with heparin or saline.

**Q4. What are the common sites for insertion of intravenous needle?**
- Hand, arm or at the bend of the elbow
- Foot or leg
- Scalp veins are used for infants.

**Q5. What are the sites used for fast transfusion?**
Elbows, groins, and necks.

**Q6. What are the sites used for slow transfusion?**
Back of the hands.

**Q7. What is the length for an intravenous injection?**
1/2 to 1/5 inch.

**Q8. What is the length for an intravenous injection?**
¼ to 3/8 inch.

**Q9. What is the largest gauge?**
14 G.

**Q10. What is the smallest gauge?**
24–26 is the smallest.

**Q11. What is the gauge for all purposes in children?**
22 G.

**Q12. What is the gauge needed for blood transfusion?**
18–20 G sometimes 16 G is used.

**Q13. What are the large bore or trauma lines used to deliver large volumes of fluids fastly in emergency situations?**
12–14 G.

**Q14. What are the drugs that should be administered only by intravenous infusion and not by intramuscular route?**
- Diazepam
- Antimetabolites
- Potassium chloride
- Sodium bicarbonate
- Contrast for radiological investigations.

**Q15. What are the uses of intravenous needles?**
- Intravenous infusion of drugs and fluids
- Collection of blood samples
- Diagnostic aspiration in pleural effusion, empyema and ascitic tap.

**Q16. What is the amount of air embolism that is harmless and life-threatening?**
- About 30 mL can dissolve into the circulation and is harmless
- 3–8 mL/kg body weight can be life-threatening.

**Q17. What is blowing of vein?**
During insertion of the needle the needle may injure the side of the vein and injure the walls in blood leak.

**Q18. What is the duration for which the intravenous needle can be changed to prevent infections?**
The needle should be changed every 72–96 hours.

**Q19. What is the precaution to be taken when you remove an intravenous needle?**
Pressure should be applied at the site to puncture after removing the needle.

**Q20. What is ported cannula?**
Ported needles have an injection port on the top which can be used to deliver medicines.

**Q21. What are the uses of intravenous needles?**
Intravenous administration of fluids and drugs.

## Venflon (Fig. 2.10)

Parts of venflon are as follows:
- Catheter
- Needle
- Needle grip
- Luer lock plug
- Luer connector
- Valve
- Flashback chamber
- Injection port cap
- Hub wings
- Bushing.

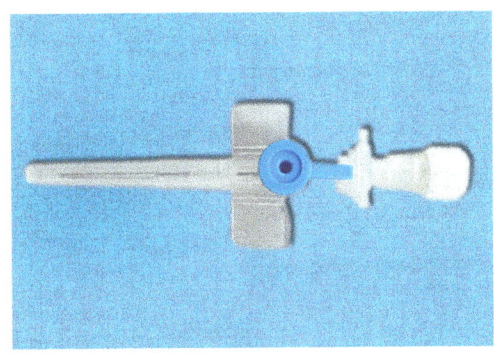

**Fig. 2.10:** Venflon.

Cannula color size code.

| Color code | Gauge | External diameter | Length (mm) | Flow rate (mL/min) | Time duration to infuse 1,000 mL (minutes) |
|---|---|---|---|---|---|
| Orange | G-14 | 2.0 | 45/55 | 250–300 | 3.5 |
| Gray | G-16 | 1.8 | 45/55 | 140–240 | 6 |
| White | G-17 | 1.5 | 45 | 140 | 7 |
| Green | G-18 | 1.2 | 45 | 90–120 | 10 |
| Pink | G-20 | 1.0 | 33 | 55–80 | 15 |
| Blue | G-22 | 0.9 | 25 | 22–50 | 22 |
| Lime yellow | G-24 | 0.7 | 19 | 20–23 | 35 |
| Violet | G-26 | 0.6 | 19 | 10–15 | 60 |

### Sizes of Commonly used Venflon (Fig. 2.11)

- Orange: 14 G
- Gray: 16 G
- Green: 18 G
- Pink: 20 G
- Blue: 22 G
- Yellow: 24 G
- Violet: 26 G

Larger number represents smaller cannula.

- Cannula or inner needle is the hollow tube which should be removed after the cannula enters the vein
- Trocar or external plastic/polyethylene—outer sheath covering the needle.

### Advantages of Venflon

- Avoids injury to the blood vessel
- Blunt tips
- Bruising will be less
- Cost-effective
- *Duration of indwelling time*: Longer
- Easy insertion
- Fragile and small veins can be easily penetrated
- *Good mobility*: Mobility of the patient need not be restricted
- Healthcare associated infection (HAI) is less
- *Injuries less*: Risk of needle stick injuries will be minimal.

## QUESTIONS

Q1. What are the four factors to be considered before using venflon?
   1. Needle gauge
   2. External diameter
   3. Length of the cannula
   4. Flow rate.

Q2. What is the largest gauge and smallest gauge?
   Orange 14 G is the largest and Violet 26 G is smallest.

Q3. What is the gauge of orange venflon?
   14 G.

Q4. What is the gauge of blue venflon?
   22 G.

Q5. What is the gauge of green venflon?
   18 G.

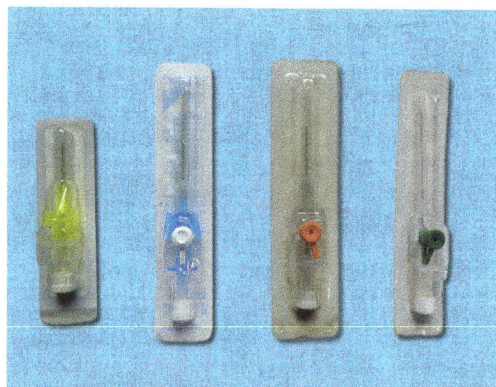

**Fig. 2.11:** Venflon color code.

**Q6. What is the smaller diameter of venflon?**
Smaller diameter is 0.7 mm.

**Q7. Which type of venflon is used in newborns?**
Yellow venflon is used for newborns.

**Q8. What is the advantage of venflon?**
Prevents needle stick injuries.

**Q9. What is the procedure of insertion of venflon?**
The catheter is introduced into the vein using a needle. The needle should be removed while the cannula remains in place.

**Q10. What are the complications of venflon?**
- Air embolism
- Arterial puncture
- Bone infection (osteomyelitis)
- Blockage
- Cannula embolism
- Damage to nerve
- Extravasation of medicine into surroundings
- Fluid overload
- Gangrene/necrosis due to extravasation
- Hemorrhage
- Hematoma
- *Injuries*: Needle stick injuries
- Infiltration
- *Infections*: Insertion site infection/phlebitis.

**Q11. What is the gauge of violet venflon?**
26 G.

**Q12. What is the gauge of orange venflon?**
14 G.

## Scalp Vein Set (Fig. 2.12)

- Butterfly set/winged infusion set
- 18–27 gauge bores are available.

### Parts of Scalp Vein Set

- Hypodermic needle
- Bilateral flexible wings

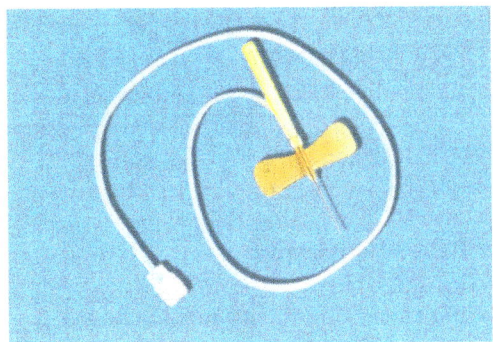

**Fig. 2.12:** Scalp vein set.

- *Connector*: A flexible transparent tube which is about 20–35 cm long. This helps in attaching the vein set to another devices like syringes, infusion pumps, etc.

The butterfly is held by its wings between the thumb and the index finger at a point very close to the needle.

### Advantages of Scalp Vein Set over a Straight Needle

- *Attachment easy*: Butterfly shaped wings will help in easy attachment to the skin
- *Better flow*: Thin wall needle will facilitate better flow
- *Comfort*: More comfort for the patient during the transfusion
- *Duration*: Will be useful for long duration infusion
- *Easy access*: Superficial veins can be accessed easily
- Flexible tube will be helpful in reaching more body surface
- Flash or flashback of blood into the transparent tube (confirms the tube is in the blood vessels)
- Gauge is small and less painful
- *Handling easy*: Butterfly shaped wings will help in easy handling
- *Injury less*: Short beveled siliconized needle will be useful to prevent traumatic cannulization
- Increased patient movement is possible.

## Disadvantages of Scalp Vein Set

- Cost of the butterfly set is more
- Difficult to collect large amount of blood
- Duration of drawing blood is longer due to small lumen
- Dead space is more due to long tube and results in drug wastage
- Expensive as compared to intravenous needles
- Flow rate slow due to small lumen
- Gauge small
- Hemolysis due to small lumen
- *Injuries*: Needle stick injuries are common
- *Infections*: Transmission of infectious diseases like human immunodeficiency virus (HIV) and viral hepatitis.

## Disadvantage of 25G and 27G Butterfly Needles

They may cause hemolysis or clot blood samples which predisposes to wrong blood tests.

## Lumbar Puncture Needle (Fig. 2.13)

Lumbar puncture needle will have a stylet inserted into the needle. Lumbar puncture needle types are as follows:
- Lumbar puncture needle 18–20 G
- 20–22 G spinal needle with stylet
- 22 G lumbar puncture needle is used for young infant
- 20 G lumbar puncture needle is used for older infant.

Length of the lumbar puncture needles:
- 1.5 inch for children younger than 12 years
- 3.5 inches for children more than 12 years of age.

## Lumbar Puncture Procedure

**Precautions:** Fundus examination should be done to rule out papilledema which will be present in presence of increased intracranial tension. Lumbar puncture is contraindicated in such cases as this will predispose to medullary coning and cardiorespiratory arrest. Computed tomography (CT) scan of brain should be taken. Clinical features of increased intracranial pressure should be observed. In shock states, lumbar puncture should be avoided.

## Method

### Position of the patient

- *Lateral recumbent position*: Place the patient in the lateral position. The vertebral column should be parallel to the bed. The transverse axis of the back should be vertical. Flex the hips, back, and neck and clean the site. The chin should touch the chest. Keep the shoulders and hips aligned, that is perpendicular to the examining table in the recumbent position. This will prevent rotation of spine. Lateral position with the patient lying flat with lumbar spine well flexed. Flex up the legs, bend the head and neck towards the knees, and place the patient in the lateral position. The vertebral column should be parallel to the bed. The transverse axis of the back should be vertical.
- *Upright sitting position*: This is used in very stout patients and deformities of spine. The child can sit up with dorsal and lumbar spine flexed as much as possible. The child should sit on the bed with legs over the side and with the back and neck

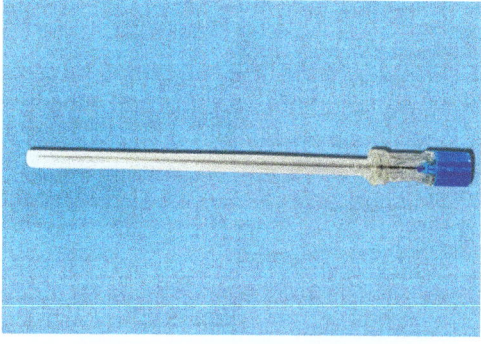

**Fig. 2.13:** Lumbar puncture needle.

bend forwards. If the lumbar puncture is done in sitting position the child should be put in lateral position once the needle is inserted successfully.

## Site of Puncture

- Subarachnoid space below the level of the spinal cord between L3 and L4
- Line joining the upper part of the iliac crest generally runs across the space between L3 and L4
- The lumbar puncture is done at this space, but also can be done one space higher or lower
- In newborn babies, the needle should be inserted in between L4 and L5
- Between L3 and L4 in older children
- Between L4 and L5 in younger children.

## Procedure

Skin should be sterilized with 1% iodine in 70% surgical spirit. Local anesthetic agent 1% lignocaine is injected into the skin between the spinous process and then injected into the interspinous ligament. A sterile towel with a small hole to cover the lumbar area is usually not used. The needle should be kept perpendicular to the transverse line of the back.

Insert a spinal needle with bowelled edge facing towards the cranium in the line of the spine. The needle will separate the fibers of the dura mater which runs vertically. Thus headache will be prevented. The needle should be placed perpendicular to the horizontal line. Advance the needle in the direction of umbilicus. The needle enters the spinal subarachnoid space of the lumbar sac below the level of spinal cord. In adults, the spinal cord will reach up to the lower border of first lumbar vertebra. A line joining the highest point of the iliac crests will run across the interval between 3rd and 4th lumbar spinous processes. The spinal level in children will be lower.

## Points to be Noted

- Cerebrospinal fluid (CSF) pressure should be observed before the fluid is collected.
- Note the color of the fluid and the force with which the fluid rushes out.
- The stylet should be removed as the needle is advanced. If no fluid is obtained the needle should be rotated. Still if no fluid is obtained, the needle should be inserted into the space between L3 and L4. Tapping at higher levels will increase the risk of injury to spinal cord.
- Collect the fluid in two bottles and a culture bottle.
- One should be sent to biochemical analysis.
- Second should be placed in the room and see for cob web formation by next day.
- The culture bottle should be sent to microbiology for culture.
- If the subarachnoid space is not entered there will be no rise of fluid level on applying pressure over the neck.
- To confirm that there is spinal block, the abdomen can be compressed by an assistant with the palm of the hand. This will result in considerable rise in the fluid level in the manometer.

## Indications for Lumbar Puncture

Indications for lumbar puncture are diagnostic and therapeutic.

- Diagnostic
  - Absolute
    - Suspected central nervous system (CNS) infections
    - Meningitis
    - Subarachnoid hemorrhage
  - Relative
    - Neurosyphilis
    - Demyelinating diseases
    - Guillain-Barré syndrome (GBS)
    - Neurodegenerative disorders like subacute sclerosing panencephalitis (SSPE) and multiple sclerosis
    - Unexplained coma
    - Paraneoplastic syndromes
    - Measuring the CSF pressure, study of CSF dynamics, blocks, etc.
    - Leukemia to rule out CNS secondaries.

- Therapeutic
  - Spinal anesthesia
  - Intrathecal methotrexate in acute lymphocytic leukemia with CNS secondaries
  - Amphotericin for fungal infections
  - Management of posthemorrhagic hydrocephalus in newborn
  - Injection of contrast media in myelography or cisternography.

## Contraindications for Lumbar Puncture

- Anticoagulant therapy
- Bleeding disorders
- Brain tumors
- Blood dyscrasias like hemophilia (signs of bleeding disorder), blood dyscrasias like hemophilia (signs of bleeding disorder)
- Coagulation disorders
- Cerebral edema
- *Convulsions*: Recent convulsions within 30 minutes or prolonged convulsions lasting for more than 30 minutes
- Increasing coma
- *Deformities of spine*: Marked spinal deformity
- Epidural abscess in the spinal cord
- *False localizing sign*: Sixth nerve palsy
- Focal neurological signs like hemiparesis, monoparesis, extensor plantar, and ocular palsies
- Focal seizures/focal tonic seizures
- Glasgow coma scale less than 13 or deteriorating level of consciousness
- Hydrocephalus
- Herniation of brain
- *Infection*: Local infection/skin sepsis
- *Increased intracranial tension*: Signs of increased intracranial tension (altered papillary responses, absent Doll's eye reflex, decorticate or decerebrate posturing, abnormal respiratory pattern, papilledema, hypertension, and bradycardia)
- Intracranial space occupying tumors and posterior cranial fossa tumors
- Neck retraction
- Papilledema
- Retinal hemorrhage
- Spinal dysraphism
- Spinal block
- Signs of spinal cord compression
- Spontaneous subarachnoid hemorrhage
- Strong suspicion of meningococcal meningitis like typical rash
- State of shock
- Thrombocytopenia
- Unequal pupils
- Unstable patient (irregular pulse, blood pressure, and respiration).

## Relative Contraindications for Lumbar Puncture

Thrombocytopenia is a relative contraindication.

## Complications of Lumbar Puncture

- Abducens nerve palsy
- Bleeding
- Back pain and localized pain (if intervertebral disk is pierced)
- *Cardiorespiratory arrest*: Cardiorespiratory status may be compromised especially in small infants when the trunk and neck are flexed.
- Dry tap
- Dizziness
- Emesis (vomiting)
- *Epidermoid tumor—intraspinal epidermoid tumor*: Performing lumbar puncture without stylet can predispose to implantation of core of epidermis into the subarachnoid space which may develop as an epidermoid tumor in later life.
- Fatal tonsillar herniation may result in sudden collapse and cardiorespiratory arrest. Sudden drop of pressure but rapid release of CSF may cause herniation which can be fatal
- *Gastrointestinal problems*: Nausea and vomiting
- *Headache*: Post-lumbar puncture headache
- *Infection*: Meningitis, osteomyelitis (vertebral bone)
- *Injury*: Traumatic tap.

## QUESTIONS

**Q1. What are the advantages of smaller gauge needle?**
Smaller gauge needle will decrease the risk of spinal fluid leak and headache.

**Q2. What are the causes of dry tap?**
- Faulty technique
- Improper positioning
- Needle block.

**Q3. What is traumatic tap?**
If the lumbar puncture is not done properly it may injure the surrounding structures and result in blood in the tap.

**Q4. What are the causes of traumatic tap?**
Puncture of epidural vein or venous plexus.

**Q5. How to interpret traumatic lumbar puncture?**
The culture, sugar level will not be altered by traumatic tap. Also Gram stain may not be affected. For every 400 red blood cell (RBC)/mm$^3$ there will be 1 white blood cell (WBC).

**Q6. What should be done if there is traumatic tap?**
The lumbar puncture can be done at a higher level, one space higher, if there is blood in the CSF, abandon the procedure.

**Q7. When can you repeat the lumbar puncture again?**
The lumbar puncture can be repeated after 48 hours.

**Q8. What are the causes of bloody tap?**
- Subarachnoid hemorrhage
- Injury to spinal vessel
- Bleeding diathesis

**Q9. How will you differentiate between traumatic tap and subarachnoid hemorrhage?**
The CSF collected by lumbar puncture can be kept for some time. In case of traumatic tap the supernatant fluid will be clear. In subarachnoid hemorrhage supernatant fluid will be xanthochromic.

**Q10. How will you differentiate between traumatic tap and blood stained CSF?**
Collect the CSF in two bottles. If the staining clears off it may be due to traumatic rupture. If the staining is uniform it may be due to blood stained CSF. On microscopic examination macrophages and crenated RBCs will be seen.

**Q11. What is cobweb formation?**
In tuberculous meningitis when the CSF collected is kept in a container a cobweb like precipitate will be formed.

**Q12. What will be the complication if the lumbar puncture is done when there is an increased intracranial tension?**
There will be tonsillar herniation of the brain into the foramen magnum causing pressure over the brainstem resulting in sudden collapse and sudden death.

**Q13. What will you examine before performing a lumbar puncture?**
Clinically examine for bulging fontanel if they are open. A bulging fontanel will indicate an increase intracranial tension.

Fundoscopic examination to rule out papilledema, which is again an indication of increased intracranial tension.

**Q14. What will you do if the CSF fluid is gushing out through the lumbar puncture needle?**
Immediately stop the procedure and pullout the needle. If not there will be a risk for herniation of brain into the foramen magnum.

**Q15. What are the causes of xanthochromia?**
- Subarachnoid hemorrhage
- Jaundice
- Tumor near cauda equina

- High protein content (GBS and spinal block).

**Q16. What are the normal features of CSF to be observed during a lumbar puncture?**
- Flow
- Volume
- Appearance
- Protein
- Sugar
- Chloride.

**Q17. What are the normal features of CSF?**
- *Color*: Colorless
- *Flow*: Normal not under tension
- *Volume*: 120-150 mL
- *Appearance*: Clear
- *Cells*: <5 mm³ (up to 120 mg/dL in newborn)
- *Protein*: 20-40 mg% (up to 120 mg/dL in newborn)
- *Sugar*: 40-60 mg%
- *Chloride*: 720-750 mg
- *Specific gravity*: 1.001
- *Daily*: 1,500 mL formed.

**Q18. In how many percentage of cases initial Gram staining will reveal an organism?**
In 68-80% of cases initial Gram staining will reveal an organism.

**Q19. What are the contents that are more in CSF than in blood?**
Chloride and magnesium.

**Q20. What are the conditions in which CSF protein is increased?**
- Meningitis
- Encephalitis
- GBS
- Spinal cord compression
- Tumor.

**Q21. What are the conditions in which CSF glucose is increased?**
- Diabetes mellitus
- Encephalitis
- Intravenous glucose.

**Q22. What are the conditions in which CSF glucose is decreased?**
Meningitis.

**Q23. What are the conditions in which CSF bicarbonate is decreased?**
Meningitis.

**Q24. What is Cotton's law?**
In meningitis, the substances that are low in the CSF than in the blood will increase, except for sugar.

The substances that are more in the CSF than blood will become decreased.

**Q25. What is disease mimicking meningitis?**
There will be clinical signs of meningitis in certain conditions like tumor, abscess, cranial hemorrhage, etc. Performing lumbar puncture in these conditions can predispose to herniation. A CT scan should be done to rule out such conditions. At the same time a normal CT scan does not mean it is safe to perform a lumbar puncture.

**Q26. What are the signs and symptoms of cerebral herniation?**
- Glasgow coma scale less than 8
- Unilateral or bilateral abnormal pupil size and reaction
- Abnormal Doll's eye movement
- Abnormal tone like decorticate/decerebrate rigidity, and flaccidity
- Tonic posturing
- Respiratory abnormalities like hyperventilation, Cheyne-Stokes respiration, apnea, and respiratory arrest
- Papilledema.

**Q27. How long will the cellular and biochemical changes will remain unchanged after the start of antibiotic treatment for meningitis?**
44-68 hours.

**Q28. When will the CSF culture will become negative after parenteral antibiotics are given in meningococcal and pneumococcal meningitis?**
CSF culture will become negative 2 hours in meningococcal meningitis.

# BIOPSY NEEDLES

## Liver Biopsy Needles
- Vim Silverman
- Menghini

## Trucut Needle (Fig. 2.14)

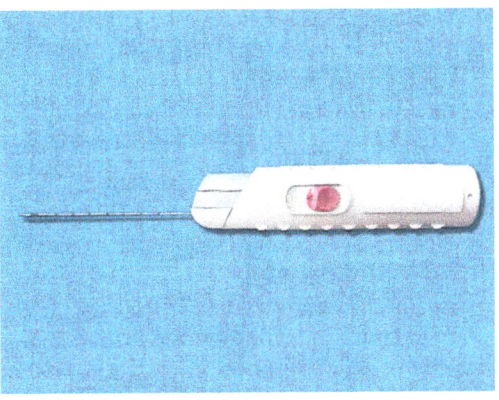

Fig. 2.14: Trucut needle.

It is designed to obtain a tissue of high quality with minimal trauma to the patient. Uses of trucut needle are:
- Liver biopsy
- Renal biopsy
- Breast, lung, prostate, and thyroid biopsies.

### Liver Biopsy

**Procedure of liver biopsy:** Palpate the liver in the midaxillary line. The skin is cleaned in the midaxillary line in the tenth space. Local anesthesia should be injected up to the capsule of the liver. The needle should be advanced into the liver. The outer hollow needle is introduced further and rotated through 360°. A small incision is made in the skin. The needle with a stylet is inserted medially until it is felt to enter the liver. The stylet is withdrawn and the split needle is introduced. It should be advanced into the liver.

### Indications for liver biopsy
- Chronic hepatitis
- Cirrhosis
- Hepatomegaly

CSF findings in normal and other various conditions.

| Condition | Cells | Glucose | Protein | Culture | Other features |
|---|---|---|---|---|---|
| Normal (newborn) | <20 lymphocytes, no RBCs | 2/3rd of blood sugar | <120 mg/dL | Negative | |
| Normal (children) | <5 lymphocytes, no RBCs | 2/3rd of blood sugar | <40 mg/dL | Negative | |
| Pyogenic meningitis | Increased number of neutrophils | <2/3rd of blood sugar | Increased | Positive | |
| Partially treated pyogenic meningitis | Increased neutrophils/ lymphocytes | Normal or low | Normal or high | Negative | |
| Tuberculous meningitis | Increased number of lymphocytes | Low | High | Negative | Cobweb formation |
| Viral meningitis | Increased | Normal In mumps sugar will be low | Normal | Negative | |

- Hemochromatosis
- Direct (conjugated) hyperbilirubinemia evaluation
- Wilson's disease
- Metabolic disorders
- Infiltrative disorders
- Storage disorders
- Neonatal cholestasis
- Wilson's disease
- Evaluation of recurrent or chronic conjugated hyperbilirubinemia
- Evaluation of liver status after liver transplantation
- Evaluation of type and extent of drug-induced liver injury
- Evaluation of portal hypertension.

**Contraindications of liver biopsy:** Absolute contraindications of liver biopsy are:
- Angiomatous malformation of liver
- Pyogenic abscess of liver
- Biliary tract infection
- Biliary obstruction
- Hydatid cyst of liver
- Prolonged prothrombin time more than 3 seconds over the control
- Prolonged PTT
- Platelet count less than 50,000/mm³.

Relative contraindications are:
- Ascites
- Intrahepatic biliary radical dilatation
- Subdiaphragmatic abscess
- Infections of right side pleura and lung.

**Complications of liver biopsy**
- *Air leak*: Pneumothorax
- Arteriovenous fistula
- *Bile leaks*: Intrathoracic biliary leaks/intraperitoneal biliary leaks and bile peritonitis/hemobilia
- Capsular bleeding
- Subcutaneous emphysema
- Hematoma
- Hemothorax
- Infection (bacteremia, sepsis, and abscess formation)
- Injury to intra-abdominal organs
- Local pain/pleural pain
- Sedation-related problems
- Biopsy of other organs like lung, gallbladder, kidney, and colon.

## QUESTIONS

**Q1. What are the types of needles used for liver biopsy?**
- trucut needle (trucut liver biopsy is the most commonly used in children)
- Menghini needle
- Vim Silverman needle.

**Q2. What is the liver biopsy needle commonly used in children?**
Trucut needle.

**Q3. What are the types of liver biopsy?**
- Percutaneous liver biopsy
- Transjugular liver biopsy.

**Q4. What are the steps to be taken before performing liver biopsy?**
- Complete blood count
- Prothrombin time
- Partial thromboplastin time (PTT)
- Blood grouping and cross matching
- Ultrasonogram
- Vitamin K should be given 3 days before liver biopsy.

**Q5. What is the position of the patient used for liver biopsy?**
- Supine position
- In some cases this can be done in sitting position.

**Q6. What is the anesthesia used for liver biopsy?**
Local anesthesia or ketamine.

### Renal Biopsy

Types of renal biopsy are:
- Native renal biopsy
- Transplant renal biopsy
- Blind renal biopsy
- Imaging-guided renal biopsy.

**Precautions for renal biopsy:** The position and number of functioning kidneys should be identified using an X-ray or ultrasonogram. If needed an intravenous pyelogram should be done.

**Procedure for kidney biopsy:** Place the child in prone position with the face turned to one side, arms abducted, and forearms beside the head. Done under general anesthesia, but can be done under local anesthesia. Place a rolled up towel under the abdomen which will make the access to the kidney easier. The kidney is located using an ultrasonogram and the skin is marked. The biopsy needle should be inserted under ultrasonogram guidance and biopsy should be obtained. The biopsy specimen should be obtained from the lower pole of the kidney as the adrenals are present on the upper poles.

### Indications for renal biopsy

- Progressive renal disease
- Nephrotic syndrome
  - Frequent relapse of nephrotic syndrome
  - Steroid resistant nephrotic syndrome
- Isolated persistent hematuria
- Unexplained proteinuria
- Chronic renal failure
- To assess the activity and renal involvement of systemic lupus erythematosus (SLE), hemolytic uremic syndrome (HUS), and Henoch–Schönlein purpura (HSP).
- Renal mass
- Following transplacent rejection.

### Contraindications for kidney biopsy:

- Absolute contraindications
  - Bleeding diathesis
  - Congenital anomalies
  - Single kidney
  - Horse shoe kidney
  - Bilateral contracted kidney
  - Uncontrolled bleeding diathesis, coagulation defects
  - Severe refractory hypertension
  - Small shrunken kidneys
  - Obstructed kidneys
  - Reflux nephropathy
  - Severe refractory hypertension
  - Polycystic kidney disease
- Relative contraindications
  - Congenital anomalies like horse shoe kidney
  - Skin infections at the biopsy site
  - Aneurysms over the biopsy site
  - Azotemia
  - Uremia
  - Pregnancy
  - Urinary tract infections
  - Acute pyelonephritis
  - *Patients on certain medications*: Warfarin and heparin
  - *Drugs*: Antiplatelet drugs and anticoagulants.

Hydronephrosis, arteriovenous fistula, and cystic kidney disease will increase the risk.

### Complications of renal biopsy:

- Arteriovenous fistula
- Blood clot resulting in urinary retention
- Bleeding
- Clot colic
- Perinephric hematoma
- Hematuria (mild usually resolves in 48 hours)
- Infection
- Pain.

### Evaluation before biopsy:

- Detailed history
- Bleeding diathesis
- *Laboratory evaluation*: Blood count and platelet count
- Coagulation profile
- Blood grouping
- Rh typing
- Ultrasonogram.

# QUESTIONS

**Q1. What are the indications for open biopsy?**
Solitary functioning kidney.

**Q2. What is the position used for renal biopsy?**
- *For native renal biopsy*: Prone or lateral position
- *For transplant kidney*: Supine position.

**Q3. What is the recent advance in renal biopsy?**
Transjugular renal biopsy. The needle can be passed through the renal vein.

## Bone Marrow Biopsy Needle
- Salah and Klima (Fig. 2.15).
- Salah is with guard.

### Parts of Bone Marrow Biopsy Needle
- Needle
- Trocar
- Cannula
- Guard will prevent penetration of the needle and injury to the viscous. The gauge should be adjusted according to the site of bone marrow biopsy. 21 G lumbar puncture needle can be used for infants. 18 or 19 G marrow needle with a short bevel should be used for older children.

### Bone Marrow Aspiration
Bone marrow aspiration is drawing of the liquid content of the bone marrow.

**Procedure for bone marrow aspiration:** The child should lie down in prone position or on his sides. Under aseptic preparations the tip of the trocar and cannula should be introduced through a nick made in the skin surface. The bone should be pierced with some pressure. The needle is inserted directly perpendicularly to the bone. As the needle enters the marrow, a feeling of giving way will be felt. There will be a sudden lack in resistance. The needle will stand without support. The stylet should be removed and marrow aspirated by suction using a 10 mL syringe.

A firm pressure should be applied after the removal of the needle to prevent oozing of blood from the site.

### Sites to Perform Bone Marrow Aspiration/Biopsy
Bone marrow aspiration can be done at the following sites:
- Anterior superior iliac crest can be used for children above 2 years of age. A point 1 cm below the iliac crest about 1–2 cm posterior to the mid-axillary line.
- Posterior superior iliac spine for children below 2 years of age. The upper third of the medial aspect of the shaft of tibia, proximal tibia, and 1–2 cm below the tibial tuberosity.
- Sternum, just above or below the manubriosternal line. This site is not recommended in children.
- Lumbar spinous processes in the mid-line (rarely).

### Advantage of Selecting Posterior Superior Iliac Spine to Study the Bone Marrow
Posterior superior iliac spine is the safest site for bone marrow study. Both bone marrow aspiration and bone marrow biopsy can be done at the posterior superior iliac spine.

### Indications for Bone Marrow Aspiration Needle
- Diagnostic:
  - Aplastic anemia
  - Bone marrow failure (myelodysplastic syndrome)
  - Bone marrow studies to diagnose leukemia and storage disorder
  - Cancers (malignancy and leukemia)

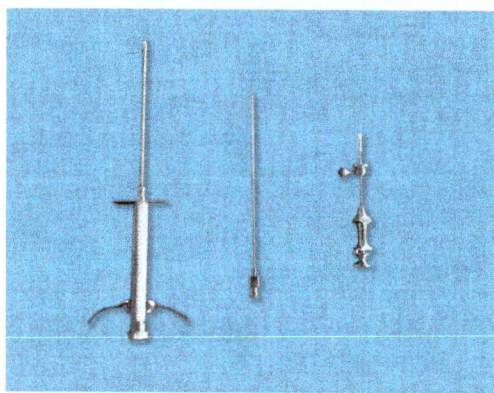

**Fig. 2.15:** Salah and Klima needle.

- Hematological disorders [evaluation of anemia and thrombocytopenic purpura (ITP)]
- Hyperplastic marrow in hemolytic anemia
- Infections (typhoid, malaria, and kala-azar)
- *Marrow infiltration*: Myeloproliferative disorders, storage disorders (Gaucher's disease, and Niemann-Pick disease)
- Osteopetrosis
- Secondaries in the bone in neuroblastoma, metastasis in nonhematopoietic malignancies.
- Staging and monitoring therapy in primary diseases of bone like anemia, leukemias, lymphomas, myeloma, and myelofibrosis
- Storage disorders
- Idiopathic thrombocytopenic purpura.
❖ Therapeutic:
  - Intraosseous infusion of fluid to correct dehydration
  - Blood transfusion
  - Bone marrow transplantation.

## Contraindications for Bone Marrow Aspiration/Biopsy

❖ Bleeding disorders
❖ Infection at biopsy site
❖ Osteomyelitis
❖ Thrombocytopenia.

## Bone Marrow Trephine Biopsy

Jamshidi needle (Fig. 2.16) is the one commonly used.

**Sites:** Proximal tibia 1-2 cm below the tibial tuberosity.
❖ Sternum
❖ Iliac crest

**Procedure of bone marrow trephine biopsy:** An incision should be made in the skin Jamshidi Swain trephine needle can be used to get a bone marrow biopsy. Aseptic preparation of the skin should be done. The skin should be incised using a scalpel. The needle is inserted directly perpendicularly to the bone. As the needle enters the marrow a feeling of giving way will be felt. The needle will stand without support. The stylet should be removed and the needle should be advanced further with clock wise and anticlockwise movements.

The needle can be pulled out with rotation movements. The specimen can be removed from the needle with a probe.

## Complications of Bone Marrow Trephine Biopsy/Intraosseous Transfusion

❖ Blockage of the needle by marrow
❖ Breaking of the needles within the marrow
❖ Incomplete penetration of the cortex
❖ Penetration of posterior bone cortex
❖ Damage to the growing plate resulting in shortening of the limb can occur if tibial tuberosity is choosed for biopsy
❖ Excessive bleeding
❖ Extravasation of fluid
❖ Hematoma
❖ Hemorrhage
❖ Infection of the marrow
❖ Injury to great vessel can occur during sternal puncture
❖ Infection
❖ Local pain
❖ Local swelling
❖ Necrosis of skin
❖ Over penetration
❖ Complication due to sedation like allergic reaction and arrhythmias.

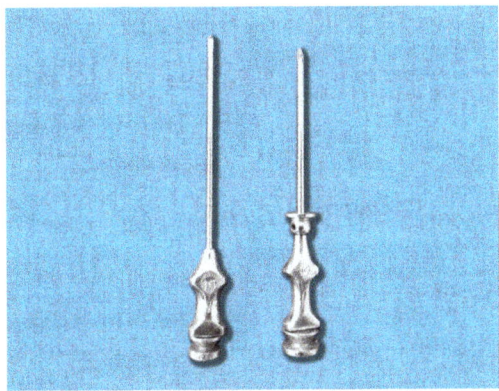

**Fig. 2.16:** Jamshidi bone marrow needle.

## QUESTIONS

**Q1. What is the difference between bone marrow aspiration and bone marrow biopsy?**
Bone marrow aspiration is drawing of liquid content of the bone marrow whereas biopsy is sampling of solid portion of the bone marrow.

**Q2. What is the therapeutic indication for bone marrow needle?**
Intraosseous transfusion of fluids in severe dehydration.

**Q3. What are the features of incomplete penetration of the cortex?**
The needle is not fixed well or the needle is under the skin.

**Q4. What are the causes of dry tap?**
- Aplastic anemia
- Myelofibrosis
- Carcinomatous infiltration of marrow
- Leukemia

**Q5. What is the preferred site for bone marrow aspiration/biopsy at various age groups?**
- Any age anterior and posterior superior iliac spine and iliac crest
- Birth to 2 years–anteromedial aspect of tibia

**Q6. What is the preferred site for bone marrow intraosseous transfusion at various age groups?**
Anteromedial aspect of tibia.

**Q7. Can bone marrow aspiration or biopsy done at sternum?**
In children sternum should be avoided for bone marrow aspiration.

## Biopsy Gun (Fig. 2.17)

- 14 G
- 18 G
- Automated devices like biopsy gun (automatic biopsy guns) are used instead of trucut needles

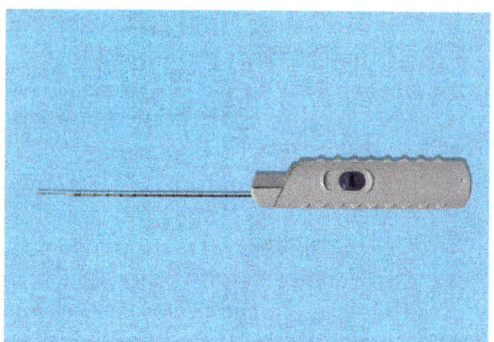

**Fig. 2.17:** Biopsy gun.

- These are used for automatic extraction of tissue samples.

### Uses
It is used in the ultrasound guided biopsy for kidney and liver specimens.

### Indications
- For diagnosis of glomerular, tubulointerstitial, and small blood vessels
- Evaluation of proteinuria, hematuria, and small vessel disease
- Renal manifestations of systemic disease.

### Renal Biopsy Procedure
- Written informed consent
- 16 G or 18 G size needles are used
- Aseptic precautions should be taken
- Under ultrasound guidance biopsy can be done
- *Short anesthesia*: IV ketamine 1–2 mg/Kg can be used
- *Site*: Lower edge of 12th rib and the lateral border of sacrospinalis
- The junction of the medial 2/3rd and lateral 1/3rd of the horizontal line joining the tip of the 12th rib with the vertebral column.

### Advantages
- Accurate than trucut biopsy
- Biopsy specimen obtained will be qualitatively and quantitatively superior than trucut needle

- Convenient
- Control with one hand easy to use by one hand cocking mechanism
- Complications are less as compared to conventional techniques
- Duration of procedure will be less, time required to take biopsy is less
- Easy to use, more complicated movements used for conventional biopsy are not needed
- Failure rate less
- Finer needle/smaller gauge needle can be used, 18 G instead of 14 G or 15 G in trucut
- Gross hematuria is not seen, which is common with trucut biopsy
- Hospital stay will be less
- Injury to the tissue less severe.

### *Disadvantages*

Ultrasonogram is needed.

### *Complications*

- Hematuria
- Arteriovenous fistula
- Perirenal/perinephric hematoma
- Flank pain
- Hematocrit decreases
- Complications are less as compared to conventional tech.

### *Follow-up*

Repeat ultrasound after 24–48 hours.

## SYRINGES

- 2 mL, 5 mL, 10 mL syringes
- 20 mL syringes.

## Parts of Syringes

- Nozzle
- Needle hub
- Piston/plunger
- Barrel made of glass or plastic with graduated marks indicates volume of fluid in syringe
- Needle with protective cover
- The plunger can be pulled or pushed into the hollow barrel.

## Uses

- Injecting fluids and medicines
- Withdrawal of fluids
- Collection of blood for investigations.

## Insulin Syringe (Fig. 2.18)

### *Parts of Insulin Syringe*

There are three parts:
1. Needle 6 mm
2. Barrel
3. Plunger

The barrel is marked with units of insulin.

### *Needles Used*

- 28 G and 29 G needles are ½ inch long
- 30 G and 31 G needles are shorter 5/16 inches.

### *Volume of Syringes*

- Half unit scale 3/10 cc (0.3 cc) syringe will hold a maximum up to 25 units of insulin smallest unit measures ½ unit.
- 0.3 cc syringe will hold a maximum up to 30 units of insulin marked with 5 units increments smallest unit measures 1 unit.
- 0.5 cc syringe will hold a maximum up to 50 units of insulin marked with 10 units increments.

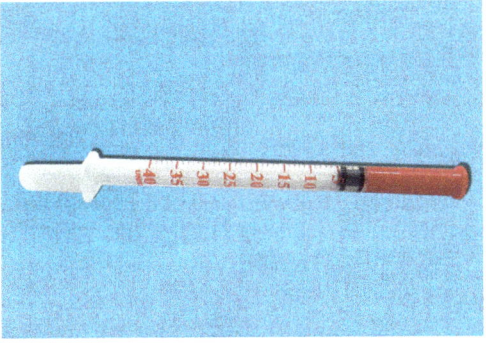

**Fig. 2.18:** Insulin syringe.

- 1 cc syringe will hold a maximum up to 100 units of insulin marked with 10 units increments.
- Smallest syringe should be used for the dose required. This is because the measuring lines will be apart and will be easy to measure the dose.
  - 1 unit = 0.01 mL
  - 2 units = 0.02 mL
  - 1 mL is equal to 1 cc
- 0.25 or 0.33 mL syringe is used for children.
- Two scales of measurement
  - U-100 system is standard for human insulin where 1 mL will contain 100 units of insulin
  - U-40 insulin where 1 mL will contain 40 units of insulin
- The insulin vial will be available as U-100 and U-40
- The unit is 0.01 mL.

### Advantages of Insulin Syringes
- Low dead space
- Less pain
- Fine gauge needle
- Low complications.

### Precautions
The unit calibration on the syringe must be matched against the strength of the insulin used.

## QUESTIONS

**Q1.** How many cc is equal to one unit of insulin?
0.01 mL.

**Q2.** Which insulin syringe is better for children?
0.25 or 0.33 mL syringe is better for children.

### Tuberculin Syringe
- 1 cc syringe white or metal pistol
- Graduations 0.01 mL and 0.5 mL
- Length of needle ½ inches
- Needle gauge 27.

### Uses
- To administer Bacillus Calmette-Guérin (BCG)
- Purified protein derivative (PPD) for Mantoux.

**Q. What are the differences between tuberculin syringe and insulin syringe?**

| Features | Tuberculin syringe | Insulin syringe |
|---|---|---|
| Uses | Tuberculin test | Insulin administration |
| Markings | Grade 0–100 | Grade 0, 40, 80, 100 |
| Barrel | Smaller in diameter for less volume | |
| Needle | For intradermal injection | Longer than for tuberculin syringe for subcutaneous injection |
| Uses | Administration of PPD in tuberculin test Test dose of penicillin | Administration of insulin |

The calibrations into units are seen in both syringes, but one unit of insulin is not same as one unit of TB antigen. Hence, insulin syringe cannot be used in place of tuberculin syringe and vice versa.

## TUBES

### Nasogastric Feeding Tubes/Infant Feeding Tube/Nasogastric Tube

*Nasogastric Tube (Fig. 2.19)*
- Made of polyethylene
- Disposable after single dose
- Sterilized by Gamma rays.

**Types:**
- Polyurethane or silicone
- Polyvinyl chloride

**Various sizes:**
- Neonates: 5–8 F
- Young children: 12–16 F

# Instruments and Procedures

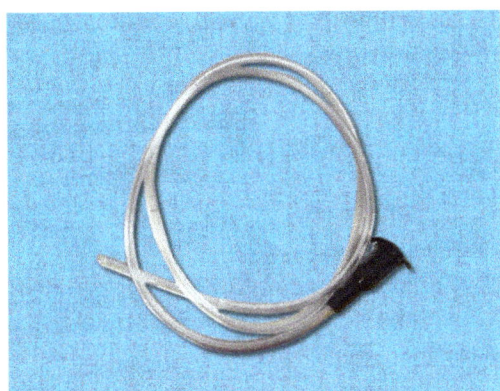

**Fig. 2.19:** Nasogastric tube.

## Uses:
- Prevent distension of abdomen in neonatal resuscitation.
- Air will be pushed into the stomach causing distension of stomach, pressure on the diaphragm compromising ventilation.
- Regurgitation of stomach contents predisposing to aspiration into the lungs.

## Size of Nasogastric Tubes
**Infant feeding tubes:**
- Size for newborn weighing less than 2,000 g is 5 F/6 F
- Size for newborn weighing more than 2,000 g is 7 F/8 F
- Age between 1 year and 2 years: 7 F/8 F
- Age after 3 years: 9 F.

**Length of nasogastric tubes to be inserted:**

The length to be inserted can be measured by measuring the distance between the tip of the nose and the tragus and then from the tragus to the xiphisternum (usually 16–17 cm in the newborn).

## Precautions
- Always measure the length of the tube to be inserted.
- Lubricate the tube before insertion.
- Confirm the position of the tube before administration of fluids or medicine through the tube.

**The indications for tube feeds in newborn:**
- Babies not sucking
- Sucking at the breast for more than 20 minutes
- Babies becoming tired quickly
- Tube feeding may be adopted for babies who are too ill to suckle or have a condition like cleft palate.

**Contraindications for nasogastric tube:**
- Aspiration risk
- Aberrant right subclavian artery
- Alkali ingestion
- Bleeding disorders
- Clotting/coagulation disorders
- Discomfort
- Epistaxis
- Esophageal varices or stricture or obstruction
- Fractures: Fracture base of skull, neck, and facial fractures
- Gastrointestinal stricture
- Gastric stasis
- Gastroesophageal reflux disease (GERD)
- High-risk group for aspiration
- Injury to nose: Nasal injuries
- Irritation of throat
- Intestinal obstruction (tube feeding is contraindicated).

**Complications of nasogastric tube:**
- Aspiration of gastric contents: Pulmonary aspiration
- Air leak syndromes: Pneumothorax
- Bleeding: Nasal bleeding (epistaxis)
- Blockage of the tube
- Breakage of tube
- Collapse of lung
- Coiling of the tube in the mouth
- Damage to soft tissue
- Damage to ciliary epithelium in the nose
- Dislodgement of tube
- Empyema
- Erosion of nose
- Esophageal injury/perforation
- Esophageal stricture

- Faulty insertion (right lower lobe bronchus, lungs, intracranial, and trachea)
- Fistula formation: Aortoesophageal fistula
- Gastroesophageal reflux in prolonged use
- Gland infection (parotid)
- Hemorrhage (pulmonary)
- Hydrothorax
- Hematemesis due to injury to arteries
- Isocalothorax: Enteral feed hydrothorax
- Infections: Pneumonitis, pneumonia, empyema, sinusitis, and sore throat
- Intravascular penetration
- Intrapulmonary feeding

## Features of Abnormal Placement of the Infant Feeding Tube

- Air leak
- Bradycardia
- Cyanosis
- Coughing
- Dyspnea (breathing problems)
- Emesis (vomiting).

## Ryle's Tube (Fig. 2.20)

- Nontoxic and nonirritant PVC
- Silastic material, more costly and less harmful to the mucosa
- Corrosion resistant stainless steel balls
- Guides the passage of tubing during intubation
- Four holes on the lateral side for effective aspiration and administration
- Marked 50 cm, 60 cm, and 70 cm from the tip
- Smooth low friction surface for easy intubation
- X-ray opaque throughout the length and the position can be confirmed radiologically
- *Length*: 105 cm
- *Sizes*: 6, 8, 10, 12, 14, 16, 18, 20, 22, and 24 F.

### Uses of infant feeding tubes/indications for Ryle's tube:

- Diagnostic:
    - Aspiration of gastric contents in poisoning
    - Bleeding into the gastrointestinal (GI) tract evaluation
    - Contrast studies: Barium contrast administration into GI tract
    - Choanal atresia
    - Duodenal atresia
    - Diagnostic motility studies for determination of motor activity of GI tract
    - Esophageal patency can be tested to rule out tracheoesophageal fistula (TEF)
    - Fistula: TEF types diagnosis
    - Gastrointestinal bleeding to measure the blood volume
    - Gastric lavage: Meconium
    - Resting gastric juice for *Tuberculous bacilli*
    - Giardiasis diagnosis can be done by passing the tube into the duodenum.
- Therapeutic:
    - Aspiration of gastric contents to empty the stomach.
    - Bowel irrigation.
    - Bag and mask ventilation (BMV) for more than 2 minutes. If BMV is continued for more than 2 minutes, air would enter the stomach and cause distension. It is better to insert a nasogastric tube to decompress stomach.
    - Coma patients to prevent aspiration.
    - Drug administration.
    - Decompression of GI tract in neonatal resuscitation before bag and mask ventilation, and intestinal obstruction to

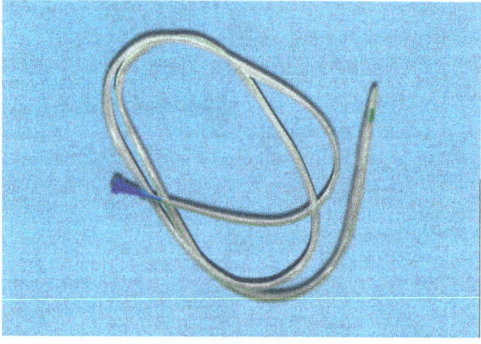

**Fig. 2.20:** Ryle's tube.

prevent distension of stomach in certain conditions like diaphragmatic hernia.
- Enteral feeding/gavage feeding.
- Feeding: Intragastric feeding/nutrition in low birth weight/preterm babies that cannot suck effectively at the breast or take oral feeds or who are too ill to suckle or have a condition like cleft palate, lower cranial nerve palsies, and in unconscious patients.
- Gastric wash in poisoning:
- Gastric drainage.
- Infant feeding tubes are also used for urinary catheterization, umbilical vein cannulation, and suction of endotracheal tube in intubated child.

## QUESTIONS

**Q1. What are the sizes of orogastric feeding tubes?**
- The nasogastric tube used to feed a baby is usually size 6-10 F.
- Two sizes are available:
  1. 3.5 F/5 F/6 F for infants weighing less than 2,000 g
  2. 8 F for infants weighing more than 2,000 g.

**Q2. What are the sizes of orogastric feeding tubes for neonates?**
5-8 F.

**Q3. What are the sizes of orogastric feeding tubes for young children?**
12-16 F. The nasogastric tube used to feed a baby is usually size 6-10 F.

**Q4. How will you calculate the length of the nasogastric tube to be inserted?**
- The length to be inserted can be measured by measuring the distance between the tip of the nose and the tragus and then from the tragus to the xiphisternum (usually 16-17 cm in the newborn).
- The length of the tube should be measured from the philtrum to the tragus and then from tragus to xiphisternum before inserting it.

**Q5. How will you insert a nasogastric tube?**
Lubricate the first 2-4 cm of the tube. Ask the patient to swallow as you advance the tube. If any resistance is felt the tube can be rotated and advanced.

**Q6. What are the precautions for nasogastric tube insertion?**
- Should be flushed regularly to avoid occlusion by building up of foods or medicines
- Position should be checked at least once a day
  - After coughing, retching or vomiting
  - When there is discomfort or reflux
  - Signs of respiratory distress.

**Q7. What are the ways by which the position of nasogastric tube can be checked?**
- By taking X-rays
- Testing the pH of the aspirate
- Introducing air into the tube and auscultating over the epigastrium may not be a reliable test.

**Q8. What is the method of insertion of nasogastric tube?**
- The nasogastric tube used to feed a baby is usually size 6-10 F. The tube should be inserted into the nose with the head slightly raised. The position of the tube should be verified by auscultating the abdomen while pushing air into the tube.
- The outer end of this tube should be connected to a syringe. Milk can be poured into this syringe and allowed to flow into the stomach by gravity. Start with 10 mL/kg/day and gradually increase the amount by 10 mL/kg every day.

**Q9. How will you insert a feeding tube?**
The tube should be lubricated with saline. Flex the neck slightly. The tube should be inserted through one of the nostril or mouth. The tube should be lubricated and slided into the nostril along the base of the nose. Assist by swallowing.

The tube should be advanced slowly up to the desired length. The tube should be fixed to the cheek or upper lip using an adhesive tape.

**Q10. How far a feeding tube should be inserted?**
Measure the distance from the tip of the nose/philtrum of the mouth to the tragus of the ear and from there to the xiphisternum. The tube should be inserted through one of the nostrils or mouth. The tube should be advanced slowly up to the desired length.

**Q11. How will you check that the tube is inside the stomach?**
By pushing air into the tube using a syringe auscultate over the abdomen.

**Q12. How will you confirm that the tube is in the stomach and not in the respiratory tract?**
After insertion, the clinician should push air and auscultate over the stomach area to check its position. Aspiration of gastric contents will show low pH.

Check X-ray abdomen is the procedure to confirm that the tube is in the stomach.

**Q13. What are the indicators of nasogastric tube in the respiratory tract?**
- Tube placed under water shows bubbling of air
- Tube placed near a mirror fogs the mirror
- A feather or cotton placed at the mouth of the tube moves with each respiration
- Safety checks to ensure that the tube is not in the respiratory tract.

**Q14. What precaution will you take while removing the tube from the patient?**
Pinch the tube at the one end and remove the tube. This will prevent dripping of stomach contents in the tube. A continuous negative suction can be applied by syringe to prevent trickling of contents into the trachea.

**Q15. What is the amount of feeds to be given?**
Tube feeding should be given in accordance to the stomach capacity. For instance, stomach capacity on first day is 10 mL per kg of body weight.

**Q16. What are the complications of naso/orogastric feeding?**
- Aspiration can occur if the tube is not in the stomach.
- To prevent this, the position of the tube should be checked before each feed.
- Air will be pushed into the stomach causing distension of stomach, pressure on the diaphragm compromising ventilation.
- Regurgitation of stomach contents predisposing to aspiration into the lungs.

**Q17. How often the naso/orogastric tube should be changed?**
- The orogastric tube can be left for 3–4 days.
- The nasogastric tube should be changed from one nostril to other once a day. The nasogastric tube should be changed every 24–48 hours.
- Polyurethane or silicone tubes can be used for 30 days.
- Polyvinyl chloride can be used for 1–2 weeks.

**Q18. What are the indications for withdrawing the tube?**
- Coughing
- Cyanosis
- Respiratory distress
- Gasping

**Q19. What is the procedure of oral insertion of tube?**
- During newborn resuscitation the tube should be inserted through the

mouth and not through the nose, so the airway is not obstructed.
- Insert the tube through the mouth or through the nose through one of the nostrils.
- If inserted through mouth fixation may be difficult and cause more gagging.
- If inserted through nostrils fixation will be easy, but it may cause airway obstruction as the newborns are obligatory nasal breathers.
- Aspirate the stomach contents from the stomach before each feed. If 50% of the feed is present, skip one feed. If more amount is present then avoid feeding through the tube. Parenteral feeds may be considered.
- Change the tube every 24–48 hours. After each feed give about 2 mL of distilled water. Allow the feeds to flow into the stomach by gravity. Do not push the milk into the tube.

**Q20. How long the tube can be kept in situ?**
For newborns it can be kept for 3–4 days and for older children it can be kept or 5–6 days.

**Q21. What is the advantage of infant feeding tube/nasogastric tube in neonatal resuscitation?**
Prevent distension of abdomen in neonatal resuscitation.

**Q22. What are the precautions taken after insertion of nasogastric tube?**
Aspirate the stomach contents from the stomach before each feed. If 50% of the feed is present, skip one feed. If more amount is present then avoid feeding through the tube. Parenteral feeds may be considered.
  Change the tube every 24–48 hours. After each feed give about 2 mL of distilled water. Allow the feeds to flow in to the stomach by gravity. Do not push the milk in to the tube.

**Q23. What are the advantages of polyuretahane or silicone feeding tube?**
- Polyuretahane or silicone feeding tube will not be affected by gastric acid.
- Can be used for up to 6 weeks.
- Polyvinyl chloride (PVC) tubes can be used up to 2 weeks only.

**Q24. What are the fine bore feeding tubes?**
Gauge less than 9 causes less discomfort.

**Q25. What are the advantages of fine bore feeding tubes?**
- Less risk for sinusitis
- Pharyngitis
- Esophageal erosion.

## Intercostal Drainage Tube

The intercostal drainage tubes are flexible plastic tubes inserted into the pleural space or mediastinum through the chest wall. These are used to remove air, blood, chyle, effusion, fluid, pus, etc. from the intrathoracic space.

### Different Sizes of Tubes used for Intercostal Drainage

- Newborn: 12–14 F
- Infants: 14–16 F
- School age: 16–24 F
- Adolescents: 28–32 F

Intercostal drainage bag is used to collect the drained fluid.

### Indications for Pleural Tap (Thoracocentesis)

- Diagnostic
  Pleural effusion: Serous, purulent, blood or chyle, and transudate or exudates
- Therapeutic
  - To drain large pleural effusion causing respiratory embarrassment
  - Massive or rapid collection of pleural fluid
  - Empyema
  - Pneumothorax (tension pneumothorax)
  - Pyopneumothorax
  - Hemothorax
  - Chylothorax
  - Instillation of drugs, especially in pleural malignancy
  - Postoperative drainage.

## Indications for Intercostal Drainage according to the Fluid in Pleural Cavity

- Presence of gross pus in the pleural space
- Loculated pus
- pH less than 7
- Glucose less than 40 mg/dL.

## Indications for Intercostal Drainage in Pneumothorax

- Symptomatic patient
- Bilateral pneumothorax
- Pneumothorax in a patient on ventilator
- Tension pneumothorax.

## Two Techniques

- Blunt insertion: Blunt dissection technique
- Trocar technique.

## Precautions

- The chest wall should be percussed and a site with maximal dullness should be selected. Under strict aseptic precautions the needle should be inserted into the pleural space while providing steady negative pressure.
- Pleural aspiration can be done using a syringe. A wide bored needle should be used as a thick pus will get obstructed in small needles.
- The intercostal drainage tube should be inserted into the pleural space. The tube should be directed inferiorly and posteriorly. The neurovascular bundle will be present at the inferior border of the ribs. To avoid injury to the neurovascular bundle the tube should be inserted adjacent to the upper border of the lower ribs.
- The drainage bottle should be placed below the level of chest to avoid flow of fluid into the pleural cavity.
- The fluid in the tube will be fluctuating. If there is a block, the fluctuation of fluid will be absent.
- Throughout the procedure, a closed drainage system should be maintained, any break in the system will result in sucking of air on to the pleural cavity.
- X-ray should be taken to check the position and resolution of pneumothorax.

## Complications of Pleural Tap

- Air leak: Pneumothorax
- Air embolism
- Bleeding
- Chylothorax
- Diaphragmatic paralysis
- Death due to vasovagal shock
- Dysrhythmias
- Emphysema (subcutaneous)
- Empyema thoracis
- Esophageal perforation
- Fistula–bronchopleural fistula: There is bubbling from the drainage tube. The tube should be kept in place until bubble stops
- Fasciitis: Necrotizing fasciitis
- Gut injury/gastric injury
- Hydropneumothorax
- Hemothorax
- Hematoma
- Hypoproteinemia
- Horner's syndrome due to injury to second order preganglionic neurons
- Injection site infection or introduction of infection
- Injury to intercostal artery, vein or nerve
- Injury: Organ injury to lung, spleen, liver, stomach, and diaphragm
- Injury to neurovascular bundle
- Infections: Pneumonia and osteomyelitis
- Improper position of the tube, kinking, clogging, dislodgement of disconnection of the tube
- Pleural shock
- Unilateral pulmonary edema due to re-expansion.

## Technical Problems

- Blocked drain
- Malposition of tube
- Drain dislodgement.

## QUESTIONS

**Q1. What is the site of intercostal drainage in pleural effusion?**
The tube should be inserted in the 5th to 8th intercostal space in the posterior axillary line.

**Q2. What is the site of intercostal drainage in pneumothorax?**
The intercostal tube should be inserted at the site of second intercostal space in the midclavicular line. Insert the tube anteriorly towards the apex.

**Q3. What are the precautions to be taken in intercostal drainage?**
- The drain should be always kept below the level of the patient
- Do not keep the drain clamped as air may enter and predispose to pneumothorax.

**Q4. What is thoracocentesis?**
It is a procedure of insertion of a needle into the pleural space for removal of fluid or air from the pleural cavity.

**Q5. What are the complications of rapid pleural tap?**
Acute noncardiogenic 26 G smallest pulmonary edema.

**Q6. What is the indication for decortication?**
When the drainage is present for more than 14 days.

**Q7. What are the contraindications for pleural tap?**
- Local skin infection
- Coagulopathy

**Q8. How will you verify if the intercostal drainage tube is functioning?**
The fluid column in the tube will be moving up and down.

**Q9. What are the points to be noted while inserting an intercostal tube?**
The following steps should be followed while inserting an intercostal tube:
- The tube should be inserted in between 5th and 7th intercostal space in the midaxillary line for pleural effusion. In pneumothorax the tube should be inserted in the second intercostal space in the midclavicular line.
- The tube should be lying 5–10 cm in the pleural cavity.
- The puncture in the chest should be directed towards the suprasternal notch.

**Q10. What are the different methods used for thoracostomy?**
- Direct puncture
- Trocar and cannula
- Trocar and chest tube.

**Q11. How will you remove an intercostal tube?**
Removal of the intercostal tube: The tube should be clamped. The tube should be pulled out rapidly at the same time a sterile dressing should be applied immediately after removal of the tube. A large wound should be sutured if present.

**Q12. When will you remove the intercostal tube?**
- When the drainage is below 10 mL/day for 3 days or no pus or air is draining
- No air bubbling is seen for more than 24 hours
- When the lung is fully expanded
- No recollection radiologically
- When you suspect bronchopleural fistula
- When there is block in the tube
- If the drainage is present for more than 14 days decorticating may be needed.

**Q13. What are the causes of failure of ICD?**
- Improper positioning of the intercostal tube
- Presence of bronchopleural fistula
- Loculation of fluid or pus
- Thickening of pleura resulting in nonexpansion of lungs
- Inappropriate use of antibiotics
- Kinking of the ICD tube
- Block of the ICD tube
- Improper tube size.

**Q14. What is the safe zone for insertion of ICD?**
The region bordered by
- Lateral border of pectoralis major
- Anterior border of latissmus dorsi and a horizontal line inferior to axilla
- Horizontal line superior to the nipple.

**Q15. What are the indications, contraindications and complications of ICD?**
*ICD indications*:
- Air in the pleural cavity—pneumothorax
- Blood in the pleural cavity—hemothorax
- Bronchopleural fistula
- Chylothorax
- Direct monitoring of intrapleural pressure
- Drainage of thoracic cavity after cardiothoracic surgery
- Empyema
- Fluid in pleural cavity—pleural effusion
- Gas in the pleural space
- Hydrothorax
- Hydropneumothorax
- Injury to chest wall (Penetrating injury)

*ICD contraindications*:
- Adhesions
- Bullae (pulmonary)
- Coagulopathy refractory to treatment
- Diaphragmatic hernia
- Empyema caused by acid fast organisms like *Mycobactreium tuberculosis*

*Complications of ICD*:
- Air leak syndromes
- Bleeding
- Breathing difficulties
- Cardiac injury
- Chronic pain
- Cough
- Cardiac injuries
- Cardiogenic shock
- Diaphragmatic injury/perforation
- Dislodgement of tubes
- Edema—reexpansion pulmonary edema
- Empyema
- Emphysema (subcutaneous)
- Faulty positioning of the tube (subdiaphragmatic sucutaneous position)
- Great vessels injury (Aortic injury)
- Hemorrhage
- Infection
- Injuries to viscera—to lungs, liver, spleen, thoracic aorta, heart
- Injury to blood vessels—axillary, intercostal, pulmonary, internal mammary.

**Q16. What are the causes of failure of expansion of lung after insertion of ICD tube?**
- Blockage of tube
- Insertion of tube into other spaces.

**Q17. What will you suspect when there is bubbling from the drainage tube? What is the management?**
- bronchopleural fistula
- The tube should be kept in place until bubble stops.

## Intravenous Extension Tube (Fig. 2.21)

❖ This tube is connected between the intravenous needle and the intravenous fluid container bottle.
❖ Length: 150 cm.

### Advantages

❖ Easy to do procedures on the patients
❖ Risk of needle stick injuries will be less
❖ Increased safety to healthcare personnel.

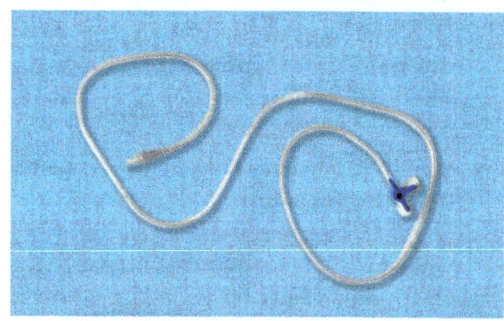

**Fig. 2.21:** Intravenous extension tube.

## Disadvantages

The flow rate will be reduced. A 14 G extension tube will function similar to 18–20 G. Hence, it is used for patients who does not require volume resuscitation.

## Endotracheal Tubes (ET Tube) (Fig. 2.22)

Should be uniform in diameter throughout the length of the tube. A black line at the tip is known as vocal cord guide. The endotracheal tube should be inserted up to a point so that vocal cord guide should be placed at the vocal cords. Tubes with cuff at the level of vocal cord guides are available, but not used in neonatal resuscitation. The tubes will be marked in centimeters, which will help to identify the distance inserted from the tip of the tube. Uniform diameter endotracheal tubes (2.5, 3.0, and 3.5 mm internal diameters). Appropriate size should be selected. Murphy's eye is the hole present on the side of the ET tubes. This will function as a vent which prevents complete obstruction of the airway when the primary opening of the ET tube is blocked. Two types of tubes are present. A straight tube with two side holes and a curved tube with a single hole.

## Types of Endotracheal Tube

- According to the material:
  - Sterile disposable tube—recommended
  - Metal tube (previously used and not used now)
- Diameter wise:
  - Uniform diameter tube—recommended
  - Tapered end tube—not recommended

- Blades:
  - Straight used for infants less than 1 year of age and when epiglottis is floppy
  - Curved used for older children.

## Features of the Tubes

- Nonirritating material
- Uniform diameter throughout.

## Various Sizes of Endotracheal Tube

Various sizes for various ages: 2 mm, 2.5 mm, 3 mm, 3.5 mm, and 4 mm.

## Endotracheal Tube Size used for Babies

Endotracheal tubes size 2.5 mm, 3 mm, 3.5 mm, and 4 mm.

According to gestational age:

| Gestational age (weeks) | Size (mm internal diameter) |
|---|---|
| <30 | 2.5 |
| 30–34 | 3.0 |
| >35 | 3.5 |

According to weight:

| Weight | Tube size mm (diameter) | Gestational age (weeks) |
|---|---|---|
| >1 Kg | 2.5 | >28 |
| 1–2 Kg | 3.0 | 28–34 |
| 2–3 Kg | 3.5 | 34–38 |
| >3 Kg | 3.5–4 | >38 |

## Depth of Insertion

Can be calculated by using the formula:
Insertion depth at lip in centimeters = Weight in kilograms + 6 cm

The length of the tube that has to inserted from the lip should be as follows:

| Weight of the infant (kg) | Endotracheal tube to be inserted from the lip |
|---|---|
| 1 | 7 |
| 2 | 8 |
| 3 | 9 |
| 4 | 10 |

At these lengths the tip of the tube inserted will be in the midtrachea. If it is inserted

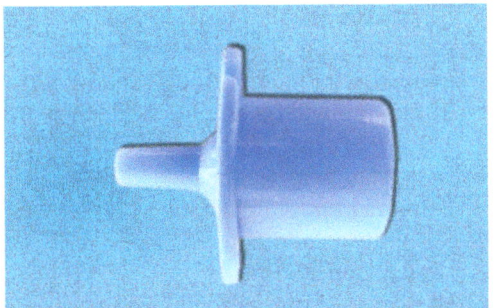

**Fig. 2.22:** Endotracheal tube universal adaptor.

further the endotracheal tube may enter one of the main bronchus. Shorten the endotracheal tube by 4 cm beyond the lips.

**Endotracheal tubes of various sizes:** Endotracheal tubes with metal stylet to prevent kinking. These tubes are tapered at the distal end in sizes ranging from 2.5 mm, 3 mm, 3.5 mm, and 4 mm.

| Birth weight (g) | Gestational age (weeks) | Endotracheal tubes size of internal diameter (mm) | Depth of insertion from the upper lip (cm) |
|---|---|---|---|
| <1,000 | <28 | 2.5 | 6–7 |
| 1,000–2,000 | 28–34 | 3 | 7–8 |
| 2,000–3,000 | 35–38 | 3.5 | 8–9 |
| >3,000 | >38 | 3.5–4 | 9–10 |

Metal stylet should be avoided because of the trauma they may cause during intubation. The length of the tube should be shortened to 13 cm to eliminate the dead space. A flexible stylet should be inserted into the tube to facilitate easy insertion of the tube into the trachea. The stylet should not extend beyond the end of the endotracheal tube.

## Stylet for Intubation (Fig. 2.23)

- Malleable metal rods to give certain shape to aid in the navigation of the tube.
- Endotracheal tubes are floppy and will not maintain normal curvature during intubation and need stylet to facilitate insertion.

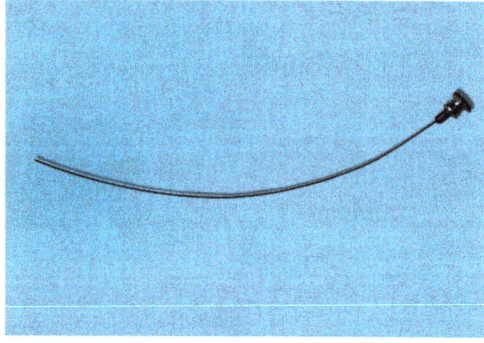

**Fig. 2.23:** Stylet for intubation.

- This will suit the pediatric and adult endotracheal tubes. Longer stylet are used for adult tubes.

## Endotracheal Intubation

If spontaneous respirations do not immediately follow the removal of fluid and particulate matter, an endotracheal tube is introduced through the glottis.

- *Oral intubation*: It is advantageous because of the relative ease with which it can be inserted. Oral intubation should be used in emergencies.
- *Nasal intubation*: It should be done as elective procedure. In emergencies oral intubation should be done. Nasal intubation has less chance of slipping. The tube is inserted into the nose and visualized in the oropharynx. The tube can be guided into the glottis using a McGill forceps. Do not use a stylet for nasotracheal intubation.

Confirmation of the position of the trachea is also done by carbon dioxide detectors.

### Indications

- Aspiration of thick meconium: Tracheal suction as in meconium aspiration syndrome (MAS)
- Birth asphyxia management: Neonatal resuscitation
  - If the bag and mask ventilation is ineffective (poor chest rise)
  - Prolonged pressure ventilation is required
  - If tracheal suction is needed (meconium aspiration)
- Chest compression requirement is a relative indication. When chest compression is needed, ventilation through endotracheal intubation will be helpful to increase the efficacy of positive pressure ventilation.
- Diaphragmatic hernia
- Extreme premature babies
- Respiratory failure
- General anesthesia
- Hypotensive shock

- Mechanical ventilation
- In laryngomalacia to prevent collapse or obstruction of larynx
- Drugs administration through trachea: Need for surfactant therapy. Intubation will be useful to administer epinephrine directly into the trachea.

## Procedure

Patient should lie in supine position. Place a folded towel behind the shoulders so that the neck is extended. Hold the laryngoscope in the left hand, press the hyoid bone posteriorly this will close the esophagus. Now view the glottis area. Insert a tube of appropriate size. Check for air entry on both sides.

## Warning:

- The vascular bundle runs at the inferior surface of the ribs. Inserting the tube at the inferior border will injure the vessels or nerve. Hence, the tube should be inserted at the upper border of the lower ribs.
- Child may collapse due to vasovagal shock. Give injection atropine before the procedure.

## Confirm the Position of the Tube

The position of the tube can be confirmed by one of the following ways:
- Confirm the tube position by auscultation of breath sounds. It should be heard equally on both sides of the chest. If the sounds are heard only on one side, there is a possibility of the tube entering one of the bronchi. The tube should be withdrawn a little so that the tube reaches the bronchus before bifurcation.

If the endotracheal tube has been inserted too deeply, it will pass directly into the right main stem bronchus. Delivery of oxygen is therefore confined to the right lung, and insufflations cause expansion in the right chest, with little or no visible excursion on the left. Breath sounds are absent on the left, whereas on the right they are loud and clear. This discrepancy can be determined more accurately by an assistant who listens with a stethoscope.

This being the case, the endotracheal tube should be withdrawn slightly until breath sounds are equal on each side of the chest. Take an X-ray chest to confirm good ventilation and expansion of the lung. Shorten the endotracheal tube by 4 cm beyond the lips.
- Symmetrical chest wall movements.
- Absence of fog in the tube or on a mirror placed at the outlet of the tube.
- Absence of sounds over the stomach or absence of gastric dilatation.
- Exhaled $CO_2$ detection will be helpful in confirming the tracheal position of the endotracheal tube. This will be helpful when the clinical assessment is equivocal. However, inadequate pulmonary expansion decreased pulmonary blood flow and small tidal volumes will influence the interpretation of the exhaled $CO_2$ concentration.

Also improvement in color, heart rate, and activity of the baby will be an indirect evidence for the correct position of the tube.

## Contraindications for Endotracheal Intubation

There are many conditions in which the use of endotracheal tubes are contraindicated.
- Airway obstruction
- Severe trauma to the airway
- Cervical spine injury

## Complications of Endotracheal Intubation

- Apnea due to laryngeal stimulation
- Bradycardia due to laryngeal stimulation
- Cardiac arrest
- Displacement of loose tooth
- Edema of the airway
- Failure of equipment
- *Glottis*: Subglottic stenosis
- Hypoxia
- Injury to mouth and oropharynx, aggravation of pre-existing trauma, airway

Complications associated with endotracheal and predisposing causes.

| Complications | Predisposing causes | Management |
|---|---|---|
| Hypoxia | Delay in intubation Malposition or displacement of the tube | Preoxygenate with bag and mask, provide free flow oxygen, attempt of intubation should be limited to 20 seconds |
| Bradycardia/apnea | Hypoxia | Preoxygenate with bag and mask, provide free flow oxygen |
| Contusions/lacerations of gums, tongue, airway | Rough handling, too long or too short blade, improper techniques of insertion | Select appropriate sized blades Adequate training |
| Pneumothorax | Over ventilation of one lung | Proper positioning of the endotracheal tube |
| Perforation of trachea or esophagus | Vigorous attempt or stylet protruding beyond the tube | Gentle attempt and proper placement of stylet |
| Obstruction of endotracheal tube | Kink in the tube | Suction of the tube or replacement of the tube |
| Infection | Introduction of organisms | Clean and sterile techniques |

trauma (lacerations, edema, and airway perforation).

## Malposition of the Endotracheal Tube

The tube may not be in trachea. This should be suspected when the following features are present:
- Air noises present on auscultation over the stomach on injecting air into the stomach
- Breath sounds not heard over the lungs
- Chest rise absent
- Distension of abdomen
- Exhaled $CO_2$ detection does not indicate presence of exhaled $CO_2$
- Fog absent in the tube or on a mirror placed at the outlet of the tube
- Gastric dilatation present
- Heart rate does not increase, no clinical improvement, with cyanosis and bradycardia persisting.

## QUESTIONS

**Q1. How will you calculate the size of endotracheal tube?**

The size of the uncuffed endotracheal tubes can be calculated by using the following formula:

$$\frac{\text{Age in years}}{4} + 4$$

The size of the cuffed endotracheal tubes can be calculated by using the following formula:

$$\frac{\text{Age in years}}{3} + 4$$

**Q2. How will you calculate the length or depth of endotracheal tube?**

The length of the endotracheal tubes can be calculated by using the following formula:

$$\frac{\text{Age in years}}{2} + 12$$

Internal diameter of the tube × 3
Uncuffed tubes are used up to the age of 8 years

**Q3. Why uncuffed tubes are used up to the age of 8 years?**

Up to the age of 8 years the cricoid cartilage will act as a natural cuff.

**Q4. What is the formula used for endotracheal tube size?**

<6 years:

$$\frac{\text{Age}}{3} + 3.5$$

>6 years:

$$\frac{Age}{4} + 4.5$$

For children more than 1 year the following formula is used

Internal diameter =

$$\frac{16 + \text{Child's age in years}}{4}$$

**Q5. What are the precautions to select the tube size?**
One size smaller and one size larger than the required size should be available before starting the intubation.

## Endotracheal Tube Universal Adaptor

Sizes available are:
- 16 mm
- 18 mm

## Oxygen Tube (Fig. 2.24)

- *Length*: 210 cm long tube with star lumen
- *Two sizes*: Adult and pediatric sizes
- This is used to ensure continuous flow of oxygen
- The lumen is star shaped to avoid accidental blockage.

## CATHETERS

Catheters are thin, flexible tubes that can be inserted into the body cavity, duct or vessels for treating diseases or performing surgical procedures. The process of insertion of a catheter is known as catheterization.

### Suction Catheters

- Size 12 or 14 F
- Suction catheters should be attached to the suction apparatus.

### Uses

Suction oral cavity, nose, and stomach.

### Foley's Catheter (Fig. 2.25)

- Named after Frederic Foley who produced the original design in 1929
- Self-retaining catheter
- The Foley's catheter is made of silicon or ordinary rubber.
- Two lumen one for inflating the balloon, second for draining urine.
- Inflatable bag near the end with a capacity of 5–30 mL on distension with water will be used to hold the tube at the internal meatus.

### Parts

- Urine drainage port
- Balloon port
- Bladder opening
- Balloon.

### Sizes

5 to 26 fr (5 fr, 6 fr, 8 fr, 10 fr, 12 fr, 14 fr, 16 fr, 18 fr, 20 fr, 22 fr, 24 fr, 26 fr).

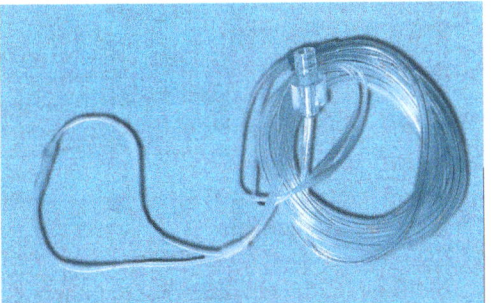

**Fig. 2.24:** Oxygen tube.

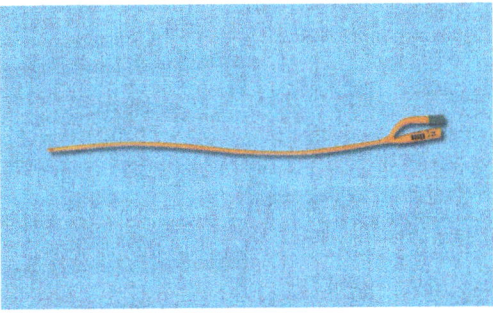

**Fig. 2.25:** Foley's catheter.

## Uses
- To collect urine sample
- Monitoring urinary output.

## Method
Flexible tube passed through the urethra into the bladder. It is an indwelling urinary catheter which will be retained. It has two lumens; one with open at both ends for the drainage of urine which runs down the length and second is having a valve on the outside end which connects to a balloon at the tip. The balloon can be inflated by injection of sterile water into the tube the balloon lies in the bladder, the tube will not slip.

## Indications
Foley's catheter is used in the drainage of urine from the following patients:
- Anesthetized patients
- In comatosed patients
- Patients with urinary incontinence
- Urinary obstruction and neurogenic bladder
- Before and after hysterectomy
- Before and after cesarean section.

## Contraindications
- Foley's catheter should not be used in persons who can urinate normally
- Pelvic fracture.

## Disadvantages
- The lumen is small
- Semi-rigid and cannot overcome serious urethral obstruction without the aid of metal introducer
- Due to its softness, it will collapse if firm suction is applied, so it is not recommended in cases with bleeding or clot obstruction
- Uneven distension of the balloon with angulation of the tip may interfere with drainage.

## Complications
- Hematuria
- Hospital acquired urinary tract infections
- Injury
- Urethral stricture
- Damage or rupture of urethra
- Urine flow may be blocked
- Balloon may not inflate
- If the catheter is pulled before balloon is deflated severe complications can occur, even death can occur.

## Malecot Catheter (Silicone)
Reusable, self retaining catheter which is radiopaque made of India rubber has a flower at the tip which helps to retain the catheter in place thereby preventing accidental removal.
- Uses bladder drainage
- Intercostal drainage in empyema
- Self-retaining catheter
- Two or four winged female catheter.

## Parts
Malecot wings are useful for enhanced drainage of the urine and retain the catheter.

## Indications
- Gastrostomy feeding
- The catheter is used for drainage following:
  - Perinephric drains in renal surgeries and bladder surgeries
  - Intercostal drainage in empyema.

## Contraindications
- Urethral injuries
- Urethral obstruction
- Bladder neck mass causing obstruction
- Cancer prostate

## Advantages
- Reuseable
- Radiopaque.

## Problems Associated with Foley's Tube
- Activity restriction
- Abscess formation
- Bleeding/Hematuria
- Bacteriuria
- Biofilms on the catheter due to collection of microorganisms on the indwelling urinary catheter

- Catheter-associated UTI (CAUTI)/septicemia
- Calculi (Bladder stones)
- Cancer (in long-term catheter use)
- Damage to urinary tract—Injury or erosion of the urethra/kidney
- Encrustations (mineral deposition within the biofilm)
- Epididymitis
- False passage in the urethra
- Fistula
- Fever

## QUESTIONS

**Q1. What are the various sizes of Malecot catheters?**
Sizes: 10, 12, 14, 16, 18, 20, and 22 F

**Q2. Is the advantage of silicone catheter to latex catheters?**
Silicone tubes are soft and preferred over latex catheters.

**Q3. What is the use of malecot wings?**
- Malecot wings will help in enhanced drainage of the urine and retaining the tube in position.
- Prevents accidental removal.

**Q4. Why Malecot catheter is known as female catheter?**
Initially this is used in females.

## Central Venous Catheter (Fig. 2.26)

- Central line or central venous line
- A radiopaque, transparent catheter.

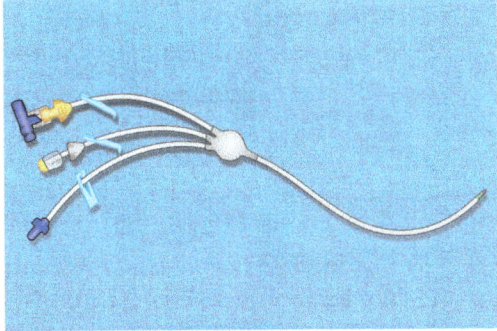

**Fig. 2.26:** Central venous catheter.

### Types of Central Venous Catheters

- *Peripherally inserted central catheter (PICC) line*: Where the venous catheter is inserted into a vein in the arm
- *Tunneled catheter*: Where the catheter is passed under the skin
- *Implanted port*: The catheter is left entirely under the skin.

### Veins used for Central Venous Line

This catheter is placed into a larger vein like:
- Internal jugular vein in the neck
- Superior vena cava or right atrium
- Subclavian vein or axillary vein in the chest
- Femoral vein in the groin
- Umbilical vein.

### Sizes

- 3.5 F for low birth babies
- 5 F for term babies
- 8 F for older children.

### Indications for Central Venous Line

- Administration of hypertonic and irritant solutions
- Blood collection for frequent sampling/monitoring
- Blood gas monitoring
- Blood pressure monitoring (continuously) in newborn
- Central venous pressure monitoring
- Cardiac catheterization
- Chemotherapy
- *Drugs*: Hypertonic saline, amiodarone, 10% dextrose, sodium bicarbonate, calcium, inotropes, etc.
- Dialysis
- Exchange blood transfusion
- Fluid administration
- Glucose (concentrated) transfusion
- Hemofiltration
- Inotropes infusion
- Inferior vena cava (IVC) filter placement
- Parenteral nutrition for more than 1 week duration.

## Contraindications

- Coagulopathy
- Obstructed veins
- Stenosis of veins.

## Advantages of Central Venous Line

- Hypertonic and irritant solutions will get rapidly diluted
- The catheter can be left in place for a longer time to infuse long-term medicine.

## Complications of Central Venous Catheters

- Air leak syndrome—pneumothorax
- Arteriovenous fistula formation
- Bleeding
- Blood clots
- Blocked line by kinking
- Catheter blockage
- Chylothorax
- Duct (thoracic) injury
- Embolism (air)
- Erosion of vessels
- Failure of the procedure
- Fracture/fragmentation of the catheter
- Guidewire-induced arrhythmia (supraventricular)
- Hemothorax
- Hematoma
- Infection
- Injury to artery/veins/vena cava/right atrium by guidewire/dilator
- Interruption of blood flow to intestines, kidney or liver or limb
- Shifting of catheter
- Thrombosis.

## Care of the Central Venous Line

- Change the dressing
- Flush the catheter
- Keep the site dry.

## Precautions

- Central lines should not be used for taking blood samples, blood transfusion or drug administration.
- The risk for pneumothorax is more with subclavian than internal jugular vein. The risk for arterial injury, hematoma formation, catheter related infections are higher with internal jugular vein.
- Umbilical vein catheterization can predispose to venous thrombosis and extraperitoneal portal hypertension.
- Radiological-guided insertion will be associated with less complications like infections, pneumothorax, etc.
- Rate of complications in umbilical vein catheterization is twice that of umbilical artery catheterization
- Arterial catheters are more safer than venous catheters
- The complications in arterial catheter is directly proportional to the duration of indwelling catheter, but no such relation is seen in venous catheters.

## QUESTIONS

**Q.1 What are the contraindications for umbilical catheter?**
- Infections like omphalitis, necrotizing enterocolitis, and peritonitis
- Abdominal wall defects like omphalocele, gastroschisis, and umbilical fistula.

**Q2. What are the advantages of umbilical artery or vein catheterization?**
- Provides a quick access to the central circulation
- Avoids repeated needle pricks for collection of blood samples
- Blood pressure can be measured
- Intravenous transfusions
- Exchange transfusion.

**Q3. What is the size of umbilical catheter?**

| Weight | Catheter size (F) |
|---|---|
| <1,500 Kg | 3.5 |
| 1,500–3500 Kg | 5.0 |
| >3,500 Kg | 8.0 |

**Q4. Why analgesics/anesthesia is not needed for umbilical cauterization?**
It is because umbilical cord had no pain sensation.

**Q5. What is the formula to calculate the desired umbilical catheter?**
- Desired umbilical vein catheter can be calculated by the formula: Desired length in centimeters = 1.5 × baby weight in Kg
- The umbilical catheter tip should lie at the level of the ductus venosus and the IVC just above the level of diaphragm. This level lies approximately at T9–T10.

# BAGS

These are special sterile bags used for collection and temporary storage of urine, pus, fluid in the cavities, etc. These bags will be connected to the drainage tubes. The bags are made of vinyl material and are having markings to measure the fluid collected in the bag.

## Intercostal Drainage Bag
- One-way valve at the inlet
- Outlet
- *Contents*: Water, saline or dextrose can be used.

### Indications
To collect fluid from intercostal tube.

### Complications
- Air leak
- Emphysema (subcutaneous)
- Infection
- Hemorrhage
- Re-expansion pulmonary edema
- Injury to organs—liver, spleen, and diaphragm.

### Precautions
- Should be attached to underwater seal drainage system, which allows the air to escape and will not allow it to re-enter
- Clamping of the outlet may predispose to tension pneumothorax
- In air leaks, moderate suction should be done
- Always keep the bag below the level of the patient.

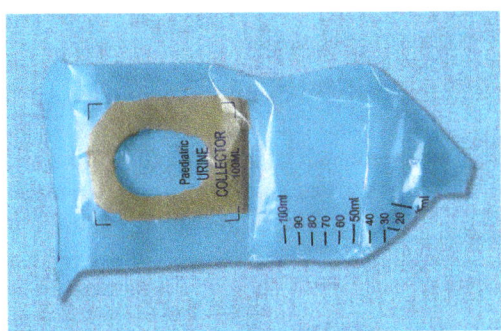

**Fig. 2.27:** Infant urine collection bag.

## Urinary Bag
- Sterile, disposable collecting bags
- Used to collect urine from urinary catheters
- Contains antireflux flap system, which will prevent back flow of urine
- Should be made of transparent material so that the quantity and quality of the urine can be observed
- The bag should be printed with calibrations to measure the volume of urine that gets collected
- When the bags gets filled the urine should not leak.

### Types
- Urinary bag without outlet
- Infant urinary bag 100 mL capacity (Fig. 2.27).

### Indications
- Retention of urine
- Urinary incontinence.

### Complications
Urinary tract infections.

### Precautions
The drainage bag should be changed at least once in a month.

# QUESTIONS

**Q1. What are the indications for change of urinary bag early?**
- Bad
- Odor

- ❑ Clouding
- ❑ Discoloration of bag

**Q2. How will you clean the urinary bag?**
- ❑ One part of bleach and 10 parts of water. This bleach solution should be poured into the urinary bag and agitated for 30 seconds. The fluid should be drained out.
- ❑ One part of vinegar can be added to three parts of tap water.

## INFUSION SETS

### Infusion Set/Transfusion Set

*Parts of Infusion Set*
- ❖ Drip chamber
- ❖ Fluid filter
- ❖ Air inlet
- ❖ Soft tube
- ❖ Terminal connector
- ❖ Luer lock or luer slip

### Intravenous Fluid Infusion Set (Fig. 2.28)
- ❖ Made of polyethylene
- ❖ Sterilized by using gamma rays
- ❖ Disposable after single use.

There are of two types:
1. Macrodrip set
   - ❖ These are the common sets
   - ❖ 15 drops per minute will provide 1 mL
   - ❖ *Use*: To infuse large volume of fluid.
2. Microdrip set
   - ❖ 60 microdrops = 1 mL
   - ❖ 60 drops per minute will provide 1 mL
   - ❖ *Use*: To infuse small volume of fluid.

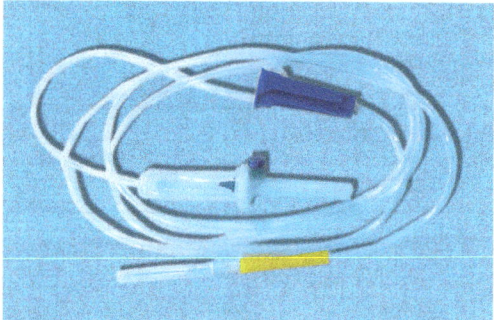

**Fig. 2.28:** Intravenous fluid infusion set.

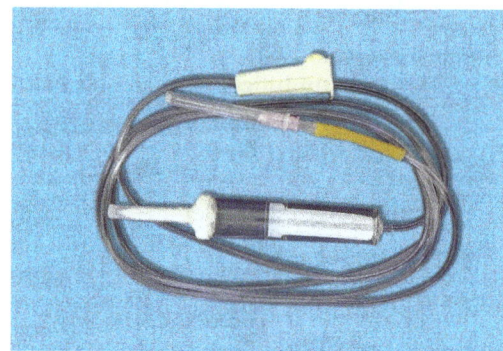

**Fig. 2.29:** Blood transfusion set.

### Blood Transfusion Set (Fig. 2.29)

Blood transfusion set will have additional strainer to strain clots or coagulated blood products.
- ❖ 15 drops per minute will provide 1 mL
- ❖ *Uses*: Transfusion of blood or blood products and to infuse blood and blood products.

## QUESTIONS

**Q1. What are the uses of infusion sets?**
- ❑ For intravenous fluid administration
- ❑ For blood and blood products transfusion
- ❑ For administration of drugs like antimetabolites
- ❑ Parenteral nutrition
- ❑ Infusion of parenteral fluids
- ❑ Administration of some medications, which require slow rate of infusion.

**Q2. How to calculate the amount of fluid to be given?**
- ❑ Each 1 mL contains 15 macrodrops
- ❑ Each 1 mL contains 60 microdrops
- ❑ Suppose you have to give 100 mL in 1 hour
- ❑ *No. of Macrodrops*:
  - ➤ 100 × 15 in 60 minutes
  - ➤ That is 1,500/60 = 25 drops per minute
- ❑ *No. of Microdrops*:
  - ➤ 100 × 60 in 60 minutes
  - ➤ That is 6,000/60 = 100 drops per minute.

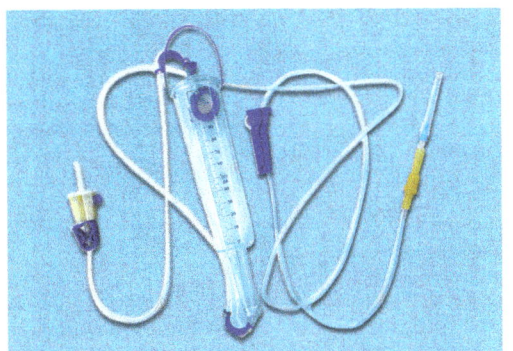

Fig. 2.30: Measured volume infusion sets.

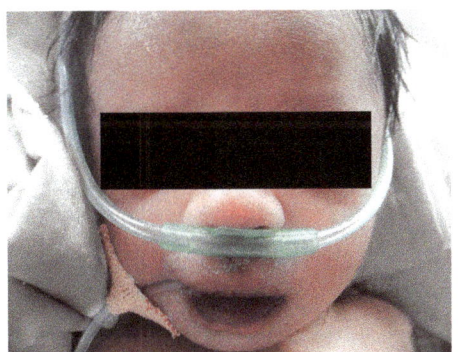

Fig. 2.31: Nasal cannula.

In other words, the amount of intravenous fluid in mL to be given in 1 hour will be equal to number of microdrops. Dividing the number of microdrops per minute by 4 will be equal to the number of macrodrops per minute.

## Measured Volume Infusion Sets (Fig. 2.30)
- Made of polyethylene
- Graduated with marking up to 110–150 mL
- Sterilized by using gamma rays.

### Uses
Used to infuse smaller measured volume of fluid in a given time.

### Advantages
- Accurate flow rate
- Automatic shut off valve will prevent air embolism
- Bulb self-sealing for extra medication
- C-clamp or roller type facilitates easy control and adjustment of flow rates
- Disposable after single use
- Efficient
- Flow rate will be uniform
- Fluid administration: Precise
- Use of measured volume infusion sets will prevent overhydration.

## OXYGEN DELIVERY SYSTEMS
Oxygen should be supplied through the mask. Oxygen delivery systems are as follows:
- Nasal cannula
- Nasal catheter
- Oxygen hood
- Oxygen tent
- Oxygen mask.

Oxygen administration may lead to retrolental fibroplasia and bronchopulmonary dysplasia. Oxygen should not be given more than needed.

## Nasal Cannula (Fig. 2.31)
Nasal cannula is a tube with one end split into two prongs which can be placed in the nostrils. This is used to deliver a mixture of air and supplemental oxygen or increased airflow. Nasal cannula can produce 24% to 40% oxygen, 1-6 liter per minute of $O_2$.

### Advantages
- Easy to use
- Cost is low
- Disposable
- The functions of the upper respiratory tract like humidification, warmth, and physical defense mechanisms will be maintained normally.
- Required oxygen will be 1 L/min.

### Disadvantages
- Dislodged easily
- Effectiveness low in mouth breathers of blocked nose
- Concentration of oxygen delivered will be 30–35%.

## Nasal Oxygen Catheter
It is a catheter used to deliver supplemental oxygen into the nose of a patient with hypoxia.

This is 40 cm long. The sizes are 8 Fr, 10 Fr, 12 Fr, 14 Fr, 16 Fr, 18 Fr.

### How will you Calculate the Length of the Tube to be Inserted?

The distance can be calculated by measuring the distance between the nose to the nasion. Required oxygen flow 1 L/min.

### Advantages

Patients on these catheter can eat, drink or talk while using the catheter Decreases the risk of rebreathing carbon dioxide.

### Disadvantages

- The functions of the upper respiratory tract like humidification, warmth, and physical defense mechanisms will be partially cutoff.
- The chance of blockage is high.
- Concentration of oxygen delivered will be 35–40%. Nasal passage will become dry.

## Nasopharyngeal Oxygen Catheter

It is a catheter used to deliver supplemental oxygen into the nasopharynx to a patient with hypoxia. The length of the tube inserted should be equal to the distance measured between the ala nasi and the tragus.

### Advantages

- This will be more comfortable for the child.
- This can be used even when the child is on the mother's lap.

### Disadvantages

- Nasal block
- Intolerance
- The physical defense provided by the upper respiratory tract will be absent.
- The chance of blockage by pharyngeal secretions is high.
- Concentration of oxygen delivered will be 45–60%.

## Oxygen Hood (Fig. 2.32)

- This is a transparent plastic shell cover used to cover whole of the face.

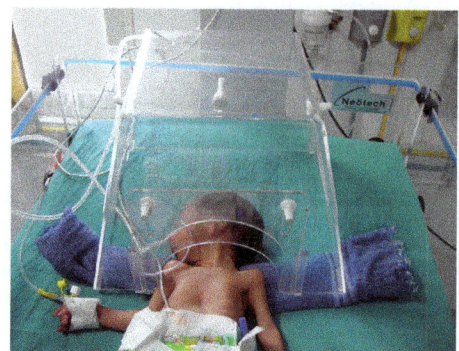

**Fig. 2.32:** Oxygen hood-side view.

- Do not cover the space between the hood and the neck as carbon dioxide is removed through this space. Also, this will allow the child to breath some room air.
- The side doors should be closed.
- The neck opening should be adjusted by sliding down the door.
- The oxygen level should be adjusted to maintain oxygen saturation in between 90% and 93%.

### Advantages

- It is comfortable for the baby
- Avoids direct flow of cold oxygen
- Chest and abdomen can be assessed
- Though high concentration of oxygen of 5 L/min is required, the amount of oxygen concentration delivered to the baby will be only 30%.

### Disadvantages

- cannot be used in the baby resting on the mother's lap.
- Continuous use will result in accumulation of carbon dioxide inside the hood.
- Sweating of the baby.

### Precautions

The system should be checked every hourly for proper functioning.

## Oxygen Tent

It is a tent-like enclosure made of transparent bendable plastic material in which the air supply can be enriched with oxygen. The tent can be placed over the head and shoulders or over the entire body.

## Advantages

- Access to patient is easy—the patient can be seen and monitored
- Broken nose patients can use this Comfortable
- $CO_2$ can be washed out quickly
- Drinking is easy
- Eating is easy
- Facial burns patients can use this
- Good control
- Higher level of oxygen can be provided
- Humidification is easy
- Inexpensive.

## Disadvantages

- Accidental fire can occur
- Bedsores can occur
- Blurring of the view due to mist formation inside the tent
- Concentration of oxygen is lost when the tent is opened
- Duration for cleaning is more
- Drying of mucosa can occur
- Epistaxis can occur
- Feeding is difficult
- Feeling of isolation by the patient
- Gas flow obstruction if tent compresses the face
- High volumes of oxygen is required
- High levels of oxygen cannot be achieved
- Hot as temperature control is not possible.

## Oxygen Mask (Fig. 2.33)

Oronasal mask will cover the nose and mouth whereas the full face mask will cover the entire face. Exhalation ports are present at the sides through which the $CO_2$ is exhaled. Oxygen masks can provide moderate oxygen of about 40% to 60% oxygen, 6-10 litres per minute of $O_2$.

- Transparent silicone masks
- Ensure tight air seal around the nose and mouth
- While delivering air or oxygen.

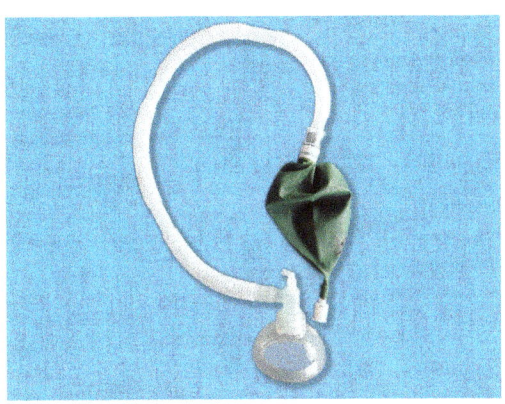

**Fig. 2.33:** Oxygen mask.

## Precautions

Grip should be soft to avoid more pressure.

## Advantages

- Visual inspection of breathing can be done.
- As the masks are disposable there is no need for sterilization
- Face can be visualized for assessing the patient
- Patient can see others during treatment and is useful in patients with claustrophobia who are afraid of lose space.

## Disadvantages

- Claustrophobia feeling
- Dryness of nose
- Expired air will mix with inspired air as there is no one way valve
- Facial skin irritation
- Gas flow is interrupted can result in Suffocation
- Humidity is lacking
- Interfere with eating and talking.

## Non-rebreather Mask (Fig. 2.34)

This is used to assist in delivery of oxygen to the patient.

Non-rebreather mask (NRB) allows delivery of high concentrations of oxygen—Oxygen range: Non-rebrether mask will provide 90-100% of oxygen at an oxygen flow rate of 12-15 liters per minute of oxygen.

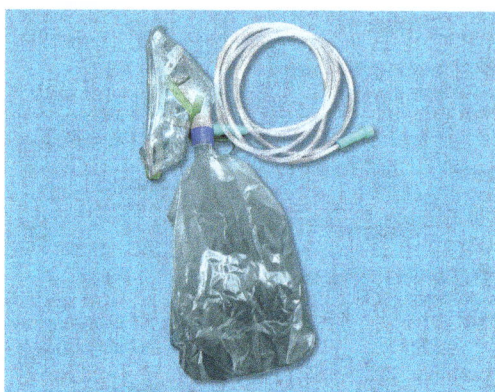

**Fig. 2.34:** Non-rebreathing mask with oxygen reservoir.

**Types:** There are two types:
1. With valve
2. Without valve.

**Parts:**
- Oxygen reservoir
- Exhalation port
- High flow will increase the oxygen levels
- Oxygen source.

**Uses:** This can be used in condition requiring high concentration of oxygen, chronic airway obstruction, smoke inhalation, and carbon monoxide poisoning.

### Oxygen Reservoir Bag

The oxygen reservoir bag is made of soft and transparent plastic. This will store oxygen which will allow deep breathing without waste of oxygen.

*Advantages*
- Helps to provide more oxygen concentration to 100%
- Increases $FiO_2$
- Increases the efficiency and patient comfort.

## PEDIATRIC BREATHING CIRCUIT

These are the assembly of components which are used to connect the patient's airway to the anesthetic machine.

### Jackson Rees (JR) Circuit

- Allows gas to be delivered from the machines to the patient
- This connects the patient's airway to the machine providing artificial breathing atmosphere
- Flow inflating ventilation device.

*Parts*
- Adjustable popoff valve to prevent over pressure
- Adopters
- Breathing tube
- Corrugated tubes for connecting components
- $CO_2$ absorber
- Fresh gas entry port
- Filters
- Gas reservoir in the form of corrugated tube.

*Features of Ideal Circuit*
- Delivers oxygen in same concentration in the machine in the shortest time
- Effective elimination of $CO_2$
- Minimal dead space
- Minimal resistance.

*Fresh Gas Flow Required*
- Spontaneous
- Two to three times minute volume with a minimum of 3 L/min
- Controlled flow.

*Advantages*
- Permits easy fixation to the face
- Direct access for tracheal toilet and suction easy
- Nonirritating to the mucous membrane
- Can be used for several days
- Low resistance to breathing
- Minimal dead space
- Provides continuous positive pressure airway and 100% oxygen
- Decreases work of breathing
- Opens alveoli/airways that is collapsed during expiration

- Continuous positive airway pressure (CPAP) will reduce the preload and afterload on the heart, and work of breathing
- Improves oxygenation.

### Disadvantages
- The volume of the reservoir should be approximately equal to the tidal volume
- If it is small, ambient air may be entrained
- If it is too large, rebreathing can occur
- High gas flow required to prevent rebreathing. Fresh gas flow (FGF) of about two to three times of patient's minute volume is needed.

### Indications
- Impending respiratory failure
- Chronic obstruction of airways with respiratory failure
- Continuing airway obstruction.

## QUESTIONS

**Q1. What is JR circuit?**
Jackson Rees circuit.

**Q2. What is the use of corrugated tube?**
This will help in transfer of heat.

## NEWBORN RESUSCITATION

### DeLee Oral Mucus Trap (Fig. 2.35)

A DeLee trap is preferred for suction, which should be applied by the operator's mouth. Wall suction in delivery rooms is traumatic to neonates because it is far too forceful. If wall suction is used, it must be modulated by a regulator to a level not greater than 120 mm Hg.

### Transparent 20 cc Mucus Trap

These are sterile, disposable trap used for deeper suctioning of mucus from the mouth, airway and stomach.

## QUESTIONS

**Q1. What are the types of oral mucus trap?**
Two types are available:
1. DeLee type of mucus trap: Two types:
   i. Disposable
   ii. Autoclavable (can be reused)
2. Bulb sucker.

**Q2. What is the use of oral mucus trap?**
To clear the mouth and nose from secretions.

**Q3. Which type of oral mucus trap is preferred for suction in newborn?**
DeLee mucous trap is preferred for suction in newborn.
*DeLee trap:* A DeLee trap is preferred for suction, which should be applied by the operator's mouth.

**Q4. Which part should be sucked first?**
Suction of the nose will reflexly initiate respiration causing secretions/fluid in mouth to get aspirated. Hence, mouth should be sucked first.

**Q5. Suction should be done in which position of the baby?**
Suction can be done in the following two positions:
1. *Supine position*: Suction should be short and intermittent. Suction should not be deep and continuous touching posterior pharyngeal wall, as in that case reflex bradycardia or apnea can occur.
2. *Head-turned to one side position*: Now the secretions gravitate at the cheek from where it is sucked out.

**Q6. What should be the suction pressure for clearing oral secretions?**

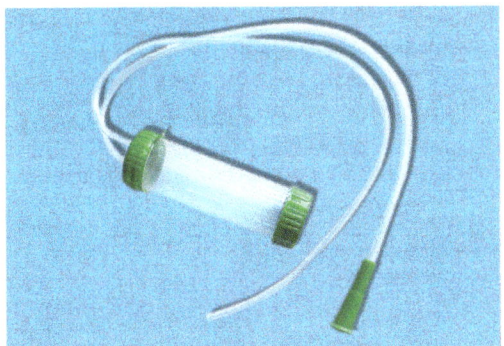

**Fig. 2.35:** DeeLee oral mucus trap.

A negative pressure of around 100 mm Hg should be applied.

**Q7. Can the commonly available wall sucker machine be used for suction in newborn?**
Wall suction in delivery rooms is traumatic to neonates because it is far too forceful. If wall suction is used, it must be modulated by a regulator to a level not greater than 120 mm Hg. The commonly used sucker machines work at much higher negative pressure (around 200 mm Hg), which can cause injury to tender mucous membrane of mouth or throat of the newborn baby. So it should not be used; however if available, slow sucker machine working at around 100 mm Hg can be used for neonates.

**Q8. At what time of resuscitation mucus trap is used?**
Mucus trap is used at the initial steps of resuscitation. The tube with hole should be inserted into the mouth of the baby and the tube with mouth piece should be inserted into the resuscitator's mouth.

## Face Masks (Fig. 2.36)

Masks of appropriate size should be used so that it covers the mouth and nose, but do not cover the eyes or overlap the chin. Round mask will effectively seal the face of a small infant whereas anatomically shaped masks will be fitting better in large term infant's face

A good mask should have a low dead space of about less than 5 mL. The rim should be cushioned so that it will facilitate a tight seal without exerting excessive pressure on the face.

The resuscitation masks will have a rim that is cushioned or noncushioned. The cushioned mask will be advantageous as the rim confirms more easily to the shape of the newborn's face and forming a seal. Also the risk for injury to eyes is low. Less pressure is needed to form a seal.

## QUESTIONS

**Q1. What are the different shapes in which the face masks are available?**
- Round shaped
- Anatomically shaped which fit the contours of the face. The most pointed part will fit over the nose.

**Q2. What are the different sizes in which the face masks are available?**
Face masks are available in:
- Large 5 inches (12.7 cm)
- Medium 4.5 inches (11.4 cm)
- Small 4 inches (10.2 cm).

**Q3. What is an ideal face mask?**
The rim of the face mask should cover the tip of the chin, mouth, and the nose, but not the eyes.

**Q4. What are the disadvantages of too large or too small masks?**
- Too large masks will cause eye injury and will not result in a good seal.
- Too small masks will occlude the nose and will not cover the mouth and nose.

**Q5. What are the types of mask?**
- *Shape*: Circular or anatomical
- Cushioned or noncushioned
- Cushion at the rim of the mask can be made of foam, rubber or inflated rim
- Circular air cushioned mask is commonly used.

**Q6. What should be an appropriate sized mask?**
An appropriate sized mask should be such that it will cover mouth, nose, and tip of chin, but not the eyes.

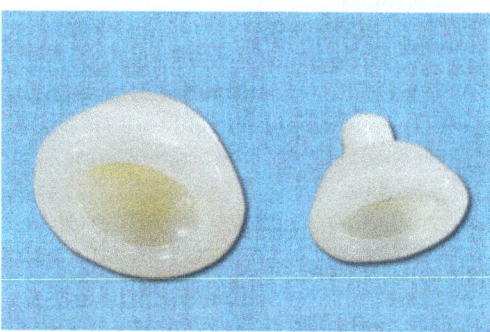

**Fig. 2.36:** Face mask.

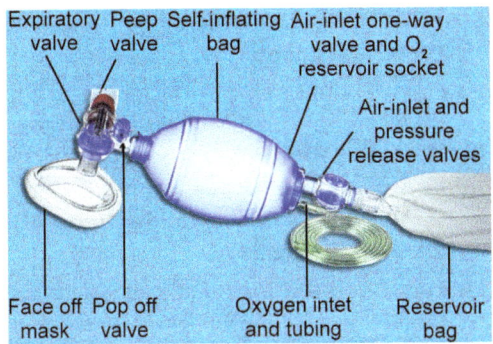

Fig. 2.37: Artificial manual breathing unit bag.

Q7. What are the advantages of cushioned mask?
- ❑ The rim confirms easily to the shape of the face
- ❑ Less pressure to the face
- ❑ Less chance of damage to the eyes.

## Artificial Manual Breathing Unit Bag (Fig. 2.37)

Handheld device compressible, self-inflating, and nonrebreathing silicone bag to provide positive pressure ventilation to patients breathing inadequately or not breathing. Artificial manual breathing unit (AMBU) bag will provide 6–7 mL/Kg/breath.

## Types
- ❖ Self-inflating bags
- ❖ Flow-inflating bags (anesthetic bags) will fill only when the oxygen flows in from the compressed source.

## Parts
- ❖ Compressible inflating bags with capacity of 200–750 mL (self-inflating/flow inflating)
- ❖ Air inlet
- ❖ Oxygen connector
- ❖ Patient outlet through which gas exits from the AMBU bag to the baby. The face mask or the endotracheal tube will be attached here.
- ❖ Fish mouth valve/inspiratory valve
- ❖ Popoff valve or pressure release valve will prevent overinflation and pneumothorax by releasing air if pressure exceeds 40 cm $H_2O$.

- ❖ Expiratory valve
- ❖ Non-rebreathing patient valve
- ❖ Oxygen reservoir
- ❖ Oxygen reservoir bag
- ❖ Face mask.

## Bag Resuscitator

This bag is attached to the inserted endotracheal tube. It receives 100% oxygen from a wall source or from a tank. Infant masks are usually supplied with this apparatus, but are of no value in resuscitation of severely depressed infants.

## Sizes
- ❖ *Bag*: Capacity of the resuscitation bags:
  - Adult: 1,600 mL
  - Infant and child: 500 mL
  - Neonate: 250 mL
- ❖ *Mask*:
  - Adult: Size 4
  - Child: Size 2
  - Infant: Size 1
- ❖ *Oxygen concentration*:
  - Room air without oxygen source: 21%
  - Oxygen source with 5–10 L: 40–60%
  - Oxygen reservoir with 15 L: 100%

## Uses
- ❖ Resuscitation of newborn when heart rate is less than 100/min
- ❖ Apnea
- ❖ Respiratory support in respiratory depression or arrest
- ❖ Ventilation of anesthetized patient.

## Method
- ❖ One hand is used to position the head and maintain the patency and the face seal
- ❖ The other hand is used to ventilate the child
- ❖ Sniffing position should be maintained if cervical spine is normal. The thumb and the index finger should be used to maintain the face seal. Ring and little finger should be placed under the angle of mandible. The middle finger should be placed under the mandibular symphysis.

## Contraindications

- Meconium aspiration syndrome in nonvigorous baby
- Diaphragmatic hernia and eventration of diaphragm as the air entering the gastrointestinal tract will cause distension of gastric and intestines in the chest causing further respiratory capacity
- Paralysis
- Complete airway obstruction.

**What are the contraindications of bag and mask ventilation?**

The contraindications to bag and mask ventilation are:

- Diaphragmatic hernia (air may enter the stomach and dilate it. As the stomach may be lying in the thorax, its dilatation will lead to further compromise the lung volume).
- Meconium aspiration syndrome with nonvigorous baby. When there is presence of meconium stained liquor and the baby is not vigorous at birth the meconium present in the oropharynx will be pushed into the trachea and lead to obstruction. After endotracheal suction, one may give bag and tube ventilation.

## Complications

- Aspiration
- Barotrauma
- Collapsed lung due to pneumothorax
- Embolism: Air embolism
- Failed resuscitation
- Gastric insufflation/rupture
- Hypoventilation
- Injury to lung by gastric acid aspiration
- Volutrauma due to overstretching, pneumothorax, and adult respiratory distress syndrome
- Mendelson's syndrome.

## QUESTIONS

**Q1. What is sniffing position?**
It is about 35° of neck flexion and 15° of head extension.

**Q2. What is the advantage of sniffing position?**
Sniffing position will prevent falling of tongue and obstructing the airway.

**Q3. What is AMBU?**
- Ambulatory manual breathing unit
- Artificial manual breathing unit
- Air mask bag unit.

**Q4. What are the types of resuscitation bags?**
There are two types of resuscitation bags available; self-inflating bags and flow-inflating bags. Self-inflating type is most commonly used for resuscitation of newborn at birth. In flow-inflating type (anesthetic bag), the bag will get filled with flow of oxygen under pressure from some compressed source. Flow-inflating bags or anesthetic bags fill only when oxygen from a compressed source flows into it. Self-inflating bags fill spontaneously after it is squeezed.

**Q5. What are the differences between self-inflating bags and flow-inflating bags?**
*Self-inflating bags*
- These bags fill spontaneously and pull air or oxygen into the bag and will remain inflated at all times.
- Pressure release valve should release at approximately 30–35 cm $H_2O$ pressure. If necessary, the bag should supply high pressure for good chest expansion. Without a compressed gas source positive pressure ventilation can be delivered. This requires an oxygen reservoir to deliver 100% oxygen.
- More training is used to use this flow inflating bag.

*Flow-inflating bags*
These bags inflate only when compressed gas is flowing into it. The use requires flow of gas into the bags inlet, adjustment of flow of gas out through the flow control valve to control and regulate pressure inflation, and creation of tight seal between the mask and face.

## Instruments and Procedures

Differences between self-inflating bags and flow-inflating bags.

| Features | Self-inflating bags | Flow-inflating bags |
|---|---|---|
| Refilling | Refills independently of gas flow because of the recoil of the bag | Refilled only by compressed gas flowing into it |
| Control valves | Pressure-release valves | Flow controlled valve |
| | Pressure-release valves will prevent delivering very high pressure | Capable of delivering very high pressure so manometer should be used to monitor the peak and end expiratory pressures |
| Peak inspiratory pressures | Peak inspiratory pressures are limited by pressure-release valves. | Can provide greater range of peak inspiratory pressures |
| Control of oxygen concentration | Flow of oxygen is unreliable | More reliable control of oxygen concentration |
| Oxygen supply | High oxygen concentrations (90–100%) requires attached oxygen reservoir | High oxygen may be delivered passively |
| Personal | Less training needed | More training needed |
| Advantages | Do not need a gas source<br>Easy to use<br>Safety pop-off valve is present | Deliver 100% oxygen at all times<br>Can deliver continuous positive airway pressure (CPAP) or positive end-expiratory pressure (PEEP) |
| Disadvantages | Will inflate even without adequate seal<br>Requires oxygen reservoir to deliver 100% oxygen | Requires a gas source and tight seal to get inflated<br>Safety pop-off valve is not present<br>More skill required |

**Q6. What are the sizes of resuscitation bag?**
Newborn, pediatric, and adult sizes are available.

**Q7. What is the type of resuscitation bag used for newborn resuscitation?**
The self-inflating resuscitation bag used for newborn resuscitation.

**Q8. What is the capacity of the resuscitation bags for children?**
200–750 mL.

**Q9. What is the capacity of the neonatal resuscitation bags?**
200–300 mL.

**Q10. What is the capacity of the resuscitation bags for children?**
Volume of bag: 750 mL.

**Q11. What should be the maximum volume of neonatal resuscitation bags?**
Volume: 500–750 mL. The bags should not have volume more than 750 mL. The bag should supply a volume of 5–8 mL/kg required by newborns.

**Q12. What is the volume of air required for neonatal ventilation?**
Term infants need 5–8 mL/Kg) 15–25 mL.

**Q13. What are the parts of neonatal resuscitation bags?**
Parts of the neonatal resuscitation bags are:
- ❑ Self-inflating bag
- ❑ Pressure manometer
- ❑ Appropriate sized masks

1. Air inlet and attachment site for oxygen reservoir. As the bad re-expands air will be sucked through this one way valve.
2. Oxygen inlet
3. Patient out let
4. Valve assembly is positioned between the bag and the patient outlet. The valve opens when the bag is squeezed releasing the oxygen/air into the patient. The valve will close when the bag reinflates during the exhalation phase of the cycle. When the bag is compressed, the valve opens and lets air flow to the patient. When the patient exhales, this valve closes and prevents exhaled air entering the bag.
5. Oxygen reservoir

6. Pressure release pop-off valve—pop off valve for pressure release. The valve will open and release the air when the pressure exceeds 40 cm of $H_2O$. This valve will prevent over inflation by releasing the air when the pressure is above 30–40 cm of $H_2O$. This will prevent excessive pressure being build up in the bag and will prevent alveolar rupture by releasing excess pressure.

**Q14. What is the percentage of oxygen provided by self-inflating bag without oxygen reservoir?**
It will be 40% (room air provides 21% and oxygen reservoir provides 100% oxygen).

**Q15. What are the points to select an appropriate sized mask?**
The mask should cover the chin, mouth, and nose. It should not cover the eyes.

**Q16. Why the bag is called as self-inflating bag?**
Because if fills automatically after it is squeezed.

**Q17. What is the type material by which the bag is made of?**
- Silicone bag: Autoclavable, e.g. Laerdal type of bag
- Rubber bag: Not autoclavable, e.g. AMBU type.

**Q18. How many valves are there in the valve assembly of Laerdal type of bag?**
There are three valves in the valve assembly:
1. Inspiratory valve opens during inspiration or squeezing the bag. This is present in the upper part of the bag.
2. Expiratory valve allows the exhaled air to go out. This is present in the lower part of the bag.
3. Pressure release valve/pop-off valve/ this is a safety valve. The set pressure limit is written on the valve. It is usually 30–40 cm of water.

**Q19. What are the structures present on the inlet side?**
- A valve that only allows entry of air or oxygen into bag on release of the bag. This valve will close tightly when bag is squeezed.
- Two inlets; a big one and a small one. The bigger one is for entry of air. Oxygen inlet connected through tube to oxygen source and air inlet is for entry of air. Oxygen reservoir is attached to air inlet.

**Q20. What is baby outlet?**
This is the other end of the bag where mask is fitted. On squeezing the bag, air/air-oxygen mixture passes through this outlet and enters the baby's mouth and nose through the mask.

**Q21. What is oxygen reservoir?**
This is the device that can be attached to the air inlet. This reserves oxygen inside it and increases oxygen delivery to the baby to about 90–100%.

**Q22. What are the types of oxygen reservoir?**
There are two types of oxygen reservoir:
1. *Open-ended*: A corrugated white tube. Corrugation increases the capacity of the tube and creates columns of oxygen.
2. *Closed-ended*: It is actually a packet or bag with some valve arrangement which allows small quantity of air to enter into the bag, apart from oxygen through the air inlet.

**Q23. What will be the percentage of oxygen delivered at the baby end, if oxygen reservoir is used or not used?**
- No reservoir, oxygen inlet not attached to $O_2$ source more than room air $O_2$ % = 21%
- No reservoir, oxygen inlet attached to oxygen source with flow rate 5–6 times more than air-oxygen mixture at baby end with $O_2$ % = 40–60%
- Reservoir in use, oxygen inlet to $O_2$ source as above more than $O_2$ % at baby end = 90–100%.

## Q24. How will you choose the mask?
A mask that covers the mouth and nose and not the eyes should be used. Also the mask should not extend beyond the ramus of the mandible.

## Q25. What is the initial pressure to be given for the initiation of breathing?
The initial pressure required to dilate the airless lung will be more. 30–40 cm of $H_2O$ will be required for the first breath.

## Q26. What is the pressure to be given after the initiation of breathing?
The pressure required for further breaths will be about 15–20 cm of $H_2O$.

## Q27. What is the advantage of using oxygen reservoir?
- Without oxygen reservoir, 40% oxygen will be delivered.
- With oxygen reservoir, 50–100% oxygen will be delivered.

## Q28. How to check that the resuscitation bag is working?
First block the mask or baby outlet by sealing with the palm of the hand and then squeeze the bag. The sealing palm will feel pressure and the squeezing hand will feel resistance. The pop-off valve will open. This will indicate that the bag is functioning. If the results are negative, there is leak somewhere, especially check the junctions and look for any crack in the bag.

## Q29. What are the indications of bag and mask ventilation in neonatal resuscitation?
If after initial steps of resuscitation any of the following is present:
- Apnea or gasping condition of the baby
- Heart rate less than 100/min even if the baby is breathing
- Persistent central cyanosis in spite of free flow of 100% $O_2$.

## Q30. What is laryngeal mask airway ventilation? What are its indications and contraindications?
Mask that fit over the laryngeal inlet have been effective in ventilating full-term infants.

*Indications*:
- Ineffective bag and mask ventilation
- Failed endotracheal intubation.

*Contraindications*:
- Small preterm babies
- Meconium stained amniotic fluid.

## Q31. What are the prerequisites of bag and mask ventilation?
- Airway should be clear of secretions
- Baby's head should be properly positioned and neck should be slightly extended
- The position of the resuscitator (doctor/nurse) either the head end of the baby or on the left side of the baby. Mask should be tightly applied. The junction of the face (skin) and the mask is the common site of leakage and ineffective positive pressure generation. Again the nasolabial furrows are particularly vulnerable sites. The resuscitation bag should be pretested to see that it is functioning.

## Q32. How should you position the baby for bag and mask ventilation?
Place the baby with neck slightly extended. Mask should cover the nose and mouth, not the eyes. Hold the mask with the thumb and index finger. The third, fourth, and fifth fingers should rest along the jaw.

## Q33. What is the rate at which a newborn should be ventilated?
The rate at which the ventilation should be done is approximately 40–60/min.

The bag is abruptly squeezed and released at a rate approximating 40 times per minute.

*Pressure*: Initial inflation pressure and initial inspiratory time.

Peak inspiratory pressure depends on the condition of the lung. The pressure can be 20–40 cm of water in the babies with diseased lungs. 15-40 cm of $H_2O$ will be adequate to achieve lung inflation. If the inflation is not adequate, check for the patency of the airway, reapply the mask and ventilate with higher pressures. If the bag is grasped in the palm of the hand and squeezed with all five fingers, pressures in excess of 60-70 cm $H_2O$ are delivered, which may result in pneumothorax. By squeezing with the thumb, index, and middle fingers only, safer and usually effective pressures of 25-35 cm $H_2O$ are delivered. Sometimes higher pressures are required initially for adequate lung expansion, necessitating use of the entire hand for bag compression.

Long inflation time for initial inflation breath is required (about 2-3 seconds)

*Rate*: 40-60/min. The bag is abruptly squeezed and released at a rate approximating 40 times per minute.

Breathe----- two -----three ----- Breathe
Squeeze------Release-----------Squeeze

Peak inspiratory pressure depends on the condition of the lung. 15-40 cm of $H_2O$ will be adequate to achieve lung inflation. 30-40 cm of $H_2O$ will be required for the first breath. If the inflation is not adequate, check for the patency of the airway, reapply the mask, and ventilate with higher pressures.

**Q34. How will you assess the effectiveness of bag and mask ventilation?**

The effectiveness of bag and mask ventilation can be assessed by:
- Observe the chest wall movements
- Auscultate for the breath sounds
- Monitor the heart rate
- Observe the skin color
- Avoid underinflation or overinflation.

**Q35. What will you do if the air entry is inadequate or absent following bag and mask ventilation?**

If the air entry is inadequate or absent following bag and mask ventilation, check for the following:
- Verify if the mask is applied properly to the face
- Verify if the airway is blocked
- Position of the head—Extreme flexion or extension should be avoided
- Apply adequate pressure to the bag.

**Q36. What are the signs of improvement with bag and mask ventilation?**

Signs of improvement are:
- *Heart rate*: Increases to normal more than and equal to 100/min
- *Color*: Improves
- Spontaneous breathing.

**Q37. When to stop bag and mask ventilation?**

The bag and mask ventilation can be stopped if any of the following is observed:
- Heart rate ≥ 100/min
- Spontaneous breathing.

**Q38. What are the complications of bag and mask ventilation?**

The complications of bag and mask ventilation are:
- Trauma to the eyes and face
- Pulmonary air leak
- Intestinal distension (elevates the diaphragm, resulting in decreased lung volume). This can be avoided by inserting a nasogastric tube into the stomach after 2 minutes of intermittent positive pressure ventilation (IPPV).

**Q39. How much pressure should be applied for squeezing the bag?**
- Squeezing pressure should be such that there is effective rise and fall of the chest wall as if the baby is having normal and easy breath.
- Initial pressure required is little more to open up the fluid filled alveoli, initial pressure = 30-40 cm $H_2O$.

- Subsequent regular ventilatory pressure (maintenance) = 15–20 cm $H_2O$.
- With diseased lung the maintenance pressure = 20–30 cm $H_2O$.

**Q40. How often the bag should be squeezed?**
- *Rate of ventilation*: 40–60 breaths per minute
- *Following the rhythm*: Two and three squeeze (breath).

**Q41. What are the causes of ineffective ventilation by bag and mask and how to correct them?**
- Mask is not adequately sealed on the face
  - *Correction*: Reapply with adequate seal
- Airway is blocked
  - *Correction*:
    - Airway (Mouth and throat) should be cleared of secretion
    - Head should be properly positioned - neck slightly extended
    - Ventilation with the baby's mouth slightly open, if necessary using an oral airway
- The bag is leaking somewhere
  - *Correction*: To check functioning of the bag, use the palm and correct the leakage
- Inadequate squeezing pressure
  - *Correction*: Adequate pressure so that effective rise and fall of chest wall can occur.

**Q42. What are the dangers of chest compression?**
- If pressed excessively over ribs: Fracture of ribs more than injury to the lung.
- If pressed excessively over xiphoid process = injury to the liver.

**Q43. How will you sterilize the parts of AMBU bag?**
The plastic valves should be sterilized using chemicals and the other parts should be sterilized using soap and water.

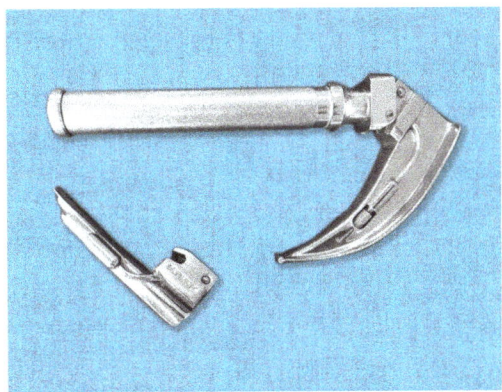

**Fig. 2.38:** Laryngoscope with straight and curved needles blades.

## Laryngoscope with Detachable Blades (Fig. 2.38)

Laryngoscope (pencil handle with attached Miller size 0 premature or size 1 infant blade). The adequacy of the light source must be ascertained during periodic routine checks of all equipment when not in use.

### Parts
- Handle with container for battery
  *Blade*: Straight or curved
  - Straight blade is used to depress the tongue, preferred in infants
  - Curved blade is used to push the epiglottis to one side preferred in children older than 8 years.

### Size of Laryngoscope
The number increases with the increase in size
- 0 for preterm
- 1 for term
- 2 for 2–10 years
- 3 for more than 10 years
- 4 for adults.

### Uses of Laryngoscope
- Bronchoscope insertion
- Cord palsy
- Direct laryngoscopy
- Esophagoscope insertion
- To visualize the epiglottis

- Endotracheal tube insertion
- Foreign body.

## Complications
- Oral trauma
- Aspiration of tooth
- Dislocation of tooth

## Sterilization of Laryngoscope
Blade wash under running water with detergent and then can be autoclaved/boiled/chemically sterilized with alcohol, gluteraldehyde/gas sterilized.

# QUESTIONS

**Q1. What are the types of laryngoscope blades?**
Laryngoscope blade can be straight or curved. Straight blades are used in infants less than 1 year old when the distance between the mouth to epiglottis is less. Curved blades can be used for children more than one year of age when the distance between the mouth to epiglottis is more.

**Q2. What are the sizes of laryngoscope blades?**
- *Size 0*: For preterm neonates
- *Size 1*: For term neonates.

The size of the laryngeal blades used are:

| Weight | Laryngeal blade |
| --- | --- |
| 1 kg | 0 |
| 2 kg | 0 |
| 3 kg | 0–1 |
| 4 kg | 1 |

| Blade size | Gestational age |
| --- | --- |
| No. 1 | Term |
| No. 0 | Preterm |
| No. 00 | Extremely preterm |

**Q3. How will you assess the length of the blade to be used?**
The length of blade to be used can be assessed by measuring the length from the angle of the mouth to the ear lobe.

**Q4. What are the differences between the straight and curved laryngoscope blades?**

| The epiglottis can be lifted up | Blade can be advanced up to vallecula. Now if the scope is lifted up the epiglottis with the cords will drop down and can be visualized |
| --- | --- |

**Q5. When do you use it?**
During direct vision endotracheal (ET) intubation.

**Q6. What are the indications of ET intubation?**
- Meconium stained liquor and the baby is not vigorous at birth
- When IPPV by bag and mask is ineffective
- When IPPV by bag and mask requirement is prolonged for more than few minutes
- IPPV in premature baby should better be by ET intubation
- When IPPV with chest compression: ET tube and bag ventilation has more efficacy than bag and mask ventilation baby with diaphragmatic hernia.

**Q7. How will you confirm the position of the tube ?**
The position of the tube can be confirmed by one of the following ways:
- Confirm the tube position by auscultation. The breath sounds should be heard equally on both sides of the chest. If the sounds are heard only on one side, there is a possibility of the tube entering one of the bronchi. The tube should be withdrawn a little so that the tube reaches the bronchi before bifurcation.

If the endotracheal tube has been inserted too deeply, it will pass directly into the right main stem bronchus. Delivery of oxygen is therefore confined to the right lung, and insufflations cause expansion in the right chest, with little or no visible excursion on the left. Breath sounds are absent on the left whereas on the right they are loud and clear. This discrepancy can be determined more accurately by an assistant who listens with a stethoscope. The tube should be withdrawn a little so that the tube reaches the bronchi before bifurcation.

Breath sounds are absent on the left whereas on the right they are loud and clear. This being the case, the endotracheal tube should be withdrawn slightly until breath sounds are equal on each side of the chest. Take an X-ray chest to confirm good ventilation and expansion of the lung. Shorten the endotracheal tube by 4 cm beyond the lips.
- ❑ Symmetrical chest wall motion
- ❑ Absence of fog in the tube or on a mirror placed at the outlet of the tube
- ❑ Absence of sounds over the stomach or absence of gastric dilatation
- ❑ Exhaled $CO_2$ detection will be helpful in confirming the tracheal position of the endotracheal tube. This will be helpful when the clinical assessment is equivocal. However, inadequate pulmonary expansion, decreased pulmonary blood flow, and small tidal volumes will influence the interpretation of the exhaled $CO_2$ concentration.

Also improvement in color, heart rate, and activity of the baby will be an indirect evidence for the correct position of the tube.

## Uses
- ❖ Helps easy endotracheal insertion
- ❖ To assist and removal of endotracheal tube during difficult situations

## Disadvantage
Trauma to the airway.

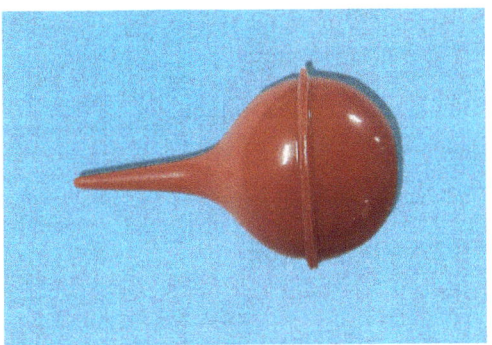

**Fig. 2.39:** Bulb Sucker.

## Bulb Sucker (Fig. 2.39)
Bulb sucker with long tapered tip will increase the suction power.

## Uses
- ❖ During resuscitation of newborn
- ❖ Aspiration
- ❖ Irrigation.

## Advantages
- ❖ Hand operated
- ❖ Cost-effective
- ❖ No electricity is needed
- ❖ Reuseable.

## Disadvantage
Sterilization is difficult.

## Precautions
First aspirate the mouth before nose. This is because if the nose is aspirated first the child will take a gasp thereby aspiration of contents in the mouth.

## Umbilical Cord Clamp (Fig. 2.40)
- ❖ It is used to clamp the umbilical cord to stop the blood flow through the cord.
- ❖ It consists of interlocking teeth which will fit together and will not reopen.
- ❖ Cord should be clamped immediately after birth or within few minutes after birth.

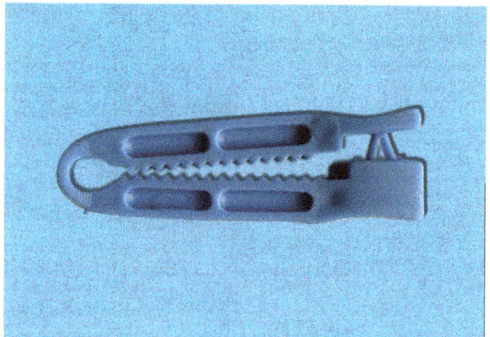

**Fig. 2.40:** Umbilical cord clamp.

## QUESTIONS

**Q1. What is the length of the umbilical cord in a normal newborn?**
50 cm.

**Q2. What is the length of the umbilical cord left before clamping?**
The length of the stump should be about 4–5 cm.

**Q3. Why the cord should be cut leaving about 4 cm only?**
The criteria is that the cut end of the umbilical cord should not touch the genitalia. The cord will falls by 7–10 days of life. The baby will void urine from second day of life. Hence, if the cord is long, it will contaminated by the urine.

The cord should not be cut too close to the abdomen as it may injure the intestinal contents protruding through the umbilicus or through umbilical hernia.

However, in the following conditions, the umbilical cord should be clamped leaving more length:
❑ Babies needing umbilical cord catheterization
❑ Babies needing intervention through umbilical cord
❑ Babies with jaundice at birth
❑ Babies not cried immediately after birth.

**Q4. What are the conditions in which more length is left before clamping the cord?**
❑ Birth asphyxia
❑ Rh incompatibility
❑ Any intervention of umbilical cord catheterization required.

**Q5. What is early cord clamping of the cord?**
Clamping of the cord within first 1 minute after birth.

**Q6. What is delayed cord clamping?**
The cord is clamped 25 seconds to 5 minutes after the delivery of the child. Clamping after 2 minutes is delayed cord clamping. About 80–100 mL of blood will get transferred from the mother to the baby in the first 3 minutes. 90% of this transfer will occur immediately within first few breaths.

**Q7. What are the advantages of delayed cord clamping?**
❑ This will increase the hemoglobin levels and iron levels in the newborn babies
❑ There will be decreased incidence of necrotizing enterocolitis (NEC)
❑ Decreased incidence of intraventricular hemorrhage
❑ Transfer of immunoglobin will decrease infections
❑ Transfer of more stem cells which will help in tissue and organ repair.

**Q8. What is the disadvantage of delayed cord clamping?**
There is increased incidence of jaundice which may require phototherapy, polycythemia may occur.

## ASTHMA DEVICES

### Inhalers (Fig. 2.41)

Depending upon the construction, cloud generation, and techniques of inhalation, there are different types of inhalers. Inhaler devices depend upon the following:
❖ Construction
❖ Aerosol cloud generation

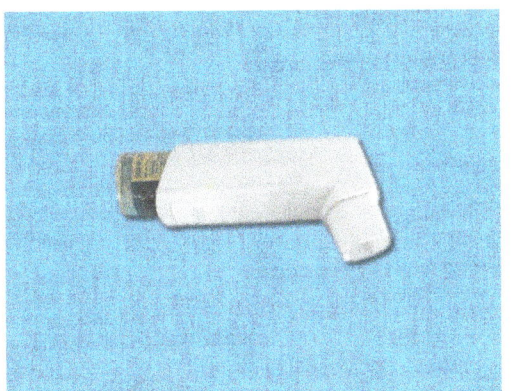

**Fig. 2.41:** Inhaler.

- Inhalation techniques
- Ease of use.

## Types
- Manually actuated pressurized metered dose inhalers (MDI)
- Breath actuated pressurized metered dose inhalers (pMDI)
- Dry powder inhalers (DPI)
- Mist inhalers
- Rotahalers
- Nebulizers.

## Advantages
- Higher local concentration of drug
- Faster action
- Minimal side effects.

## Drugs used in Inhalers
- Inhalable steroids
- Beta 2 agonists.

## Problems Associated with Inhalers
- Device dependent problems:
    - Larger particles more than 10 μm will get deposited in the mouth and throat.
    - Particles 0.5–10 μm will get deposited in the lungs
    - Smaller particles will get deposited in the lungs. However, if the particles are very small less than 0.5 μm they will get exhaled.
- Device independent problems
    - Lack of exhalation before inhalation
    - Inadequate inspiratory flow
    - Inhalation through nose.

| Age/conditions | Recommended devices |
|---|---|
| Young children | Metered dose inhaler (MDI) + LV spacer |
| >7 years | Dry powder inhaler (DPI)/Rotahaler |
| Adults | MDI |
| Patients without coordination | DPI/Rotahaler |
| Elderly | MDI + SV spacer |
| Emergency | Nebulizer |

## Rotahaler
It is a device used to deliver dry, fine medications from Rotacap capsules. Rotacaps are capsules that contain medications in very fine, dry powder forms.

## Parts of Rotahaler
- Mouth piece
- Rota chamber
- Barrel
- Grid
- Hole for inserting Rotacaps (capsule inlet)
- Air inlet.

## Method
Insert-twist-inhale

Insert the transparent end first and rotate the base of the Rotahaler so that the capsule gets separated in to two halves. Breathe out completely and place the mouth in the mouth piece and breathe slowly.

## Procedure
Insert the capsule and rotate the base of the Rotahaler. Powdered aerosols are generated once the patient inhales. Breathe in deeply and hold the breath for 10 seconds.

## Indications
Long-term use of bronchodilators in conditions like chronic asthma and chronic obstructive pulmonary disease (COPD).

### Advantages

- The medications are delivered into the lungs very effectively.
- Coordination of actuation and inspiration needed in MDIs are not required.
- It is used easily by children and elders
- Multiple inhalations can be taken
- Acceptable
- Economical.

### Precautions

- As the powder in the Rotacaps are not for oral use, they should not be swallowed.
- Cleaning using warm water.
- Store at 25°C and use for about 12 months after which it is better to use a new one.

## Metered Dose Inhaler

- It is the commonest form of device used for aerosol therapy.
- It is a pressurized inhaler in which the medications are given in the form of suspension or solution.
- Particle size less than 5 microns.

### Parts

- Canister
- Actuator nozzle
- Metering valve
- Propellant with drug suspension
- Mouth piece.

Metered dose inhaler contains drug in crystallized form or solution form with propellant and surfactant. All MDI use hydrofluoroalkane (HFA) as propellant. On actuation of MDI the aerosol is delivered at high velocity, which results in inhalation of medicine difficult. It can be overcome by using spacer or other holding chambers. This will reduce the oropharyngeal deposition of the drug. Breath holding will increase the penetration and number of particle deposited.

### Priming

- Before using a MDI, discharge 4-5 doses before starting to inhale. This will increase the adequate mixing of the propellant and medication.
- The priming should be done if the MDI are dropped or not used for a long time.

### Advantages

- Measured amount of medications can be delivered accurately
- Inhalers will have extra doses for priming
- Onset of action will be rapid
- Amount of drug needed will be less
- Systemic side effects will be less as less drug enters the systemic circulation.

### Disadvantages

- Coordination between inhalation and actuation of medicines is needed. Spacer will be useful in young children who cannot coordinate the inhalation.
- *Candidiasis*: Oral infections like candidiasis.

### Pressurized Metered Dose Inhalers

Contains drugs in crystallized or solution form, propellants under pressure and surfactant which will prevent clumping of drug crystals.

Pressurized metered dose inhalers with valve holding chamber or spacer is used for infants and under 5 years.

### Breath actuated pressurized metered dose inhalers:

These are devices used as inhalation delivery system. The following types are present.
- Pressurized metered dose inhalers
- Dry powder inhalers.

**Recent advantages:** MDIs are coming with integrated dose counters.

## Dry Powder Inhalers

- Dry powders are inhaled in powder form which results in more effective delivery of the medications to the lungs.
- The child has to generate adequate air flow velocity of 60 L/min (at least 30 L/min) to take the drug to the respiratory tract. This cannot be used to treat acute asthma.

* Multiple dose DPIs will contain cartridges with multiple doses.

## Drugs Used
* Corticosteroids
* Salbutamol
* Salmeterol
* Ipratropium bromide
* Sodium chromoglycate
* Budenoside.

## Advantages
Dry powder inhalers have several advantages over MDI, which are as follows:
* Amount of drug delivered will be more (large sized particles can be delivered as compared to MDIs)
* Breath activated
* Coordination of actuation and breathing not needed
* Convenient
* Cost-effective
* Dry powder can be used
* Easy to use.

## Disadvantages
* Cannot be used in children under the age of 5-6 years
* Do not have gas propellant
* Child has to generate adequate air flow velocity of 60 L/min (at least 30 L/min)
* Deposition into the mouth is high as there is no other interface between DPIs and the mouth, which may predispose to oral thrush and dysphonia.

## Precautions
Rinse the mouth to prevent the complications due to deposition of drug in the mouth.

## Spacer (Fig. 2.42)
* Large plastic or metal devices with a mouth piece and an inlet for aerosol inhaler.
* These are external devices that can be attached to the MDIs that allows for a better drug delivery enhanced by actuation and inhalation. The spacers will prevent deposition of drug in the mouth.
* The holding chamber should provide a distance of 10-13 cm between the pMDI nozzle and the mouth.
* Valved holding chamber and plastic holding chamber will have electrostatic charges in the chamber and attract the aerosol particles reduce the drug delivery.
* Holding chambers with polyamide material will not have electrostatic charges.

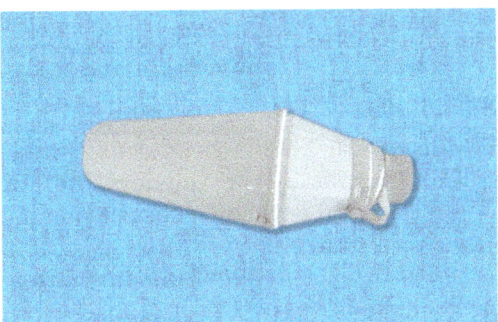

Fig. 2.42: Spacer.

## Method
Place the inhaler at the inlet and ask the child to breath from the mouth piece in and out five times.

## Precautions
* Make a tight seal between the mouth and the mouth piece so that no medicine escapes.
* Breath slowly and deeply so that more medicine reaches the airways.
* Plastic chambers will have electrostatic charges which will attract the aerosol particles thereby decreasing the drug delivery.
* Spend about 30 seconds before next use.

## Cleaning the Spacer
* Cleaning of plastic chamber with water will result in having electrostatic charges that reduce the drug delivery. Clean with warm water with detergent and allow to air dry.

- ❖ Polyamide material will overcome the electrostatic charges.

### Advantages
- ❖ Spacers will slow the speed of the aerosols coming out of the inhalers thereby preventing them getting deposited in the upper airways.
- ❖ Prevents infection in the mouth like oral candidiasis.
- ❖ Adverse/side effects of the drug less due to less deposition and absorption at the mouth.
- ❖ Coordination between the pressing the canister of the inhaler and inspiration is not needed.
- ❖ Candida infection is less.
- ❖ Easy to use.
- ❖ Reduced dose of the drug can be used.

## Nebulizers
- ❖ Drugs are administered in the form of mist inhaled into the lungs.
- ❖ Salbutamol respiratory solutions are available as 0.5% solution 5 mg/mL.
- ❖ Dose 0.05 mg or 0.01 mL/Kg diluted in 3 mL saline.
- ❖ Nebulized for a period of 5–10 minutes.
- ❖ Can be repeated at an interval of 20 minutes.
- ❖ Aerosols are a mixture of gas and solid or liquid particles. Oxygen, compressed air or ultrasonic C waves are used convert solutions or suspensions into aerosols.

### Principle
Aerosols are produced in the size of 1–5 μm in diameter.

### Types
- ❖ Conventional jet nebulizers/atomizers
- ❖ Ultrasonic nebulizers: Ultrasonic nebulizers will give uniform particles.

### Parts
- ❖ Oxygen source
- ❖ Compressor
- ❖ Mouth piece
- ❖ Outlet
- ❖ Inlet
- ❖ Jet
- ❖ Cap
- ❖ Baffle plate
- ❖ Filter.

### Drugs used
- ❖ Corticosteroids
- ❖ Salbutamol with or without ipratropium.

### Indications
- ❖ Acute asthma
- ❖ Chronic obstructive pulmonary disease
- ❖ Cystic fibrosis
- ❖ When high dose of bronchodilators are required

### Contraindications
- ❖ Should not be used for house care
- ❖ Do not use without oxygen.

### Advantages
- ❖ Delivers large doses at a faster rate
- ❖ Requires low dose.

### Disadvantages
- ❖ Acute asthma only should be treated with nebulizers
- ❖ Bulky
- ❖ Clinic or hospital setup is needed. Need trained persons to operate. Needs acute care settings and can be given only in clinics or hospitals
- ❖ Death due to hypoxia can occur due to ventilation perfusion mismatch
- ❖ Expensive
- ❖ Conventional nebulizers are not efficient and aerosol is wasted during exhalation
- ❖ Oxygen should be used to prevent hypoxia due to ventilation perfusion mismatch, especially when nebulized with short acting beta 2 agonists. Oxygen 8–10 L/min is used to drive the nebulizer medication

- Causes more noise 60 dB by jet nebulizers
- Less portable due to weight.

## Precautions

- *Amount of fluid in the nebulizer*: The total volume should not exceed 5 mL
- Bronchodilators for nebulizer should be used.
- *Combinations*: Ipratropium should never be mixed with budenoside. Salbutamol solution can be mixed with ipratropium bromide
- Diluents should be normal saline. Distilled water should not be used as diluents. Water, distilled water or any other fluid should not be used
- *Duration*: Should be completed in 5-8 minutes.

## Peak Flow Meter (Fig. 2.43)

It is a portable hand-held device to measure the peak expiratory flow rate (PEFR). It is used to monitor the lung function and the effectiveness of treatment of asthma.

## Types

- Low range peak flow meter for children.
- Standard range peak flow meter for older children and adults.

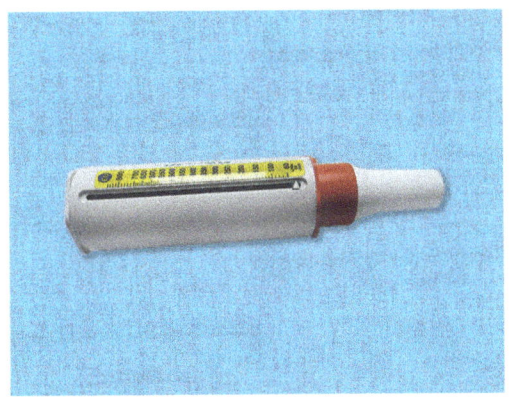

**Fig. 2.43:** Peak flow meter.

## Three Zones

| Zone | % of normal peak flow | Inference |
|---|---|---|
| Green | 80–100 | Asthma is in good control |
| Yellow | 50–80 | Signals caution |
| Red | <50% | Indicates danger zone |

## Advantages

- Patients can use by themselves
- Cost-effective
- Easy to handle.

## Disadvantages

Children aged above 5 years only can use the peak flow meter.

## Precautions

- The arrow or marker of the flow meter should be at zero before each use. The child should standup straight
- Take deep breath
- Close the lip tightly around the mouth piece to make it airtight
- The tongue should be kept away from the mouth piece
- In one breath blow out as hard and as quickly as possible
- The test should be repeated three times
- Note the highest value and not the average
- Do the test at the same time of the day.

# AIRWAYS

## Oropharyngeal/Guedel Airway (Fig. 2.44)

- To maintain or open the airway of the patient unobstructed during general anesthesia
- It will prevent the tongue from covering the epiglottis
- Prevents biting of the tongue
- Prevents airway occlusion.

## Materials

- Metal
- Plastic
- Elastomeric.

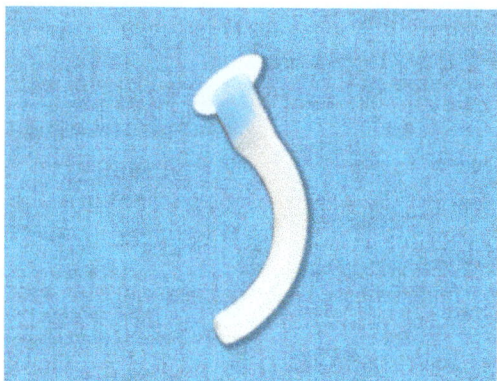

**Fig. 2.44:** Guedel oropharyngeal airway.

### Parts

It had three parts:
1. Flange
2. Body
3. Tip.

Oropharyngeal airways will prevent the tongue from falling backwards.

### Sizes

000, 00, 1, 2, 3, 4, and 5.

### Indications for Airway

* Unconscious children
* Pierre Robin syndrome
* Bilateral choanal atresia
* Large tongue obstructing the airway
* To keep the mouth open during bag and mask ventilation.

### Technique of Insertion of Oral Airway

The airway should be kept by the side of the cheeks with the flange portion at the lips. The curved tip should be up to the angle of jaw.

The oral airway should be placed in the mouth so that the concavity of the oral airway will fit into the convexity of the tongue. One end should reach the posterior pharynx and the flange should be just outside the lips.

**Measurement of airway:** The size is measured from the first incisor to the angle of jaw.

**Head tilt/Chin lift technique:** The oropharyngeal airway is inserted upside down and when the airway touches the back of the throat it should be rotated to 180°. This will help in easy insertion. In children it can be inserted using a tongue depressor.

Sizes—infant to adult:
* Children: 00, 1, and 2
* Adults: 3, 4, 5, and 6

Correct size is calculated from angle of mouth to the angle of jaw.

### Precautions

* This should be used only in unconscious patients as they will simulate gag reflex in conscious patients
* The tube can be removed once the swallow reflex appears
* Correct size should be used
* Small size may push the tongue into the posterior pharynx, causes airway obstruction
* Large size tip may press the epiglottis against the posterior pharyngeal wall, causes airway obstruction.

### Advantages

* Facilitates cardiopulmonary resuscitation
* Useful in patients with large tongue.

### Disadvantages

* Does not prevent obstruction by fluids, blood, and saliva
* Does not prevent closing of glottis.

### Complications

* Airway obstruction (if the airway is large)
* Bleeding
* Oral trauma

### Sterilization

Sterilization is done by using running water with detergent and boiling/autoclaving/chemical disinfection/gas sterilization.

## Nasopharyngeal Airway

- The tube is inserted into the nostril to secure an open airway.
- In unconscious patients, the muscles in the jaw will relax and the tongue will fall backwards and obstruct the airway.

### Sizes Available

- 6.5 mm/28 F
- 7.0 mm/30 F
- 7.5 mm/32 F
- 8.0 mm/34 F
- 8.5 mm/36 F

### Indications

When airway maintenance is required and oropharyngeal airway is contraindicated.

### Contraindication

Fracture base of skull.

### Procedure

The size is selected from the nostril to the angle of jaw. The airway is inserted until the flared end will rest on the nostril.

## MISCELLANEOUS

### Infusion Pump (Fig. 2.45)

Infusion pump is used to infuse fluids, medications, etc. through intravenous route. The rate and duration of fluid delivery can be programmed.

### Types of Pumps

- Large volume pumps
- Small volume pumps.

### Type of Infusion

- Continuous infusion
- Intermittent infusion
- Patient controlled infusion.

### Advantages

- The infusion pump can infuse fluids as little as 0.1 ml per hour.

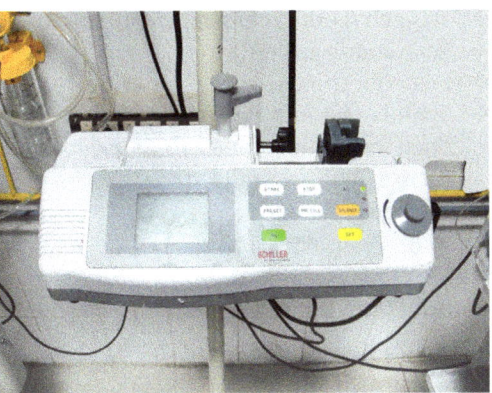

**Fig. 2.45:** Infusion pump.

- They can be used to administer fluids subcutaneously or epidurally also.
- Down pressure will detect the block to the flow or kinked.
- An up pressure sensor will detect when the bag or sensor is empty.

### Tongue Depressor (Fig. 2.46)

#### Types

- Curved or straight
- Disposable or reusable
- Metal plate or plastic.

#### Uses

- To depress the tongue and examine the throat and oral cavity for tonsils, palate, posterior pharynx, uvula, etc.

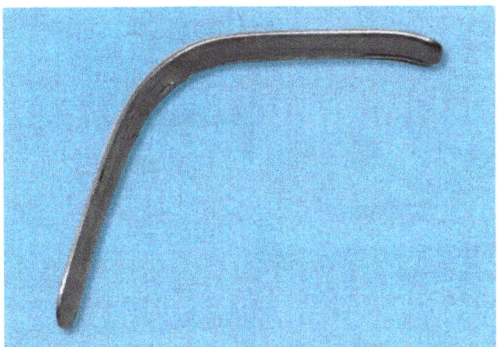

**Fig. 2.46:** Tongue depressor.

- To open mouth in unconscious patient
- To examine gag reflex
- Posterior rhinoscopy
- Spatula test in tetanus—when you try to open the mouth using a tongue depressor there will be generalized spasm
- Oral surgery
- Indirect laryngoscopy.

## Paladai (Fig. 2.47)

It is a little bowl with a spout.

### Indications

The babies who are too weak to suck from the breast can be given expressed breast milk through paladai instead of bottles.

### Advantages

- The amount of milk consumed by the babies can be monitored
- The paladai can be cleaned and sterilized easily
- It is easy to wash every time after the feeds
- Feeding using paladai will conserve energy for the baby as the energy is not spent for sucking at the breast
- Incidence of infections is low
- Milk spillage is minimal
- Increased volume of feeds can be given in less time
- Incidence of nipple confusion is less than that fed on bottles.

### Method of Feeding

The teat of the paladai with milk should be placed at the corner of the mouth. The baby will swallow the milk flowing passively from the paladai. Paladai can be sterilized by boiling for about 10 minutes before each feed.

## Prader Orchidometer (Fig. 2.48)

It is used to measure the testicular volume noninvasively.

String of 12 wooden or plastic ellipsoid beads on a string known as Prader's balls increasing in size from 1–25 mL.

These beads are compared with the testicles of the patient and the volume is read off the beads

1,2.3.4.5.6,8.10.12.15.20,25.

### Normal Volume of Testes

- Prepubertal size: 1–3 mL (yellow)
- Pubertal size: 4–12 mL (orange)
- Adult size: 15–25 mL (red).

### Uses

To distinguish between different causes of precocious puberty.

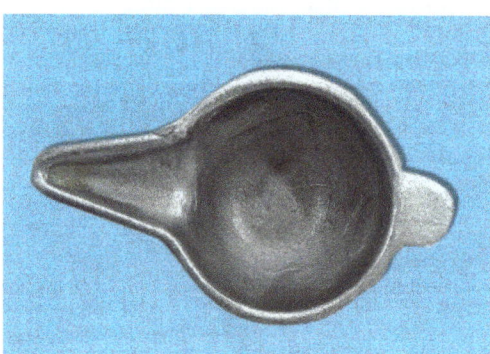

Fig. 2.47: Paladai.

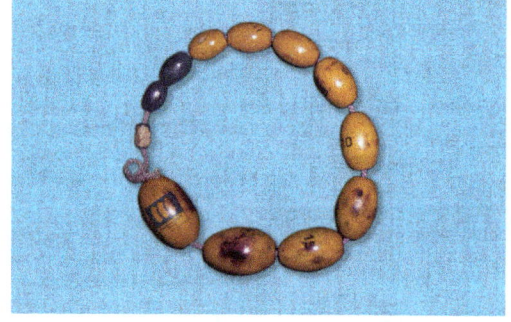

Fig. 2.48: Orchidometer measuring volume of testicles.

# QUESTIONS

**Q1. What are the causes of small testes?**
Hypogonadism (primary or secondary).

**Q2. What are the causes of large testes (macroorchidism)?**
- ❏ Fragile X syndrome
- ❏ Inherited generalized learning disability.

## 3-way Connector/3-way Stopcock (Fig. 2.49)

### Parts of 3-way Stopcock
- ❖ This has two inlets and one outlet
- ❖ Stopcock at one end and luer connectors at the other end
- ❖ Luer connectors: One rotating male luer lock with rotating nut and two female luer lock connectors
- ❖ Color coded arrows/flow indication marks on the tap.

### Advantages
- ❖ Additional lines can be connected
- ❖ *Blood pressure monitoring*: Invasive blood pressure monitoring possible
- ❖ Clear and transparent body facilitates easy visualization
- ❖ Compatible luers with any standard products
- ❖ Disposable
- ❖ Dead space will be minimal in the ports. Minimum priming volume will be needed for routine procedures
- ❖ Easy to administer medicines intermittently
- ❖ Facilitates multiple lines through single access
- ❖ Good tap rotation of 360°
- ❖ Hemodynamic pressure monitoring will be easy.

### Uses
- ❖ Ascitic tap
- ❖ Invasive blood pressure monitoring
- ❖ Exchange blood transfusion.

## Blood Culture Bottle (Fig. 2.50)

It is used for microbiological culture of blood in cases with bacteremia and septicemia. There will be specific media for aerobic and anaerobic organisms. Different types of blood culture media are:
- ❖ Glucose broth
- ❖ Bile broth
- ❖ Brain heart infusion broth
- ❖ Trypticase soy broth
- ❖ Columbia broth.

About 5–10 mL of blood is collected by venipuncture under aseptic precautions and injected into the culture media at a ratio of

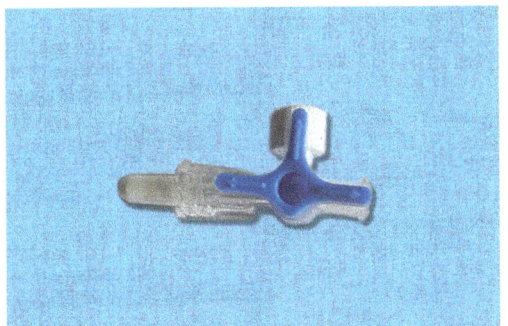

**Fig. 2.49:** 3-way connector/3-way stopcock.

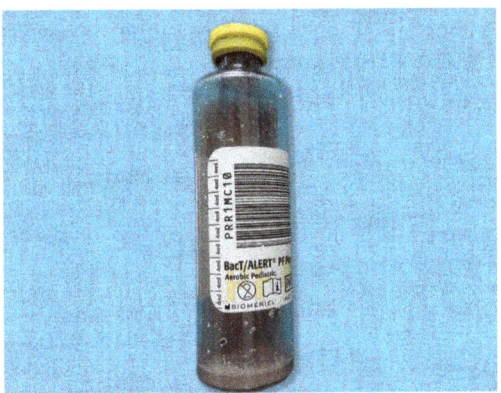

**Fig. 2.50:** Blood culture bottle.

blood to broth of 1:10. In children the ratio can be 1:5.

The blood culture bottles are incubated at body temperature (35–37°C) for about 5 days.

| Bottle top | Volume of blood required (mL) | Uses |
|---|---|---|
| Yellow top | 0.5–4 | Pediatric aerobic culture |
| Green top | 5–10 | Adult aerobic culture |
| Orange top | 5–10 | Anaerobic culture |
| Black top | 5–10 | Mycobacteria culture |
| Silver top | 3–5 | Mycoplasma culture |

Age wise recommended volume of blood to be collected for blood culture:
- Neonates: 1–2 mL
- Infants: 2–3 mL
- Children: 3–5 mL
- Adults: 10–20 mL.

## QUESTIONS

Q1. **What are the precautions to be taken before taking blood for culture?**
The top of the blood culture bottle and the venepuncture site should be cleaned with 70% isopropyl alcohol.

Q2. **How can the yield of blood culture be increased?**
- This can be done by multiple sets of cultures
- Blood can be taken at the time of increase in temperature.

Q3. **Why repeated blood culture from various sites is needed for diagnosis of infective endocarditis?**
This is because the bacteria will be released intermittently form the infective endocarditis. This also will reduce the probability of false positive culture due to skin contaminants.

Q4. **What are paired specimens?**
Blood is collected from two different sites at the same time.

Q5. **What are the changes in the culture medium indications growth of micro-organisms?**
- Hemolysis
- Presence of gas
- Turbidity
- Formation of microcolonies.

# CHAPTER 3

# Radiology—X-rays

## CHAPTER OUTLINE

- General Considerations
- X-rays Chest
- Cardiovascular System
- Respiratory System
- Abdomen
- Endocrine System
- Chromosomal Disorders
- Genitourinary System
- Hematology
- **Musculoskeletal System**
- General
- Skeleton
- Skull
- Neck
- Pelvis
- Newborn
- **Pediatric Surgery**
- Cardiovascular System
- Respiratory System
- Gastrointestinal System
- Miscellaneous

## INTRODUCTION

Reading X-rays is an important aspect of medicine. This chapter gives you the details of X-ray finding in various clinical conditions.

## GENERAL CONSIDERATIONS

### Radiology Basics—Plain, Contrast

**Q1. How X-rays are produced?**
X-rays are produced when electron beam produced from cathode (tungsten filament) strikes the anode (thermionic emission) made of tungsten.

**Q2. What are the effects of radiation on the fetus?**
Dose of 0.1 Gy (10 rad) to the embryo or fetus is recommended as a threshold dose. Radiation of 500 millirads (mrad) (limit) may lead to microcephaly, mental retardation. Now the units Sievert/Gray is followed instead of rads.

**Q3. When is therapeutic abortion recommended in radiation?**
Therapeutic abortion recommended when the radiation 0.1 Gy (10 rad) to the embryo or fetus.

Large doses of radiation are harmful to the central nervous system. There is increased incidence of leukemia and cancer in the children, when there is a history of exposure of irradiation in the antenatal period. Exposure to irradiation should be avoided in the first trimester of pregnancy.

**Q4. What is Rule of 10 for radiological exposure of any female in the reproductive age group?**

The ovulation takes place by about 14 days prior to the first day of next menstrual cycle. There is possibility that the ovum can get fertilized by a sperm that is present in the female genital tract 3–4 days before this day. Hence any exposure to radiation after this time can result in exposure of the fertilized ovum. To avoid this, the exposure to radiation should be restricted to first 10 days of the menstrual cycle.

**Q5. Where should be the X-ray film kept in posteroanterior (PA) view?**
The film should be placed against the front of the patient's chest.

**Q6. What should be the distance between the patient and the X-ray tube?**
The X-ray tube should be 2 m away from the patient.
  Proper immobilization is essential.

**Q7. What are the best positions/views to diagnose various conditions?**
Best positions to diagnose various conditions are:

| Conditions | Best positions/views |
|---|---|
| Left pleural effusion | Left lateral decubitus |
| Right pleural effusion | Right lateral decubitus |
| For mitral valve | Right anterior oblique |
| Left atrial enlargement | Barium swallow |
| Tracheal bifurcation | Left anterior oblique |
| Renal scan | Prone position |
| Barium meal in hiatal disorders | Trendelenburg position |

Best views to diagnose various conditions are:

| Conditions | Best views |
|---|---|
| Pneumothorax—foreign body | Expiratory film |
| Chest X-ray for cardiac and other respiratory problems | Inspiratory film |

**Q8. Which is the investigation of choice for sequestration of lung?**
Angiography is the investigation of choice for sequestration of lung.

**Q9. Which is the investigation of choice for minimal pericardial effusion, mitral stenosis?**
ECHO is the investigation of choice for minimal pericardial effusion, mitral stenosis.

**Q10. Which is the investigation of choice for minimal ascites?**
Ultrasonogram abdomen is the investigation of choice for minimal ascites.

**Q11. What are the views taken in children?**
a. Anteroposterior (AP) view is taken for children below 3 years with child lying in supine position.
b. X-ray lateral view with child lying in supine position
c. Erect PA view is taken for children above 3 years of age.

**Q12. What are the important views in which X-rays are taken?**

| Views | Part best viewed |
|---|---|
| Towne view | Paranasal sinuses, mastoid air cells, petrous sinus, internal acoustic meatus |
| Water view | Maxillary sinus, floor of orbit |
| Caldwell's view | Frontal sinus, ethmoidal sinus |
| Lateral view | For sphenoidal sinus |
| Lordotic | For apex lingual lobe of lung |
| Reverse lordotic | Interlobar effusion |
| Oblique | Spondylolisthesis |
| Von Rosen | Congenital dislocation of the hip (CDH) |
| Skyline | Fracture patella |
| Stryker's view | Recurrent subluxation/dislocation of shoulder |
| Lateral skull view | Sella turcica |

**Q13. What is the difference between consolidation and ground glass opacity?**
Consolidation is increase in lung attenuation with obscuring the underlying vasculature.
  Ground glass opacity is increased in lung attenuation without obscuring the underlying vasculature.

## Radiological Findings—Head to Foot

*General*
X-ray bones: Dense bones—osteopetrosis.

## Skull

- Skull X-ray:
  - Hair on end appearance—thalassemia
  - Widening of sutures—increased intracranial tension.
- X-ray changes (in the skull) in increased intracranial tension:
  - Sutures—widened
  - Erosion of posterior glenoids
  - Silver beaten appearance
  - Deep sella turcica.

## Neck

X-ray neck lateral view:
- Prevertebral space—when X-ray neck is taken with neck extended, the shadow should be more than one-half of the width of the adjacent vertebral body
- Retropharyngeal abscess
- Subcutaneous air in the neck, axilla, supraclavicular region—subcutaneous emphysema.

## Chest

X-ray chest:
- Steeple sign—hyperinflated lung with narrowing of trachea will be seen in acute laryngotracheal bronchitis. This is known as steeple sign.
- Thumb sign—observed in X-ray neck lateral views and is seen in swollen epiglottis.
- Silhouette sign—right middle lobe pneumonia homogeneous opacity in the middle and lower zone obliterating the medial border of the heart on that side.

### a. Lungs:

| X-ray findings | Diagnosis | Points |
|---|---|---|
| Homogeneous opacity in the right upper lobe | Upper lobe pneumonia | Air bronchogram will be seen |
| Haziness over the entire lung in children with lying down posture | Pleural effusion | Cardiophrenic and costophrenic angle will be obliterated |

Contd...

Contd...

| X-ray findings | Diagnosis | Points |
|---|---|---|
| Fluid level in erect posture | Pleural effusion, hydropneumothorax | Mediastinal shift to opposite side |
| Homogeneous opacity | Empyema | Cardiophrenic and costophrenic angle will be obliterated. Mediastinal shift to opposite side |
| Dilated bronchioles, linear streaking | Bronchiectasis | Honeycomb appearance |
| Air shadow between lung and pleura, hyperlucency without lung markings | Pneumothorax | Mediastinum will be shifted to opposite side. ICD should be done at second intercostal space |
| Patchy shadow | Consolidation | |
| Thick walled cavity with air fluid level | Lung abscess | |
| Miliary mottling | Miliary tuberculosis, eosinophilia | Diffuse mottling shadows |
| Hilar adenopathy | Tuberculosis, lymphomas | |
| Bilateral hyperventilation | Bronchial asthma, bronchiolitis | |
| Diffuse, fluffy infiltrate in perihilar region | Pulmonary edema | Batwing appearance, butterfly distribution |
| Kerley B lines—enlarged lymphatics in the intralobular septum | Pulmonary edema | Will be associated with cardiomegaly |
| Elevation of diaphragm | Diaphragmatic hernia, eventration of diaphragm | Congenital pulmonary adenomatoid malformation may resemble these conditions |

*Features of oligemic lung fields*:
The vascular markings will cover less than one third of the lung field

*Features of plethoric lung fields*:
The vascular markings will cover more than two third of the lung field.

### b. Heart:

| X-ray findings | Condition |
|---|---|
| Jug-handle appearance | Atrial septal defect (ASD) |
| Boot shaped heart | Tetralogy of Fallot (TOF) |
| Cardiomegaly—cardiothoracic ratio >60 (in adults 50 is significant) | • Cardiac failure<br>• Cardiomyopathy (dilated)<br>• Pleural effusion |
| Peripheral pruning of pulmonary vessels | Pulmonary hypertension |
| Money bag appearance, water bottle appearance | Pericardial effusion |
| Snowman appearance—Figure of 8 appearance | Total anomalous pulmonary venous drainage (TAPVD) |
| Egg on side appearance | Transposition of the great vessels (TGV) |
| Air around the heart | Pneumopericardium |

### c. Mediastinum:

- Causes of mediastinal widening:
  - Tuberculous hilar adenopathy
  - Tumors
  - Tumors of thymus—thymoma
  - Teratoma
  - Hodgkin's lymphoma
  - Neuroblastoma
  - Aberrant thyroid.
- Dextrocardia:
  - Dextrocardia with situs solitus: Apex will be on the right side with normally related abdominal organs
  - Dextrocardia with situs inversus: Apex will be on the right side with transposition of abdominal organs (liver and stomach).

### d. Diaphragm:

- Diaphragmatic hernia
- Eventration of diaphragm.

### Abdomen—X-ray abdomen:

- Multiple fluid levels—intestinal obstruction
- Air under diaphragm—Intestinal perforation
- Intravenous pyelogram (IVP)
- Micturating (MCU) cystourethrogram—vesicoureteral reflux.

### Upper limbs/hands:

- Phalanx—middle constriction maintained in Morquio's, mucopolysaccharidoses
- Bullet-shaped—Hurler's syndrome

### X-ray wrist:

Bone age—look for number of epiphysis
- Decreased bone age—bone age will be decreased in hypothyroidism, rickets, osteogenesis imperfecta
  - Rickets—widening of epiphysis, cupping, widening and fraying of metaphysis the distal end of long bones like radius.
  - Increased height of the physeal plate.

### Lower limbs:

X-ray lower end of femur and upper end of tibia:
- Absent epiphysis—hypothyroidism

### Vertebral column:

X-ray vertebral column: Bamboo spine in Ankylosing spondylitis due to syndesmophytes (Calcified intervertebral ligaments).

### X-ray pelvis:

Flaring of iliac crest—Down syndrome.

### Contrast studies:

- *Barium enema*: Apple core appearance of the sigmoid colon—carcinoma colon.
- Intravenous pyelography
  - Spider leg appearance—polycystic kidney
  - Thimble bladder—tuberculosis (TB) of bladder.
- Intravenous urography (IVU)
  - Flower vase appearance of ureters—horseshoe kidney
  - Golf hole ureter—TB urinary bladder
  - Cobra head deformity—in IVP—ureterocele.

## QUESTIONS

**Q1. What are the criteria for cardiomegaly in X-ray chest?**
The cardiothoracic ratio will be more than 60% in newborn babies and >50% in adults.

**Q2. What is the condition associated with box-shaped cardiomegaly?**
Ebstein anomaly.

**Q3. What are the conditions associated with decreased bone age?**
Bone age will be decreased in hypothyroidism, rickets, and osteogenesis imperfecta.

## Increased Intracranial Tension
- Separation of sutures
- Silver beaten appearance
- Erosion of glenoids
- Deepening of sella turcica

## Clinical Examination
- Fundus examination will show papilledema
- Blood pressure will be elevated
- Heart rate decreased

## Clinical Features
- Headache
- Vomiting.

## Invertogram
A plain X-ray is taken with the child held upside down about 12–24 hours after birth (Fig. 3.1).

## Lateral Radiograph of Abdomen
Lateral radiograph of abdomen (Fig. 3.2) helps to differentiate abnormal gas-filled/fluid levels containing structures such as:
- Stomach on lateral radiograph anterior transverse fluid level under left dome of diaphragm
- Duodenum is seen near colon, posterior
- Air in the bladder is seen in anterior retropubic region
- Portal vein gas shadow which is centripetally placed seen in advanced necrotizing enterocolitis (NEC).

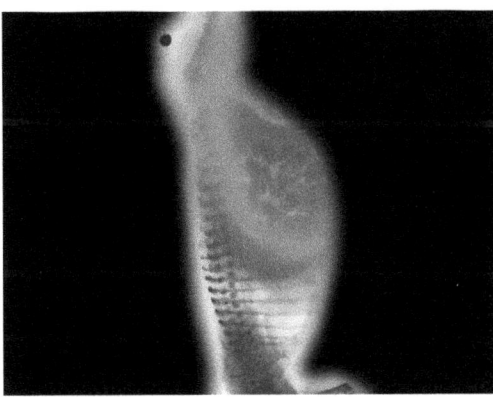

Fig. 3.1: X-ray—invertogram for anorectal anomalies.

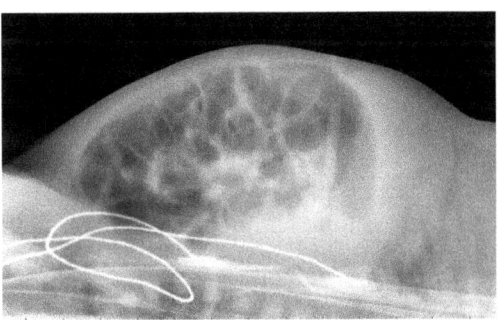

Fig. 3.2: X-ray lateral radiograph of abdomen.

## Prone Cross Table Lateral View (Fig. 3.3)
- It helps to differentiate mechanical from functional obstruction for ileus.
- It also serves an alternative to invertogram in anorectal malformations.
- Absent air indicates mechanical obstruction. Rectal gas suggests paralytic ileus.

## QUESTIONS

**Q1. How will you read a normal X-ray?**
- See for the symmetry of clavicles
- Look for bones
- Look for ventilation of lungs
- Look for the location of liver and stomach gas bubble

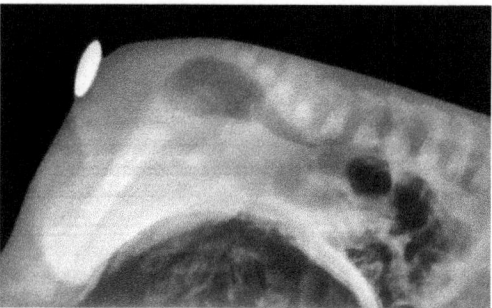

**Fig. 3.3:** X-ray—prone cross-table lateral view for anorectal anomalies.

- Identification of aorta
- Upper mediastinum
- Pulmonary parenchyma

See for the symmetry of clavicles—if the X-ray is taken in proper position, the clavicles will be symmetrical on both sides.

Pectus excavatum will result in compression of heart in the AP dimension and result in compensatory increase in transverse diameter.

Look for ventilation of lungs and assess the bilateral symmetry.

Aeration or volume of lungs can be assessed by noting the level of diaphragm in adequate inspiration, the diaphragm should be at the level of 6th rib anteriorly or 8th rib posteriorly.

*Motion artifacts*—if the exposure is not short enough, there may be patient or respiratory movements causing blurring of the diaphragmatic contour and pulmonary vascular markings.

Evaluate each anatomic portion of the lung thoroughly.

Identification of aorta—descending aorta along the left margin of the spine will indicate a left aortic arch, descending aorta along the right margin of the spine will indicate a right aortic arch.

**Q2. What is the distance between the X-ray source and the film?**
Six feet.

**Q3. In which phase of respiration will you take normal chest X ray (PA View)?**
Deep inspiration.

**Q4. What are the zones in X-ray chest?**
There are three zones:
1. *Zone I*: Upper border—apex; lower border—line joining the lower borders of the anterior ends of the second costal cartilage.
2. *Zone II*: Upper border—line joining the lower borders of the anterior ends of the second costal cartilage; lower border—4th costal cartilage.
3. *Zone III*: Upper border—below the 4th costal cartilage; lower border—lower end of the lungs.

**Q5. Do the zones represent the lobes?**
No, the zones do not represent the lobes.

**Q6. What are the differential diagnoses of an enlarged shadow at the right cardiac border?**
- Hilar node enlargement
- Right-sided aortic arch
- Manubrium sterni

End on views of the blood vessels may be misinterpreted as enlarged hilar nodes.

**Q7. How will you differentiate the hilar node from a right-sided aortic arch?**
Right-sided aortic arch will indent the right wall of trachea but the hilar node irrespective of its size will not indent the trachea.

**Q8. How will you differentiate the hilar node from a manubrium sterni?**
Medial ends of the clavicle will be away from midline in manubrium sterni.

**Q9. How will differentiate if unilateral increased translucency of lungs is due to air in the alveoli or pleural space?**
If the air is in alveoli as in emphysema, the lung markings will be seen, in pneumothorax where the air is in the pleural space, the alveolar markings will not be seen.

Hilar lymph node enlargement. This will be seen as a convex outer margin.

## Q10. What is the feature of an overpenetrated postero anterior view of X ray chest film?
The lower thoracic vertebra will be seen clearly.

## Q11. How will you differentiate between thymus shadow and mediastinal node?
Thymus shadow will be more diffuse whereas mediastinal node will be more globular.

Collapse and consolidation will confirm the shape and the site of a segment or lobe of the lung.

## Q12. How will you differentiate between thymus shadow and cardiac shadow?
In thymus enlargement, the base of the heart will be normal.

## Q13. What are the features of enlarged left atrial appendage?
- ❑ Prominent left atrial appendage at the left border of the heart
- ❑ Double shadow seen through the left atrium
- ❑ Upward displacement of the left main bronchus
- ❑ Compression of the esophagus will be evident in barium swallow study.

# X-RAYS CHEST

## Digital X-rays
Should be marked as R or L to indicate which part of the X-ray is right or left.

## Q1. How to read a normal chest X-ray?
- ❑ A systematic approach to the X-ray interpretation is essential
- ❑ Also a good understanding of the basic pathology which causes structural changes is needed to a good X-ray interpretation.

## Various Positions of X-ray Chest
- ❖ Supine
- ❖ Erect

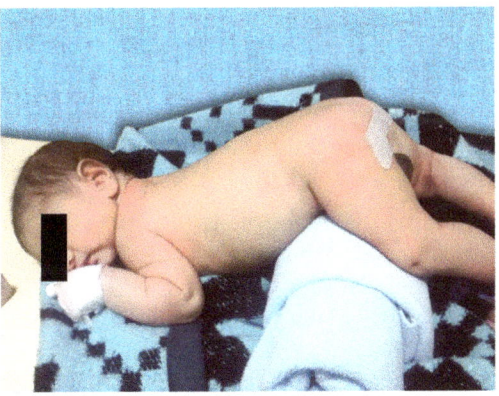

**Fig. 3.4:** Prone cross-table translateral position for anorectal anomalies and intestinal obstruction.

- ❖ Lateral
- ❖ Decubitus (right or left lateral)
- ❖ Inversion
- ❖ Prone translateral (Fig. 3.4).

## Various Projections of X-ray Chest
1. *Standard projections/views of X-ray chest*:
   - ❖ Posteroanterior view taken on full inspiration to examine the lungs, bony thoracic cage, mediastinum, great vessels
   - ❖ Lateral for retrosternal, retrocardiac and lung lesions.
2. *Additional projections*:
   - ❖ Anteroposterior view for vertebra, posterior mediastinal mass
   - ❖ Supine for patients under critical care
   - ❖ Lateral decubitus for pleural effusion
   - ❖ Expiratory view for pneumothorax
   - ❖ Lordotic view for apex of lung
   - ❖ Frontal view
   - ❖ Right anterior oblique (RAO) view/left anterior oblique (LAO) view for fractures and intrathoracic lesions.

## Following of Technical and Clinical Aspects
- ❖ Technical aspects
- ❖ Clinical aspects.

**Technical aspects:**
- ❖ Technical points to be considered in X-ray evaluation

- First evaluate the technical factors of the X-ray film
- Locate the right and left markers
- Centering—medial end of the clavicles should be equidistant from the spinous process.

1. *Position of the patient*: Is the patient straight or rotated? If the patient is straight the inner end of clavicles will be symmetrical with reference to the vertebral columns *Patient rotation*:
   - Quality of exposure or film
     - Under exposure
     - Over exposure
   - Is the film penetrated adequately?
2. *Quality of the film*: Readable quality or not, adequate inspiration, normal penetration, centered on mid chest. It should not be too white or too black in color.
   
   A quality of the film should have the following:
   - Adequate inspiration
   - Normal penetration
   - Centered on mid chest
   - Rotation—should not be rotated
   - Appropriate exposure.
3. *Penetration*: Adequate penetration should be enough to bring out the pulmonary details which are essentially the pulmonary markings. The penetration can be normal, under- or overpenetrated
   
   In normal penetration, the vertebral bodies and the disk spaces should be just visible at T8 and T9 level.
   
   The following points will indicate good penetration:
   - Pulmonary vascular markings are well brought out. Is it adequately penetrated or else the pulmonary details will not be brought out which are essentially the vascular markings.
   - Intervertebral disk spaces and vessels posterior to the heart are seen well. When the penetration is adequate, the intervertebral disk spaces and the vessels posterior to the heart are seen well.
   
   It should be adequately penetrated. Adequately penetrated films will bring out the details of pulmonary vascular markings.
4. *Degree of rotation*: Note the distance between the center of the vertebral bodies and the lateral aspect of ribs. See if the medial end of clavicle is equidistant from the midline.
   - Medial ends of the clavicle should be equidistant from each other.
   - Aeration of the lungs can be assessed by noting the level of the diaphragm.
   - In adequate respiration, the diaphragm will be at the level of the 6th rib interiorly and 8th rib posteriorly.
   - Two-thirds of the heart will lie on the left side of the chest and one-third on the right.
   - The left side of the heart will be made of left atrium and left ventricle.
   - Superior vena cava (SVC) will lie above right heart border.
   - Expiratory or inspiratory film—see if the area of interest is covered.

### Clinical aspects:

Read the film from out to in or from in to out. The anatomic parts should be thoroughly evaluated. Look at the position of clavicles. The medial ends of the clavicles should be equidistant from the midline. Look at the soft tissues and the bony cage.

### Note the Following Structures

- Bones (ribs, clavicle, scapula, spine, shoulder joint) and soft tissues (cutaneous tissue, muscles, breast)
- Bony cage
- Cardiac shadow
- Lung shadow
- Diaphragm and subdiaphragmatic area
- Mediastinum (superior mediastinum, hilum, etc.)
- Bronchial—normal/inverted/ambiguous
- Aortic arch side—left or right

- Upper abdomen: Abdominal situs—normal/inverted/ambiguous.

## Note the Following Areas
- Cardiophrenic angle
- Costophrenic angle
- Trachea
- Mediastinal shift.

*Systematic approach*—should be followed so that no part is missed. The X-ray can be evaluated in the following order:
- Extrathoracic
  - Abdomen
  - Neck
  - Soft tissues
  - Bones
- Thorax
- Mediastinum—mediastinal silhouette on each side
  - Position, size and density of each hilum
  - Thymus
  - Trachea and bronchi/tracheal position look at the trachea especially right wall
- Position and shape of diaphragm
- Costophrenic angles
- Great vessels
- Bronchial situs—normal/inverted/ambiguous
- Aortic arch left sided or right sided
- Heart—side, apex, size, contour and shape
  - Side—right/left
  - Direction of apex
  - Size—CT ratio 55-60%
  - Gross cardiac anatomy
  - Contour.

*Lung fields*—pathological conditions like consolidation, pneumonia. The minor interlobar fissure will be separating the right upper and middle lobes and will be seen running horizontally in the third and fourth right intercostal spaces.

*Lung vasculature*—plethora, oligemia, pulmonary venous engorgement.

*Diaphragm*—the level of the diaphragm will be lower on the side of the apex.

*Upper abdomen*—look for abdominal situs—normal/inverted/ambiguous. Look for free air under the diaphragm.

*Musculoskeletal*—vertebra, rib abnormalities.

*Tubes and catheters*—always compare each part with the corresponding opposite side.
- Retrocardiac space
- Abdominal situs—normal/inverted/ambiguous
- Bronchial—normal/inverted/ambiguous
- Aortic arch side—left or right.

*Look for the location of liver and stomach gas bubble*—the cardiac apex will be on the same side of the stomach and opposite side of the liver shadow. In heterotaxia, the apex will be on the right and the stomach on the left side. Midline liver will be associated with asplenia—Ivemark syndrome or polysplenia syndrome. Carefully look in a sequence the parts like soft tissues, bones, aeration of each lung in the upper, middle and lower thirds as well as medial, mid and outer thirds by comparing with the opposite sides.

Look for the vascularity in each of these zones

Look for tracheal position. The trachea should be in central position.

### Bones and soft tissues:
- Bony cage and soft tissue of thoracic wall
- Bony skeleton—look at the position of clavicles. Is the chest symmetrical? Is there any scoliosis?
- Are the ribs crowded or widely spaced? If so note the areas in which the abnormalities are noted. Look for the presence of cervical ribs. Look for erosion of ribs. Look for chest abnormalities like scoliosis.

### Bony cage:
- Look for bones
- Rib notching will be seen in older children with coarctation of aorta.

**Cardiac shadow:**

- Two-thirds of the heart will lie on the left side of the chest and one-third on the right.
- The left side of the heat will be made of left atrium and left ventricle.
- Superior vena cava will lie above right heart border.
- Heart—side—right/left
  - Direction of apex
  - Size—CT ratio 55–60%
  - Gross cardiac anatomy
  - Contour.
- Increased cardiac shadow will be seen:
  - Congestive cardiac failure (CCF)
  - Cardiomyopathy
  - Pericardial effusion.
- Dextrocardia is a condition in which heart is placed on the right side of the chest with the apex of the heart is pointing towards the right instead of normal heart pointing towards left. In isolated dextrocardia only the heart is placed on the right side with no other defects (Fig. 3.5). Dextrocardia is often associated with abdominal situs solitus or situs inversus. In this condition the right hemidiaphragm will be placed at a lower lever as compared to the left side. The apex of the heart will push down the diaphragm.
- Dextroposition is a form of dextrocardia with apex still directed to the left side (Fig. 3.6). This is a condition in which the heart is shifted to right either due to push by, diaphragmatic hernia, pleural effusion, etc. or pull due to fibrosis, collapse, etc.

**Localization of the chambers:**

*Localization of the atria:*

- The atrial situs will be the same as visceral situs. Localize the liver shadow and the stomach bubble
- Right-sided liver shadow and left-sided stomach bubble will indicate situs solitus. Situs solitus of atria will indicate that the right atria are on the right of the left atria. Situs inversus indicates liver is on the left side and the stomach bubble is on the right side (Fig. 3.7). Midline liver with variable

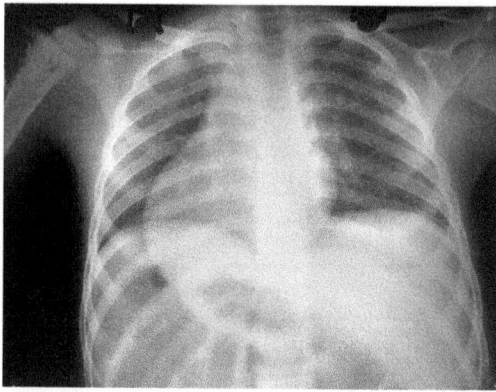

**Fig. 3.5:** Dextrocardia with situs inversus heart on the right side of the chest and apex facing right side. Note the diaphragm lies at lower level on the side of the apex.

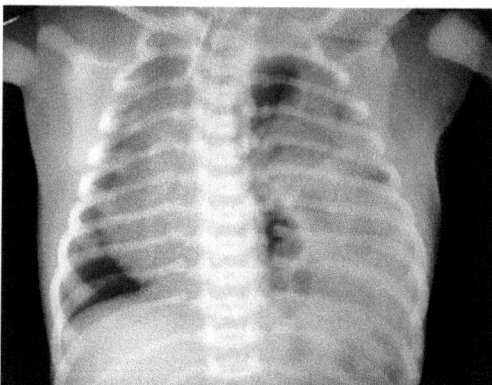

**Fig. 3.6:** X-ray dextroposition with the cardiac shadow shifted to right with apex still facing to the left side.

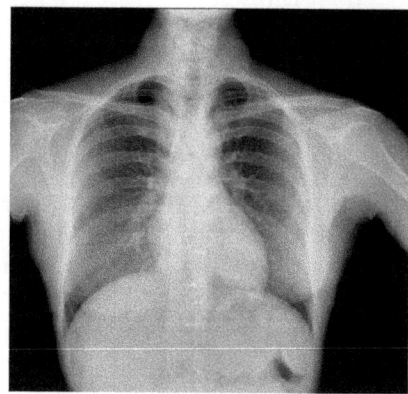

**Fig. 3.7:** Normal chest X-ray.

position of stomach will indicate—situs ambiguous—two right atria or two left atria.

*Localization of the ventricles*:
Localization of the great arteries can be determined by angiocardiography.

**Pulmonary vascular markings:**
- Increased pulmonary blood flow: When the pulmonary blood flow is increased the pulmonary arteries will be enlarged and appear to extend into the lateral third of the lung field, where they are not usually present.
  - Increased vascularity to the lung apices where the vessels are normally collapsed.
  - The external diameter of the right pulmonary artery visible in the right hilum will be wider than the internal diameter.
- Decreased pulmonary blood flow—hilum appears small, remaining lung field appears black, vessels appear small and thin.
- Normal pulmonary blood flow.

**Heart:**
- Look at the cardiac size and shape. Two-thirds of the heart lies on the left side of the chest, with one-third on the right.
- Right heart border is formed by
  - SVC
  - Right atrium
  - IVC
- Left border is formed by
  - Aortic knuckle
  - Pulmonary artery ( Main pulmonary trunk )
  - Left atrial appendage
  - Left ventricle
- On both sides trace the pulmonary artery branches which are seen fanning out through the lungs.

**Hilum:** Position, size and density of each hilum.

**Position of the heart:**
- The heart will be displaced as a whole in pleural effusion, pneumothorax, fibrosis, collapse of lung.
- In scoliosis, the heart will be displaced.
- In obesity, the heart will be lifted a upward and the apex will be tilted upward
- In adults, one-third of the heart will be lying on the right and two-thirds on the left side. In infancy, the heart is of transverse or globular and right side is equal to left side. By 5-7 years the heart will resemble the adult type.

**Shape of the heart:**
- In infancy and up to 5-7 years, the heart can be globular
- Globular shaped in pericardial effusion
  - Saber en boot or boot shaped heart in tetralogy of Fallot
  - Figure of 8 sign or snowman sign or dumbbell sign—in total anomalous pulmonary venous drainage (TAPVD)—supracardiac type
- Money bag appearance in pericardial effusion
- Scimitar-shaped in Scimitar syndrome
- Box-shaped heart in Ebstein anomaly.

**Contours of cardiomediastinum:**
- *Contours of right cardiomediastinum*:
  The following structures will form the right cardiomediastinal contour from superior to inferior:
  - Right paratracheal stripe is made up of right brachiocephalic vein and SVC
  - Arch of azygos vein
  - Ascending aorta
  - Lateral border of right atrium
  - Inferior vena cava (IVC).
- *Contours of left cardiomediastinum*:
  The following structures will form the left cardiomediastinal contour from superior to inferior:
  - Left paratracheal stripe is made up of common carotid artery, left subclavian artery and left jugular vein
  - Uppermost rounded or convex part—posterior part of transverse aortic arch (aortic knuckle or knob)
  - Below this flat or concave pulmonary conus—trunk of pulmonary artery

- Below pulmonary conus—auricle of left atrium
- Lower, largest segment—left ventricle.
❖ *Contours of anterior cardiomediastinum (lateral view)*:
The anterior border is formed by the following structures from above downward:
- Superior mediastinum—great vessels, thymus
- Transverse part or arch or aorta
- Ascending aorta
- Right ventricular outflow tract
- Pulmonary trunk
- Right ventricle
- Left ventricle.
❖ *Contours of posterior cardiomediastinum*:
- Above—left atrium and pulmonary veins
- Below—right atrium
- Diaphragmatic surface is formed by IVC, right atrium, right ventricle.

**Size of the heart:**
❖ Normal sized heart
❖ Cardiomegaly—cardiothoracic ratio will be more than 50
❖ Small heart—cardiothoracic ratio will be less than 50.

**Chamber enlargement:**
❖ In left ventricular hypertrophy, here is a prominent convexity and the heart will form an obtuse angle with the diaphragm. In right ventricular hypertrophy, the apex will be lifted up and the heart will form an acute angle with the diaphragm.
❖ Increased cardiac shadow will be seen:
- Congestive cardiac failure
- Cardiomyopathy
- Pericardial effusion.
❖ Right atrium enlargement—right border will be more convex.
❖ Left atrium enlargement—will show double contoured right border with both right and left atrial shadow.
❖ Right ventricular hypertrophy—the apex will be shifted outward and tilted up
❖ Left ventricular hypertrophy—the apex will be shifted downward and outward.

**Shape and size of aorta:**
❖ Dilatation
❖ Poststenotic dilatation
❖ Identification of aorta—descending aorta along the left margin of the spine will indicate a left aortic arch. Descending aorta along the right margin of the spine will indicate a right aortic arch.

**Pulmonary artery:**
❖ Pulmonary bay on the left border of heart will be obliterated and concave in pulmonary stenosis. For example: in tetralogy of Fallot.
❖ In pulmonary artery, dilatation the pulmonary bay on the left side will be full and convex.

**Lung shadow:**
❖ *Lungs*: View the lung on both sides starting from the apex. Both lungs will appear dark due to air in the lungs. Scan both the lungs above downward starting from the apices. Compare both sides at the same level. See if both right and left sides are equal in volume and aeration. When there is more air on one side that side will be more black and more volume.
❖ *Pulmonary parenchyma*: Look for pneumonia.
❖ Bronchopulmonary sequestration is common in right lower lung field. In this condition, a segment of the lung will be supplied by an artery arising from the descending aorta.
❖ *Ventilation of lungs*: Note the volume and aeration of both lungs. The right and left lungs will be equal in aeration and volume. Look at the volume and the degree of the aeration of the hemithorax.
- On full inspiration, anterior end of the 6th rib should cut the diaphragm.
- Posterior end of the 10th rib.
- If the expansion is more than the lung is considered as hyperinflated.
❖ *Bilateral hyperventilation*: Generalized increased translucency of the thorax with low-flattened diaphragms.

- *Unilateral increased translucency of lungs*: Patient rotation should be ruled out.
- Air in the alveoli or pleural space will result in unilateral increased translucency.
  - Obstructive emphysema
  - Compensatory emphysema.
- *Lungs*: View the lung on both sides starting from the apex. Note the volume and aeration of both lungs. The right and left lungs will be equal in aeration and volume.
- *Lung fields*: The lungs are divided into three zones for purpose of radiological examination.
  a. *Zone I (upper zone)*: This zone extends from the apex to the horizontal line drawn through the lower borders of the anterior ends of the second costal cartilages.
  b. *Zone II (mid zone)*: This zone extends from the horizontal line drawn through the lower borders of the anterior ends of the second costal cartilages to the horizontal line drawn through the lower borders of the anterior ends of the fourth costal cartilages. This will contain hilar structures of the lungs.
  c. *Zone III (lower zone)*: This zone extends from the horizontal line drawn through the lower borders of the anterior ends of the fourth costal cartilages to the base of the lungs.

Aeration of lung in the upper, mid and lower thirds also medial, mid and outer thirds Vascularity in each of the zones.

- *Apical zones*: Few consider apical zone above clavicles.
- *Lung vasculature*:
  - Plethora
  - Oligemia
  - Pulmonary venous engorgement.
- *Bat's wing appearance*: Pulmonary edema.
- Interlobar fissures will be seen.

## Diaphragm:

- Look for the position and shape of diaphragm. The shape will be distorted in diaphragmatic hernia.
- The diaphragm on both sides will not lie on the same level. Usually the left side of the diaphragm will be lying lower than the right by up to 2 cm. If the difference is more than 2 cm, elevation or depression of diaphragm should be suspected. The diaphragm will lie at a lower level at the side of the apex.
- *Position of diaphragm:* The position will be elevated in eventration of diaphragm,
  - Distinct or blurred
  - Normal position—the dome of the diaphragm will be elevated on the side opposite to apex of the heart. In normal children and adults, the right dome of diaphragm will be lying at a higher position than the left.
- The dome of diaphragm on the side of apex should be more caudal.
- *Abnormalities of diaphragm*:
  - Diaphragmatic hernia—the outline is interrupted
  - Eventration the dome lies at a higher position than normal. The outline is not interrupted
  - Tethered diaphragm shadow will be seen in fibrosis of lung or pleura pulling the diaphragm.
- *Look for costophrenic angles*: It will be obliterate when fluid is collected as in pleural effusion, empyema, hydrothorax, hemothorax.

## Mediastinum:

- Look the meditational silhouette on each side:
  - Mediastinal shadow
  - Lymph nodes.
- *Upper mediastinum*: Tumor mass—thymoma, lymphoma, neuroblastoma, teratoma.
- *Thymus*: Thymus will be normally present in infants.
  - Absent thymus will be seen in DiGeorge syndrome.
  - Thymus will shrink under severe stress.
- *Wave sign or sail sign*: Triangular-shaped inferior margin on the right side or

bilateral due to normal thymus. Normal thymus shadow up to 3 years.
- Changes in shape during respiration on steroid therapy it will shrink.

**Hilar region:**
- This will be seen as a convex outer margin.
- *Hilum*: Position, size and density of each hilum.
- Hilar lymph node enlargement—hilar adenitis
- Manubrium sterni
- Right aortic arch.

**Views:**
- Frontal view
- Lateral view should be taken to localize the lesion.
- Right lateral film will be helpful for localization of calcification of valve and right ventricular hypertrophy. The anteriorly placed right ventricle will lie close to the sternum.
- Lateral decubitus view will help in diagnosing free fluid.
- *Musculoskeletal*: The film, bones under review, can be read from outer to in or in to out
  - Vertebral/rib anomalies
  - Fractures
  - Central position
- *Mediastinum*: Look the meditational silhouette on each side.

**Tubes, catheters:**

The endotracheal tube should be 1-2 cm above the carina approximately at the level of T1-T2.

**Motion artifacts:**
- It is more common if the exposure time is prolonged. Proper immobilization is essential. The motion of the patient or respiratory movements will result in blurring of the pulmonary vessels and the diaphragm contour.
- Look under the diaphragm for free air and dilated loops.
- Always compare the opposite side for soft tissues.

- Bony skeleton.
- Position of the trachea.
- Not to miss the findings check for the following:
  - Airways—trachea, right and left bronchi
  - Bony shadows—ribs, clavicle, scapulae, spine, humerus, sternum
  - Cardiac shadow—size, shape, silhouette
  - Diaphragm
  - Effusions
  - Fields of lung
  - Gastric bubble
  - Hilar region.
- Iatrogenic—tubes, devices, valve replacements
- Soft tissues surrounding the chest wall
- Interpretation of lung shadows:
  - Black—air
  - Dark gray—fat
  - Light gray—soft tissue
  - Off white—bones
  - Bright white—metals.

## Normal Chest X-ray

Normal chest X-ray will be associated with the following findings:
- Situs solitus
- The liver and IVC lies on the right
- The stomach bubble and spleen will lie on the left
- Systemic venous atria lie on the right side and opposite to the gastric fundus.
- Viscera atrial situs
- Cardiac silhouette normal
- Cardiothoracic ratio 50
- Cardiac shape normal.

### Thymus (Sail Sign) (Fig. 3.8)

*Thymus shadow*: Triangular-shaped inferior margin of the thymus as it touches the minor fissure. This is seen in normal newborns and young children.

In normal infants, the thymus can be seen.

*Thymus sail sign* is due to normal thymus which will be seen in young children.

# Radiology—X-rays

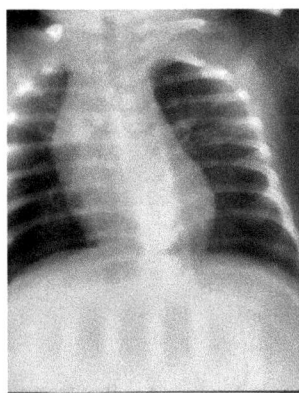

**Fig. 3.8:** Normal thymus—sail sign.

**Features of normal thymus shadow (Mnemonic—10 S's):**

- Sail like appearance on the right upper border of lung
- Soft tissue density
- Symmetrical shadow
- Smooth borders
- Shape and size will vary
- Size will vary with respiration, especially inspiration
- Scalloped or wavy contour of thymus (thymic wave sign) due to impression by anterior reflection of ribs
- Sharply demarcated, straight base caused by minor fissure
- Shift of mediastinum not present
- Silhouette sign positive
- Structures surrounding are normal bronchovascular markings on both sides, no mass effect on vascular structures or airways, no loss of lung volume, costophrenic angle free
- Spinnaker sail sign will be seen in pneumomediastinum, where thymic lobes are elevated.

## QUESTIONS

**Q1. What is the difference between thymus sail sign and spinnaker sail sign?**
Thymus sail sign is due to normal thymus and spinnaker sail sign is abnormal elevation of thymus due to pneumomediastinum.

**Q2. What is wave sign of Mulvey?**
Indentation of normal thymus by ribs resulting in wavy border. It is seen in normal children.

**Q3. What are the causes of thymus enlargement?**
- ❑ Benign causes—thymic hyperplasia, intrathymic hemorrhage, hemangioma, lymphangioma.
- ❑ Malignant causes—leukemia, lymphoma, Langerhans cell histiocytosis.

## Mediastinal Widening

Mediastinal widening usually occurs due to vascular abnormalities or mediastinal mass (Fig. 3.9).

Width more than 6 cm on an upright PA chest view, or more than 8 cm in supine AP chest X-ray.

Mediastinum chest width ratio is greater than 0.25 in children.

- *Causes of mediastinal widening*
  - Anterior mediastinum mass
  - Posterior mediastinum mass
- Tumor
- Lung-pulmonary masses
- *Vascular causes:* Vascular shadow caused by aortic aneurysm, aortic dissection, aortic unfolding, double SVC, aberrant right subclavian artery, azygos continuation of IVC
- Lymph node enlargement
- Neoplasia
- Gastrointestinal causes—achalasia, hernia
- Anthrax infection
- Mediastinal lipomatosis
- *Technical factors:* Rotation, poor inspiration, supine position, lordotic position.

Conditions associated with mediastinal widening:
- Mediastinal node enlargement
- Lung—atelectasis, lung mass
- Vessels—enlarged pulmonary arteries, unfolded aorta, double SVC, aberrant right

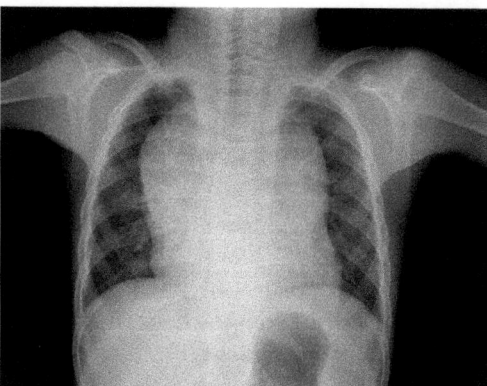

**Fig. 3.9:** X-ray mediastinal widening.

subclavian artery, azygos continuation of IVC, thoracic aortic aneurysms, aortic dissection.
- ❖ Mediastinal mass
  - Anterior mediastinal mass (lymphoma, substernal thyroid enlargement, teratoma, thymic tumors, germ cell tumors)
  - Middle mediastinal mass (lymphadenopathy, bronchogenic cyst, esophageal duplication cyst, neurenteric cyst, esophageal malignancy)
  - Posterior mediastinal mass (neurogenic tumors, neurilemmoma, neurofibroma, extramedullary hemopoiesis, paraspinal abscess)
- ❖ Multiple compartments—lymphadenopathy, lymphoma, vascular lesions.
- ❖ If the X-ray is taken with improper techniques, the mediastinum may appear widened.
- ❖ The rotation, poor inspiration, supine or lordotic position.
- ❖ In extramedullary hemopoiesis, paravertebral soft tissue shadow around the lower thoracic vertebra will be widened. This is seen in thalassemia, sickle cell anemia.
- ❖ There will be expansion of transverse process of the vertebral bodies and ribs will be present.

*Silhouette sign*: An intrathoracic opacity on chest radiograph touching the aorta, heart, and diaphragm will obliterate that border. Obliteration of borders of heart, mediastinum, and diaphragm by the opacity due to the mass if it is in anatomic contiguity.

*Hilum convergence sign*: Vessels will be converging into the hilum. If the vessels are going into the opacity, it will be a mediastinal mass.

*Cervicothoracic sign*: An opacity extending above the clavicle. It will be located in posterior mediastinum and entirely in the thorax. If the opacity disappears as it nears the clavicle, the mass will be in the cervicothoracic region partly in the thorax and partly in the neck.

*Thoracoabdominal sign*: If the margins are converging it is intrathoracic and if the margins are diverging the mass had both intrathoracic and intra-abdominal components.

## Hilar Node Enlargement

Hilar nodes are enlarged in TB (Fig. 3.10).

### Bilateral Hilar Node Enlargement
- ❖ Infections—TB
  - Mycoplasma
  - Histoplasmosis
  - Coccidioidomycosis

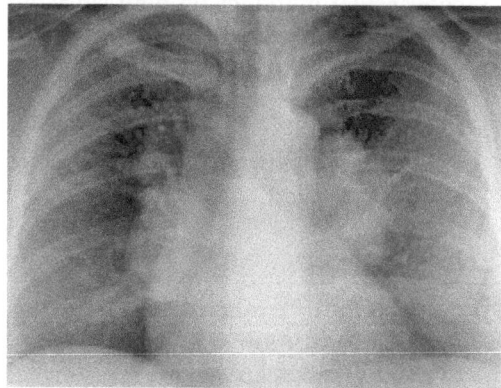

**Fig. 3.10:** Bilateral hilar adenopathy sarcoidosis.

- Malignancy
  - Hodgkin lymphoma
  - Leukemia
  - Metastasis
  - Spread from renal tumor
- Inhalational diseases
  - Silicosis
  - Berylliosis
  - Coal worker's pneumoconiosis
- Inflammatory conditions: Sarcoidosis.

## QUESTIONS

**Q1. What are the complications of tuberculous hilar lymphadenopathy?**
- ☐ Bronchopneumonia
- ☐ Bronchiectasis
- ☐ Collapse
- ☐ Dissemination—hematogenous
  - ➢ Emphysema
  - ➢ Erosion into vessels

**Q2. What is multidrug-resistant tuberculosis?**
Organisms resistant to isoniazid (INH) and rifampicin with or without resistance to other antituberculous drugs.

## Interlobar Effusion

Localized transudative interlobar pleural fluid can accumulate in the interlobar fissure.

### Radiological Findings

**Frontal view:**
- Well demarcated collection of fluid in the minor interlobar pulmonary fissure
- Right sided: Homogeneous opacity
- Intermittent appearance at same site during CCF
- Located on the course of interlobar fissures
- Lenticular contour.

**Lateral view:**
Spindle-shaped shadow within the fissure and continuous with the thickened pleura on both sides.

### Phantom Tumor or Vanishing Lung Tumor

The interlobar effusion due to cardiac failure will get resolved after fluid restriction and taking diuretics like furosemide.

This condition should be suspected in order to avoid unnecessary investigations to rule out tumors in the lung or other parts in the chest.

### Differential Diagnosis

- Pulmonary infarction
- Hydatid cyst
- Mesothelioma
- Pulmonary or metastatic masses
- Tuberculoma
- Epicardial fat.

### Discussion—Interlobar Effusion

**Causes:**

Congestive cardiac failure is the most common cause for interlobar effusion.

**Differential diagnosis for radiological shadows:**

- Exudates
  - Parapneumonic pleural effusion
  - Malignant pleural effusion
  - Hemothorax
  - Chylothorax
  - Fibrous tumors arising from visceral pleura of the interlobar fissure.
- Transudates: Renal failure.

## QUESTIONS

**Q1. What is the pathogenesis of interlobar effusion?**
There will be transudation from the pulmonary vascular space. Fluid can accumulate in the interlobar fissure whenever the amount of fluid collection exceeds the ability for reabsorption. This is also known as interlobar hydrothorax or Phantom tumor or vanishing lung tumor. There will be a local increase in elastic recoil due to adjacent partially atelectatic lung which exerts suction cup effect.

**Q2. Why interlobar effusions are more common on the right side?**

Interlobar effusions are common on the right side due to greater hydrostatic pressure on the right side in CCF as compared to left which results in impaired venous and lymphatic drainage.

## Rib Notching

The notching can be seen in superior or inferior part of the ribs.

1. *Superior rib notching*: The ribs will get eroded at the superior borders.
   - Abnormal osteoblastic activity in osteogenesis imperfecta, connective tissue disorders like rheumatoid arthritis, systemic lupus erythematosus (SLE), Marfan syndrome, Sjögren's syndrome and conditions causing local pressure effects
   - Abnormal osteoclastic activity in hyperparathyroidism, neurofibromatosis type 1 rarely when the mass is very large
   - Poliomyelitis.
2. *Inferior rib notching (Roesler sign) (Fig. 3.11)*: The ribs will get eroded at the inferior borders where the dilated vessels due to bronchopulmonary collaterals will erode the ribs. This will be seen in chest X-ray AP view. This is also known as Dock's sign.

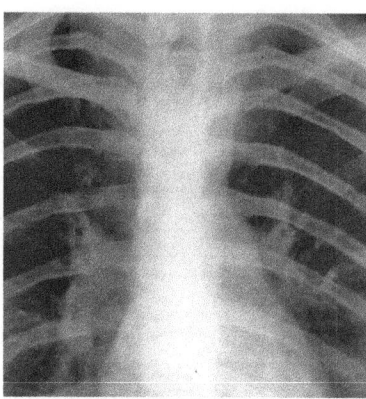

**Fig. 3.11:** Coarctation of the aorta (CoA)—inferior rib notching.

Causes of inferior rib notching (mnemonic—A-I):
- Arteriovenous malformations of the chest wall, pulmonary arteriovenous malformations
- Bronchopulmonary collaterals in coarctation of aorta, interrupted aortic arch
- Blalock-Taussig shunt (involves only upper two ribs)
- Coarctation of aorta with bronchopulmonary collaterals (4-8 ribs are involved)
- Collaterals due to subclavian artery obstruction in Takayasu disease
- Dilatation of intercostal arteries
- Enlarged venous collaterals in obstruction of SVC
- Fallot's tetralogy with bronchopulmonary collaterals
- Great vessel obstruction—superior vena caval obstruction, aortic thrombosis, Takayasu's aortitis
- Hypertrophic nerves—neurofibromatosis type 1—erosion of inferior part of ribs where the neurovascular bundle is present
- Hypertrophic polyneuropathy
- Hyperparathyroidism
- Hemolytic anemia—thalassemia
- Infections—poliomyelitis
- Intercostal neuroma
- Interrupted aortic arch.

3. Both inferior and superior rib notching will be seen in:
   - Local pressure effects—neurofibromatosis type 1. This will cause inferior rib notching and if large can also cause superior rib notching.
   - Hyperparathyroidism.

*Unilateral rib notching* may be associated with Blalock-Taussig shunt where only the upper two ribs are involved in trauma, solitary mass.

*Single rib notching* can be seen in trauma or solitary masses like neurogenic tumors, schwannoma.

*Retrosternal rib notching*: It is due to dilatation of internal mammary artery.

## QUESTIONS

**Q1. Why first and second ribs are not notched in coarctation of aorta?**
First and second intercostal arteries are supplied by superior intercostals branch of costocervical trunk

**Q2. What is Dock's sign?**
Bilateral rib notching in coarctation of aorta due to collateral circulation in the internal mammary arteries.

## Pneumomediastinum (Fig. 3.12)

It is a condition where there will be free air or gas in the mediastinum. The air may originate from the alveolus or conducting airways.

### Radiological Findings (Mnemonic—A-H)

Posteroanterior and lateral views should be taken.
- Air around the heart and mediastinum will be seen as radiolucent outline
- Air in the mediastinum
- Aortopulmonary space will be sharply defined
- Angel wing sign—air outlines the thymus
- Bronchial wall outlined by air
- Continuity of right and left mediastinum
- Continuous diaphragm sign under the cardiac shadow
- Cervical soft tissues with streak of air
- Dissection on medial border of superior vena cava left subclavian artery, left common carotid artery, right innominate artery by air extending into the neck
- Dissection of pericardial fat by air
- Double bronchial wall sign—the bronchial wall will be clearly visible between air present inside and outside of the bronchial walls.
- Extrapleural sign—air in the mediastinum will extend bilaterally in between mediastinal pleura, parietal pleura will be visualized along the left mediastinal border. The pleura will be parallel to the mediastinum and descend to the mid hemidiaphragm
- Free mediastinal air
- Gas shadow seen under surface of the heart which connects both right and left side
- Haystack sign—as the gas crosses the superior mediastinum, the heart will look like a haystack.

### Signs in Pneumomediastinum

- *Spinnaker sail sign or angel wing sign* is seen in pneumomediastinum. Thymus consists of two lobes. Free mediastinal air lifts the thymus off the heart and major vessels. Each lobe is displaced laterally outlined by air and appears like spinnaker sails.
- *Tubular artery sign*—gas outlining the major aortic branches.

### Differential Diagnosis

- Medial pneumothorax
- Pneumopericardium
- Subcutaneous emphysema
- Pneumoperitoneum
- Pneumoretroperitoneum.

### Causes of pneumomediastinum:

- Spontaneous not associated with injury
  - Rupture of marginally situated alveoli
  - Erosion of trachea by tumor
  - Extension from pneumoperitoneum

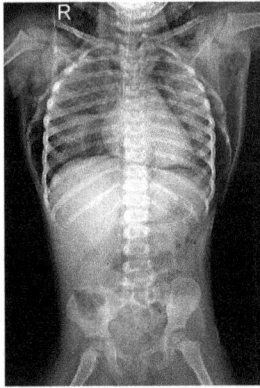

**Fig. 3.12:** X-ray—pneumomediastinum.

- Traumatic
  - Alveolar rupture
  - Bowel rupture
  - Barotrauma
  - Chest injury
  - Divers especially SCUBA divers
  - Esophageal rupture (alcoholics, Boerhaave syndrome)
  - Emphysema
  - Erosion of esophagus or trachea
  - Extension of air from pneumothorax, pneumoperitoneum, pneumoretroperitoneum
  - Fracture ribs causing lung injury
  - Gas embolism
  - High pressure environment
  - Iatrogenic following surgery
  - Iatrogenic injury to bronchus, esophagus.

**Predisposing factors for rupture of alveoli causing pneumomediastinum:**

- Aspiration pneumonia
- Bronchial asthma (status)
- Cough
- Delivery of baby
- Diabetic acidosis
- Emesis
- Exercise
- Expiratory effort against closed nose and mouth (Valsalva maneuver)
- Free-basing crack cocaine inhalation
- Fracture ribs
- Giant cell pneumonia
- Hyaline membrane disease
- Infections like measles.

## QUESTIONS

**Q1. What is Macklin effect?**
   The sequence of events during the development of pneumomediastinum is:
   ☐ Rupture of alveoli
   ☐ Air dissection along the bronchovascular sheath
   ☐ Free air reaching the mediastinum.

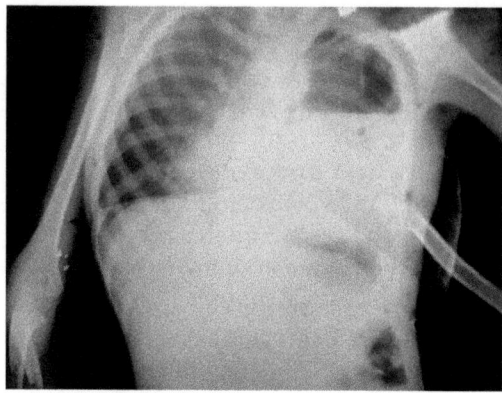

Fig. 3.13: X-ray—silhouette sign.

**Q2. What are the other areas where the air can spread?**
   ☐ Submandibular space
   ☐ Retroperitoneal space
   ☐ Vascular sheaths in the neck.

**Q3. What are the complications of pneumomediastinum?**
   ☐ Compression of great veins
   ☐ Compromise of venous return
   ☐ Hypotension
   ☐ Hypoxia due to ventilation perfusion mismatch.

### Silhouette Sign (Fig. 3.13)

Silhouette sign or loss of outline sign where the differentiation between heart borders against the adjacent lung segments are lost because it is obscured by the pathology which is in direct anatomical contact.

The borders of the organs like heart, diaphragm, etc. adjacent to the structures causing opacity will be obliterated.

## CARDIOVASCULAR SYSTEM

### Normal Heart

- *Heart position:* Major part of the heart will lie on the left side with the apex pointing toward the left. In normal heart, the right and left markings on the X-ray marked as—"R" and "L" respectively should be observed

in relation to the apex of the heart. In normal heart, the "R" marking and the liver shadow will be at the opposite side of the apex.
- *Penetration:* The vertebra should not be seen behind the heart in the posteroanterior view. If it is visible, the film may be an overpenetrated film.
- *Heart size:* Cardio-thoracic ratio (CTR) will be 50% or less.
- The diaphragm on the side of the cardiac apex will be lying at a lower level that the opposite side.
- Situs apex will be on the left side with diaphragm lying at lower level on the left side.

## Cardiac Silhouette

The normal cardiac silhouette is shown in Figure 3.14.

## Normal Heart

### X-ray—Normal Heart

Right cardiac border is formed by the following above downwards:
- Superior vena cava
- Ascending aorta
- Right atrium, which forms the major part.

*Left cardiac border* is formed by the following above downwards:
- Aortic knuckle
- Pulmonary trunk

- Left ventricle, which forms the major part.

*Cardiothoracic ratio* is the ratio of cardiac diameter (CD) to the thoracic diameter (TD). CTR is used to estimate the heart size. This is the ratio between the largest transverse diameter of the heart to the widest diameter of the chest in the posteroanterior view.

Two vertical lines are drawn down the most lateral points on each side of the heart.

$$CTR = (A + B)/C$$

Where "A" is the maximal cardiac dimension on the right of the midline and "B" is the maximal cardiac dimension on the right of the midline. "C" is the widest diameter of the chest.

Draw two vertical lines at maximum extension of both right side and left side of the heart and measure the maximum width:
- One-third lies on right
- Two-thirds lie on left
- This should be measured only in posteroanterior views.

$$CTR = a + b/c$$

"a" is the maximal width from midline to the right border

"b" is the maximal width from midline to the left border

"c" is the maximal width at the level of highest point of the right dome of the diaphragm

Normal CTR will be 0.6 in newborn babies

Normal CTR will be 0.5 in older children and adults

Supine view should not be used for measuring the CTR ratio.

Anteroposterior (AP) views should not be used for measuring CTR because of the following reasons:
- There will be magnification of cardiac shadow in AP view
- The distance between the radiational source is less.

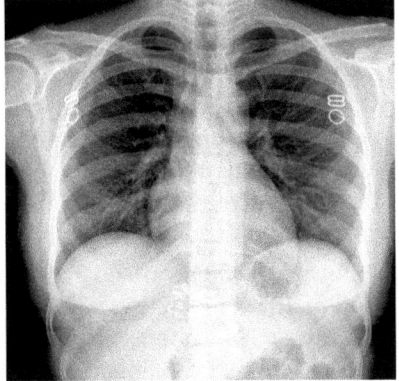

**Fig. 3.14:** Normal chest X-ray with normal heart.

Causes of false positive cardiomegaly:
- ❖ Epicardial fat
- ❖ X-ray taken in expiration.

## Heart Size

- ❖ Enlarged—congenital heart defects:
  - Myocarditis or cardiomyopathy
  - Pericardial effusion
  - Metabolic disturbance—hypoglycemia, severe hypoxemia, and acidosis
  - Overhydration or overtransfusion.
- ❖ Small.

## Position

- ❖ Two-thirds will lie on the left side in normal children and adults.
- ❖ In the midline in mesocardia, where the longitudinal axis of the heart lies in the midsaggital plane and the heart has no apex.
- ❖ Shifted to right in condition where the heart is pulled or pushed to one side.

## Abnormal Silhouette of the Heart

- ❖ Boot-shaped heart in tetralogy of Fallot (TOF)
- ❖ Egg on side appearance in transposition of the great arteries (TGA)
- ❖ Large globular heart
- ❖ Box-shaped heart in Ebstein's anomaly
- ❖ Snowman sign or appearance in TAPVD or TAPVR (supracardiac type)
- ❖ Increased or decreased pulmonary vascularity
- ❖ Dextrocardia or mesocardia
- ❖ Dextrocardia—the cardiac shadow is predominantly located in the right side of the chest
- ❖ *Dextroversion,* which is often accompanied by other cardiac malformations.

## QUESTIONS

**Q1. What is normal cardiothoracic ratio?**
Measure the width of the heart at the maximal points on both sides of midline. Also measure the maximal intrathoracic width.
The ratio between the heart and the thorax is known as CTR. The CTR in the infants will be more than 0.6. In older children and adults, it will be 0.5.

**Q2. Why cardiothoracic ratio is more in newborns?**
Cardiothoracic ratio is more in newborns because of the following factors:
- ❑ Thymic shadow
- ❑ The inspiratory expansion of lungs will be inadequate.

**Q3. When will you infer cardiomegaly on newborn and in older children and adults?**
Cardiothoracic ratio more than 50 in adults and more than 60% in newborn.

**Q4. When will you take posteroanterior (PA) view and when will you take anteroposterior view (AP)?**
For spine AP view and for heart and lung PA view.

**Q5. What are the causes of cardiomegaly?**
- ❑ Cardiac failure
- ❑ Dilated cardiomyopathy
- ❑ Pericardial effusions.

**Q6. What are the causes of peripheral pruning of pulmonary artery?**
Pulmonary hypertension.

**Q7. What is saber en boot?**
Boot-shaped heart.

**Q8. What is the cause of boot-shaped heart?**
It is due to small pulmonary artery and right ventricular hypertrophy in TOF.

**Q9. What is the view to be taken in a suspected case with isolated left ventricular enlargement?**
Lateral view will show the left ventricular enlargement.

**Q10. What are the factors used for localization of atria?**
The atria will be almost always present on the side of the liver and opposite to the fundus of the stomach.

As the sinoatrial node is always present in the right atrium P axis of the electrocardiogram (ECG) can be helpful in localization of right atria.

In situs solitus, the liver will be on the right side and stomach on the left side. In situs inversus, the liver will be on the left side and stomach on the right side.

**Q11. What are the factors used for localization of the apex of the heart?**

The diaphragm will be lying low on the side of the apex of the heart. The diaphragm is not elevated due to the liver but the dome is low on the side of the apex of the heart.

**Q12. What are the conditions associated with the following?**
- Saber en boot—boot-shaped heart
- Figure of 8
- Snowman appearance
- Money bag appearance
- Egg on side appearance.

*Saber en boot—boot shaped heart*: Due to small pulmonary artery and right ventricular hypertrophy in TOF.

*Figure of 8*—TAPVC/TAPVR return

*Snowman appearance*—TAPVC/TAPVR

*Money bag appearance*—pericardial effusion

*Egg on side appearance*—TGA

Radiological appearance and conditions associated with:

| Radiological appearance | Conditions |
| --- | --- |
| Figure of 8 appearance or snowman appearance | TAPVC/TAPVR (supracardiac type) |
| Egg on side appearance (egg-shaped heart with narrow base) | TGA |
| Globular heart | Dilated cardiomyopathy normal up to 5-7 years of age |
| Sitting duck appearance | Truncus arteriosus |

*Contd...*

*Contd...*

| Radiological appearance | Conditions |
| --- | --- |
| Box-shaped heart | Ebstein's anomaly (due to gross dilatation of right atrium) |
| Peripheral pruning of pulmonary vessels | Pulmonary hypertension |
| Bag of money appearance or money bag appearance | Pericardial effusion |
| Jug handle appearance | Atrial septal defect (ASD) |
| Saber en boot appearance | TOF |
| Leather bottle appearance | Pericardial effusion |
| Scimitar sign | Scimitar syndrome |
| Double atrial shadow Shadow within shadow | Mitral stenosis (MS) |
| Hilar dance on fluoroscopy | ASD |
| Inverted three sign on barium studies | Coarctation of aorta |
| Cardiomegaly– cardiothoracic ratio> 60 (in adults 50 is significant) | • Cardiac failure<br>• Cardiomyopathy (dilated)<br>• Pleural effusion |
| Air around the heart | Pneumopericardium |

- Congestive cardiac failure—cardiomegaly
- Pulmonary hypertension—heart size will be normal
- Prominent main pulmonary artery (MPA) segment dilated hilar vessels with clear lung fields.

## Dextrocardia (Fig. 3.15)

### Discussion

- Dexter—right
- Kardia—heart

The apex of the heart faces to the right side.

### Embryology

- Primitive cardiac loop will bend to the right by 22–23 days of gestation.
- By next 10–12 days cardiac septation will occur and the apex of heart will migrate to the right side of the thorax to lie in the left chest pointing leftward. When this migration does not occur, it results in dextrocardia.

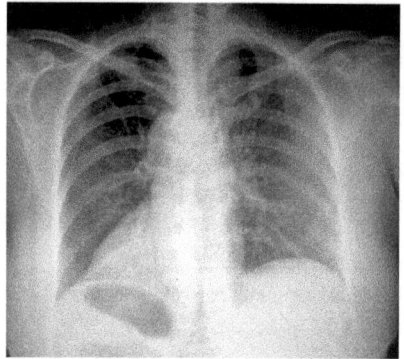

**Fig. 3.15:** X-ray of dextrocardia with situs inversus.

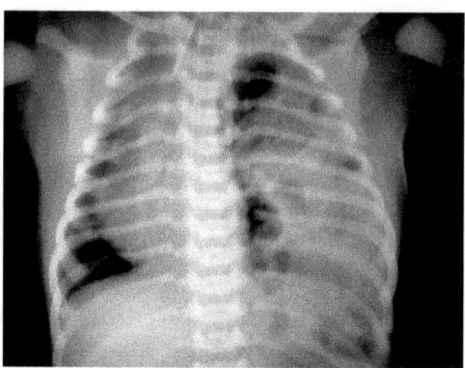

**Fig. 3.16:** X-ray of dextroposition.

- Dextroversion, dextrorotation, and pivotal dextrocardia are synonyms with dextrocardia with situs solitus.
- Dextroposition is the heart shifted right side by external means
- *Mixed dextrocardia* is dextrocardia with atrioventricular discordance.

*Types*
- Isolated dextrocardia due to embryonic arrest
- Dextrocardia associated with situs inversus.

*Causes*
- Isolated
- Situs inversus
- *Dextroposition (Fig. 3.16)*—due to intrinsic causes—pleural or lung pathology like fibrosis, pleural effusion, eventration of diaphragm, and pneumothorax. Dextroposition in conditions like fibrosis the heart is pulled to the right side and there is no rotation of the heart.
- *Dextroversion*—which is often accompanied by other cardiac malformations *Dextroversion* is location of heart on the right side without inversion of cardiac chambers. This consists of rotation of ventricles of heart like turning of a page of the book with the atria remaining in normal position.
- *Dextrocardia*—in dextrocardia, the apex of the heart faces to the right side

- *Mesocardia*—the cardiac shadow is predominantly located in the midline of the chest
- *Mirror image dextrocardia*—the anterior posterior relationship of various parts of the heart is normal but the right left orientation is reversed.

**Situs Inversus Totalis**

Situs inversus totalis is associated with mirror image of anatomic configuration of atria, lungs, and abdominal viscera.

*Radiological Findings*
- The cardiac apex will be on the right side
- The stomach will be on the right side
- The liver will be on the left side
- The diaphragm will be at lower level on the side of the apex of the heart. Hence in situs inversus, the diaphragm on the right side and will be lower than the left side
- In chest X-ray with normal heart, the diaphragm will be higher of the right side than the left. This is not due to liver on the right side, but the apex on the left side (Fig. 3.16).

## QUESTIONS

Q1. What is situs?
Situs is orientation of the cardiac atria, central bronchial pattern and anatomy of lungs, and location of upper abdominal viscera in relation to midline.

## Q2. What are the types of situs inversus?
- *Situs inversus solitus:*
  - Apex right side
  - Liver right side
  - Stomach left side
  - Dome of diaphragm on the right side lie lower that left.
- *Situs inversus totalis:*
  - Apex right side
  - Liver left side
  - Stomach right side
  - Dome of diaphragm on the right side will lie lower that left.

## Q3. What is situs solitus?
- The atrium is on the right
- Right lung is trilobed and the left is bilobed
- Liver, gallbladder, and inferior vena cava (IVC) are on the right side
- Stomach, spleen, and aorta are on the left side.

## Q4. How will you identify the side of cardiac apex?
The diaphragm will lie on the lower level at the side of the apex than the opposite side.

## Atrial Septal Defect
X-ray chest findings in ASD are:
- Apex is occupied by the dilated right ventricle
- Bilateral pulmonary plethora due to increased pulmonary vasculature
- Bilateral atrial and ventricular enlargement in large shunt due to ASD
- Border is rarely formed by ascending aorta
- Cardiac enlargement due to right atrial enlargement and right ventricular enlargement
- Dilated pulmonary trunk
- Dilatation of superior vena cava (SVC) in sinus venosus type
- Enlarged right pulmonary artery (disproportionate enlargement)
- Enlarged right ventricle
- Filling of retrosternal space due to right ventricular enlargement (in lateral view)

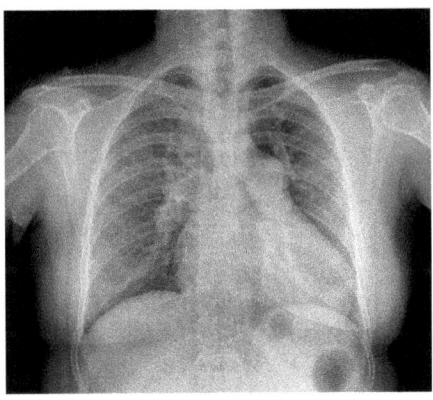

**Fig. 3.17:** Jug handle appearance in atrial septal defect.

- Gross enlargement of pulmonary artery—external diameter of right pulmonary artery is more than that of internal diameter of trachea
- Hilar dance—on fluoroscopy there is pulsation of the pulmonary arteries
- Increased pulmonary vascularity (pulmonary plethora) arteries enlarged and appear to extend into lateral one-third of lung, increased vascularity to the lung, where they appear collapsed normally
- Inconspicuous aortic shadow (so small aortic shadow)
- Jug-handle appearance (dilated right atrium, ventricle, and pulmonary arteries with less prominent aortic knuckle)
- Prominent MPA segment
- Left ventricular silhouette is seen posteriorly
- Increased prominence of right lower cardiac silhouette due to right atrial enlargement (Fig. 3.17).

## QUESTIONS

**Q1. What are the types of ASD?**
- Ostium secundum (most frequent)
- Ostium primum is located in the lower portion of the septum.
- Patent foramen ovale

- Sinus venosus type:
  - Superior vena caval type
  - Inferior vena caval type.
- Coronary sinus ASD (least common).

**Q2. What is the hemodynamics in ASD?**

The blood from SVC and IVC
↓
Right atrium
↓
Right ventricle
↓
Pulmonary arteries
↓
After oxygenation in the lungs blood enters the left atrium through the pulmonary veins
↓
Left ventricle
↓
Aorta

If the ASD is relatively large, the pressure gradient will be small. As the pressure in the left atrium is slightly higher than the right atrium, blood will flow from the left atrium to the right atrium causing volume overload to the right ventricle.

**Q3. What are the complications of ASD?**
- Atrial fibrillation
- Bacterial endocarditis (rare in ASD)
- Cardiac arrhythmias
- Decompression sickness in divers because inert gases like helium and nitrogen do not pass through the lungs where they will be exhaled
- Eisenmenger's syndrome—reversal of shunt
- Frequent lung infections—recurrent respiratory tract infections
- Heart failure—right-sided cardiac failure
- Increased risk for cerebrovascular accident or stroke
- Pulmonary arterial hypertension
- Paradoxical embolus
- These complications are seen more commonly in the adult life.

**Q4. What are the contraindications for closure of ASD?**
- Significant shunt Qp-Qs ratio 0.7 or below
- Severe pulmonary hypertension
- Irreversible pulmonary vaso-occlusive disease
- Shunt reversal—Eisenmenger's syndrome.

**Q5. Name few conditions associated with ASD.**
- Down syndrome
- Ebstein's anomaly
- Fetal alcohol syndrome
- Holt–Oram syndrome—both ostium secundum and ostium primum defects are associated
- Lutembacher syndrome—ASD with acquired mitral stenosis.

## Tetralogy of Fallot

### Radiological Findings in Tetralogy of Fallot

❖ Apex of heart lifted due to right ventricular hypertrophy the left ventricle is lifted away from the left dome of diaphragm.
  - Boot-shaped heart (Coeur en sabot) the concavity at MPA segment is due to pulmonary oligemia, underdeveloped MPA. "Boot-shaped heart" is due to hypoplasia of pulmonary truck and elevation of apex due to right ventricular hypertrophy.

❖ Conspicuously clear lung fields (black lung fields) due to pulmonary oligemia.
  - Concavity of the pulmonary artery due to pulmonary artery stenosis. A distinct concavity between the aortic knuckle and the ventricle due to hypoplasia of the pulmonary artery.
  - Cardiothoracic ratio normal—normal sized heart or small heart. No cardiomegaly

# Radiology—X-rays

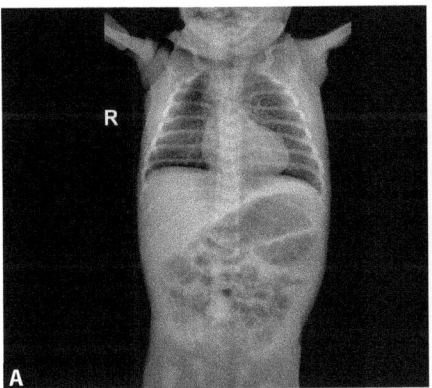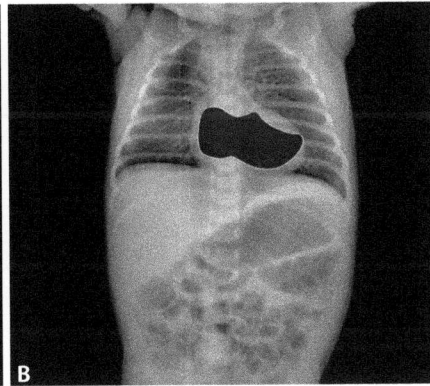

**Figs. 3.18A and B:** (A) TOF X-ray shows upturned apex due to Right ventricular hypertrophy. Pulmonary bay is obliterated due to pulmonary oligemia; (B) Boot-shaped heart in tetralogy of Fallot.

- Decreased pulmonary vascular markings (pulmonary oligemia).
- Enlargement of right atrium (occasionally)
- Enlargement of right ventricle (Figs. 3.18A and B).

## QUESTIONS

**Q1. What is Coeur en Sabot?**
Boot-shaped heart—hypertrophy of the right ventricle displacing the left ventricle upwards and to the left, there by producing the appearance of a wooden shoe with an upturned toe—the "Coeur en sabot".

**Q2. What will be X-ray finding in TOF with collaterals?**
Reticulogranular pattern of the lung fields.

**Q3. What is the cause of rib erosions in TOF?**
It is due to the erosion by the development of collaterals between systemic and pulmonary circulation.

**Q4. What is the cause of unilateral rib erosions in TOF?**
On the side of Blalock-Taussig operation due to development of collaterals.

**Q5. What is the cause of unilateral pulmonary oligemia?**
Left-sided unilateral pulmonary oligemia is due to absence of left pulmonary artery.

**Q6. What are the components of TOF?**
- ❏ Infundibular spasm
- ❏ High VSD
- ❏ Overriding of aorta
- ❏ Right ventricular hypertrophy.

**Q7. What are the abnormalities associated with TOF?**
Right-sided aortic arch is seen—25–30% of cases.

**Q8. What is the hemodynamics in TOF?**

The blood from SVC and IVC
↓
Right atrium
↓
Right ventricle
↓
Pulmonary arteries
↓
After oxygenation in the lungs
↓
Blood enters the left atrium through the pulmonary veins
↓
Left ventricle → Aorta

## Mitral Stenosis

Radiological findings in X-ray chest (postero-anterior view) in mitral stenosis:
- Aortic knob small
- Bulge of left heart border immediately below the left main bronchus
- Bedford's sign the enlarged left main bronchus can deviate the middle descending aorta to the left
- Cardiomegaly (due to right ventricular enlargement)
- Compression of carina
- Carina splayed
- Double shadow of right atrium (shadow with in the shadow) the dilated left atrium causes a shadow in the upper and outer border while that of the right ventricle causes a shadow in the lower and inner border. Posterior displacement of barium in the esophagus in a right anterior oblique view of barium swallows)
- Dilatation of the pulmonary veins (antler or inverted moustache sign) due to increased pressure in the left atrium, the apical lines are more prominent like moustaches
- Enlargement of left atrial appendage
- Elevation of the left upper lobe bronchus
- Straightening of the left border of the heart is due to the dilated left atrial appendage and the pulmonary artery. Also the aortic knuckle and left ventricle will be small. This is also called as mitralization of the heart (Fig. 3.19).
- Features of pulmonary hypertension are prominent pulmonary artery, dilatation of the pulmonary artery near the hilum and pruning of the pulmonary artery at the peripheries.
- Features of pulmonary venous congestion:
    - Kerley B lines these are fine, dense horizontal lines in the base of the lung (in the costophrenic angles) due to stagnation of the blood causing distension of the interlobular septa and the lymphatics. They can be seen up to 4 cm

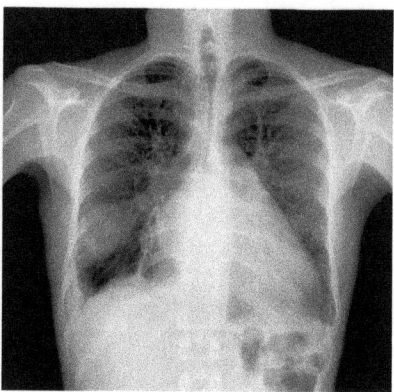

**Fig. 3.19:** Mitral stenosis with straightening of left heart border (Mitralization).

- Kerley A lines—at apex
- Kerley B lines—basal at the costophrenic angle
- Kerley C lines are fine network of interlacing linear shadows seen at the hilar or basal region.

Redistribution of pulmonary blood flow to the upper lobes will result in inverted mustache sign:
- Features of pulmonary hemosiderosis—multiple small opacities
- Calcification of the mitral valve
- X-ray chest lateral view will show double density due to left atrial enlargement
- Atrial appendage (left) prominent
- Elevation of left main bronchus due to left atrial enlargement
- *Barium studies* will show indentation of esophagus on the right by the enlarged left atrium.

## QUESTION

**Q1. What are the differences between Kerley A lines and Kerley B lines?**
Kerley A lines radiate from hilum. They are 2–6 cm in length.

Kerley B lines are seen in base of the lungs and are perpendicular to the pleura. They are 1–3 cm in length.

# Radiology—X-rays

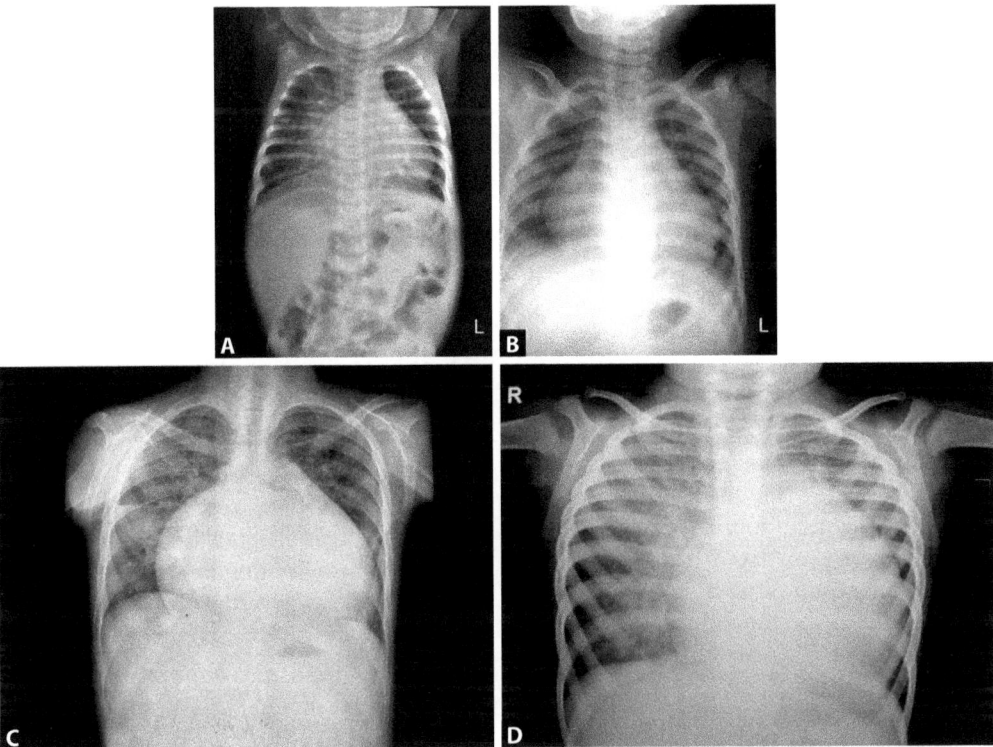

**Figs. 3.20A to D:** (A and B) Cardiomegaly; (C) Cardiomegaly—leather bottle appearance; (D) Massive cardiomegaly with pulmonary plethora.

## Cardiomegaly

### Criteria for Cardiomegaly in Adults and Children

The CTR of more than 50% in older children and adults will be considered as cardiomegaly.

In newborns a CTR of more than 60% will be considered as cardiomegaly (Figs. 3.20A to D).

### X-ray Chest Showing Cardiomegaly

Cardiomegaly may be due to involvement of any of the following structures in the pericardial sac:
* Cardiac chambers—ventricular dilatation
* Cardiac wall—ventricular hypertrophy
* Pericardial space—pericardial effusion
* Additional structures—tumors.

## QUESTIONS

**Q1. What are the causes of cardiomegaly in newborn?**
- Congestive cardiac failure (CHD with left-to-right shunts with failure)
- Myocarditis
- Dilated cardiomyopathy
- Ebstein's anomaly
- Endocardial cushion defects
- Hypertrophic cardiomyopathy
- Pericardial effusion
- Pulmonary hypertension.

**Q2. What are the radiological features of cardiac failure?**
- Cardiomegaly
- Pulmonary congestion.

**Q3. What is congestive heart failure (CHF)?**

Congestive heart failure is a clinical syndrome in which the heart is unable to supply an output sufficient to meet the metabolic requirement of the tissues.

## Transpositions of Great Vessels

Aorta and pulmonary artery arise from inappropriate ventricles. This is due to failure of development of spiral septum, which separates the truncus into aorta and pulmonary artery to follow a spiral course (Fig. 3.21).

- ❖ Aorta lies anterior to pulmonary artery, pulmonary artery located posteriorly
- ❖ Aorta lies in the midline (midline aorta)
- ❖ Bulge along the upper left cardiac border produces by inverted aorta and right ventricular outflow tract. Ascending aorta with convexity to the right
- ❖ Border or left ventricle will be more straight than usual
- ❖ Cardiomegaly (after 2 weeks of life) due to right heart enlargement
- ❖ Convexity of right atrial border
- ❖ Decreased size of aorta
- ❖ Enlargement of left atrium (if VSD is present)
- ❖ Egg on side or egg of a string appearance
- ❖ Great arteries arise from ventricles in parallel fashion

Hypoplastic thymus—narrow superior mediastinum due to hypoplastic thymus, hyperaeration, abnormal relationship of aorta, and pulmonary artery.

- ❖ Increased pulmonary flow
- ❖ Juxtapositioning of the atrial appendages—right atrial appendage lying above the left atrial appendage.

## QUESTIONS

Q1. **What is corrected TGA?**
Transposition of the great arteries (TGA) with inversion of ventricles.

Q2. **What are the conditions associated with TGA?**
- ❑ Ventricular septal defect
- ❑ Pulmonary stenosis.

Q3. **What is the medical treatment for TGA?**
Prostaglandin E 1 administration to maintain the ductus arteriosus patent.

Q4. **What is the surgical treatment for TGA?**
Rashkind procedure balloon septoplasty creating an ASD. Mustard operation an intra-atrial baffle is created thereby diverting the pulmonary venous return to the right ventricle and systemic venous return to the left ventricle.

## Total Anomalous Pulmonary Venous Return (TAPVR) or Total Anomalous Pulmonary Venous Connection (TAPVC) or Total Anomalous Pulmonary Venous Drainage (TAPVD)

Total anomalous pulmonary venous return type I supracardiac type.

### Radiological Findings

- ❖ Abnormal soft tissue shadows
- ❖ Bilateral lungs will be clear:
  - Cardiomegaly
  - Dumbbell sign
  - Enlarged vertical vein

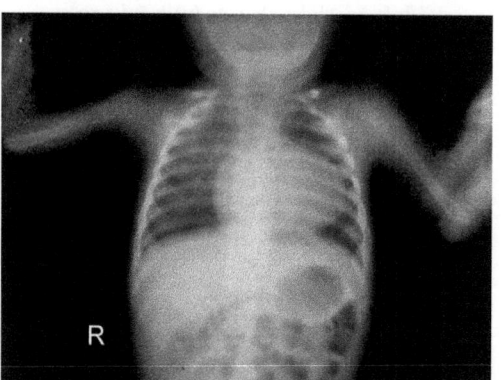

**Fig. 3.21:** Egg on side appearance.

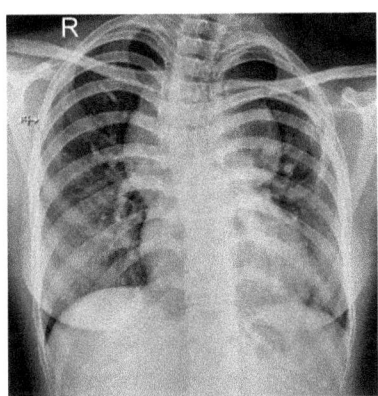

**Fig. 3.22:** Figure of 8 appearance in total anomalous pulmonary venous return.

- Figure of 8 appearance—bilateral paratracheal shadows due to dilatation of right vena cava, innominate vein and ascending vertical vein (Fig. 3.22)
- Increased pulmonary vasculature.
- Figure of 8 sign or snowman sign or dumbbell sign or cottage leaf of bread heart
- Heart and the superior mediastinal structures will resemble snowman
- Entire pulmonary blood flow is directed to the right atrium via superior vena cava.
- Three prominent vessels will form the head of the snowman:
  1. Prominent SVC on the right
  2. Innominate vessels, left brachiocephalic vein superiorly in the midline above the heart
  3. Dilated vertical vein on the left side.
- The enlarged right atrium of the heart forms the body of the snowman.

## QUESTIONS

**Q1. What is snowman in snow storm sign?**
Supracardiac TAPVC with pulmonary plethora.

**Q2. What is the defect in TAPVC?**
It is due to the failure of common pulmonary vein to join the posterior wall of left atrium.

**Q3. What are the conditions associated with TAPVC?**
TAPVC is associated with the following:
- Asplenia
- Atrial septal defect—patent foramen ovale
- Arteriovenous malformation (pulmonary)
- Bronchopulmonary sequestration
- Congenital pulmonary adenomatoid malformation (CPAM).

**Q4. What are the types of TAPVC?**
- Supracardiac
- Cardiac
- Infracardiac
- Mixed.

## Coarctation of Aorta

### X-ray Findings in Coarctation of Aorta

- Aortic knob—large for age and convex
- Ascending aorta prominent
- Bilateral rib notching—rib notching between fourth and eighth ribs. This will be seen later and is rare under 5 years of age. Unilateral right rib notching is seen, if the coarctation of aorta (COA) is distal to brachiocephalic trunk and proximal to the origin of left subclavian artery or right sided aortic arch with aberrant left subclavian artery. Unilateral left rib notching is seen, if the COA is associated with aberrant right subclavian artery arising after the coarctation (Fig. 3.23)
- Cardiomegaly—heart size may be normal or increased due to left ventricular enlargement
- Dilatation of ascending aorta may be seen
- Dilatation of descending aorta (poststenotic dilatation)
- Dilatation of right atrium, right ventricle, and left atrium
- Dock sign—rib notching
- E or reverse three sign—mirror image of E sign in the barium filled esophagus. It is due to indentation of the barium filled

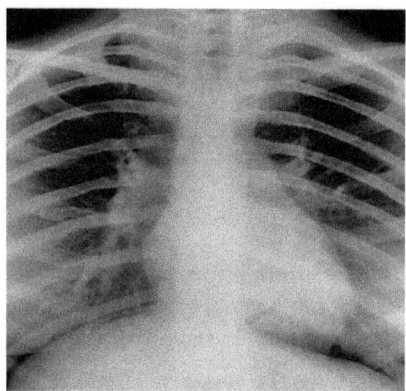

**Fig. 3.23:** Coarctation of aorta inferior rib notching.

esophagus by the left subclavian artery and distal aorta
- Erosion of ribs due to collaterals (rarely the erosions may be seen from the age of 2 years)
- Figure of three sign in overpenetrated films. It is due to dilatation of the left subclavian artery and distal aorta and pinching at the site of coarctation
- Flat and small aortic knuckle
- Pulmonary congestion may be present
- Left ventricle will be normal in size.

## QUESTIONS

**Q1. What are the three adaptive mechanisms in a case with coarctation of aorta?**
- Elevation of systolic blood pressure in the aortic segment proximal the coarctation
- Vasoconstriction in the arterioles to maintain an high diastolic pressure
- Development of collaterals.

**Q2. What are the blood pressure changes in a case with coarctation of aorta?**
- Both systolic and diastolic pressures will be elevated in the upper limbs
- Systolic pressure will be low and diastolic pressure will be high in the lower limbs
- Rib erosions are seen over the posterior part of the ribs. Rib erosions are rare before 6 years of age.

**Q3. What are the sites in which rib erosions are seen in COA below the left subclavian artery?**
Between third and eight ribs, it is rarely seen above second or below ninth ribs.

**Q4. What are the sites in which rib erosions are seen in COA at the level of the left subclavian artery obliterating it?**
Rib erosions will not be seen on that side but will be seen on the opposite side.

**Q5. What are the sites in which rib erosions are seen in COA anomalous origin of the subclavian artery in the right side?**
Rib erosions will not be seen on the right side, but will be seen on the left side.

**Q6. In which condition of COA lower ribs will be eroded?**
In COA, in the abdominal aorta.

**Q7. What is the cause of retrosternal notching?**
It is due to dilatation of internal mammary artery.

**Q8. What are the defects associated with COA?**
- Bicuspid aortic valve
- Ventricular septal defect
- Atrial septal defect
- Transposition of great vessels
- Hypoplastic mitral valve.

**Q9. What is the syndrome associated with coarctation of aorta?**
Turner's syndrome.

**Q10. What are the complications of coarctation of aorta?**
- Aneurysms—mycotic
- Berry aneurysms
- Bleeding in subarachnoid space
- Congestive cardiac failure
- Dissection of aorta
- Endocarditis.

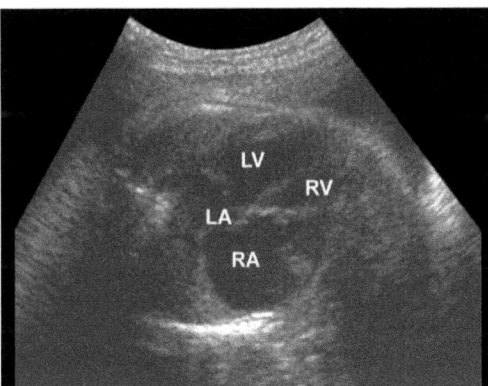

**Fig. 3.24:** Ebstein X-ray anomaly on ECHO picture.

## Ebstein Anomaly

There will be downward displacement of the septal and posterior leaflet of dysplastic tricuspid valve. This results in atrialization of right ventricle.

### Ultrasonogram of Ebstein X-ray Anomaly (Fig. 3.24)

- Atrial enlargement—right atrial enlargement
- Aortic root small
- Box like cardiomegaly
- Compression of adjacent lungs
- Cardiothoracic ratio is more (even up to >95%)
- Calcification of tricuspid valve can occur
- Diminished pulmonary vascular markings
- Distorted right ventricle
- Dilated right ventricle
- Dilated right ventricular outflow tract
- Extreme cardiomegaly
- Elongated right atrium
- Funnel-like cardiomegaly.

## QUESTIONS

**Q1. What is Ebstein's anomaly?**
Ebstein's anomaly is a condition where there is atrialization of right ventricle due to malposition of tricuspid valve leaflet.

**Q2. What is the teratogenic agent that can cause Ebstein anomaly?**
Lithium given to the mother during antenatal period can cause Ebstein anomaly in the fetus.

## RESPIRATORY SYSTEM

### Infections

#### Pneumonia

**Radiological findings of pneumonia:**

- Alveolar infiltrates, patchy of varying size
- Atelectasis
- Consolidation
- Haziness
- Heart border will not be seen clearly
- Patchy shadows are not limited by interlobar fissures (in lobar pneumonia, the shadows will be limited by interlobar fissures)
- No loss of lung volume
- No mediastinal shift.

*X-ray features* vary upon the causative agents.
The radiological findings will give a clue to the etiology of pneumonia (Table 3.1).

**Bilateral involvement:**

| | |
|---|---|
| Interstitial pneumonia | Viral |
| Interstitial pneumonia in immunosuppressed host | *Pneumocystis carinii* |

Pneumonitis in the right upper lobe may be seen in aspiration (Fig. 3.25).
Interstitial reticular opacities may be seen.
Viral infections will predominantly affect the airways.
Round pneumonia will be seen as round shadow. It is seen in *Mycoplasma pneumonia*.

## QUESTIONS

**Q1. What are the features of group B streptococcal (GBS) pneumonia?**
Group B streptococcal (GBS) is the most common organism causing pneumonia in newborns.

**Table 3.1:** X-ray showing radiological findings in various types of pneumonia.

| Types of pneumonia | Radiological changes |
|---|---|
| Pneumococcal pneumonia caused by *Streptococcus pneumoniae* | • Acute lobar pneumonia<br>• Air bronchogram<br>• Small synpneumonic effusion<br>• Cavitation rare<br>• No loss of lung volume |
| *Haemophilus influenzae* | Lobar consolidation with pleural effusion |
| Aspiration | • Right upper lobe pneumonia<br>• Heterogeneous opacities |
| Tuberculous | • Hilar adenopathy<br>• Bronchopneumonia<br>• Cavitations<br>• Upper lobe pneumonia |
| Chemical pneumonitis | Lower lobe pneumonia |
| Partial bronchial obstruction | Right middle lobe |
| *Staphylococcus aureus* | • Abscess (multiple small)<br>• Bilateral involvement<br>• Cavitation<br>• Decreased lung volume<br>• Effusions (early and large)<br>• Empyema, resolution slow<br>• Fibrosis (residual) can occur<br>• Pneumatocele |
| *Klebsiella pneumoniae* (Friedlander's pneumonia) | • Abscesses<br>• Air bronchogram<br>• Air crescent sign (mass within a mass) due to lung necrosis<br>• Bronchopneumonic pattern<br>• Cavitation<br>• Displacement of adjacent structures<br>• Extensive lobar consolidation<br>• Edema<br>• Effusion<br>• Fissure (oblique) bulges interiorly and inferiorly (bulging fissure sign) due to increased volume (gangrene is a complication)<br>• Ground-glass opacity<br>• Homogenous parenchymal consolidation<br>• Increased lung volume<br>• Right side is commonly affected<br>• Upper lobe is commonly involved |
| *Mycoplasma pneumonia* | • Patchy/nodular/peribronchial consolidation<br>• Homogenous opacities<br>• Slow progression to sublobar or lobar consolidation |

The radiological findings will resemble hyaline membrane disease (HMD).

**Q2. What is the difference in radiological finding between group B streptococcal GBS pneumonia and hyaline membrane disease (HMD)?**

The lung volume will be increased in GBS whereas it will be decreased in HMD.

**Q3. What is Loeffler's pneumonia?**

It is also known as eosinophilic pneumonia and is due to allergic reaction to variety of agents like drugs, worm infestations, etc. This is characterized by widespread

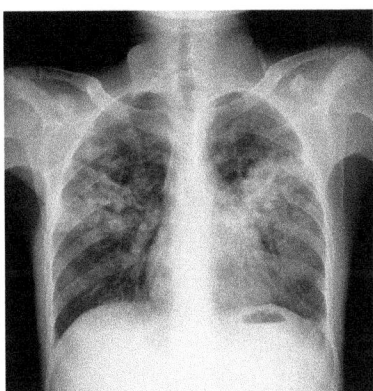

**Fig. 3.25:** Bilateral consolidation.

transitory pulmonary infiltrates resembling military mottling. Localized pneumonic consolidation may be seen in few cases. This condition is associated with eosinophilia.

**Q4. What are the risk factors for *Klebsiella pneumonia*?**
- Alcoholics
- Antimicrobial therapy
- Bacteremia
- Cancer patients
- *Comorbidities*—kidney disorders, chronic liver disease
- Diabetes
- Dialysis patients
- Elderly
- Fluoroquinolones (ciprofloxacin)
- Graft functions delayed (organ transplantation)
- Hospital-acquired
- Immunodeficiency
- Invasive devices, catheters (urinary, central, venous), procedures, and ventilators
- Intensive care unit stay.

Limit use of antibiotics like fluoroquinolones, cephalosporins, carbapenems, colistin, metronidazole, and vancomycin.

## Consolidation

Consolidation is a region of normally aerated lung tissue filled with liquid. Consolidation is a radiological sign. The alveolar space contains fluid instead of air. The fluid can be water, pus, fluid, or blood.

### Radiological findings in consolidation:
- Air alveologram
- *Air bronchogram*—As alveoli is filled with fluid, the air in the bronchus will be clearly visualized
- Borders (upper) will not be clear
- Coalescent opacities
- Confluent, cloud-like opacities
- Costophrenic and cardiophrenic angles will be free
- Dense opacity
- Diffuse consolidation
- Extension to the pleural surface
- Fleeting/labile changes
- Haziness or white lung at the affected part of the lung
- Ill-defined opacities
- Margins may be limited by fissure (unlike pneumonia where the shadows are not limited by fissures)
- Normally aerated pulmonary parenchyma
- No loss of lung volume
- No mediastinal shift.

### Consolidation of right upper lobe (Figs. 3.26 and 3.27):
- Dense opacity in the right upper lobe
- No shift of mediastinum
- Air bronchogram
- Upper border will not be clear
- Lower border is formed by horizontal fissure
- Silhouette sign is positive

### Clinical findings in consolidation of right upper lobe (Fig. 3.28):
- No shift in the mediastinum
- Chest expansion will be diminished on the affected side
- Percussion will be dull
- Vocal fremitus will be increased
- Bronchial breath sounds
- Medium, late, or pan-inspiratory crackles
- Vocal resonance will be increased.

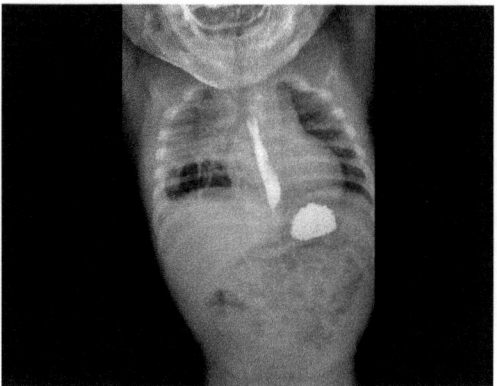

**Fig. 3.26:** Gastroesophageal reflux (GER) with right upper lobe consolidation due to aspiration.

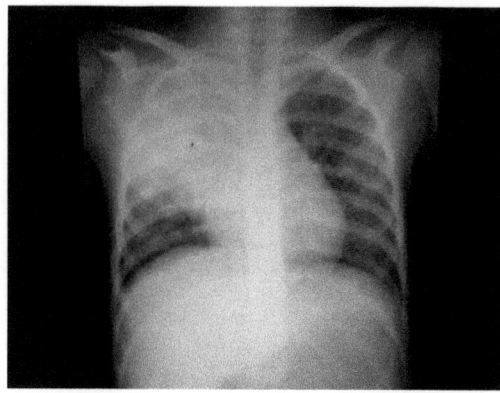

**Fig. 3.28:** Right upper lobe consolidation.

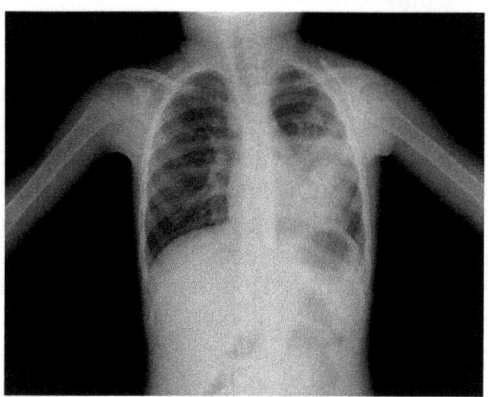

**Fig. 3.27:** Left lingular consolidation with air bronchogram

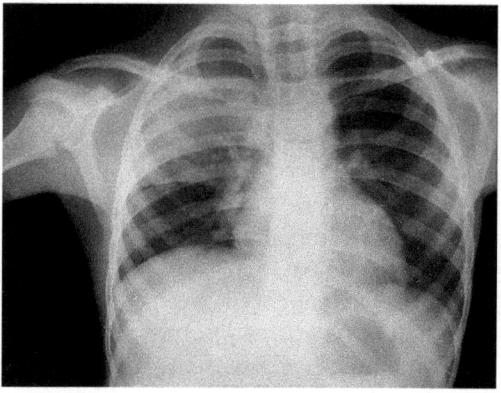

**Fig. 3.29:** Right middle lobe consolidation with well-defined margins at the right fissure.

## QUESTIONS

**Q1. What is the CT scan finding in consolidation?**

CT angiogram sign—vessels can be seen through the consolidation.

**Q2. What are the differences between ground-glass opacity and consolidation?**

In ground-glass opacity, there will be increase in lung attenuation without obscuration of underlying vessels. But in consolidation, increase in lung attenuation with obscuration of underlying vessels.

**Lobar consolidation:** Lobar consolidation is due to collection of inflammatory exudates within the intra-alveolar space (Fig. 3.29).

The consolidation will be confined to one lobe. The alveolar spaces in the lobe of lungs are filled with fluid like exudates, transudate, or blood. Peripheral wedge-shaped shadow in the medial segment of the middle lobe or lingular lobe will be seen.

**Radiological features:**
- Air bronchogram due to air in the bronchus
- Bronchi will be spared
- Bulging fissure sign may be seen with fissures are convex outward
- Confined to particular lobes (lobar pattern)

- Defined margins at the fissures or ill-defined borders at early stages due to spread through pore of Kohn
- Expansion decreased on the affected side due to atelectasis with collapse
- Fissures will limit the opacity
- Homogenous opacification.

**Radiological findings in middle lobe syndrome:**
- Opacificaton of right lobe
- Air bronchograms
- Atelectasis
- Right middle lobe collapse may be associated
- Indistinct right heart border.

**Lateral X-ray:** Wedge-shaped opacity extending anteriorly and inferiorly from the hilum (seen in lateral film).

**Differential diagnosis:**
- Pneumonia
- Pulmonary edema
- Atelectasis
- Pneumonia.

# QUESTIONS

**Q1. What is bulging fissure sign?**
The fissures will be seen bulging out due to fluid in the alveoli.

**Q2. What is Brock syndrome?**
It is atelectasis of right middle lobe of lung—middle lobe bronchiectasis (Brock syndrome). The right middle lobe bronchus is externally compressed by the enlarged lymph nodes or collateral or internally compressed by right middle lobe bronchus.

**Q3. Why right middle lobe is commonly involved?**
The right middle lobe is commonly involved because:
- It is surrounded by lymph nodes
- It originates in a narrow slit-like lumen (fish mouth appearance even in normal children)
- The right middle lobe bronchus runs a long course. The right middle lobe is separated from the upper and lower lobes by fissures and lacks collateral ventilation.

**Q4. What is the most common cause of lobar pneumonia?**
Bacterial infection especially pneumococcal pneumonia due to *Streptococcus pneumoniae*.

Other organisms like *Klebsiella, Legionella, Haemophilus influenzae,* and *Mycobacterium tuberculosis* also can cause lobar pneumonia.

**Q5. What are the four stages of lobar pneumonia?**
1. Stage of congestion in the first 24 hours
2. Stage of red hepatization of consolidation due to extravasation of red blood cells into the alveoli
3. Stage of gray hepatization appears as the red cells in the alveoli disintegrate
4. Stage of resolution where complete recovery occurs.

**Q6. What are the complications of lobar consolidation?**
- Parapneumonic effusion
- Empyema.

**Q7. What is middle lobe syndrome?**
Obstruction will cause atelectasis which results in wedge-shaped opacity best seen in lateral X-rays of chest.

Right middle lobe syndrome—endobronchial obstruction is the most common cause of middle lobe syndrome.

**Q8. What is the difference between pneumonia and lobar pneumonia?**
In pneumonia, there will be patchy area of consolidation. In lobar pneumonia, entire lobe or lung will be affected.

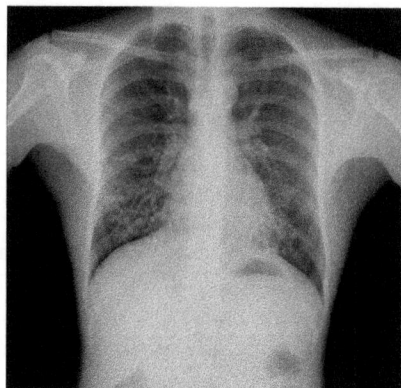

**Fig. 3.30:** Bronchiectasis left lower lobe.

### Bronchiectasis (Fig. 3.30)

X-ray findings in bronchiectasis:

X-ray of chest:

- *Railroad tracks*—Marked linear streaking and loss of volume (crowding of ribs)
- Atelectasis (due to mucous plugging)
- Bronchovascular markings are less clear or lost. Normal at other parts of lung
- Bronchial wall thickening
- Branching band shadows pointing toward the hilum
- Beaded appearance in varicose bronchiectasis
- Crowding of bronchi due to loss of lung volume/atelectasis
- Cystic spaces more than 2 mm (sometimes may contain air-fluid levels)
- Curvilinear opacities due to peribronchial thickening
- Dilated of air-filled bronchi
- Density in the background is increased
- *Emphysema*—Compensatory overinflation of other uninvolved segments of the lung
- End on view of dilated bronchi—ring shadows
- Fluid may be seen in cystic bronchiectasis
- Foreign body, if radiopaque can be seen
- Gloved finger appearance
- Honeycomb appearance may be seen only in advanced severe cases. Multiple cystic lesions of varying sizes, seen as circular or polygonal translucent areas surrounded by dense and linear shadows.
- Tram-track opacity or signet ring sign—Linear lucencies
- Clustered cysts in cystic bronchiectasis, thick-walled bronchi appear much larger, and appear like large ring shadows.
- No mediastinal shift.

**Discussion—bronchiectasis:** Abnormal persistent dilatation of bronchial tree is due to destruction of the elastic and muscular components of the bronchial walls.

Three mechanisms result in bronchiectasis:
1. Airway obstruction
2. Infection
3. Fibrosis

High-resolution computed tomography (HRCT) is the most sensitive test.

## QUESTIONS

**Q1. What is bronchiectasis?**

It refers to permanent dilatation of the bronchi due to inflammatory destruction of bronchial and peribronchial tissues. There will be a persistent and irreversible destruction, distortion, and dilatation of bronchioles of more than 2 mm in diameter.

**Q2. What are the infections associated with bronchiectasis?**
- ❑ Measles
- ❑ *Bordetella pertussis* (whooping cough)
- ❑ Endobronchial tuberculosis
- ❑ Bronchitis.

**Q3. What are the causes of bronchial obstruction?**
- ❑ *Luminal causes.*
  - ➤ Intraluminal foreign body
  - ➤ Aspiration of foreign body.
- ❑ *On the wall of the tracheobronchial tree:*
  - ➤ Bronchial asthma
  - ➤ Tumors.
- ❑ *Outside the wall*:
  - ➤ Lymph nodes
  - ➤ Left atrial enlargement

- Aneurysms
- Allergy.

**Q4. What are the predisposing factors for bronchiectasis?**
- Aspiration
- Abnormal vessels causing compression of the airways, infection, and bronchiectasis
- Alpha-1 antitrypsin deficiency
- Allergic bronchopulmonary aspergillosis
- *Bronchial tree abnormalities*—Congenital disorders
- Cystic fibrosis
- Drug abuse (prone for aspiration)
- Exposure to toxic gases that damage lung tissue
- Foreign body aspiration
- Gastroesophageal reflux disease (GERD)
- Genetic disorders
- *Gas exposure*—Toxic gases like chlorine gas, ammonia
- Host immunodeficiency
- *Infections*—Measles, tuberculosis

**Q5. What are the syndromes predisposing to bronchiectasis?**
- Agammaglobulinemia
- Patterson-Brown syndrome
- Chandra-Khetarpaul syndrome
- Immunodeficiency syndromes
- Immotile cilia syndrome
- Kartagener's syndrome
- Macleod syndrome
- Middle lobe syndrome
- Mounier-Kuhn syndrome (tracheobronchomegaly)
- Swyer-James syndrome
- Williams–Campbell syndrome (defect in bronchial development)
- Yellow nail syndrome
- Young syndrome.

**Q6. What is the gold standard test for diagnosis of bronchiectasis?**
Bronchography.

**Q7. What are the bronchography findings in bronchiectasis?**
Four types of bronchiectactic changes (saccular, cylindrical, fusiform, or varicose will be seen) and failure of peripheral tapering of the bronchi.

Pruned tree appearance–less peripheral pooling in the terminal bronchioles.

**Q8. What are the features of Kartagener's syndrome?**
Dextrocardia, situs inversus, and sinusitis.

**Q9. What are the features of young syndrome?**
- Obstructive azoospermia
- Infertility
- Sinusitis
- Bronchiectasis.

**Q10. What are the features of yellow nail syndrome?**
- Lymph edema
- Pleural effusion
- Discolored nails.

**Q11. What are the features of Williams–Campbell syndrome?**
This will be associated with defective cartilage development.
- Short stature
- Thoracic deformity
- Bronchiectasis.

**Q12. What are the features of Mounier-Kuhn syndrome?**
- Tracheobronchomegaly
- Bronchiectasis.

**Q13. What is pseudobronchiectasis?**
Pseudobronchiectasis usually follows whooping cough. There will be cylindrically dilated bronchus in bronchography. It is due to bronchial dilatation without destruction in certain conditions like tracheobronchitis. This condition is reversible, unlike bronchiectasis, where it is irreversible. Bronchography repeated after few months will show normal studies.

**Q14. What is reversible bronchiectasis?**
See pseudobronchiectasis.

**Q15. What are the types of bronchiectasis?**
- True bronchiectasis
- Pseudobronchiectasis (or) reversible bronchiectasis.

**Q16. What is bronchiectasis sicca?**
In this condition (dry), there is no production of sputum. Persistent cough with hemoptysis is present.

**Q17. What is Brock's syndrome?**
Middle lobe bronchiectasis—(Brock's syndrome). The right middle lobe bronchus is compressed by the enlarged tuberculous lymph nodes.

The right middle lobe is commonly involved because it is surrounded by lymph nodes and it originates in a narrow slit-like lumen. Also, the right middle lobe bronchus runs a long course, the right middle lobe is separated from the upper and lower lobes by fissures, and lacks collateral ventilation.

**Q18. What are the segments that are commonly involved in bronchiectasis?**
- Left lower lobe segments
- Right middle lobe
- Lingular segment of the left upper lobe
- Right lower lobe.

**Q19. What are the factors that predispose to left lower lobe bronchiectasis?**
- Left main bronchus is two-thirds the size of the right main bronchus
- Left main bronchus crosses the mediastinum at an acute angle behind aorta
- Superior and posterior basal segments of the left lobe are always in dependent position.

**Q20. What are the factors that predispose to right middle lobe bronchiectasis?**
- Right middle lobe bronchi arise in an acute angle and then bend forward
- Common sites where the enlarged hilar node presses the bronchus.

**Q21. What are the complications of bronchiectasis?**
- Abscess (lung abscess)
- Brain abscess (metastatic abscess to the brain through vertebral plexus of veins)
- Cavity formation (small cysts fuse to form cavity)
- Consolidation
- Cor pulmonale
- Diarrhea (antibiotic associated)
- Empyema
- Failure to thrive
- *Failure*—Cardiac and respiratory failure
- Gangrene of lung
- Hemoptysis (massive)
- Honeycomb appearance
- *Infections*—Pyemia and septicemia
- Pneumothorax
- Pyothorax
- Pleurisy
- Pericardial effusion
- Pulmonary osteoarthropathy
- Recurrent exacerbation leading to pneumonia and atelectasis
- Recurrent pneumonia
- Amyloidosis (rare).

**Q22. What is the best investigation to diagnosis subtle bronchiectasis?**
High-resolution CT scan. Bronchograms are not used now.

**Q23. What are the medical managements of bronchiectasis?**
- Treat respiratory infections
- Prolonged antibiotic therapy
- Postural drainage.

**Q24. What are the contraindications of postural drainage?**
- Intracranial disease
- Cardiac diseases
- Spinal disease (postoperative).

**Q25. What are the features of increasing severity of bronchiectasis?**

- Change in quantity (increase) and quality of sputum—becoming yellow, purulent, and foul smelling.
- Systemic features like fever.

**Q26. What are the surgical managements of bronchiectasis?**
- Removal of the lobe is done if the lesions are localized and the remaining lung is normal and not responding to treatment or associated with a foreign body or with localized anatomical defects.
- Localized lesion progressing despite medical management—segmental or lobar resection.
- *Lung transplantation*—If the involvement is bilateral, extensive and not responding to medical therapy.

**Q27. What are the good prognostic factors in bronchiectasis?**
- Absence of rhinosinusitis
- Unilateral bronchiectasis
- Lower lobe sessions
- Younger age
- Absence of obstructive lung disease
- Presence of treatable causes like foreign body, congenital cyst.

**Q28. What are the indications for surgery in bronchiectasis?**
- Localized disease
- Life-threatening hemorrhage
- Anatomical obstruction of the bronchi and suppurative lesions
- When foreign body cannot be removed by bronchoscopes.

**Q29. What are the steps to prevent bronchiectasis?**
- Removal of foreign body at early as possible
- Postural drainage
- Early treatment of primary infections
- Immunization against measles, whooping cough
- Treatment of other predisposing causes like gastroesophageal reflux, vascular rings, etc.

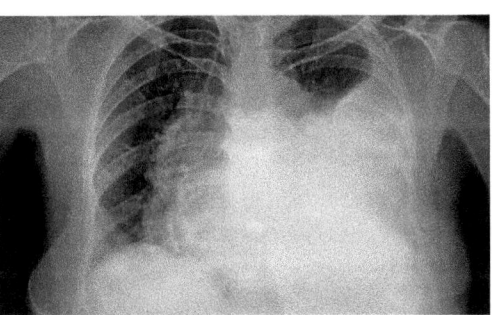

**Fig. 3.31:** Empyema thoracis left side.

### Empyema Thoracis (Fig. 3.31)

It is a condition with collection of pus in the pleural space.

**Radiological findings:**
- Asymmetric homogenous opacity with highest level in the axilla
- Bronchovascular markings will be absent
- Bulging and widening of intercostal spaces
- Biconvex/lenticular in shape
- Curvilinear enhancement of chest wall boundary due to inflammatory hyperemia of pleura
- Costopherenic and cardiophrenic angle will be obliterated
- *D-sign*—Bulging out of the chest wall is seen in loculated pleural fluid bulging
- Displacement of mediastinum to opposite side
- Elliptical shape with well-delimited borders
- Fluid between enhancing thickened parietal pleura and visceral pleura (split pleura sign)
- Gas bubbles in pleural space by gas forming organisms (Fig. 3.32).

**Differential diagnosis:**
- Pleural effusion
- Parapneumonic effusion
- Malignant effusion
- *Lung abscess*—Peripheral pulmonary abscess.

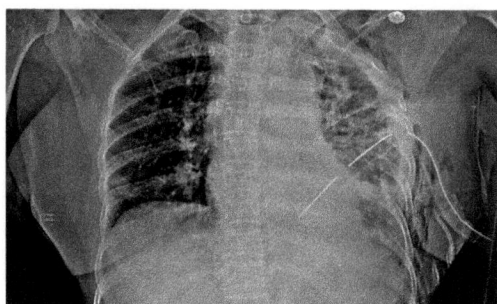

**Fig. 3.32:** Empyema left side after intercostal drainage tube insertion.

Differences between empyema and lung abscess

| Features | Empyema | Lung abscess |
|---|---|---|
| Shape | Lentiform | Round |
| Angle with chest wall | Obtuse angle | Acute angle |

Differences between empyema and pleural effusion

| Features | Empyema | Pleural effusion |
|---|---|---|
| Parts affected | Unilateral | Usually bilateral |
| Symmetry | Asymmetric | Symmetric |
| Upper border | Biconvex/lenticular shape forms obtuse angle with chest wall | Crescentic in shape (transudate or sterile pleural effusion) |

## QUESTIONS

**Q1. What is empyema thoracis?**
It is accumulation of pus in the pleural space.

**Q2. What is empyema necessitans?**
The pus will get collected under the skin of the chest wall and will be communicating with the empyema thoracis. This will result in a swelling in the chest wall. Cough impulse will be present.

**Q3. What is Hoover's sign?**
It refers to decreased movements on the affected side.

**Q4. What are the organisms causing empyema?**
- *Gram positive*—*Streptococcus pneumoniae, Staphylococcus aureus,* and *Streptococcus pyogenes*
- *Gram-negative*—*Escherichia coli, Pseudomonas, Klebsiella pneumoniae, Haemophilus influenzae,* and *Proteus.*

**Q5. What are the stages of empyema?**
- Exudative phase lasts for 1–3 days
- Fibrinopurulent phase from 4 days to 14 days
- Organizing phase beyond 14 days.

**Q6. What is the stage of parapneumonic effusion?**
Stage of exudative phase is known as parapneumonic effusion.

**Q7. What are the causes of failure to improve with treatment?**
- *Antibiotics*—Inadequate dose, poor penetrance
- Inadequate drainage
- Multiple loculations.

**Q8. What are the precipitating factors of empyema?**
- Abscess rupture into the lungs
- Bacterial pneumonia
- Catheter-based infection in indwelling catheters
- *Drainage*—Intercostal drainage/Thoracocentesis
- Esophageal perforation
- Extension of nonpleural infection like mediastinitis, abdominal infection
- *Infections*—Pulmonary infection, subdiaphragmatic abscess/septicemia
- Iatrogenic/surgery
- Injury/trauma
- Spontaneous pneumothorax.

**Q9. What are the complications of empyema?**
- Arthritis
- Brain abscess
- Empyema necessitans
- Loculated empyema
- Meningitis
- Osteomyelitis of ribs

- ❏ Pyopneumothorax
- ❏ Purulent abscess
- ❏ Peritonitis
- ❏ Pyopericardium
- ❏ Septicemia.

**Q10. What are the complications following treatment of empyema?**
- ❏ Subcutaneous emphysema
- ❏ Bronchopleural fistula.

**Q11. What are the long-term complications of empyema?**
- ❏ Restrictive lung disease
- ❏ Pleural thickening
- ❏ Fibrothorax.

**Q12. What is the view to be taken to diagnose minimal fluid?**
Lateral decubitus with patient lying on the affected side.

**Q13. What is VATS?**
Video-assisted thoracoscopic surgery.

## Lung Abscess (Fig. 3.33)

It refers to localized circumscribed collection of pus in the lungs.

### Radiological findings:
- ❖ Air-fluid levels
- ❖ Cavity with thick wall and irregular lumen
- ❖ Circumscribed shadow with collection of pus

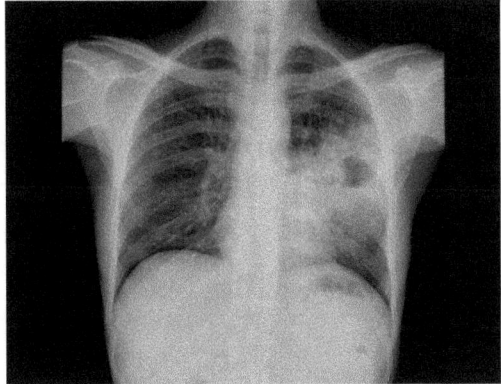

**Fig. 3.33:** Lung abscess left side.

- ❖ Central lucency
- ❖ Dense opacity.

### Differential diagnosis:
- ❖ Pneumonia
- ❖ Stomach or bowel loops in the chest cavity
- ❖ Empyema

| Features | Lung abscess | Empyema |
|---|---|---|
| Angle with chest wall | Present | Not present |
| Lung parenchyma | Destroyed | Displaced |
| Dimensions of fluid | Rounded configuration | Longer AP dimension |

- ❖ Infected bronchogenic cyst or emphysematous bulla
- ❖ Pulmonary infarction and neoplasm (cavitating bronchogenic carcinoma).

### Discussion:
- ❖ Localized collection of pus that leads to formation of cavity with a thick wall
- ❖ Liquefactive necrosis of lung
- ❖ Form cavities more than 2 cm
- ❖ Pus filled cavity.

### Etiology:
- ❖ *Infective causes*—Pneumonia
- ❖ *Noninfective causes*—Necrosis within a tumor, bronchogenic carcinoma, metastasis, and Wegener's granulomatosis.

### Site of abscess:
- ❖ Lower lobe in anaerobic infections, dependent parts, poorly ventilated, poorly drained bronchopulmonary segments. Usually associated with air-fluid levels.
- ❖ Upper lobe well ventilated, well drained, *Mycobacterium tuberculosis* is an obligate aerobe.

### Types of abscess:
- ❖ Primary pneumonia with lung abscess occurs in previously normal lungs.
- ❖ Secondary pneumonia with lung abscess occurs in lungs with underlying pathology like bulla, cyst, bronchiectasis,

and sequestrated lung. Abscess is due to existing lung pathology—necrotizing pneumonia, and due to other causes like vascular septic emboli, rupture of extrapulmonary abscess into the lungs.
- Preexisting solid mass like bronchogenic carcinoma, metastasis, and Wegener's granulomatosis.

**Predisposing conditions:**
- Aspiration
- Bronchial obstruction
- Bacteremia spread to lungs
- Bronchopneumonia (necrotizing)
- Convulsions
- Cystic fibrosis
- Congenital defects (bronchoesophageal fistula, pulmonary sequestration)
- Drowning
- Diabetes mellitus
- *Dental problems*—Severe periodontal disease
- Extraction of teeth
- *Emboli*—Septic pulmonary emboli from infective endocarditis
- *Fistula*—Tracheoesophageal fistula
- Gastroesophageal reflux
- General anesthesia
- Granulomatosis with polyangiitis
- Gingival disease
- Hygiene of oral cavity is poor
- Hepatic abscess extended to lung
- Immunodeficiency
- Inhalation of foreign body
- Infective endocarditis
- Infections of lung incompletely treated (Staphylococcal, *Klebsiella pneumoniae*)
- Injury to lung (penetrating lung injury)
- Iatrogenic—Instrumentation.

**Complications of lung abscess:**
- Amyloidosis (rare)
- Bacteremia
- Bronchiectasis
- Brain abscess (metastatic infection)
- Cachexia
- Cavity formation
- Drain through communication to bronchus
- Empyema
- Fistula (bronchopleural fistula)
- Generalized infection
- General condition deterioration
- Gangrene of lung
- Hemoptysis
- Hemorrhage.

**Clinical features of lung abscess:**
- Acute, tender clubbing
- Bad breath
- *Cough*—Productive
- Chills
- Chest pain
- Cachexia
- Difficulty in breathing
- Expectoration
- Fever
- Foul smelling sputum
- Fatigue
- General condition deterioration
- Hemoptysis.

## QUESTIONS

Q1. What are the differential diagnoses for hyperlucency with fluid level?
- ☐ Hydropneumothorax
- ☐ Hollow parenchymal lesion
- ☐ Lung cavity
- ☐ Abscess
- ☐ Lung cyst.

Q2. What are the differential diagnoses for hyperlucency with pneumatocele?
- ☐ Bleb
- ☐ Bullae
- ☐ Bronchiectasis
- ☐ Cystic adenomatoid malformation of lung
- ☐ *Cysts*—Hydatid cyst.

Q3. What are the differential diagnoses for hyperlucency with fluid level?
- ☐ *Fluid level inside the lung*—Lung abscess
- ☐ *Fluid level outside the lung*—Hydropneumothorax.

**Q4. What are the differential diagnoses for hyperlucency with ring shadows and cavity?**
- ❏ *Thick-walled cavity*—Lung abscess
- ❏ *Thin-walled cavity*:
  - ➢ Pneumatocele
  - ➢ Bullae
  - ➢ Bronchiectasis
  - ➢ Cyst.

## Bronchiolitis

It is a condition with small airways obstruction due to viral infections.

### Radiological findings:
- Air trapping
- *Atelectasis*—Segmental/subsegmental
- *Attenuation*—Mosaic attenuation
- Bilateral symmetrical involvement
- Bulging intercostal spaces
- Bilaterally symmetrical findings
- Bronchovascular makings are prominent with no collapse or consolidation
- Centrilobular solid nodes (tree-in-bud pattern)
- Diffuse opacities
- Diffuse hyperinflation of lungs
- Equal distribution of opacities between upper and lower lobes
- Flattening of dome of diaphragm
- Ground glass nodules (in hypersensitivity to bronchiolitis)
- Hyperinflation of lungs
- Heterogeneous and homogenous opacities typically peripheral in distribution
- *Infiltrates*—Patchy or peribronchial infiltrates
- Increased peribronchial thickening in perihilar regions
- *Lateral view*—Anteroposterior diameter is increased.

### Differential diagnosis:
- Asthma
- Allergic conditions
- Bronchopneumonia
- Congestive cardiac failure
- Cystic fibrosis
- Emphysema
- Foreign body in trachea.

### Discussion:
- Acute inflammation of bronchioles.
- It is the most common cause of infection in infants.

**Causative agent:** Caused by respiratory syncytial virus, parainfluenza virus, and adenovirus, respiratory syncytial virus is the most common cause of bronchiolitis.

**Age group:** 2 months to 2 years with a peak incidence of 6 months.

### Clinical findings:
- Anteroposterior diameter is increased
- Apnea (common in infants < 2 months)
- Breathing problems
- Bulging intercostal spaces
- Cough
- Cyanosis in severe cases
- Dyspnea
- Decreased activity
- Expiratory wheeze
- Fever
- Feeding difficulties
- Flaring of nose
- Grunting
- *Hoover's sign*—Severe chest wall recession
- Irritability
- Intercostal/subcostal recession
- Increased respiratory rate.

## QUESTIONS

**Q1. What are the causative agents?**
- ❏ Respiratory syncytial virus
- ❏ Adenovirus
- ❏ Parainfluenza virus
- ❏ Rhinovirus.

Respiratory syncytial virus is the most common cause of bronchiolitis in about 50–90% of cases.

**Q2. What is the age group in which bronchiolitis is common?**
Age group—2 months to 2 years with a peak incidence of 6 months.

**Q3. What are the complications of bronchiolitis?**
- *Air leak syndrome*—Pneumothorax, pneumomediastinum
- Acute respiratory failure
- Bronchial asthma/hyperreactive airway disease
- *Bacterial infections (secondary)*—Septicemia
- Congestive cardiac failure due to hypoxia
- Convulsions
- Dehydration (increased insensible loss due to tachypnea, low intake, etc.)
- Encephalopathy due to hypoxia
- Fluid overload with hyponatremia due to syndrome of inappropriate antidiuretic hormone secretion (SIADH).

**Q4. What is the management of bronchiolitis?**
Depends upon the severity of bronchiolitis:
*Mild bronchiolitis*:
- Supplemental oxygen
- Adequate hydration.

*Severe bronchiolitis*:
- Ventilatory support is indicated in the following conditions
- Apnea
- Clinical deterioration with worsening respiratory distress
- Hypercapnia
- Respiratory acidosis
- Bradycardia or tachycardia more than 200 beats/min
- *Poor perfusion*:
  - Ventilation may be needed for 3–4 days. High frequency ventilation will be more useful than mechanical ventilation
- Surfactant replacement may be needed.
- *Ribavirin aerosol*:
  - Ribavirin will inhibit DNA and RNA synthesis. This can be sued in the following high-risk children.
- Preterm babies, babies with bronchopulmonary dysplasia, and immunodeficiency
- Steroid use of dexamethasone is not found to be useful
- Bronchodilators
- Epinephrine 0.01 mL of 1 in 1,000 adrenaline is diluted with 3 mL of normal saline and nebulized over 5 minutes
- Immunotherapy
- Nebulization with salbutamol. Nebulization with ipratropium bromide was not found to be useful
- Antibiotics can be given in the presence of bacterial infections. Antibiotics should be given in children with fever, toxicity, leukocytosis, increased neutrophils and band count, and X-ray showing evidence of pneumonia.

**Q5. What is the prognosis of bronchiolitis?**
Radiological improvement will be seen within 9 days.

**Q6. What are the measures for prevention of bronchiolitis?**
- *Respiratory syncytial virus (RSV) vaccination*—Live attenuation vaccine can be given in newborn period
- Subunit vaccine
- Respiratory syncytial virus immunoglobulin 750 mg/kg
- *Monoclonal antibody*—Humanized RSV. Monoclonal antibody Palivizumab 15 mg/kg/month may decrease the incidence but not cost effective.

**Q7. What are the differences between bronchial asthma and bronchiolitis?**

Differences between bronchial asthma and bronchiolitis:

| Features | Bronchial asthma | Bronchiolitis |
|---|---|---|
| Age | Any age common after 1 year of age | Common from 2 months to 5 months that can occur up to 2 years of age |
| Precipitating factors | Infection, external allergens like house dusts, pollens | Infection |
| Fever | Moderate to severe, throughout the illness | Mild to moderate. Fever at the onset of illness |
| Toxic look | Alert active, not toxic | Toxic |
| Predominant finding | Wheezing | Crackles |
| Eosinophil count | Increased eosinophil count in blood and nasal secretions | No rise in eosinophil count |
| Serum immunoglobulin E (IgE) level | High | Normal |
| Response to therapy | Responds to bronchodilators/aerosol therapy | Will not respond to bronchodilators/aerosol therapy |
| Recurrence | Recurrent attacks | Usually single episode, rarely second episode |

**Q8. What is the best investigation for bronchiolitis?**
High-resolution computed tomography scan (HRCT) at the end of inspiration will show homogenous attenuation.

**Q9. Why children are more prone for bronchiolitis?**
It is due to smaller airways in children.

**Q10. What is the prognosis?**
Radiological improvement will be seen within 9 days.

## Pleural Effusion

Pleural effusion is the collection of serous fluid in the pleural cavity, the space between the parietal and visceral pleura.

### Radiological Features

It depends upon the amount, type of fluid, nature (free or loculated), patient's position, and radiographic projection.

❖ *Posterior-anterior view in erect position*:
  ▪ Apical opacity (apical capping) in large effusions
  ▪ Blunting of lateral costophrenic angle
  ▪ Black air-filled space devoid of lung markings will be seen lateral to the lung margin
  ▪ *Concave upper border toward the lung*—Meniscus sign. The upper margin of the opacity is concave that extends high laterally and medially (the apex of the meniscus may be slightly lower than the actual upper limit because the fluid is laterally tangential to the X-ray beam). The depth of the penetration increases attenuation of the radiation.
  ▪ Cardiophrenic angle will be obliterated when fluid collection is more
  ▪ Displacement of trachea and mediastinum to opposite side
  ▪ Diaphragmatic inversion on the left side (inferomedial displacement of stomach, air bubble, and colonic gas shadow)
  ▪ Ellis line/curve highest level in the axilla (meniscus-shaped upper border with density higher medially and lateral than at the center)
  ▪ Fluid in the horizontal/oblique fissures

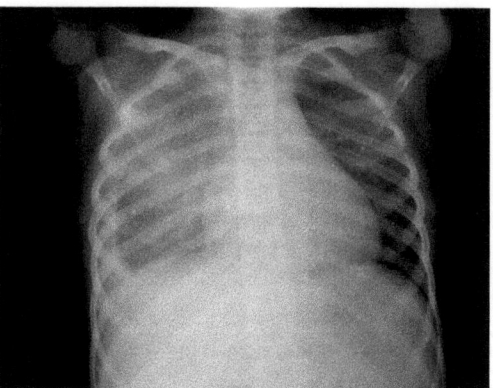

**Fig. 3.34:** X-ray taken in supine position right-sided pleural effusion showing haziness over the right lung.

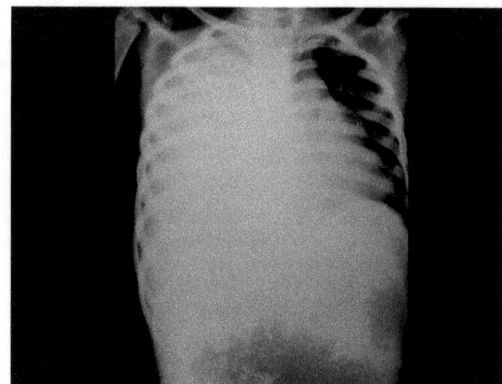

**Fig. 3.36:** Massive right pleural effusion showing mediastinal shift to left side.

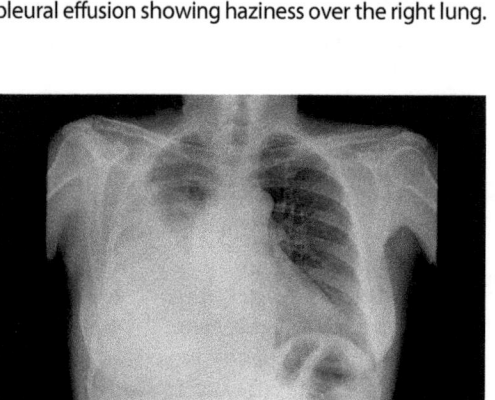

**Fig. 3.35:** Moderate right pleural effusion.

- Gap between the gastric air bubble and lower lobe air will be increased
- Heart border will be obliterated on the side of pleural effusion
- Homogenous opacification (Fig. 3.34)
- Hemidiaphragm will be obliterated on the side of pleural effusion (Silhouette sign)
- No air bronchogram (Figs. 3.35 and 3.36).

❖ *Look for loculated effusions*:
- *Subpulmonic effusion*—Collection of fluid below the diaphragm will lead to elevation of diaphragm. The diagnosis is confirmed by X-ray (left lateral decubitus).

❖ *Lateral decubitus*—Dependent layering of fluid
- Tracheal and mediastinal shift will be seen in massive effusions
- Even 50–75 mL can be demonstrated radiologically in lateral decubitus which can be seen as linear opacity separating the lung from the parietal pleura
- Obliterate posterior costophrenic angle.

❖ *Supine view*:
- Asymmetric density with haziness of lung increased on the side of pleural effusion
- Pulmonary vascular structures are visible and not obscured or silhouetted
- 175 mL of pleural fluid is required to produce notable changes in supine film.

(Ellis curve: The level of dullness raises in the axilla as compared to the anterior and posterior levels. This is because the parietal and visceral pleura are lying much closer at the lateral surfaces than on the other sides. Hence due to the capillary action, more fluid rises at the lateral part of the pleural surfaces. This gives rise to a raised radiographic shadow at the lateral parts).

The amount of fluid necessary to elicit pleural effusion clinically and radiologically is as follows:
- 200–300 mL of pleural fluid is needed to diagnose clinically and radiologically in posteroanterior (PA) view
- Mild effusion up to 4th rib
- Moderate effusion up to 2nd rib
- Massive effusion above 2nd rib
- Up to 500 mL may present without apparent changes in the X-ray chest frontal view.

## Differential Diagnosis
- Agenesis or aplasia of lung
- Atelectasis
- Bronchopneumonia
- *Consolidation*—Massive
- Collapse of lung
- *Cancers*—Non-Hodgkin lymphoma
- Chylothorax
- Diaphragmatic hernia/rupture
- Empyema
- *Excision of lung*—Pneumonectomy
- Ewing sarcoma
- Fibrothorax
- Foreign body obstruction
- Gastrothorax
- Hydrothorax
- Hemothorax
- Hypoplasia of lung
- Infusothorax (chemothorax) complication of central venous catheter malposition with tip in the pleural space
- *Intubation problems*—Right or left main bronchus intubation
- Massive tumor.

## QUESTIONS

**Q1. What is interface sign?**
It is seen in pleural effusion. Interface between the spleen and the pleural fluid will be less sharp than that of between the liver spleen and ascites.

**Q2. What is bare area sign?**
It is seen in pleural effusion. The peritoneal ligament prevents ascitic fluid from extending over the entire posterior surface of the liver, whereas in pleural space, the pleural fluid may extend over the entire posterior costophrenic recess behind the liver.

**Q3. What is the amount of pleural fluid that can obliterate the posterior costophrenic sulcus?**
75 mL will obliterate the posterior costophrenic sulcus.

**Q4. What is the amount of pleural fluid that can obliterate the posterior costophrenic angle in the upright film?**
175 mL will obliterate the posterior costophrenic angle in the upright film.

**Q5. What is the amount of pleural fluid that can obliterate costophrenic angle?**
200–500 mL posterior and then lateral costophrenic angles will be obliterated.

**Q6. What are the radiological findings in loculated pleural effusion?**
In loculated effusion the collection of fluid will be seen in the minor fissure with opacity showing smooth margins and the shape of the shadow will be biconvex.

**Q7. What are the radiological findings in main stem bronchus obstruction causing opacification of the hemithorax?**
Abrupt cutoff of main stem bronchus.

**Q8. What is the cause of apical opacity (apical capping) in large effusions?**
- Small lung volume at the apex
- Fluid lateral and superior to the lung.

## Pneumothorax

### X-ray Findings
X-ray erect posture. The radiological features are:
- Chest infections
- Absent lung markings on the side of pneumothorax beyond the lung markings
- Black due to increased radiolucency on the affected side

- ❖ Collapsed lung on the affected side is seen as a homogenous opacity at the hilum
- ❖ Collapsed lung with translucent air shadow without any lung or vascular markings will be seen lateral to the collapsed lung
- ❖ Cardiac border seen to a greater extent toward the diaphragm
- ❖ Costophrenic angle, deep, lucent
- ❖ Distinct lateral margin of the collapsed lung will be clearly seen on the affected side
- ❖ Displacement of mediastinum to the opposite side
- ❖ Depressed ipsilateral hemidiaphragm
- ❖ *Deep lateral sulcus sign* in supine film. The air will rise anteriorly and inferiorly resulting in the costophrenic angle on the side of pneumothorax lying more inferiorly than the opposite side (depressed costophrenic angle)
- ❖ *Double diaphragm sign*—In supine film due to interface of the dome of diaphragm and anterior costophrenic sulcus and hemidiaphragm
- ❖ Deep sulcus sign (subpulmonic pneumothorax), deep costophrenic sulcus on supine film
- ❖ Expansion of rib cage
- ❖ Edge of the lung will be more than 2 mm from the chest wall
- ❖ Flattening of ipsilateral diaphragm
- ❖ Gas collects in the apex in erect films
- ❖ Herniation of lung across the midline
- ❖ *Hyperinflation/hyperlucency*—The side will be more volume and more black
- ❖ Intercostal spaces will be widened
- ❖ Tension pneumothorax will be associated with herniation of lung across the midline, widened intercostals spaces
- ❖ Thin line of collapsed visceral pleura is the best single sign (Figs. 3.37 to 3.39).

Q. **How will you take an X-ray for a small pneumothorax?**
An expiratory film taken after full expiration will be helpful in small pneumothorax.

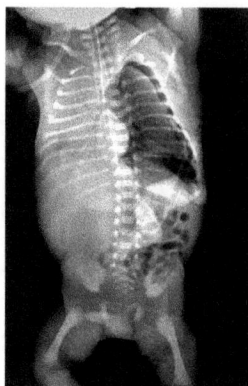

**Fig. 3.37:** Left-sided pneumothorax with collapsed lung margins.

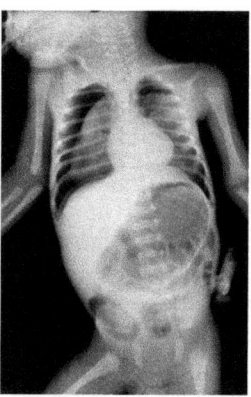

**Fig. 3.38:** Bilateral sided pneumothorax with collapsed lung margins.

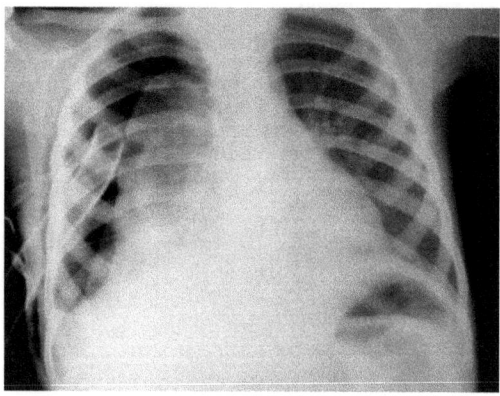

**Fig. 3.39:** Pneumothorax with intercostal drainage tube insertion and collapse of right lung.

## Differential Diagnosis

- Artifacts
- Asthma, acute exacerbation
- *Breast*—Overlapping breast margin
- Congenital lobar emphysema
- Chronic obstructive pulmonary disease (COPD), acute exacerbation
- Diffuse cystic lung diseases
- Emphysema
- Esophageal perforation
- *Fistula*—Bronchopleural fistula
- Giant bullous emphysema
- Hyperlucent hemithorax
- Intrathoracic herniation of stomach
- Swyer-James syndrome
- Poland syndrome
- Pulmonary embolism (Westermark sign).

## QUESTIONS

**Q1. What is primary pneumothorax?**
Pneumothorax is due to rupture of apical subpleural blebs without any clinically or radiologically apparent underlying lung disease.

**Q2. What is secondary pneumothorax?**
It refers to pneumothorax due to underlying lung disease.

**Q3. What are the differences between primary pneumothorax and secondary pneumothorax?**

| Features | Primary pneumothorax | Secondary pneumothorax |
|---|---|---|
| Underlying lung disease | Absent | Present |
| Prognosis | Better | Poor due to underlying lung disease |

**Q4. How will you differentiate between pneumothorax and emphysema?**
In emphysema, the pulmonary vessel markings will be seen. In pneumothorax, no vessel markings will be seen. Also in pneumothorax, the collapsed lung will be seen as a white shadow through the black background of air.

**Q5. What are the types of pneumothorax?**
- Closed pneumothorax
- Open pneumothorax
- Tension pneumothorax.

**Q6. What is closed pneumothorax?**
This is usually due to rupture of an emphysematous bulla. The opening in the pleura closes and the communication between the lung and the pleural space is closed. The symptoms will not be severe. The intrapleural pressure will be lower than that of the atmospheric pressure. Opening of the lung is small. It heals spontaneously.

**Q7. What is open pneumothorax?**
Opening remains patent. Pressure in pleural cavity is equal to that of atmospheric pressure.

**Q8. What is tension pneumothorax?**
Valvular type air enters pleural space during inspiration but cannot escape. This leads to entrapment of large volume of air in the pleural space. The pressure in the pleura will exceed the atmospheric pressure. Dyspnea will be very severe. There will be mediastinal shift, which will be progressive. Central cyanosis may be present. This is a medical emergency.

**Q9. What are the causes of pneumothorax?**
*Traumatic*:
- Assisted ventilation
- Accidents
- Barotrauma (mountain climbing, scuba diving)
- Broken ribs
- *Chest injury*—Blunt injury or penetrating/nonpenetrating wounds
- Cardiothoracic surgery
- Contact sports like football, hockey
- Deceleration injury
- Damage to lungs by procedures like lung biopsy, central line placement

- Endoscopic perforation of esophagus
- Fighting
- Fall from height
- Gunshot injury
- *Iatrogenic*—Tracheostomy, central venous catheter, and ventilator
- Irradiation of thorax.

*Spontaneous*:
*Primary spontaneous pneumothorax* occurs in persons with no underlying lung disease.

Risk factors for primary spontaneous pneumothorax:
- Alpha-1 antitrypsin deficiency
- *Build*—Thin people
- Cigarette smoking
- *Drug abuse*—Cannabis
- Ehlers–Danlos syndrome
- Family history of pneumothorax
- *Gender*—Male
- *Height*—Tall people
- Homocystinuria.

*Secondary spontaneous pneumothorax* occurs in persons with underlying lung problems.

Risk factors for secondary spontaneous pneumothorax:
- Asthma
- Anaerobic infections
- Blebs (subpleural)
- Congenital cyst (rupture of a tension cyst in the lung)
- Chronic bronchitis
- Cystic fibrosis
- Chronic obstructive pulmonary disease (COPD)
- *Connective tissue disorders*—Marfan's syndrome, Ehlers–Danlos syndrome
- Congenital lung disorders
- Congenital lobar emphysema
  - Congenital pulmonary adenomatoid malformation
  - Cancer lung
  - Diffuse emphysema
  - Emphysematous bullae
- Endometriosis of diaphragm (catamenial pneumothorax)
- Foreign body
- Fungal infections
- *Granulomatous disease*—Sarcoidosis
- Histiocytosis X
- Hyaline membrane disease
- *Infections*—Necrotizing pneumonia, lung abscess (rupture of suppurative disease of lung), staphylococcal infection, Pneumocystis carinii pneumonia, and tuberculous lesion in the lung
- Interstitial lung disease
- *Infarction*—Pulmonary infarction.

**Q10. What is coin test?**
*Positive coin test*—A metallic coin is placed on the chest wall anteriorly or posteriorly, over the affected part. This coin is tapped by another coin and auscultated by placing the diaphragm of the stethoscope on the opposite side. In patients with pneumothorax, a high-pitched, tympanitic metallic sound will be heard. This should be always compared with the normal side.

**Q11. What are the complications of pneumothorax?**
- Atelectasis of lung
- *Air leak to mediastinum*—Pneumomediastinum
- Bronchopleural fistula
- *Cardiac arrest*—Pneumopericardium
- Collapse of lung
- Displacement of intercostal tubes
- Emphysema (subcutaneous/surgical emphysema)
- *Fatal complications in tension pneumothorax*—Shock, cardiac arrest, and respiratory failure
- Hydropneumothorax
- Hypoxia
- Hypotension
- *Infections*—Empyema thoracis, pyopneumothorax

- *Iatrogenic complications*—Emphysema, injury to lung, myocardium, and other organs, hemothorax, injury to neurovascular structures
- Thickened pleura
- Re-expansion pulmonary edema
- Recurrence of pneumothorax.

**Q12. How will you treat tension pneumothorax?**

Treatment of tension pneumothorax is by intercostal drainage at the second intercostal space 1 cm away from the sternal border or in the fourth intercostal space in the anterior axillary line.

**Q13. What is the difference between congenital lobar emphysema and tension pneumothorax?**

The margins of collapsed lung will be seen in pneumothorax which will be absent in congenital lobar emphysema.

## Hydropneumothorax (Fig. 3.40)

It is a condition associated with abnormal presence of both air and fluid within the pleural space.

### X-ray Findings

- Air-fluid levels
- Borders between air and fluid will be well defined

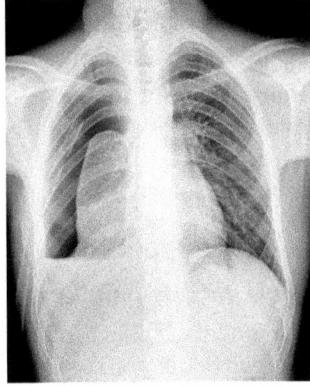

**Fig. 3.40:** Hydropneumothorax right side. Horizontal fluid level extending across the whole length of right hemithorax and right side pleura visible. Right pneumothorax seen above the fluid level.

- costophrenic angle/cardiophrenic angle—obliteration
- Dense opacity on the side of hydropneumothorax
- Displacement of mediastinum to opposite side
- Extension of horizontal fluid level across the whole length of hemithorax
- Edge of the collapsed lung will be seen
- Fluid shadow shifts with change in position
- Grayness (uniform) of entire hemithorax with absence of lung markings (in supine film).
- Horizontal fluid level.

### Differential Diagnosis

- Pyopneumothorax
- Hemothorax
- Lung abscess
- *Pneumothorax*—Meniscus sign will be absent in hydropneumothorax.

### Causes of Hydropneumothorax

Hydropneumothorax can occur as complications of the following conditions:
- *Abscess*—Lung abscess rupture
- *Biopsy*—Transbronchial biopsy
- Chest tube insertion (iatrogenic)
- *Chest infections*—Tuberculosis
- Cystic lung disease
- Chest injuries
- Cancers (pleural mesotheliomas, angiosarcomas)
- *Clostridium welchii* infections
- Connective tissue disorders
- Dermatomyositis
- *Echinococcus granulosus* infection (hydatid)
- Infections (*Staphylococcus*, *Pneumococcus*, and *Klebsiella*)
- Injury/trauma to the thorax
- *Iatrogenic*—Intercostal aspiration/drainage.

## QUESTIONS

**Q1. What is hydropneumothorax?**

Hydropneumothorax is the presence of both air and fluid within the pleural space.

**Q2. What is the difference between hydropneumothorax and pyopneumothorax?**

The fluid in hydropneumothorax will be serous and the fluid in the pyopneumothorax will be pus. The meniscus sign along the chest wall seen in pleural effusion is not seen in hydropneumothorax. This is because of the increase in intrathoracic pressure by trapped air that obliterates the fluid interface.

**Q3. What are the clinical features of hydropneumothorax?**
- Acute onset of respiratory insufficiency
- Anorexia
- Breathlessness
- Breath sounds are absent
- Cough
- Chest pain aggravated by deep breathing
- *Constitutional symptoms*—Weight loss, malaise, and anorexia will be seen
- Dyspnea
- Expansion of hemithorax
- Fullness of chest.

**Q4. What are the clinical signs of hydropneumothorax?**
(4 S)
- Straight line dullness
- Succussion splash
- Shifting dullness
- Sound of coin.

## Pneumatoceles (Fig. 3.41)

It refers to thin-walled air-filled cysts in the lung parenchyma.

### Causes

**Infectious causes:**
- Staphylococcal pneumonia
- Streptococcal pneumonia
- *Haemophilus influenzae*
- *Escherichia coli*
- Group A streptococci
- *Klebsiella pneumonia*

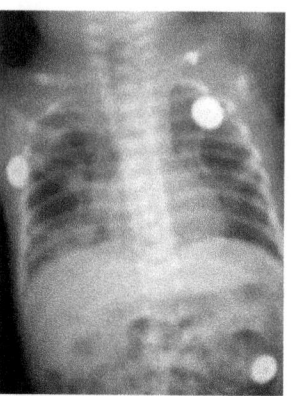

**Fig. 3.41:** Pneumatoceles.

- Adenovirus
- Tuberculosis.

**Noninfectious causes:**
- Trauma
- Positive pressure ventilation
- Hydrocarbon ingestion.

## QUESTIONS

**Q1. What are the differences between abscess and pneumatocele?**

The following are features of pneumatoceles that will help to differentiate from lung abscess (Table 3.2):
- The wall are thin
- Contains little or no fluid
- Smooth inner margins
- May be symptomless.

**Q2. What are the complications of pneumatocele?**
- Pneumothorax
- Secondary infection.

## Collapse—Right Upper Lobe

### Radiological Findings in Collapse
- Airless segment of collapsed lung
- Blurring heart borders on the side of collapse
- Bronchial cutoff sign due to endobronchial obstruction
- Crowding of ipsilateral ribs

**Table 3.2:** Showing the differences between pneumatocele and lung abscess.

| Features | Pneumatocele | Lung abscess |
| --- | --- | --- |
| Clinical symptoms | Symptomless | Fever, dyspnea |
| Walls | Thin | Thick |
| Fluid | Little or absent | Present |
| Inner margins | Smooth | Irregular |

- Crowding of air bronchogram, pulmonary vessels
- Dense homogenous opacities
- Displacement of trachea to the side of collapse
- Flattening of hemidiaphragm
- *Golden S-sign*—When hilar mass is combined with collapse of the right upper lobe
- Hyperlucency of other parts of lung
- Hemidiaphragm obscured (silhouette sign—loss of normal silhouette)
- Interlobar fissure pulled toward the collapse
- Ipsilateral hemidiaphragm will be elevated
- Juxtaphrenic peak
- Loss of lung volume
- Mediastinal shift to the side of collapse
- No air bronchogram
- Obscured mediastinum, cardiac outline
- Prominent pulmonary artery on the opposite side as whole cardiac output pass through single artery.

*The radiological features depend upon the lobe involved*:
- *Right upper lobe collapse*:
  - Displacement of mediastinum to the right
  - Elevation of horizontal fissure
  - Elevation of right hilum
  - *Golden S-sign*—When hilar mass is combined with collapse of the right upper lobe
  - Hyperinflation of right middle and lower lobe
  - Right juxtaphrenic peak
  - *Silhouette sign*—Loss of normal silhouette of right paratracheal stripe.

## Differential Diagnosis

- Consolidation of right upper lobe
  - Mass in the upper part of thorax.
- *Right middle lobe collapse*:
  - Blurring of right heart border—Silhouette sign—Loss of normal silhouette of right heart border
  - Horizontal fissure will not be visible as rotates down
  - Triangular opacity in the anterior aspect of the chest (in lateral view).
  - Consolidation of right middle lobe.
- *Right lower lobe collapse*:
  - Opacity at the base of the right lung
  - Crowding of ipsilateral ribs
  - Displacement of mediastinum to the right
  - Right hilum is depressed
  - *Silhouette sign*—Loss of normal silhouette of right hemidiaphragm.
- Consolidation of right lower lobe
- Pulmonary mass
- Posterior mediastinal mass
- Pulmonary sequestration.
- *Left upper lobe collapse*:
  - Hazy opacity with more opacity near the midline fading out inferiorly
  - Blurring of left heart border
  - Left hilum drawn upward
  - Left main bronchus almost horizontal
  - Left lower lobe bronchus almost vertical
  - Peaked or tented left hemidiaphragm (juxtaphrenic peak sign)
  - *Silhouette sign*—Loss of normal silhouette of aortic knuckle.
  - Consolidation of left upper lobe.
- *Left lower lobe collapse*:
  - Triangular opacity
  - Crowding of ipsilateral ribs
  - Displacement of mediastinum to the right
  - Elevation of left hemidiaphragm

- Loss of outline of descending aorta
- Loss of normal left hemidiaphragmatic outline
- Left hilum is depressed
- *Silhouette sign*—Loss of normal silhouette of hemidiaphragm and descending aorta.
❖ Consolidation.
❖ *Lingular lobe collapse*: Silhouette sign—Loss of normal silhouette at left heart border.
❖ Effusion.

## QUESTIONS

**Q1. What are the causes of collapse?**
- ❑ *Intraluminal*:
  - ➢ Aspiration of foreign body
  - ➢ Mucous plugging.
- ❑ *Mural*: Bronchogenic carcinoma
- ❑ *Extrinsic compression*: Hilar mass.

**Q2. How will you differentiate between collapse and empyema presenting as unilateral opacity?**
- ❑ *Collapse*—The mediastinum will be shifted to the same side of the collapse.
- ❑ *Empyema*—The mediastinum will be slightly shifted to the opposite side of the empyema.

## Bilateral Hyperventilation

### Asthma

**Radiological findings in asthma:**
❖ Air trapping during expiration
❖ Atelectasis due to mucous plugging
❖ Bilateral hyperventilation/hyperinflation
❖ Bronchial wall thickening
❖ Peribronchial cuffing
❖ Diffuse increased reticular pattern
❖ Differential ventilation (large segments hypoventilated and small segments hyperventilated)
❖ Pulmonary edema (rarely)
❖ Flattening of diaphragm.

In some patients, the X-ray of chest will be normal.

**Differential diagnosis for asthma:**
❖ Aspiration
❖ Bronchiolitis obliterans
❖ Cardiac asthma
❖ Dysfunction of vocal cord (factitious asthma)
❖ Eosinophilic pneumonia
❖ Foreign bodies in the airway
❖ *Granulomatosis*—Bronchocentric.

### Bilateral Hyperventilation

Excessive ventilation of the lungs is beyond requirement to achieve normal arterial blood gases. Both lungs will be more black and more voluminous. Both lungs will be equal in aeration. The diaphragm will be depressed.

## QUESTIONS

**Q1. What are the conditions associated with bilateral hyperventilation?**
Bilateral hyperventilation will be seen in the following conditions:
Generalized increased translucency of the thorax with low flattened diaphragms will be seen in the following conditions:
- ❑ Asthma
- ❑ Bronchiolitis
- ❑ Compensatory hyperventilation in metabolic acidosis
- ❑ Cystic fibrosis
- ❑ *Central upper airway obstruction*—Tracheal obstruction (vascular ring, tracheal foreign body)
- ❑ Diabetic ketoacidosis
- ❑ *Drugs by central action on brain*—Aspirin overdose
- ❑ Exercise
- ❑ Fever
- ❑ *Granulomatous disorders*—Bronchocentric granulomatosis
- ❑ Gas exchange poor as in pulmonary edema, pulmonary embolism

- High altitude
- Hyperventilation syndrome
- Hysterical hyperventilation
- Hypoxia
- Iatrogenic hyperventilation
- *Inspiratory effort more*—Normal children with a large inspiratory effort
- *Anxiety*—Psychological disorders.

**Q2. What are the complications of hyperventilation?**

Respiratory alkalosis.

**Q3. What are the factors influencing the respiratory drive?**
- Elasticity of lungs
- Resistance in airways
- pH
- Carbon dioxide ($CO_2$)
- Oxygen ($O_2$).

**Q4. What is the differential diagnosis for hyperlucency with attenuated lung markings?**

Emphysema.

**Q5. What are the differential diagnoses for hyperlucency with absent lung markings?**
- Bullae
- Pneumothorax.

## Emphysema

There will be overinflation of alveoli. The lung tissue will be destroyed resulting in impairment of exchange of gases.

It is also known as obstructive lung disease because the air flow during exhalation is slowed.

Destruction of lung tissue around small airways.

## Congenital Lobar Overinflation

Congenital lobar overinflation (previously known as congenital lobar emphysema)
- Radiological findings
- Abnormal lung lobe
- Blood vessels are widely separated. Blood supply will be normal
- Congenital condition common in the left upper lobe
- Contralateral displacement of mediastinum/mediastinal shift to opposite side
- Distension or overdistension of the lobe of the lung
- Enlarged or overexpanded lung lobe due to increased lung volume due to overinflation
- Flattening of diaphragm
- Grossly enlarge one or more lung lobes
- Hyperlucent lung segment
- Hemidiaphragmatic depression
- Herniating to opposite side
- Hazy mass like density immediately after birth (due to fluid)

*Ipsilateral atelectasis*—compressive atelectasis of adjacent lung especially the lower lobes.

Lateral film will show posterior displacement of heart.

*Common lobe involved*—left upper lobe followed by right middle lobe and right upper lobe. Lower lobes are rarely involved.

### Types of Emphysema in Foreign Body Obstruction

- Obstructive emphysema
- Compensatory emphysema.

### Obstructive emphysema

**Discussion:**

When a foreign body obstructs partially, the air will be trapped in one lung. This will result in enlargement of the lung. This is known as obstructive emphysema (Figs. 3.42A and B).

X-ray showing obstructive emphysema is due to air trapping and due to partial obstruction by the foreign body.

Picture of foreign body is removed from the respiratory tract.

### Compensatory emphysema:

When one lung is absent or affected, the other lung will enlarge as a compensatory

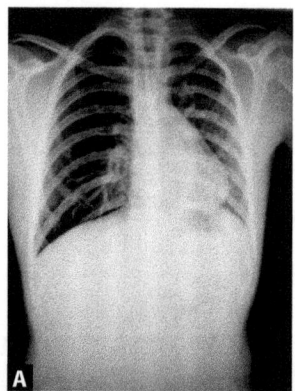

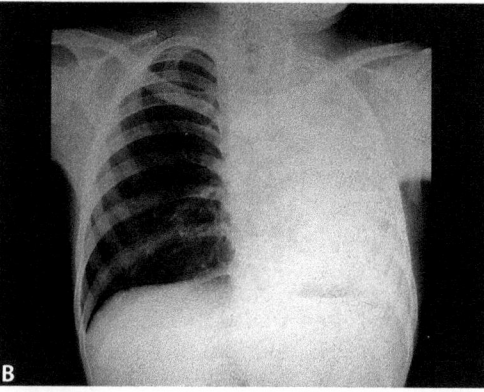

**Figs. 3.42A and B:** (A) Obstructive emphysema—right side due to foreign body obstruction; (B) Compensatory emphysema.

mechanism. This is known as compensatory emphysema.
- Emphysema occurs due to compensation to loss of lung volume on the opposite lung or lobes of same lung.
- When one lung or part of one lung is consolidated or fibrosed or collapsed, the remaining parts or other lung will show increase in vital capacity.
- Distended and no destruction.

Compensatory emphysema is seen in the following conditions:
- Fibrosis
- Collapse
- Consolidation.

### Compensatory vs Obstructive Emphysema

A foreign body in the bronchus may cause partial or total obstruction. When the obstruction is total, there will be collapse on the affected side. This will result in compensatory expansion of other lung known as compensatory emphysema. When the obstruction of the respiratory tract is partial, air will be trapped distal to the obstruction resulting in obstructive emphysema.

## QUESTIONS

Q1. **What are the predisposing factors for emphysema?**
- ☐ Air pollution
- ☐ Bronchial asthma
- ☐ Bronchiolitis
- ☐ Cystic fibrosis
- ☐ Cigarette smoking
- ☐ Dust
- ☐ Fumes (chemical)
- ☐ Genetic—alpha-1 antitrypsin deficiency.

Q2. **What is barrel chest?**
The chest will be rounded, barrel-shaped chest which is due to long-term overinflation of the lungs. Anteroposterior to transverse ratio will be 1:1. It is usually seen in patients with emphysema.

### Pulmonary Edema (Figs. 3.43A and B)

It is collection of excess fluid in tissue and air spaces in the lungs.

Abnormal accumulation of fluid is seen in the extravascular compartments of the lung.

### Radiological Features of Pulmonary Edema

- Air bronchograms
- *Batwing appearance*—Air space opacification in the batwing distribution (Fig. 3.44)
- Bilateral pleural effusion (usually bilateral)
- *Cardiac silhouette increased*—Increased cardiothoracic ratio
- Diffuse fluffy alveolar infiltrates
- Dilated azygous vein

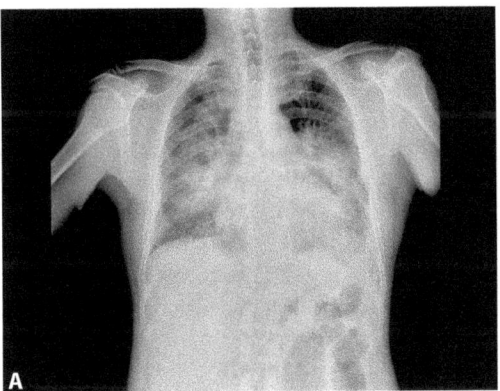
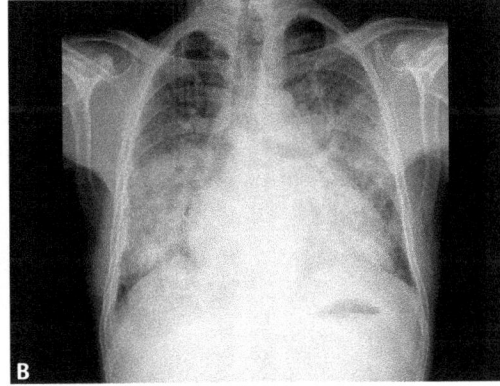

**Figs. 3.43A and B:** Pulmonary edema (Batwing appearance, alveolar edema, cardiomegaly, diversion of blood to upper lobe, effusion).

- Edema—pulmonary alveolar edema
- Fluid in the interlobar fissures is seen as thickening of major and minor fissure
- Haziness in perihilar region
- Inverted mustache sign
- Kerley A, B, and C lines
- Vanishing tumor (Disappears after diuretic administration).

*Kerley lines* are named after Sir Peter James Kerley.

Kerley A lines are seen less commonly than Kerley B or C lines. These are longer, measuring from 2 cm to 6 cm. These lines course from the periphery to the hilum. These are due to anastomotic channels between peripheral and central lymphatics in the lungs.

Kerley B lines are short, less than 1 cm in length, thin, linear, and transverse strips of opacities seen in interstitial pulmonary edema (Fig. 3.45). They will course from the hilum toward the periphery of the lungs. They will be seen when the pulmonary wedge pressure is 20–25 mm Hg or more.

Kerley B lines are seen in the periphery of the lungs perpendicular to the pleural surface (Fig. 3.46). They can be seen in any part of the lungs but are usually seen in the base of the lungs.

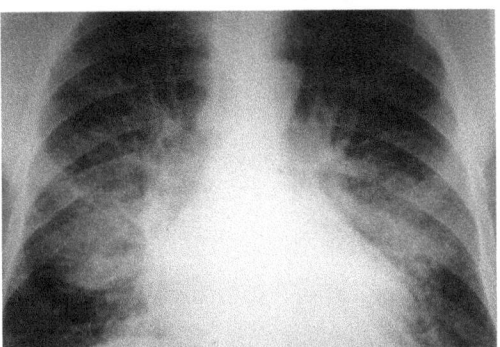

**Fig. 3.44:** Pulmonary edema: batwing appearance.

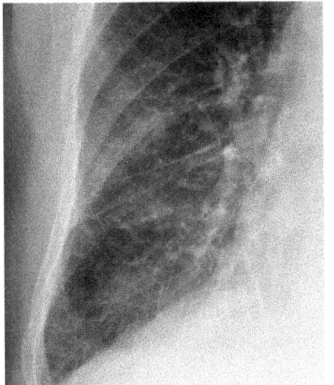

**Fig. 3.45:** Kerley B lines.

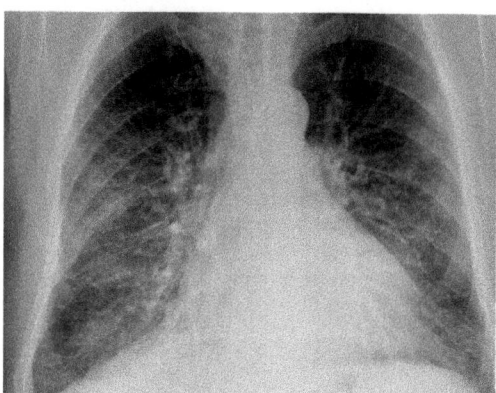

**Fig. 3.46:** Kerley B lines (anteroposterior view).

Also known as Fleischner's lines/septal lines/interlobular lines.

Kerley C lines are short fine lines seen throughout the lungs and do not reach the pleura. They also do not course radially away from the hilum. These are rarely seen. These are due to thickening of anastomotic lymphatics.

Kerley D lines are septal lines resembling Kerley B lines seen in the lateral chest X-rays. They are seen in the retrosternal area.

Q. What are Kerley B lines? What are the causes of Kerley B lines?

Thin, linear pulmonary opacities due to interstitial pulmonary edema caused by fluid or cellular infiltration into the interstitium of lungs.

Kerley B lines are due to edematous, thickened interlobular septa.

Bases of lung at costophrenic angles in anteroposterior (AP) view.

Substernal area in the lateral films.

Parallel to one another at right angles to the pleura.

## Causes for Kerley B Lines

- *Atypical infections*—Mycoplasma pneumonia
- Alveolar cell carcinoma
- *Cancers*—Lymphangitis carcinomatosis, malignant lymphoma
- Coal worker's pneumoconiosis
- *Congestive cardiac failure*—Mitral stenosis, left ventricular failure (LVF)
- Distension of lymphatics due to obstruction
- Pulmonary edema
- Interstitial pulmonary fibrosis
- *Granulomatous disease*—Sarcoidosis
- Hemosiderin deposition caused by recurrent pulmonary edema
- *Infections*—Viral pneumonia.

## Features of Kerley Lines

| Features | Kerley A lines | Kerley B lines | Kerley C lines |
|---|---|---|---|
| Site | Do not bifurcate or follow normal branching pattern of bronchi and vessels | Bases of lung at costophrenic angles periphery of the lungs perpendicular to the pleural surface | Throughout the lungs and do not reach the pleura |
| Character | Longer lines | Short, sharp, and small horizontal | Fine interlacing lines |
| Length | 2–6 cm | Less than 2 cm, 2 mm in diameter | |

## Discussion

The radiological findings will depend upon the sites of collection of fluid.

Interstitial edema—Peribronchial cuffing, Kerley lines, and thickening of interlobar fissures.

*Alveolar*—Air bronchograms, batwing distribution

*Interlobar*—Vanishing pulmonary pseudotumor

Upper lobar pulmonary venous diversion/stag's antler sign

Pulmonary venous engorgement.

*Differential Diagnosis for Pulmonary Edema*
- ❖ Diffuse pneumonia
- ❖ Massive aspiration
- ❖ Pulmonary hemorrhage.

## QUESTIONS

**Q1. What are the causes of pulmonary edema?**
- ❏ Increased hydrostatic pressure
- ❏ Increased permeability
- ❏ Diffuse alveolar damage.

**Q2. What are the types of pulmonary edema?**
Types of pulmonary edema are:
- ❏ Cardiogenic pulmonary edema
- ❏ Noncardiogenic pulmonary edema.

**Q3. What are the causes of cardiogenic pulmonary edema?**
- ❏ Cardiac failure
- ❏ Cardiac arrhythmias
- ❏ Fluid overload
- ❏ Cardiomyopathy
- ❏ Myocarditis.

**Q4. What are the causes of noncardiogenic pulmonary edema?**
It is seen in cases with injury to lung parenchyma or vasculature.
Causes of noncardiogenic pulmonary edema:
- ❏ Altitude high—Pulmonary edema usually above 8,000 feet (2,400 meters)
- ❏ Aspiration
- ❏ Acute respiratory distress syndrome (ARDS)
- ❏ Acute asthma
- ❏ Air embolism
- ❏ Antisnake venom administrating
- ❏ Allergic alveolitis
- ❏ Blunt trauma to lungs
- ❏ Congestive cardiac failure
- ❏ Disseminated intravascular coagulation
- ❏ Near drowning
- ❏ Dengue infections (viral infections)
- ❏ Drugs
- ❏ Exposure to toxins
- ❏ *Embolism*—Pulmonary thromboembolism
- ❏ Fluid overload
- ❏ *Fire accidents*—Inhalation of smoke
- ❏ Generalized convulsions
- ❏ High altitude
- ❏ *Head injury*—Neurogenic pulmonary edema
- ❏ Heroin-induced/heroin overdose
- ❏ *Hypovolemic shock*—Capillary permeability increased in shock
- ❏ *Infection*—Sepsis (capillary permeability increased in sepsis)
- ❏ Inhaled toxins like ammonia, chlorine
- ❏ Inhalation of smoke
- ❏ *Injury/trauma to lungs*—Transfusion-induced lung injury
- ❏ *Iatrogenic*—Postintubation, negative pressure pulmonary edema, and oxygen therapy
- ❏ Reperfusion pulmonary edema.

**Q5. What are the clinical and radiological differences between cardiogenic and noncardiogenic pulmonary edema?**

Clinical differences between cardiogenic and noncardiogenic pulmonary edema:

| Features | Cardiogenic pulmonary edema | Noncardiogenic pulmonary edema |
|---|---|---|
| Pathogenesis | Increased pulmonary capillary pressure | Increased capillary permeability of alveolar capillary barrier |
| Type of edema | High pressure, low permeability edema | Low pressure, high permeability edema |
| Pulmonary capillary wedge pressure (PCWP) | >20 mm Hg | <18 mm Hg |
| Associated conditions | Hypertension | *See* Answer for Q4 |

*Contd...*

Contd...

| Features | Cardiogenic pulmonary edema | Noncardiogenic pulmonary edema |
|---|---|---|
| Pulmonary artery diastolic to wedge pressure gradient | <5 mm Hg | >5 mm Hg |
| Type of fluid | Transudate | Exudates |
| Edema fluid to plasma protein ratio | <0.5 | >0.7 |
| Response to diuretics | Good | No response |

Radiological differences between cardiogenic and noncardiogenic pulmonary edema in X-rays:

| Features | Cardiogenic pulmonary edema | Noncardiogenic pulmonary edema |
|---|---|---|
| Causes | Cardiac causes resulting in increased hydrostatic pressure | Noncardia cases resulting in changes in capillary permeability due to direct or indirect pathologic insult. Low alveolar pressure, neurogenic edema |
| Bronchovascular markings | Prominent, opacities involve central and peripheral lungs | Batwing pattern |
| Kerley B lines | Present | |
| Air bronchogram | Not seen | Air bronchogram seen |
| Mediastinal widening | Present due to increased vascular pedicle width | Not seen |
| Lung volume | Decreased | Normal or increased |
| Cardiomegaly | Present | Not seen |
| Pleural effusion | May be present | Absent |
| Peribronchial cuffing | Present | Not seen |

Q6. **What is vanishing tumor?**
The collection of fluid in the interlobar regions will appear like a tumor in the X-rays. When diuretics like frusemide is given, the fluid will disappear with the shadow will disappear. This is known as vanishing tumor.

Q7. **What is inverted mustache stage—antler sign or hands-up sign?**
In normal X rays the lower pulmonary vessels will be larger than the upper due to gravity. In cardiac failure the distended pulmonary vessels in the upper part of the lungs will appear like mustache in the X rays.

Q8. **What is the drug of choice for treatment of pulmonary edema?**
Furosemide.

Q9. **What are the causes for pulmonary venous congestion?**
Hazy and indistinct margin of the pulmonary vasculature.

*Causes*:
- Left ventricular failure
- Obstruction to pulmonary venous drainage
- Hypoplastic left heart syndrome
- Mitral stenosis
- Total anomalous pulmonary venous return (TAPVR)
- Cor triatriatum.

Q10. **What is the difference between Kerley lines and blood vessels?**
The Kerley-lines are prominent laterally at costophrenic angle and become thinner as it proceeds toward the hilum. The blood vessels are wide at the hilum and narrows down toward the periphery.

## Pulmonary Plethora

- Area of blood vessels more than normal—extends into the peripheral one-third of lung
- Prominent vessels below the crest of the diaphragm, vessels below the 10th posterior rib

- Blood vessels will be visible in the outer one-third of the lungs. More than six vessels in the peripheral one-third of the lungs
- Both upper and lower zone vessels are prominent
- Cardiomegaly may be seen
- Convex bulge of the pulmonary artery segment on the left cardiac border
- *Dilated descending pulmonary artery trunk*—Right descending pulmonary artery (RDPA) diameter more than 16 mm and is more than that of trachea
- Diameter of pulmonary arteries more than that of accompanying bronchus
- End on vessels more than two times that of accompanying bronchus
- Enlargement of pulmonary vessels due to increased flow
- *Equal distribution in upper and lower part of lungs*—Recruitment of upper lobe vessels. Differential flow between the upper and lower lobe will be lost and there will be equal flow in both upper and lower parts.
- End on view of pulmonary vessels in hilar region more than 3–5 vessels
- *Five or more peripheral vessels*—More than five vessels in the peripheral one-third of the lungs
- Generalized mottling may be seen in infants and children
- Hilar vessels are uniformly enlarged. More than three to five ends on view will be seen.
- Increased vascular markings.

## Causes of Pulmonary Plethora

### Without cyanosis:
- High output states (anemia, thyrotoxicosis)
- Left to right-sided shunt [ventricular septal defect (VSD), atrial septal defect (ASD), patent ductus arteriosus (PDA), atrioventricular septal defect, coronary artery fistula into the right heart, aortopulmonary window, and partial anomalous venous connection].

### With cyanosis:
- Transposition of great vessels
- Total anomalous pulmonary venous return (TAPVR)
- Truncus arteriosus
- Double outlet right ventricle without pulmonary stenosis
- Double inlet right ventricle without pulmonary stenosis.

# QUESTION

Q. **What is the difference between pulmonary plethora and pulmonary edema?**
In pulmonary plethora, there will be enlarged pulmonary vessels with clear and sharp margins. With the development of pulmonary edema, the pulmonary vessels will become indistinct.

## Normal Pulmonary Vasculature
- Air trapping areas of mosaic attenuation during inspiration that persist on expiration
- Increase in attenuation during expiration is normal
- Apical parts have less vascular markings than lower part of lungs. When the X-ray is taken in upright position, the lungs markings will be seen more in the lower part than the upper part of the lungs
- Asymmetry at the hilar region
- Gradual tapering toward the periphery
- Vascular markings are more prominent in the lower lungs than the upper (in X-ray in upright position). Lower lobe vessels are two to three times larger than upper vessels
- Vascularity of left lower lung is less than that of right lower lung
- Normally, the right descending pulmonary artery is equal to that of the diameter of trachea
- The left pulmonary artery and left hilum are 1 cm above the right pulmonary artery
- The arteries and bronchial branches are almost same diameter with a ratio of 1.2:1.

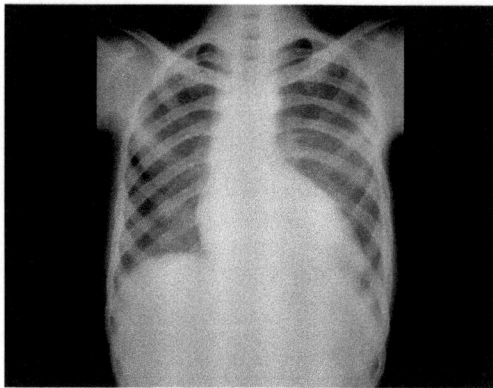

**Fig. 3.47:** Pulmonary oligemia.

### Abnormalities in Pulmonary Vasculature

* Pulmonary oligemia (Fig. 3.47)
* Pulmonary plethora
* Pulmonary artery hypertension
* Pulmonary venous hypertension.

**Pulmonary oligemia:**

**Radiological findings:**

* Appearance of overpenetrated film with oligemic lung fields (hyperlucent)
* Bronchial or other collateral vessels enlarged
* Concave or absent main pulmonary artery (MPA)
* Decreased size of pulmonary artery and veins
* Decreased density of hilar vessels
* *Expiratory air trapping*—In air trapping, low attenuation is maintained

* Enlarged right atrium (tricuspid regurgitation)
* *Four or less peripheral vessels*—Peripheral arteries are not visible. Less than four vessels in the peripheral one-third of the lungs.

## QUESTION

Q. **What are the conditions associated with pulmonary oligemia?**
  ❏ Pulmonary atresia
  ❏ Pulmonary stenosis
  ❏ Ebstein's anomaly
  ❏ *Intracardiac right to left shunts*—Tetralogy of Fallot
  ❏ Pericardial effusion
  ❏ Constrictive pericarditis
  ❏ Pulmonary embolism
  ❏ Right-sided heart failure.

### Miliary Mottling

Multiple small 1–4 mm pulmonary nodules scattered throughout the lung.

### Radiological Findings

* Miliary nodules
* Hyperinflation
* Slightly lower lobe predominance (Figs. 3.48A and B).

### Discussion

* The nodules will be of size less than 5 mm and 1–4 mm in size of pulmonary nodules.

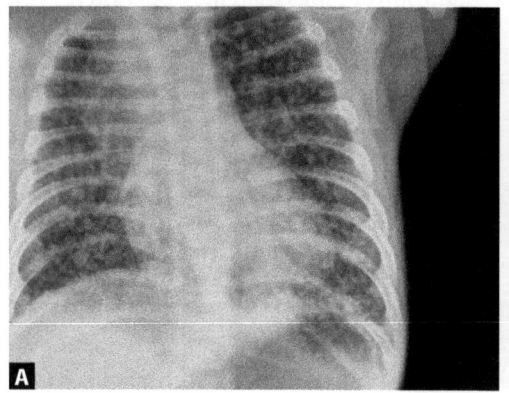
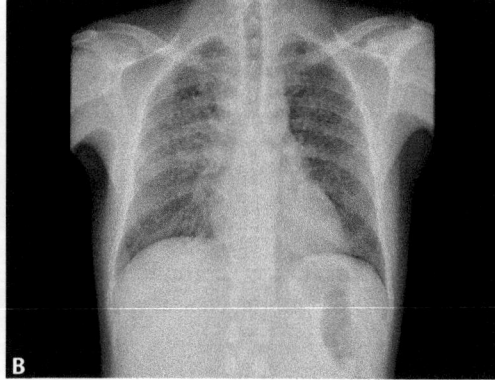

**Figs. 3.48A and B:** Miliary mottling.

They will be scattered throughout the lungs
- Hematogenous dissemination
- Generalized granulomatous lesions
- Immunodeficiency.

### Differential Diagnosis
- Eosinophilia
- Infections—Miliary tuberculosis, disseminated tuberculosis, viral pneumonitis
- Hypersensitivity pneumonitis
- Pneumoconiosis—Silicosis
- Histiocytosis
- Sarcoidosis
- Pulmonary hemosiderosis
- Langerhans cell histiocytosis (LCH)
- Pulmonary alveolar proteinosis
- Miliary metastasis (thyroid, renal cell carcinoma, malignant melanoma, trophoblastic disease.

Q. **What are the conditions associated with miliary mottling shadow in X-ray of chest?**

Miliary shadow in X-ray of chest is seen in the following conditions:

*Common conditions*:
- Miliary tuberculosis (Figs. 3.49A and B)
- Streptococcal pneumonitis
- Tropical eosinophilia.

*Rare causes*:
- Histoplasmosis
- Sarcoidosis
- Pneumoconiosis
- Hemosiderosis
- Varicella pneumonia
- Silicosis
- Hyperparathyroidism
- Blastomycosis
- Coccidioidomycosis
- Varicella zoster virus.

*Very rare causes*:
- Pulmonary alveolar lithiasis
- Pulmonary alveolar proteinosis
- Metastasis from thyroid carcinoma
- Gaucher's disease
- Histiocytosis X (eosinophilic granuloma).

### Discussion
- Tropical eosinophilia
- Miliary tuberculosis.

**Tropical eosinophilia:**
- Fluffy reticulonodular shadows especially in the midzones and bases
- Hilar adenopathy may be seen.

*Lung metastasis* is due to widespread hematogenous spread of tuberculosis. It is millet-like spread of tuberculosis bacilli as evidenced by chest X-ray (Fig. 3.50).

### Fibrosis of Lung
This is common in adults following secondary tuberculosis.

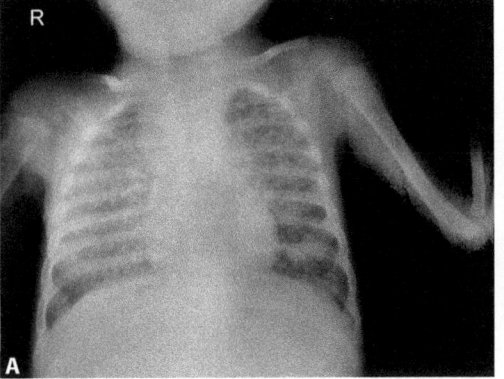 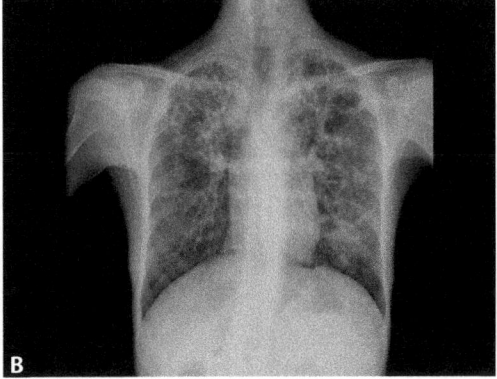

**Figs. 3.49A and B:** Miliary tuberculosis.

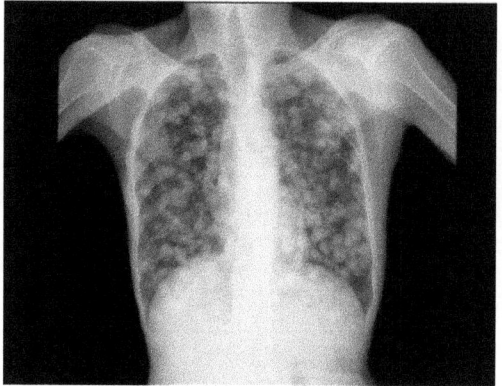

**Fig. 3.50:** Lung metastasis.

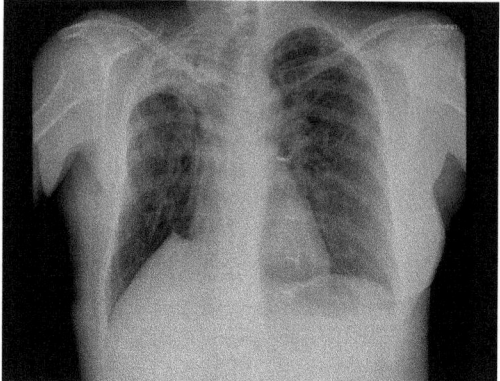

**Fig. 3.51:** Fibrosis: tenting of diaphragm and crowding of ribs.

## *Radiological Findings in Fibrosis*

- Airless segment of collapsed lung
- Blurring heart borders on the side of collapse
- Bibasilar subpleural reticulations
- Crowding of ipsilateral ribs
- Crowding of air bronchogram, pulmonary vessels
- Dense homogenous opacities
- Displacement of trachea to the side of fibrosis
- Flattening of hemidiaphragm on the side of fibrosis
- Ground-glass appearance
- Honeycombing
- Hyperlucency of other parts of lung
- Interlobar fissure pulled toward the fibrosis
- Ipsilateral hemidiaphragm will be elevated
- *Loss of lung volume*—Decreased total lung capacity
- Mediastinal shift to the side of fibrosis
- Nodules
- No air bronchogram
- Obscured mediastinum, cardiac outline
- Reticulation
- Septal thickening
- Tenting of diaphragm (Fig. 3.51)
- Loss of lung volume, tenting of diaphragm.

## *Differential Diagnosis*

- Asbestosis
- Adult respiratory distress syndrome
- Autoimmune disorders
- *Bacterial infections*—Tuberculosis
- Cystic fibrosis
- Connective tissue disorders
- Collagen vascular diseases
- *Drugs*—Methotrexate
- Eosinophilic pneumonia
- Combined emphysema and fibrosis
- *Granulomatous disorders*—Sarcoidosis
- Hermansky-Pudlak syndrome
- Hypersensitivity pneumonitis
- Inhaled substances like coal, silica
- Irradiation
- *Immune disorders*—Autoimmune conditions
- *Iatrogenic*—Drugs
- Idiopathic.

## Clinical Features in Pulmonary Fibrosis

- Crackles
- Dry cough
- Exertional dyspnea
- Digital clubbing.

## Subpulmonic Effusion (Fig. 3.52)

- The fluid collection will not be visible in supine position
- The fluid collection will be between the visceral pleura and the parietal pleura over the diaphragm. The shadow of the diaphragm will not be visible
- The visceral pleura will look like diaphragm

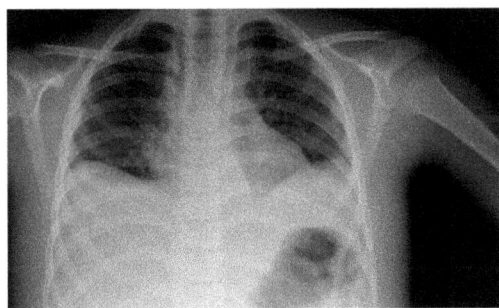

**Fig. 3.52:** Subpulmonic effusion.

- The distance between the left base of lung and the gastric bubble will be increased
- The dome will appear to be elevated
- In supine position, the fluid will move to dependent parts and the elevation will disappear.

### Differential Diagnosis
- Eventration of diaphragm
- Diaphragmatic paralysis
- Hepatomegaly on the right side
- Subdiaphragmatic abscess on the left side
- Splenomegaly on the left side.

## Foreign Body Aspiration

### Radiological Findings
- The volume will be more and the color will be darker on the side of emphysema
- The radiological findings will depend upon the site of obstruction
- The obstruction can obstruct the central, right, or left main bronchus
- The obstruction can be partial or total
- When the foreign body partially obstructs the airway, there will be air trapping on the side of obstruction. This will result in obstructive emphysema. When the foreign body totally obstructs the airway, the air inside the lung will be absorbed and there will be collapse on the side of obstruction. The other lung will expand which results in compensatory emphysema.

### Compensatory Emphysema
When the foreign body totally obstructs the right bronchus, the lungs will collapse on the right side as the air in the lungs will get absorbed. The lung on the other side will expand resulting in compensatory emphysema.

### Obstructive Emphysema
When the foreign body partially obstructs the right bronchus, the lungs will hyperinflate on the right side as the air in the lungs will get trapped during expiration.

In obstruction on one side of bronchus when X-ray is taken in inspiration and expiration, the mediastinum will be seen shifting from one side to the other side.

Plain X-ray may not show the foreign body if the object is radiolucent like onion peel, groundnuts, buttons, seeds, food particles.

**Radiological findings:**
- *Central partial obstruction*—Bilateral hyperventilation with equal volume on both side but increased volume on both sides. The diaphragm will be depressed on both sides
- *Right partial obstruction*—Right obstructive emphysema
- *Left partial obstruction*—Left obstructive emphysema
- *Right total obstruction*—Left compensatory emphysema
- *Left total obstruction*—Right compensatory emphysema.

| X-ray features | Diagnosis |
|---|---|
| • Haziness over the entire lung in children with lying down posture<br>• Fluid level in erect posture | Pleural effusion |
| Air shadow between lung and pleura | Pneumothorax |
| Patchy shadow | Consolidation |
| Miliary mottling | Miliary tuberculosis, eosinophilia |
| Hilar adenopathy | Tuberculosis, lymphomas |

*Contd...*

*Contd...*

| X-ray features | Diagnosis |
|---|---|
| Bilateral hyperventilation | Bronchial asthma, bronchiolitis |
| Mediastinal widening | Posterior mediastinal tumors—Neuroblastoma |
| Elevation of hemidiaphragm | Diaphragmatic hernia, eventration of diaphragm |

*Radiological findings in various respiratory system disorders.*

*Radiological findings depending upon the etiology in respiratory system disorders.*

| X-ray features | Etiology |
|---|---|
| Acute lobar pneumonia with complete resolution | Pneumococcal pneumonia |
| Right upper lobe pneumonia | Aspiration |
| Upper lobe pneumonia and cavitations | Tuberculous |
| Lower lobe pneumonia | Chemical pneumonia |
| Right middle lobe | Partial bronchial obstruction |
| Multiple small abscesses | Staphylococcal/Klebsiella pneumonia |

## Lung Patterns in X-ray of Chest

Basic six types of opacities in chest X-rays:
1. Air space opacity—consolidation
2. *Linear or septal*—Pulmonary edema
3. *Reticular opacities*—Usual interstitial pneumonia (UIP)
4. *Nodular opacities*—Infective causes like tuberculosis
5. *Reticulonodular shadows*—Sarcoidosis, lymphangitis, and spread of carcinoma
6. Ground-glass opacity in hyaline membrane disease

## Silhouette Sign (Fig. 3.53)

The cardiac borders will be obliterated by the shadow of any mass or fluid or node adjacent to the cardiac shadow.

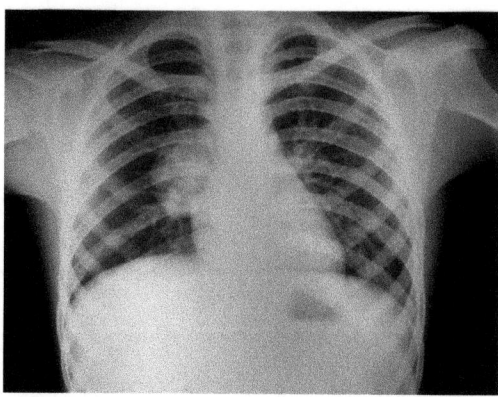

**Fig. 3.53:** Right hilar shadow-silhouette sign.

## QUESTIONS

**Q.1 Name few conditions that may produce silhouette sign.**
- ❏ Hilar adenopathy
- ❏ Mediastinal mass
- ❏ Pulmonary plethora.

**Q.2 How will you differentiate between emphysema and pneumothorax?**
In emphysema, the lung vascular markings will be seen whereas in pneumothorax, the lung markings will be absent.
 In pneumothorax, the collapsed lung will be seen on the side of pneumothorax.

## ABDOMEN

### X-ray Abdomen

*Evaluation of X-ray Abdomen*

Evaluation of X-ray abdomen in a newborn should be done in the following order:
- ❖ First focus on the relatively fixed structures like stomach and rectum.
- ❖ This should be followed by examination of solid organs like liver and spleen.

*Views*
- ❖ Supine
- ❖ Decubitus views
- ❖ Prone translateral
- ❖ Supine translateral
- ❖ Erect view.

## How to Read an X-ray Abdomen?
- First fix a hollow viscus like stomach and then move to others hollow viscus like intestines and rectum
- This should be followed by solid organs like liver, spleen, etc. This should be followed by study of bowel gas pattern.
- Diaphragmatic leaflets
- Bony structures
- Soft tissues.

## Analysis of Bowel Gas Pattern
Abnormal intraluminal and abnormal extraluminal gas.

### Abnormal intraluminal gas:
- Airless opaque nondistended abdomen—esophageal atresia without fistula
- Excessive bowel gas with abdominal distention when there is obstruction to the forward movement of gas.

**Q1. How to differentiate between the abdominal gaseous distention due to paralytic ileus and mechanical obstruction?**

In paralytic ileus, the distention will be uniform. No differential distention of the gastrointestinal (GI) tract will be seen. All portions of the GI tract will dilate in proportion to each other. The colon may appear larger than the small bowel. The dilated bowel loops are less orderly and look disorganized.

*Mechanical obstruction*: The bowel proximal to obstruction will be dilated and the part distal to obstruction will be collapsed. No proportional distention of entire gut.

The number of loops dilated will depend upon the site of obstruction.

If the obstruction is more proximal, less number of loops will be distended and it is more distal more number of distended loops will be seen.

### Abnormal extraluminal gas:
Intramural gas is due to loss of integrity of intestinal mucosa. Its intramural air will be seen as a linear or curvilinear collection of gas within the bowel wall.

Extraintestinal gas—pneumoperitoneum will indicate a hollow viscus perforation.

Pneumoperitoneum will be seen as increase translucency which diminishes the hepatic density and will outline the falciform ligament. This will result in football sign.

*Left lateral decubitus*: In esophageal atresia, the nasogastric tube will be coiled in the upper pouch.

Distention of stomach will be seen in hypertrophic pyloric stenosis and duodenal obstruction.

## Evaluation of X-ray Abdomen in a Newborn
Evaluation of X-ray abdomen in a newborn should be done in the following order:
- First focus on the relatively fixed structures like stomach and rectum.
- This should be followed by examination of solid organs like liver and spleen.

## Bowel Gas Pattern
The gas may be abdominal intraluminal or abdominal extraluminal. The extraluminal may be intramural or extraintestinal.

The time required for the swallowed air to reach various parts of the GI system is given below:

| Part of the GI tract | The time required for the swallowed air |
|---|---|
| Stomach | 30–60 minutes |
| Duodenum | 30–60 minutes |
| Jejunum | 2–4 hours |
| Ileum | 4–6 hours |
| Colon | 12–18 hours |
| Rectum | 24 hours |

Decreased bowel gas will be seen in conditions in which swallowing is affected like central nervous system (CNS) depression, prematurity also in conditions like prolonged nasogastric aspiration or repeated vomiting there will be diminished bowel gas.

Absent air shadow will be seen in conditions associated with anatomic discontinuity like esophageal atresia without fistula.

**Q1. When the abdomen is opaque, how will you differentiate whether it is due to airless abdomen or fluid-filled abdomen?**

In airless abdomen, the abdomen will not be distended. In fluid-filled abdomen, the abdomen will be distended.
- Excessive bowel gas with abdominal distention
- Obstruction is functional or organic.
- Paralytic ileus
- Mechanical ileus.

**Q2. How will you differentiate between the paralytic ileus and mechanical ileus?**

In paralytic ileus, the abdominal distention will be uniform. All the GI tract will dilate in proportion to each other.

In mechanical ileus, there will be differential distention of the GI tract. The GI tract proximal to the obstruction will be dilated and the part distal to the obstruction will be collapsed.

**Diaphragm**
- Bony structures
- Soft tissues.

**Q3. What is invertogram?**

It is used to study anorectal anomalies. The X-ray should be taken with the baby held upside down and a coin placed at the anal dimple. This is used to diagnose anorectal anomalies.

Prone translateral view is used to diagnose anorectal anomalies, intussusception.

## Intestinal Obstruction

### Radiological Findings in Intestinal Obstruction (Mnemonic A-I) (Figs. 3.54 and 3.55)

- Air fluid levels more than two in same loops of bowel but at different levels

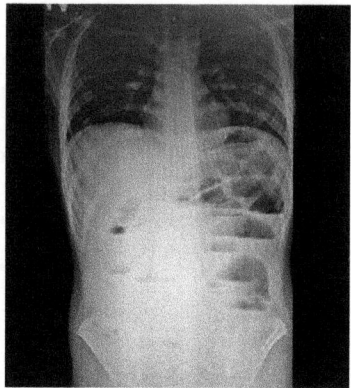

**Fig. 3.54:** X-ray—intestinal obstruction.

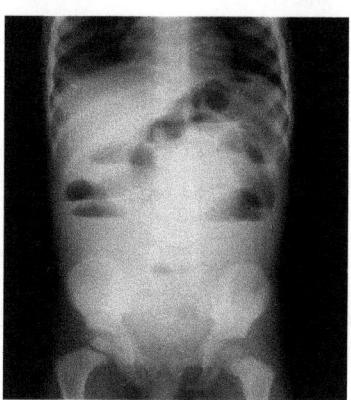

**Fig. 3.55:** X-ray multiple fluid levels.

- Absence of gas shadow in the rectum—prone translateral view will show absence of gas shadow in the rectum
- Bowel wall thickened
- Central dilated loops
- Distended loops of bowel proximal to obstruction
- Dilatation of bowel greater than 2.5–3 cm
- Edematous valvulae conniventes will be visible
- Fluid-filled bowel
- Gasless abdomen in high-grade mechanical obstruction
- Height of air fluid levels will be different in the same loop with greater than 2 cm difference
- Increased length—2.5 cm in length
- Increased small bowel—colon diameter ratio greater than 0.5.

# QUESTIONS

**Q1. What are the signs in intestinal obstruction?**
String of beads sign—small pockets of gas shadow within fluid-filled bowel.

**Q2. What are the types of intestinal obstruction?**
- Small bowel obstruction
- Large bowel obstruction.

**Q3. What are the radiological features of small bowel obstruction?**
- Central dilated loops
- Distended loops of bowel proximal to obstruction
- Dilatation of bowel greater than 2.5–3 cm (three or more)
- Edematous valvulae conniventes will be visible.

**Q4. What are the radiological features of large bowel obstruction?**
- Colonic distention proximal to obstruction
- Collapse of distal colon, small bowel will be distended if the duration of obstruction is long
- Colonic dilatation (large bowel >6 cm)
- Cecum limit of 9 cm.

**Q5. What are the findings in ischemic colon?**
- Intramural gas
- Portal vein gas.

## Gastroesophageal Reflux (Fig. 3.56)

Gastric acid reflux from the stomach into the esophagus due to lax esophageal sphincter.

### Radiological Findings

- Plain radiograph will not be useful.
- Barium meal study will show reflux of barium into the esophagus.
- Aspiration of contents into the lungs may result in aspiration pneumonia.

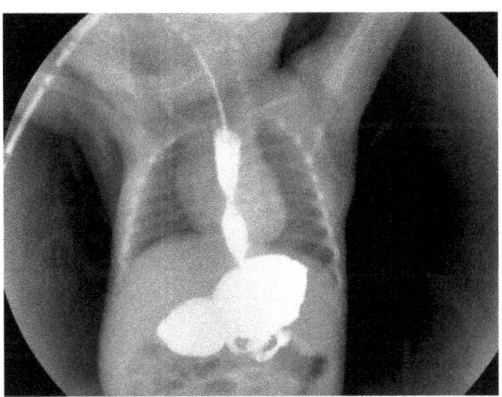

**Fig. 3.56:** X-ray—gastroesophageal reflux.

# QUESTIONS

**Q1. What is GERD?**
Gastroesophageal reflux disease.

**Q2. What are the risk factors and aggravating for gastroesophageal reflux?**
- Aspirin intake
- Beverages like alcohol/coffee
- Cigarette smoking
  - Connective tissue disorders—scleroderma
  - Delayed gastric emptying
  - Excess weight/obesity
  - Food habits—fatty food or fried foods
  - Gestational period (pregnancy)
  - Hiatus hernia
  - Intake of increased quantity of feeds
  - Junk foods.

**Q3. What are the complications of gastroesophageal reflux?**
- Aspiration pneumonia
- Barrett's esophagus
- Cancer esophagus
- Chronic cough
- Dysphagia
- Esophageal stricture
- Esophageal ulcer
- Fibrosis lung.

**Q4. What is Angle of His?**
It is the angle at which esophagus enters the stomach.

## X-ray Abdomen

Distal gut is airless at birth. Air takes 6–8 hours before reaching colon.

**Q1. How will you differentiate between small and large intestine?**

| Features | Small intestine | Large intestine |
|---|---|---|
| Location | Central location | Peripheral |
| Valvulae conniventes | Valvulae conniventes present | Absent |
| Haustrations | Absent | Haustrations present |
| Diameter | 2.5–3 cm | >5 cm |

**Q2. What are the causes of gasless abdomen?**
- ❑ The absence of gas can involve part of abdomen or total
- ❑ Total absence of gas
- ❑ Part of abdomen:
  - ➢ Acute pancreatitis
  - ➢ Annular pancreas
  - ➢ Congenital hypertrophic pyloric stenosis
  - ➢ Duodenal atresia
  - ➢ Mesenteric infarction
  - ➢ Tracheoesophageal fistula
  - ➢ Esophageal atresia.

**Q3. Plain X-ray abdomen should be taken in erect or supine position to diagnose intestinal perforation?**
Erect posture will be helpful in diagnosing perforation with air under diaphragm.

**Q4. What are the X-ray findings in normal abdomen?**
Normal X-ray of abdomen will show the following:
- ❑ Shadow of the stomach just below the left dome of the diaphragm
- ❑ The transverse colon can be traced to the splenic flexure and then down to the left colon
- ❑ Rectal air shadow will be seen in the pelvis.

**Q5. How will you differentiate an intra-abdominal swelling from a parietal swelling?**
The properitoneal pad of fat will be seen as a translucent black line. In parietal swelling, this line will be displaced inward. In intra-abdominal swelling this line will be displaced outward.

**Q6. What are the radiological findings in ascariasis?**
Distinct curvilinear opaque shadows within an air-filled bowel loop
Distinct small round opacities will represent end on view of the worms.

**Q7. What is the most common cause of abdominal pain in children?**
Worm infestation especially ascariasis.

**Q8. What are the radiological findings in lead poisoning?**
- ❑ Plain X-ray will show lead lines at the metaphyseal end of long bones
- ❑ Sclerotic margins of both iliac bones.

**Q9. What is the radiological finding in duodenal atresia?**
- ❑ Single air bubble or dilated stomach—duodenal atresia
- ❑ Double bubble sign—duodenal atresia.

**Q10. What is the radiological finding in IHPS?**
- ❑ Infantile hypertrophic pyloric stenosis (IHPS)—plain X-ray will show a large stomach bubble. There will be a paucity of in the rest of the abdomen.
- ❑ Ultrasonogarm will be diagnostic which will show thick pyloric mass.

**Q11. What is string sign?**
In doubtful cases, barium study should be done which will show narrow pyloric canal.

**Q12. What is double bubble sign?**
Duodenal atresia—a plain X-ray of the abdomen will show stomach and first part of the duodenum is the only part of the intestine filled with gas.

## Intussusception

Intussusception is a condition where one segment of intestine telescopes into another loop of intestine causing intestinal obstruction.

**Q1. What is colon cutoff sign?**
Colon cutoff sign—convex shadow inside the transverse colon near the splenic flexure.

**Q2. What are the causes of multiple fluid levels in the abdominal X-ray?**
- Multiple fluid levels will be seen in the following conditions:
  - Intestinal obstruction
  - Postdiarrheal ileus.
- If the transverse colon and rectum are visualized, intestinal obstruction is unlikely.

**Q3. How will you take prone translateral views?**
The child will lie in prone position. X-ray cassette is placed vertically by the side of the patient. The X-ray beam should be shot horizontally across the patient centering on S1 vertebra. This will show air in the rectum in the presacral space.

Prone translateral view should not be taken immediately after per rectal examination, as air will enter during insertion of fingers into the rectum. This will result in air in the rectum. Prone translateral view should be taken after 6 hours after per rectal examination.

**Q4. How will you differentiate duodenal atresia and atresia at more lower part of the intestine?**
In lower atresia, there will be more bowel loops filled gas with appearance of air-fluid levels and a gasless abdomen, which is due to unfilled distal intestine abdomen.

Distal gut is airless at birth. Air takes 6–8 hours before reaching colon.

**Q5. What are the radiological findings in intestinal gangrene?**
X-ray abdomen supine view will show mottled appearance and will be seen in necrosis of the bowel wall.

**Q6. What are the radiological findings in Intestinal perforation?**
Erect posture will show air under the diaphragm.

**Q7. What is the cardinal clinical sign of intestinal perforation?**
Obliteration of the liver dullness.

**Q8. What is the radiological feature of intestinal perforation in X-ray abdomen supine position?**
Liver density of will be decreased.

**Q9. What are the radiological findings in paralytic ileus?**
- Uniform distention of abdomen
- X-ray abdomen in supine position will show uniformly dilated stomach and intestines
- Prone translateral view will show presence of rectal gas shadow.

**Q10. What are the radiological findings in meconium ileus?**
- Distended loops with soap bubble or ground glass appearance in terminal ileum
- Calcification of will be seen in meconium ileus
- Free passage of dye in the terminal ileum.
- Multiple pellets in the colon.

**Points to know:**
1. In distal gut obstruction like Hirschsprung's disease, meconium plug syndrome, paralytic ileus, no air fluid levels will be visualized but there will be an increased amount of air throughout the gut.
2. Fetal meconium peritonitis—calcification. Predisposing conditions—mucoviscidosis—cystic fibrosis.
3. Barium swallow studies will be useful in diagnosis gastroesophageal reflux, hiatus hernia, pyloric stenosis.

## Tuberculosis of Intestine

Involvement of abdominal organs due to infection by *Mycobacterium tuberculosis* can involve any part including intestines, lymph nodes etc.

### Radiological Findings in Abdominal Tuberculosis

**Plain X-ray abdomen:**

- Air under diaphragm (due to complications like perforation)
- Bowel loops dilated
- Calcified nodes
- Dilatation of terminal ileum
- Enteroliths
- Features of intestinal obstruction
- Ground glass appearance due to ascites
- Granulomas
- Hollow viscus perforation
- Complications like intussusceptions

**Barium contrast:**

- Bowel wall thickening
- Cecum in the subhepatic region
- Deep fissures
- Enterocutaneous fistula
- Flocculation of barium
- Rapid intestinal transit
- Hypersegmentation of barium
- Hour glass stenosis—due to stenosis of lumen with smooth, stiff corners, segmental dilatation of bowel loops
- Precipitation of barium
- Loss of symmetry in fold pattern
- Sinus tracts.

**Barium enema:**

- Thickened ileocecal valve
- Inverted umbrella sign or Fleischner's sign—thickened ileocecal valve with narrowing of terminal ileum with or without wide gaping of ileocecal valve.
- Purse string stenosis localized stenosis opposite to ileocecal valve, with rounded off smooth colon
- Subhepatic cecum—cecum conical, shrunken and pulled up due to contraction and fibrosis of the mesocolon.
- Ulcers—double contrast studies will show ulcers.

## QUESTION

**Q1.** What are the types of abdominal tuberculosis?
- Luminal
- Peritoneal
- Nodal
- Hepatosplenic
- Ulcerative type—non-filling of terminal ileum, ascending colon, and caecum due to hypermotility
- Hyperplastic type long narrow vertical filling defect of terminal ileum, ascending colon.

## ENDOCRINE SYSTEM

### Hypothyroidism

*Radiological Finding in a Newborn with Hypothyroidism*

- X-rays of lower end of femur and upper end of tibia show delayed formation of epiphysis (Figs. 3.57 to 3.60).
- X-ray of knee joint for epiphyseal formation (upper tibial and lower femoral) shows epiphysis stippling or dysgenesis.
- X-ray foot—cuboidal epiphysis will be absent or epiphyseal stippling/dysgenesis.
- X-ray left wrist for formation of the carpal bones will show delayed bone age.
- X-ray skull large fontanels, wide sutures, intersutural bones (Wormian bones).
- Enlarged sella turcica, round, erosion and thinning rarely.

*Radiological Findings in Hypothyroidism*

- Appearance of epiphysis delayed
- Beaking of 12th thoracic or 1st and 2nd lumbar vertebra
- Cardiomegaly
- Deformities of ribs
- Epiphyseal stippling or dysgenesis—multiple foci of ossification
- Pericardial effusion (rarely)
- Formation of teeth delayed.

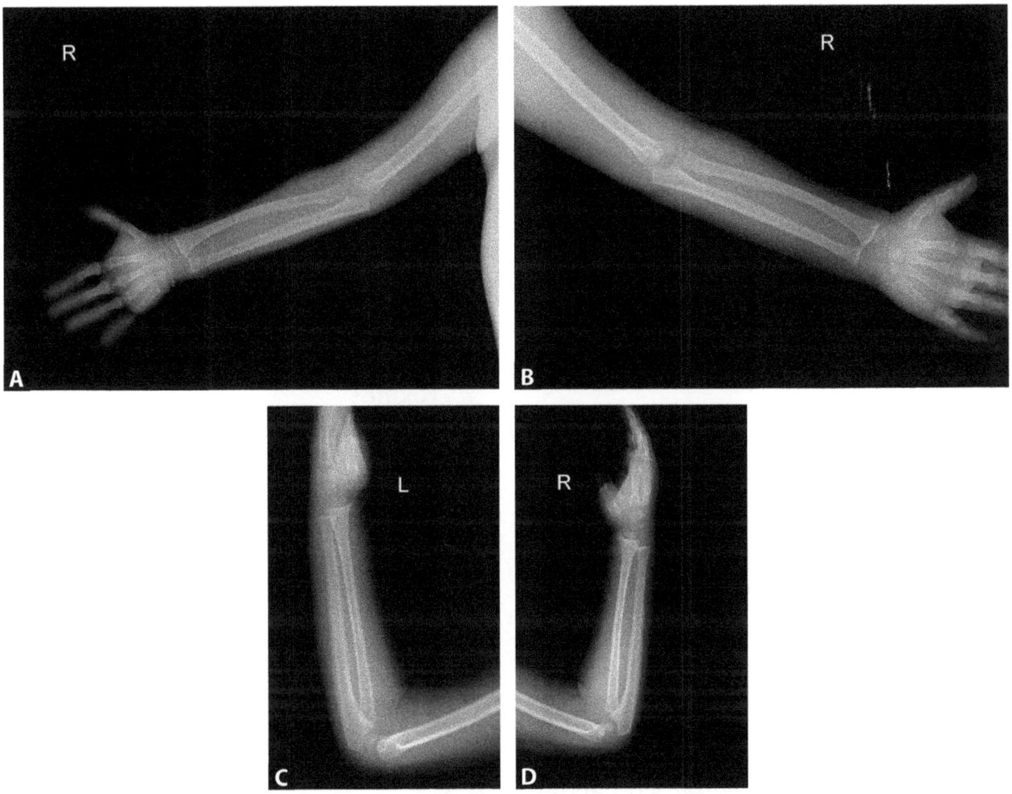

**Figs. 3.57A to D:** Hypothyroidism—14 years.

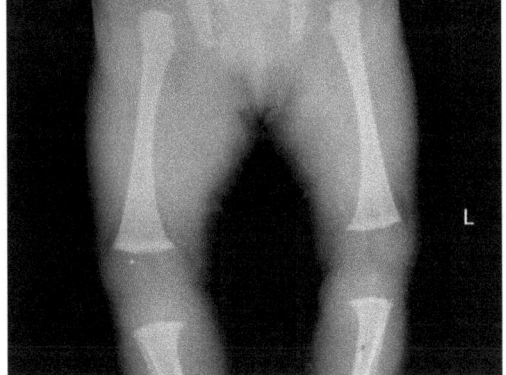

**Fig. 3.58:** Absence of epiphysis at the lower end of femur in hypothyroidism.

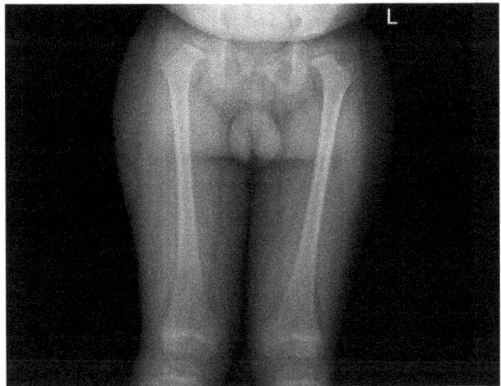

**Fig. 3.59:** Epiphyseal dysgenesis.

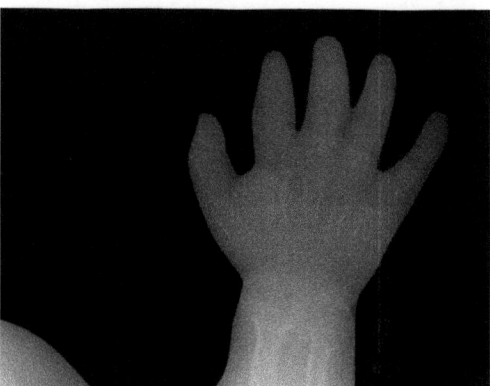

**Fig. 3.60:** X-ray showing delayed bone age.

## QUESTIONS

**Q1. What are the conditions associated with absent epiphysis at lower end of femur at birth?**
- Hypothyroidism
- Preterm.

**Q2. How will you classify hypothyroidism?**
Hypothyroidism is classified as:
- *Primary hypothyroidism*: It occurs due to a defect in the thyroid gland. There is increased secretion of thyroid-stimulating hormone (TSH).
- *Secondary hypothyroidism*: It occurs due to decreased secretion of TSH, which is due to a defect in the pituitary gland (hypopituitarism).
- *Tertiary hypothyroidism*: It is characterized by a deficient TSH secretion due to deficient thyrotropin-releasing hormone (TRH) secretion from the hypothalamus.

**Q3. How will you screen a newborn for hypothyroidism?**
*TSH screening of newborn*:
Every newborn baby should be screened for congenital hypothyroidism as delay in treatment results in irreversible mental retardation. Routine screening of TSH levels is done in the spot blood samples obtained on third days preferably before 7 day after birth. Tandem mass spectroscopy is helpful in diagnosing hypothyroidism in newborn from a small sample of blood.

**Q4. What is TMS ?**
Tandem mass spectroscopy. With a drop of blood screening of about 250 metabolic disorders can be done by this method.

**Q5. How will you treat hypothyroidism?**
L-thyroxine supplementation.

**Q6. What is the earliest side effect of thyroxine?**
Diarrhea.

**Q7. What is the part of the body for X-ray evaluation for epiphyseal dysgenesis in a 9-year-old child?**
Epiphyseal dysgenesis in the head of the humerus.

## CHROMOSOMAL DISORDERS

### Down Syndrome

*Radiological Features in Down Syndrome*

*Skull*:
Hypoplasia of base of skull, facial bones, and middle phalanx of 5th finger.

*Chest*:
- Absent ribs—X-ray chest—only 11 pairs of ribs.
- Two or three ossification centers of manubrium
- Hypersegmented sternum.

*Hands*:
Accessory epiphysis at base of 2nd metaphysis.

*Pelvis* (Fig. 3.61):
- Abnormal ilial index. Pelvis iliac wings broad and flared, with acetabular iliac angle reduced, resulting in an abnormal ilial index.
- Coxa valga (dysplasia of pelvis with shallow acetabular angle)
- Developmental dysplasia of hip (DDH)
- Mickey mouse pelvis—flared iliac wings.

*X-ray spine*:
- To rule out atlantoaxial dislocation
- Hypoplastic posterior arch of C1.

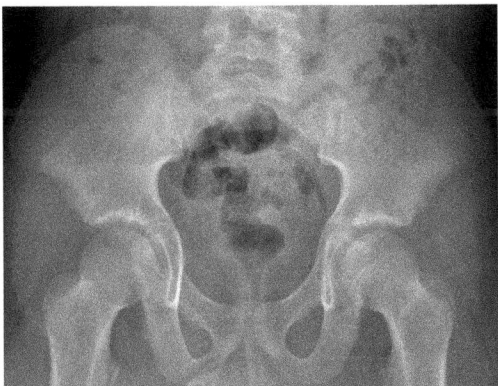

**Fig. 3.61:** *X-ray pelvis.* Down syndrome—Outward flaring of ilia (elephant ear appearance), Prominent anterior superior iliac spine and flattened acetabular roof.

## Radiological Changes in Down Syndrome

- Anterior atlantodental interval (AADI) increased. Atlantoaxial dislocation/instability (increased laxity between atlas and odontoid process, the distance between anterior arch of atlas and the odontoid process will be more than 4.5 mm at the age of 3 or more years)
- Anorectal anomalies
- Bony anomalies—absent ribs—only 11 pairs of ribs will be present
- Congenital cardiac defects—atrioventricular septal defect (AVSD), endocardial cushion defects
- Duodenal atresia (double bubble sign)
- Diaphragmatic hernia
- Esophageal atresia
- Flaring of iliac wings (Mickey mouse appearance of pelvis due to flaring of iliac crest)
- Gastrointestinal anomalies
- Hypersegmented sternum (two or three ossification centers of manubrium)
- Hypoplastic posterior arch of C1
- Intestinal obstruction
- Infections
- Joint dislocation
- Knee cap instability (knee deformed) frequent falls.

## QUESTIONS

**Q1. What is the incidence of Down syndrome?**
Incidence—1 in 700 newborns.

**Q2. What are the chromosomal abnormalities seen in Down syndrome?**
An extra 21 chromosome is present which is of maternal or paternal origin.
1. Nondisjunction—most common (94%). In most cases, the origin is maternal, especially when the mother is more than 30 years old.
2. Translocation (13, 14, 15 ≥21) (4%)
3. Mosaicism—2% (normal and abnormal cell lines)
    - Maternal age independent—where the age of conception is less than 30 years. Translocation is the most common cause in these cases.
    - Maternal age dependent—trisomy 21 is common in these cases.

**Q3. What are the abnormalities seen in cardiovascular system in a case of Down syndrome?**
- Congenital heart disease (CHD) in 40-60% of the children.

Common defects are:
- Atrial septal defects (ASDs)
- Aortic regurgitation
- Aberrant (retroesophageal) right subclavian artery
- Balanced/unbalanced AVSD
- Complete AVSD
- Conotruncal anomalies
- Coarctation of aorta
- Double outlet right ventricle
- Patent ductus arteriosus (PDA). Rarely
- Endocardial cushion defects/Atrioventricular canal defects (A-V canal defects)
- Fallot's tetralogy (TOF)—occasionally.
- Ventricular septal defect (VSD).

**Q4. What are the abnormalities seen in gastrointestinal system in Down syndrome?**

- ☐ Anal atresia
- ☐ Annular pancreas
- ☐ Biliary atresia
- ☐ Celiac disease
- ☐ Duodenal atresia
- ☐ Distention of abdomen (due to hypotonia)
- ☐ Divarication of recti
- ☐ Eruption of teeth delayed
- ☐ Fistula—tracheoesophageal fistula
- ☐ Gastric outlet obstruction—pyloric stenosis
- ☐ Hirschsprung's disease
- ☐ Intestinal atresia
- ☐ Imperforate anus
- ☐ Malabsorption
- ☐ Umbilical hernia may be present.

**Q5. What are the neuropsychiatric abnormalities seen in Down syndrome?**
- ☐ Alzheimer disease
- ☐ Autism spectrum disorder
- ☐ Behavior disorders
- ☐ Convulsions
- ☐ Developmental delay
- ☐ Depression.

## GENITOURINARY SYSTEM

### Renal Calculus

- ❖ Anywhere in the course of urinary tracts.
- ❖ Plain kidney, ureter, and bladder (KUB) film.

## QUESTIONS

**Q1. What is nephrocalcinosis?**
Formation of stones within the kidney.

**Q2. What is nephrolithiasis?**
Stones with in the collecting system.

**Q3. What is the difference between dystrophic calcification and metastatic calcification?**
- ☐ Dystrophic calcification is calcification occurring in abnormal tissue.
- ☐ Metastatic calcification occurs in normal tissues.

**Q4. What is the cause for metastatic calcification?**
Metastatic calcification occurs when the solubility product of calcium and phosphate or oxalate exceeds the normal values.

**Q5. What are the types of nephrocalcinosis?**
Cortical and medullary nephrocalcinosis.

**Q6. What are the causes of cortical hypercalcinosis?**
- ☐ Chronic glomerulonephritis
- ☐ Oxalosis
- ☐ Alport syndrome

**Q7. What are the causes of medullary hypercalcinosis?**
- ☐ Hyperparathyroidism
- ☐ Renal tubular acidosis type 1, distal
- ☐ Medullary sponge kidney

**Q8. What are the causes of radiopaque stones?**
- ☐ Calcium oxalate
- ☐ Calcium phosphate
- ☐ Triple phosphate (struvite)

**Q9. What are the causes of radiolucent stones?**
- ☐ Uric acid
- ☐ Cystine
- ☐ Xanthine

**Q10. What are the disadvantages of radiographic evaluation of renal stones?**
- ☐ Size less than 3 mm may be obscured by colonic or superimposed bone structures.
- ☐ It will not provide information about the obstruction.
- ☐ Sensitivity only 62%.
- ☐ Specificity only 67%.
- ☐ Other shadows of pelvis (phleboliths and appendicoliths may be confused of renal stone)

**Q11. What are the advantages of ultrasonographic evaluation of renal stones?**
- ☐ Available in all places
- ☐ Bedside examination can be done
- ☐ Clear image of soft tissues
- ☐ Drugs for sedation not required

- ❏ Diagnosis accurate
- ❏ Dynamic visual images
- ❏ Easy to use
- ❏ Expenses—less
- ❏ Ionizing radiation is avoided
- ❏ Noninvasive
- ❏ Painless
- ❏ Reproducible
- ❏ Real-time images
- ❏ Safe procedure.

**Q12. What are the disadvantages of ultrasonographic evaluation of renal stones?**
- ❏ Dependent on skilled personnel for interpretation
- ❏ Image resolution less—can miss stones less than 0.5 mm
- ❏ Patient cooperation needed
- ❏ It will be difficult to interpret renal stones in the following conditions:
  - ➢ Abnormalities of renal tract
  - ➢ Air or bowel gas will prevent visualization of structures
  - ➢ Bone penetration poor
  - ➢ Body habitus abnormal
  - ➢ Congenital abnormalities
  - ➢ Deep-seated stones. If distance is more, image resolution will be poor
  - ➢ Duplications
  - ➢ Ectopic kidneys
  - ➢ Ectopic ureters
  - ➢ Fatty patients. As ultrasound has limited penetration in obese persons
  - ➢ Genitourinary abnormalities
  - ➢ Horseshoe kidneys
  - ➢ Interposed bowel gas.

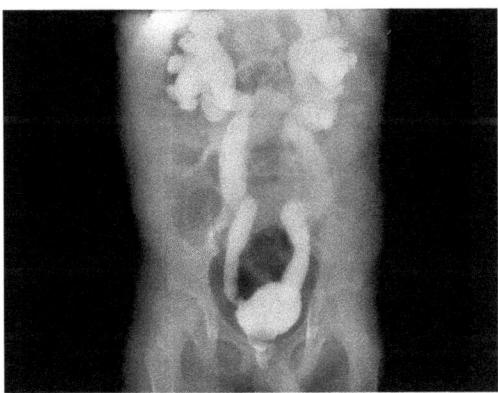

**Fig. 3.62:** Bilateral hydroureteronephrosis (HUN).

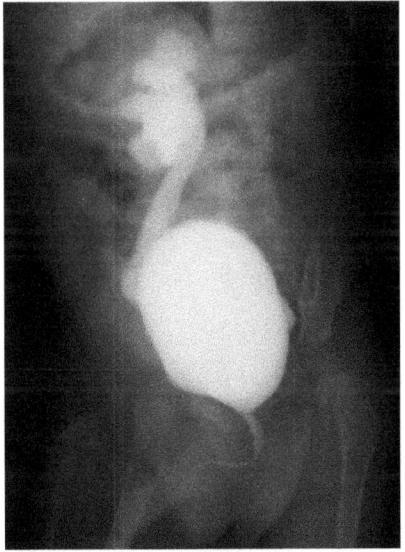

**Fig. 3.63:** Right HUN.

## Hydronephrosis (Figs. 3.62 and 3.63)

Hydronephrosis is a condition caused by obstruction to the ureters. This may be due to renal stones, infections, obstruction by tumors, enlarged prostate, etc.

### Grading

- ❖ *Grade I*: Reflux into a nondilated distal ureter
- ❖ *Grade II*: Reflux into the upper collecting system without dilatation
- ❖ *Grade III*: Reflux with blunting of calyceal fornices dilated ureter
- ❖ *Grade IV*: Reflux into a grossly dilated ureter
- ❖ *Grade V*: Massive reflux.

### Causes of Hydronephrosis

Obstruction at pelviureteric junction, ureters, bladder neck, urethra.

### Congenital causes

- ❖ Posterior ureteric valve
- ❖ Ectopic ureterocele

- ❖ Congenital urethral strictures
- ❖ Prune belly syndrome
- ❖ Anterior urethral valves
- ❖ Aberrant ureteric artery
- ❖ Neuromuscular bladder
- ❖ Neuromuscular defect at pelviureteric junction, ureter or bladder neck-phimosis
- ❖ Urethral diverticulum

**Acquired causes**
- ❖ Clot, stones, tumor, fibrosis
- ❖ Vesicoureteric reflux
- ❖ Hypertrophy of verumontanum
- ❖ Meatal stenosis
- ❖ Retroperitoneal fibrosis
- ❖ Iatrogenic—inadvertent suturing of ureter during surgery
- ❖ Carcinoma cervix
- ❖ Prostate enlargement

**Complications of Hydronephrosis**
- ❖ Renal atrophy
- ❖ Renal impairment
- ❖ Renal failure

# HEMATOLOGY

## Thalassemia

### Radiological Changes in Thalassemia
- ❖ Medullary portion of the bone is widened and the bony cortex is thinned out with a coarse trabecular pattern in the medulla.
- ❖ X-ray of the metacarpals, ribs and vertebra will show thinning of cortex.
- ❖ X-ray skull—hair-on-end appearance (thalassemia) elongated trabeculae in widening of diploic spaces. It shows hair-on-end appearance (Figs. 3.64 and 3.65). This is due to widened diploic spaces in the skull. The frontal bone appears thickened, starting in the nasal region of the frontal bone and extending symmetrically over the parietotemporal regions but sparing the occiput. This gives the appearance of bossing.
- ❖ Thickened calvarium

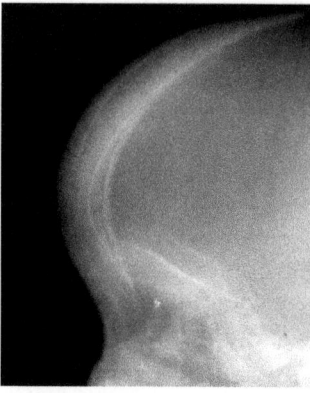

**Fig. 3.64:** X-ray—hair-on-end appearance in thalassemia.

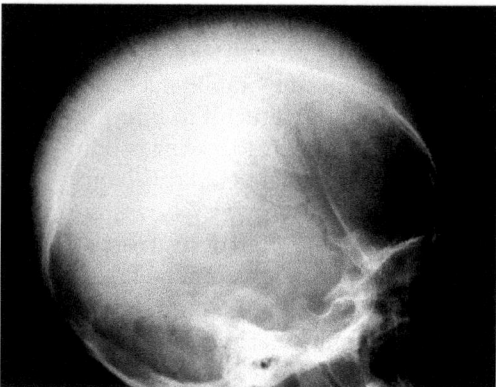

**Fig. 3.65:** X-ray skull—hair-on-end appearance.

- ❖ Pneumatization of the sinuses is delayed and the maxilla appears overgrowth with prominent malar eminences.
- ❖ X-ray bone changes are seen after 1 year.
- ❖ Widened diploic space.
- ❖ X-ray hand—reticular pattern in metacarpals (after 4 months)
- ❖ X-ray chest—reticular pattern in ribs
- ❖ X-ray chest—rib-within-a-rib appearance
- ❖ General—fractures
- ❖ Generalized osteoporosis.

### Radiological Findings in Thalassemia (Mnemonic—A-H)
- ❖ **A**ir in the frontal, maxillary, sphenoid sinuses decreased as it is filled with marrow
- ❖ **B**roadened bones
- ❖ **B**ossing of skull

- Coarse trabecular pattern in medulla
- Cortex thinned out (metacarpals, ribs and vertebra)
- Diploic space widened
- Dental malocclusion
- Epiphysis fuse prematurely
- Enlargement of bones due to expansion of bone marrow
- Fractures
- Generalized loss of bone density (osteoporosis)
- Hair-on-end appearance.

## QUESTIONS

**Q1. What is the age of presentation of thalassemia?**
Thalassemia usually presents after the age of 6 months.

**Q2. Why thalassemia presents after the age of 6 months?**
It is due to the presence of fetal hemoglobin in the early infancy.

**Q3. What is the cardinal feature of thalassemia?**
Progressive pallor.

**Q4. What are the complications of thalassemia?**
Mnemonic—A-L:
- **A**menorrhea—secondary amenorrhea
- **B**one density—reduced (osteoporosis)
- **C**holelithiasis (common in thalassemia intermedia patients)
- **C**ardiac failure/arrhythmias
- **D**ilated cardiomyopathy
- **D**elayed puberty
- **D**iabetes
- **E**ndocrine problems—hypothyroidism, hypoparathyroidism, hypogonodism
- **E**nlarged spleen
- **F**atal arrhythmias
- **F**erritin levels increased
- **G**rowth retardation—short stature
- **H**ypersplenism
- **H**ormonal problems—poor growth, short stature, delayed puberty, secondary amenorrhea
- Hemosiderosis
- **I**mpaired glucose intolerance
- **I**ron-related organ dysfunction
- **I**nfertility
- **J**oint problems—pain
- **K**idney problems—glomerulopathy/tubulopathy
- **L**iver complications—hepatitis.

**Q5. What are the complications due to iron overload in thalassemia?**
- Cardiovascular system (CVS)—pericarditis, cardiac failure, ventricular ectopics
- Liver—hepatomegaly, rarely cirrhosis
- Endocrine—pancreas—diabetes mellitus
  - Adrenal crisis
  - Delayed development of secondary sexual characters.

**Q6. What are the causes of cardiac failure in thalassemia?**
- Persistent hypoxia
- Volume overload
- Cardiomyopathy due to hemosiderosis.

## QUESTIONS RELATED TO INVESTIGATIONS

**Q1. What are the causes of anemia in thalassemia?**
- Hemoglobin production impaired
- Hemolysis
- Hemodilution
- Hemolysis due to hypersplenism
- Ineffective erythropoiesis.

**Q2. What are the peripheral smear findings in thalassemia?**
- Mnemonic—THALASSEMIA:

| | |
|---|---|
| T | **T**arget cells<br>**T**ear drop cells |
| H | **H**ypochromia<br>**H**owell-Jolly bodies<br>**H**elmet cells |
| A | **A**nisocytosis |
| L | **L**eptocytes (large, thin, hypochromic, macrocytes) |

| A | **A**nisocytosis |
|---|---|
| S | **S**chistocytosis Shape variations—poikilocytosis, cigar-shaped cells |
| S | **S**tippling (basophilic) |
| E | **E**rythroblasts—early, intermediate and late |
| M | **M**icrocytosis |
| I | **I**ncreased fetal hemoglobin (HbF) Immature nucleated red blood cells (RBCs)/reticulocytosis |
| A | **A**nemia |

- Normoblasts
- Polychromasia.

**Q3. What are the conditions associated with microcytic hypochromic anemia?**
Mnemonic—TALIPES MICRO:
- Thalassemia
- Atransferrinemia (congenital atransferrinemia)
- Lead poisoning
- Infections—chronic infections/diseases
- Pyridoxine deficiency
- E-Hemoglobin E disorder
- Sideroblastic anemia
- Myeloproliferative disorder
- Iron deficiency anemia
- Copper deficiency
- Renal failure
- Others—congenital defect in iron transport.

**Q4. Why ethmoid cells are spared in thalassemia ?**
It is because ethmoid cells lack bone marrow.

## QUESTIONS RELATED TO TREATMENT

**Q1. What is the optimum level in which the hemoglobin should be maintained?**
9–10 g/dL.

**Q2. What should be the interval between two transfusions?**
2–4 weeks.

**Q3. How many units of blood can be given in one sitting?**
Two, three or more units may be associated with interactions between units. Also the risk of reactions will be high.

**Q4. What is the amount of iron present in 1 mL of packed RBC?**
0.8 mg.

**Q5. How will you treat thalassemia major?**
- Repeated blood transfusions
- Folic acid 5 mg daily
- Antibiotic to treat infections
- Avoid oral or parenteral iron
- Iron chelators
- Splenectomy if needed.

**Q6. How will you treat thalassemia minor?**
No transfusion will be required. Reassurance and genetic counseling should be given.

**Q7. What is hypertransfusion?**
Blood hemoglobin is maintained at 10–12 g/dL.

**Q8. What is hypotransfusion?**
Blood hemoglobin is maintained at 6–10 g/dL.

**Q9. What is supertransfusion?**
Blood hemoglobin is maintained at 12–14 g/dL.

**Q10. What is the aim of iron chelation therapy?**
To keep the serum ferritin level below 1,000 µg/L. Persistence of increase serum ferritin in the range of greater than 2,500 µg/L will be associated with cardiac complications.

**Q11. What are the indications for splenectomy in thalassemia?**
The indications for splenectomy in thalassemia are:
- The requirement of excessive transfusion (PRBC more than 220 mL/kg/year)
- Evidence of hypersplenism

- Massive splenomegaly leading to persistent abdominal discomfort, dragging pain, early satiety.

**Q12. What are the vaccines that should be given before splenectomy?**
- Pneumococcal
- Meningococcal
- *Haemophilus influenzae*

These should be given at least 4 weeks before splenectomy.

**Q13. What are the problems in a child subjected to splenectomy?**
Malaria will be more severe and the mortality is high.
Infection with *Streptococcus pneumoniae* is very high.

**Q14. Name few iron chelators.**
- Desferrioxamine 25–50 mg/kg/day given by subcutaneous infusion by a pump over 5–7 hours. This should be given at least 5 days in a week.
- Deferiprone 50–75 mg/kg.

**Q15. What is the definitive treatment that cures thalassemia?**
Stem cell therapy (bone marrow transplantation with HLA-matched sibling donor).

**Q16. Can thalassemia patients get married?**
Yes, fertility has been reported.

## MUSCULOSKELETAL SYSTEM

### GENERAL

### Bone Age

At birth, X-ray knee shows appearance of epiphysis at the lower end of femur and the upper end of tibia.

From 2 to 8 years bone age is determined by examining the X-ray of the left wrist. Note the number of carpal bones and their appearance. The left hand is chosen for taking the X-ray because most people are right handed and are prone to have developed injuries, which can give abnormal shadows.

Later X-ray of the elbow is taken for assessment of bone age.

### Various Age of Appearance of Epiphysis

Age of appearance of epiphysis is as follows:

| Epiphysis | Age of appearance |
|---|---|
| Capitulum | 2 years |
| Radial head | 4 years |
| Internal epicondyle | 6 years |
| Trochlea | 8 years |
| Olecranon | 11 years |
| External epicondyle | 13 years |

**How will you calculate bone age with an X-ray of wrist showing carpal bones?**

By the age of 6 months, ossification centers for the carpal bones, i.e. capitate and hamate appear. It is easy to remember the number of ossification centers in wrist, which is equal to the age in years plus one.

Number of ossification centers in wrist = Age (years) + 1

Thus, a child of 2 years should have three ossification centers. From 1 year to 8 years, bone age is determined by examining carpal bones in the X-ray of the left wrist as follows:

| Age (year) | X-ray—number of ossification centers = Age + 1 |
|---|---|
| | Carpal centers appear by 2 months of age |
| 1 | 2 (capitate and hamate) |
| 2 | 3 |
| 3 | 4 |
| 4 | 5 |
| 5 | 6 |
| 6 | 7 |

### Number of Ossification Centers in Wrist According to Age

The number of carpal bones and their appearance is noted. X-ray left hand is taken because most people are right handed and are prone to injuries, which can give abnormal shadows. Wrist is an area where multiple bones can be seen together. Also, this part can be visualized easily with low radiation X-rays.

## Bone Age in Infancy and Childhood

*Bone age* is based on, when ossification centers appear and when the epiphyseal–diaphyseal union occur.

| Neonatal age | Part of body |
|---|---|
| 22–26 weeks | Os calcis and talus |
| 31–39 weeks | Distal epiphysis of the femur appears |
| 34 weeks of gestation to 5 weeks postnatally | Proximal epiphysis of the tibia |
| 37 weeks of gestation to 8 weeks postnatally | Cuboid |
| 36 weeks of gestation to 16 weeks postnatally | Proximal end of humerus |

A full-term newborn has the following five radiologically demonstrable ossification centers:
1. Distal end of femur
2. Proximal end of tibia
3. Talus
4. Calcaneum
5. Cuboid.

Infants—lower end of the knee joint and upper end of tibia.

| Age | Part of body |
|---|---|
| At birth | Knee joint, ankle, and wrist |
| 6 months of age | Capitate and hamate appear |
| 3–9 months | Shoulder |
| 1–12 years | X-ray wrist of the left hand |
| 12–14 years | Elbow and hip |

## QUESTIONS

**Q1. What are the conditions in which bone age is delayed?**

*Delayed bone age:* Osseous development will be delayed in:
- Hypopituitarism
- Hypothyroidism
- Malnutrition
- Constitutional dwarfism
- Chronic disease
- Male hypogonadism.

Bone Age is delayed than the chronological age in case of constitutional delay. Markedly delayed in hypothyroidism and hypopituitarism.

**Q2. What are the conditions in which bone age is advanced?**

Bone age is advanced in the following conditions:
- Genetic short stature
- Trisomy 21
- Chondrodystrophy.

**Q3. What are the conditions in which bone age is accelerated?**

Bone age is accelerated in:
- Sexual precocity
- Obesity.

## Battered Baby Syndrome (Shaken Infant Syndrome and Nonaccidental Trauma)

### Radiological Findings
- Multiple fractures
- Occult fractures
- Spiral factures
- Fractures of various ages. Older fractures will be associated with callus formation or healed fractures.

### Differential Diagnosis
- Osteogenesis imperfecta
- Road traffic accidents
- Metaphyseal dysplasia (irregular metaphysis will resemble corner fractures)
- Caffey's disease (will show periosteal reactions)
- Menkes disease (corner fractures).

## QUESTIONS

**Q1. What are the common sites of fractures in battered baby syndrome?**
- Acromion fractures
- Base of skull—occipital impression fractures
- Chest—ribs especially posterior ribs
- Sternum
- Dorsal spinous process fractures
- Diaphyseal fractures
- Extremities—bucket handle fractures (large bone fragment avulsed), corner fractures (small piece of bone avulsed due to shearing forces on the growth plate)
- Egg shell fractures—multiple
- Fractures crossing sutures.

**Q2. What are the views to be taken Ia case of battered baby syndrome?**
- Towne view for occipital fracture
- Lateral cervical and thoracolumbar spine
- Chest X-ray
- Ribs left and right oblique views
- Abdominal X-ray
- Left and right humer, hand, femur, tibia or fibula, dorsoplantar feet—anteroposterior (AP) view.

**Q3. What are the factors associated with battered baby syndrome?**
- Age of child less than 2 years
- Broken family
- Child dependent child—totally dependent or nonambulatory
- Delay seeking medical attention
- Explanation not compatible with injuries—the fractures cannot be explained by a pattern of injury and incompatible history and injury
- First borne children
- Gender—Female babies
- Handicapped children
- Fractures—Multiple fractures of various ages.

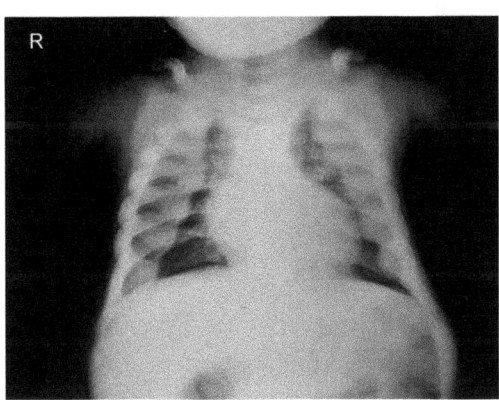

**Fig. 3.66:** Rachitic rosary (beading of ribs).

## SKELETON

### Rickets

#### Radiological Changes in the Bones in Rickets (Fig. 3.66)

- Beading of ribs (Bulbous enlargement of costochondral junctions) and soft tissue swellings around growth plates due to hypertrophied cartilage example costochondral bumps (rachitic rosary).
- Cortex indistinct
- Corticomedullary distinction lost
- Decreased bone density due to lack of osteoid mineralization
- Epiphysis—metaphysis distance increased due to delayed mineralization in the zone of provisional calcification at metaphysis
- Generalized osteopenia
- Generalized reduction in bone density due to decreased quantity of osteoid
- Uncalcified osteoid causes an appearance that the diaphysis is separated from the periosteum

#### X-ray Wrist Shows

**Epiphysis:**
- Delayed appearance of epiphysis
- Epiphyseal plates irregular and widened
- Borders are indistinct

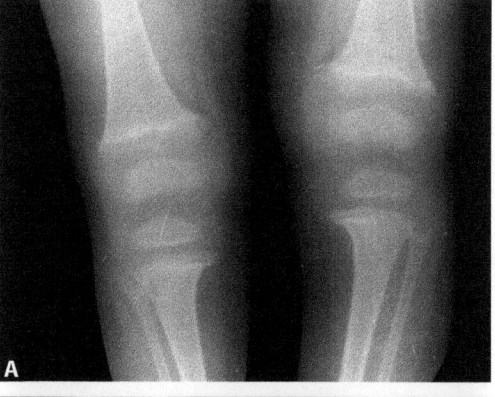

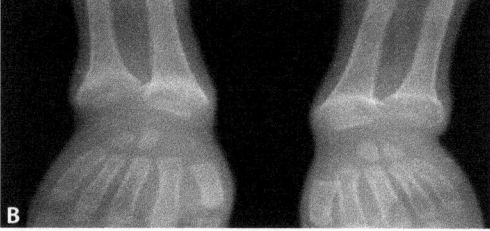

**Figs. 3.67A and B:** X-ray of knee joint showing cupping, widening and fraying. Also note decreased bone density.

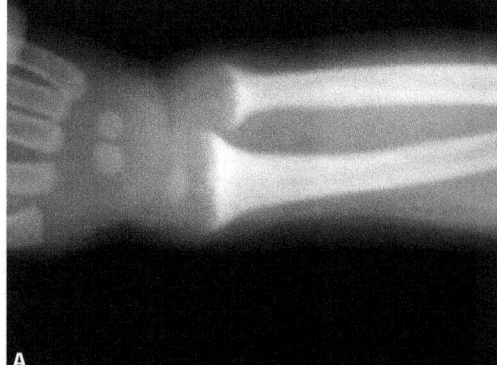

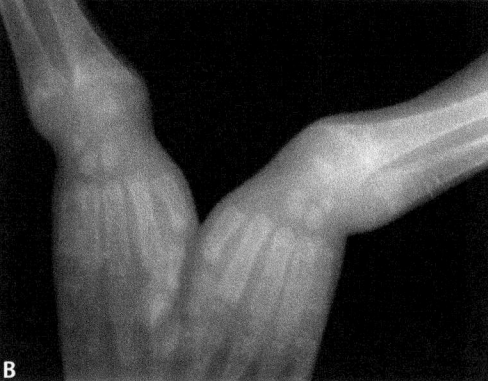

**Figs. 3.68A and B:** (A) X-ray wrist in rickets; (B) X-ray showing widening of wrist.

- Fraying at the margins at the end of the epiphysis of the bone due to lateral bulging of osteoid tissue (Figs. 3.67A and B).
- Flared epiphysis
- Height of the epiphysis to the end of shaft is increased due to lack of calcification of the newly formed bone (uncalcified osteoid).
- Physeal plate: Growth plate widening

### Metaphysis of Rapidly Growing Bones

- Widening of metaphyseal end of bone: Splaying—
- Coarse trabecular structure in metaphysis
- Cortex thin
- Cupping of metaphysis due to protrusion of cartilaginous cells in to the poorly mineralized metaphysis
- Flaring of metaphysis
- Fraying of metaphysis margin Indistinct metaphyseal margin (Irregular margins of metaphysis trumpeting) due to disorganization of spongy bone in the metaphyseal region
- Irregular calcification
- Loss of normal provisional zone of calcification (Figs. 3.68A and B)
- Metaphyseal spur
- Paint brush metaphysis (irregular, frayed, cupped metaphyseal margins)

### Diaphysis

- Anterior bowing
- Bending of long bones
- Coarse trabeculation-rarefaction of the bones (density is decreased and trabeculae will be prominent)
- Champagne glass appearance

- Double contour appearance of the shaft of radius (due to subperiosteal osteoid formation)
- Decreased bone length

### Radiological changes in growth plate

- Growth plate widening due to increased cartilaginous cells
- X-ray of ankle shows cupping and widening of the lower end of the tibia and fibula.
- X-ray skull—widening of sutures and bossing of skulls. Failure of calcification of cartilage and endochondral ossification hence it is seen in the metaphysic of growing bones.
- Pelvis—Triradiate pelvis with protrusion of hip and spine into the pelvis with protrussioacetabuli

### Healing rickets

- Radiological features of healing rickets—a dense provisional zone of calcification in the metaphysis called white line of Rickets
- Uncalcified osteoid causes an appearance that the diaphysis is separated from the periosteum
- X-ray of ankle shows cupping and widening of the lower end of the tibia and fibula.
- X-ray skull—widening of sutures and bossing of skulls.

Failure of calcification of cartilage and endochondral ossification hence it is seen in the metaphysic of growing bones.

## QUESTIONS

**Q1. What is the cause for widening of joint space?**
Due to absence of provisional zone of calcification.

**Q2. What is the cause of bowing legs?**
The long bones are weak and will be bending due to weight bearing.

**Q3. What is the cause of widening of wrists?**
The long bones are weak and will be bending due to weight-bearing while crawling.

**Q4. What are the radiological changes that indicate recovery with treatment of rickets with vitamin D?**
Appearance of provisional zone of calcification adjacent to metaphysic.

**Q5. What are the types of rickets?**
- Vitamin D deficiency rickets
- Vitamin D dependent rickets
- Vitamin D resistant rickets
- Renal rickets
- Nutritional rickets.

**Q6. What are the types of rickets?**
- Hypocalcemic rickets
- Hypophosphatemic rickets.

**Q7. What is oncogenic rickets?**
Certain tumors are substances that will cause phosphaturia.

**Q8. What is tumor rickets?**
It is oncogenic rickets.

**Q9. What is atrophic rickets?**
In severe protein energy malnutrition (PEM), the bones are not growing and hence the radiological changes are not seen.

1 IU = 0.025 μg of cholecalciferol
400 IU = 10 μg of cholecalciferol

*Treatment*:
- Oral single dose 600,000 IU units
- Maintenance dose 400–800 IU
- Oral calcium 30–75 mg/kg/day for 2 months.

**Q10. What are the skull changes in rickets?**
- Basilar invagination
- Calvarial demineralization
- Craniotabes
- Craniostenosis—premature
- Delayed tooth eruption.

**Q11. What are the spine changes in rickets?**
- Biconcave vertebral bodies
- Scoliosis
- Triradiate pelvis.

## Mucopolysaccharidosis

Radiological features:
- ❖ *Head:*
    - Atlantoaxial subluxation
    - Big or large skull
    - Calvarial thickening
    - Dolichocephalic skull
    - Diploic space-thick
    - Early or premature closure of sagittal suture
    - Flattened mandibular condyles
    - Generalized osteoporosis
    - Hyperostosis of cranium
    - Irregular anterior aspect of vertebral bodies
    - J-shaped enlarged sella turcica (saddle shaped in normal)
    - Mandibular angle wide
    - Poorly developed mastoids and paranasal sinuses.
- ❖ *Chest*—AP diameter increased (Fig. 3.69):
    - Broad clavicle—short and widened. Medial one-third of clavicle thickened
    - Costochondral beading
    - Deformities—pectus carinatum
    - Failure of fusion of sternal segments
    - Glenoid cavities flattened

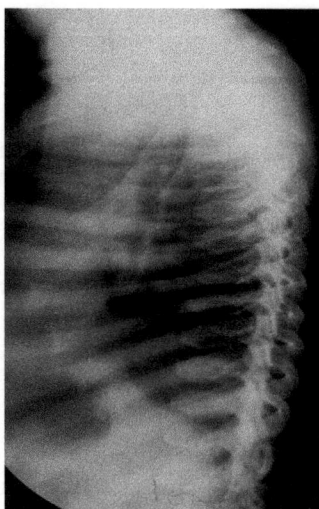

**Fig. 3.69:** Vertebra shows middle beaking in mucopolysaccharidosis.

- Ribs are spatulated, narrowed at vertebral ends and broad, and flat at sternal ends
- Oar-shaped or paddle-shaped ribs.
- ❖ *Hands (Figs. 3.70A to D):*
    - Bullet-shaped phalanges
    - Cortical thinning
    - Deformed, small, and carpal bones
    - Expansion of metaphysis
    - Flattening of glenoid cavity
    - Growth plates of distal radius and ulna are slanted toward each other curved
    - Hypoplastic terminal pharynges
    - Irregular widening of long bones
    - Irregular carpal bones
    - Metacarpal—middle constriction of metacarpal lost. Poorly modeled metacarpal bones, expansion of the medullary cavities, and pointed base of metacarpals
    - Phalanges-short and wide proximal and middle phalanges.
    - Proximal ends of metacarpals are tapering.
- ❖ *Long bones:*
    - Coarse trabeculation due to deposition of metabolites in the bone marrow
    - Constriction of humeral neck resulting in varus deformity
    - Constriction of femoral neck resulting in varus deformity
    - Diaphyseal and metaphyseal expansion more pronounced in the upper limbs than the lower limbs
    - Epiphyseal ossification delayed
    - Fragmentation of epiphysis
    - Flat foot
    - Genu valgum
    - Heterogeneous bone density
    - Irregular carpal bones
    - Joints enlarged.
- ❖ *Spine (Figs. 3.71A and B):*
    - Atlantoaxial subluxation
    - Anterior beaking—lower, anterior beaking in hurler, and middle anterior beaking in Morquio

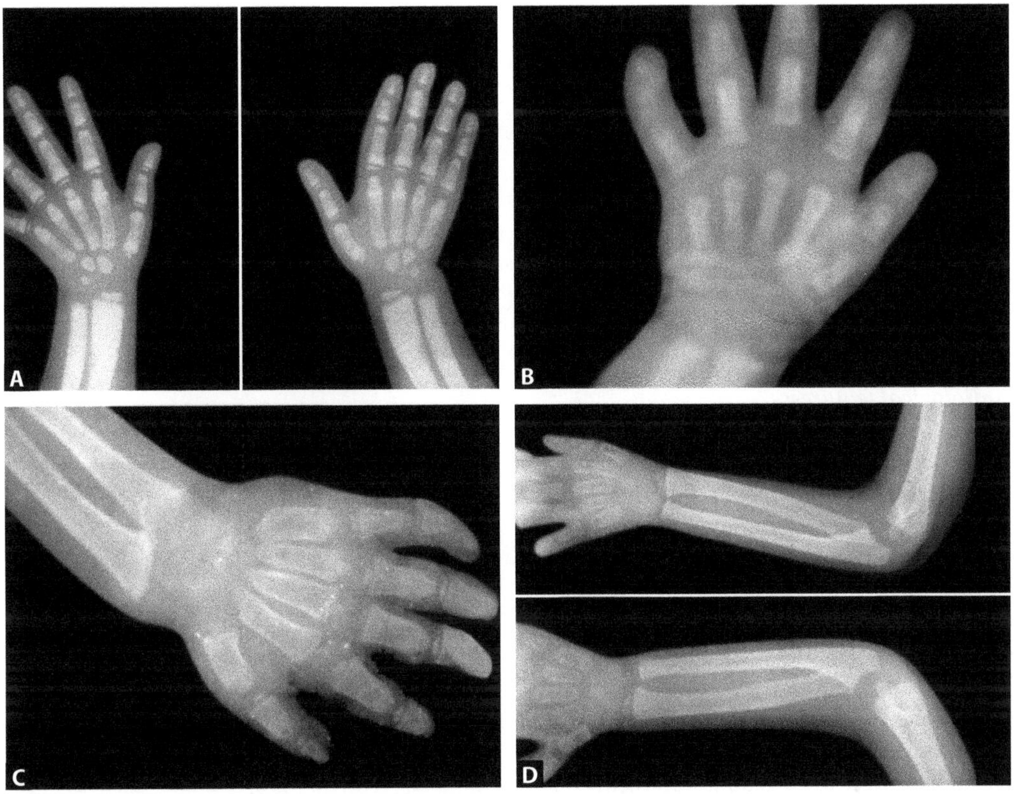

**Figs. 3.70 A to D:** (A and B) MPS; (C) MPS bullet-shaped metacarpals; (D) showing delayed bone age with absent carpal bones. Note proximal tapering of metacarpals in mucopolysaccharidosis.

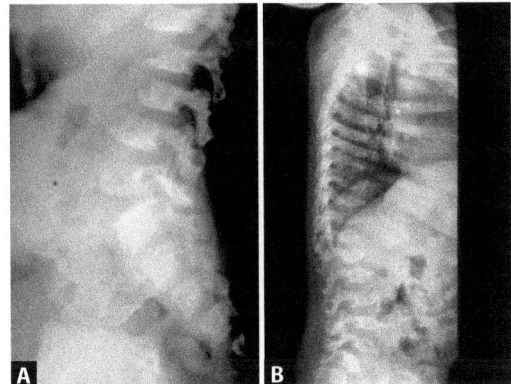

**Figs. 3.71 A and B:** X-ray of spine—vertebra showing inferior beaking in mucopolysaccharidoses.

- Bullet shaped vertebra
- Craniocervical junction narrow
- Deformities—dysostosis multiplex
- Exaggerated lumbar lordosis (hyperlordosis)
- Flattened vertebra (platyspondyly), decreased height
- Gibbus
- Hypoplasia or absence of odontoid process
- Intervertebral disk space is increased
- Kyphoscoliosis
- Vertebral body ovoid (thorax and lumbar).

❖ Pelvis:
  - Acetabular roof—shallow, wide, oblique, superior acetabulum is underdeveloped
  - Acetabular cavity enlarged
  - Broad iliac wings
  - Coxa valga

- Constricted iliac bones
- Coxofemoral joint space increased
- Dysplastic femoral head
- Elongated pelvic inlet
- Flaring of iliac bones
- Goblet-shaped pelvis
- Hip dysplasia
- Ilium is narrow in the lower part
- Ilium tapers inferiorly
- Iliac wings rounded.

## Hurler's

*Radiological features:*
- Skull—J-shaped sella
- Vertebra body ovoid (thorax and lumbar)
- Anterior beaking—lower and anterior
- Gibbus—thoracolumbar junction
- Ribs are spatulated, paddle-shaped thick anteriorly, and thin posteriorly
- Flaring of iliac bone
- Shallow acetabula and slanting irregular acetabular roof
- Tapering of proximal ends of metacarpals
- Irregular widening of long bones
- Radius curve toward ulna sloping articular surfaces of the distal radius and ulna that face each other
- Metacarpal—middle constriction of metacarpal lost
- Delayed skeletal maturation.

## Morquio

- Joint laxity and short stature appear by 1 year
- Corneal clouding
- Short neck, genu valgum, and flat feet
- Unstable knee joint, large elbow, and wrist joint.

### X-ray features:

- Flat vertebra
- Atlantoaxial subluxation
- Mid-facial hypoplasia
- Anterior beaking—anterior projection from vertebra (middle)—almost all vertebra affected
- Hypoplasia of odontoid
- Long bone shortened
- Metaphysis appear irregular—metacarpals are short and with conical tapering
- Middle construction will be maintained in Morquio
- Wide acetabulae with progressive subluxation or dislocation of femoral heads.

## QUESTIONS

**Q1. What are the radiological differences between Hurler and Morquio?**

| Features | Hurler (MPS IH) | Morquio (MPS IVA and IVB) |
|---|---|---|
| Radiological | Inferior beaking of lumbar and lower thoracic vertebra | Middle beaking of all vertebra |
| Middle constriction in the phalynx | Middle constriction is lost in the phalynx—Bullet shaped | Middle constriction maintained |
| Metacarpals in the hands | Short, proximal hypoplasia, or tapering | |

(MPS: mucopolysaccharidosis)

**Q2. What are the complications of mucopolysaccharidosis?**
- ❑ Abnormal curvature of spine and abnormal gait
- ❑ Breathing problems
- ❑ Cardiac problems
- ❑ Deformities
- ❑ Eye problems.

**Q3. What are the treatment options available for mucopolysaccharidosis?**
- ❑ Allogeneic bone marrow transplantation
- ❑ Gene therapy
- ❑ Enzyme replacement.

## Scurvy

*Radiological Findings in Scurvy (Fig. 3.72)*
- Beading of ribs—scorbutic rosary
- Dense zone of provisional calcification

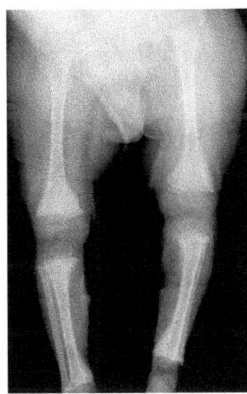

**Fig. 3.72:** Radiological findings in Scurvy.

- Enlarged metaphysis
- Fine cortex
- Flaring of metaphysis
- Generalized osteopenia
- Hemorrhages—subperiosteal hemorrhage
- Periosteal reaction
- Scurvy line—a lucent band between sclerotic provisional zone and spongiosa
- Silver lining of epiphysis.

### Signs in Scurvy

- *Corner sign of Park:* Projection of the white line laterally away from the limit of the shaft will lead to formation of spur or marginal cleft.
- Ground glass appearance of the shaft (due to rarefaction)
- *Pelkan's sign or Pelkan's spur* is due to fracture of the metaphyseal corner.
- *Pencil point cortex:* Thinning of the cortex
- *Pseudoparalysis of parrot* (other conditions—syphilis and osteomyelitis)
- *Signet-ring sign:* Signet-ring appearance of epiphysis (ring like epiphysis). The rarefied epiphyseal centers may be sharply outlined, which is termed signet ring
- *Trümmerfeld zone of lucency in the metaphysis (fragmented metaphysis):* Trümmerfeld zone is rarefaction proximal to the white line of Frankel beneath the zone of provisional calcification
- Subperiosteal hemorrhages
- *White metaphyseal line of Frankel:* The zone of provisional calcification at the epiphyseal ends of long bones will be thickened. White line of Frenkel is due to increased density at the ends of long bones.
- *Wimberger's ring sign:* Small epiphysis surrounded by a sharp sclerotic rim.

Bony changes are more around the knee joint.

### Discussion

Scurvy is due to vitamin C deficiency. Vitamin C is essential for collagen synthesis. Collagen is seen in skin, bone, joint, and blood vessels.

## QUESTIONS

**Q1. What are the bones in which the changes of scurvy are seen better?**
- ❑ Distal end of femur
- ❑ Proximal end of tibia and fibula
- ❑ Distal end of radius and ulna
- ❑ Proximal end of humerus
- ❑ Sternal end of ribs.

**Q2. What is scurvy line?**
This is the lucent transverse band between the heavier spongiosa deeper in the shaft and the sclerotic provisional zone.

**Q3. What are the changes seen during recovery?**
- ❑ Cortex becomes thicker
- ❑ Spongiosa becomes more clearly defined
- ❑ The transverse band of diminished intensity in the metaphysic will become normal
- ❑ Cortex will get mineralized.

**Q4. What are the sources of vitamin C?**
- ❑ Fresh fruits will contain vitamin C
- ❑ Citrus fruits—lemon and orange
- ❑ Amla.

**Q5. What are the clinical features of vitamin C deficiency?**
- ❑ Appetite decreased
- ❑ Bleeding tendency—increased
- ❑ Bone pain—pseudoparalysis
- ❑ Costochondral separation—beading of ribs (scorbutic rosary)
- ❑ Delayed healing of wounds
- ❑ Ecchymosis
- ❑ Fever
- ❑ Fractures
- ❑ Gum bleeding and spongy gums
- ❑ Hematuria
- ❑ Hemorrhages
- ❑ Irritable child
- ❑ Joint pain and swelling.

**Q6. What is Barton's disease?**
Scurvy associated with rickets.

## Osteogenesis Imperfecta (Brittle Bone Disease)

Genetic disorders of collagen type I production resulting in increased bone fragility and decreased bone mass density.

Type I collagen is present in bone, dental enamel, sclera, skin, blood vessels tendons, and ligaments.

### Radiological Features

- ❖ *General*:
  - Osteoporosis
  - Thinning of cortex
  - Popcorn calcification.
- ❖ *Head*:
  - Basilar invagination
  - Wormian bones.
- ❖ *Chest*:
  - Pectus excavatum
  - Pectus carinatum.
- ❖ *Spine*:
  - Kyphoscoliosis.
- ❖ *Vertebra*:
  - Compression fractures
  - Codfish vertebra
  - Platyspondyly.
- ❖ *Pelvis*:
  - Protrusion of acetabulum
  - Coxa vara.

### Mnemonics (A to Z)

- ❖ Acetabular protrusion
- ❖ Angulation of bones
- ❖ Basilar invagination
- ❖ Bowing of long bones
- ❖ Bucket handle fracture (complete)
- ❖ Callus formation
- ❖ Cortical thinning
- ❖ Corner incomplete fracture
- ❖ Codfish vertebra
- ❖ Compression fractures of vertebra
- ❖ Carinatum—pectus
- ❖ Deformities growth recovery lines
- ❖ Excavatum—pectus
- ❖ Flat vertebra—universal platyspondyly—all vertebra will be flat
- ❖ Fractures or healing fractures
- ❖ Generalized osteoporosis
- ❖ Gracile long bones radius, tibia, and fibula (overtabulated bones)
- ❖ Hyperplastic calcification
- ❖ Kyphoscoliosis
- ❖ Long bones fractures and deformities
- ❖ Multiple fractures
- ❖ Normal vertebra and pelvis (in type III)
- ❖ Osteopenia
- ❖ Popcorn calcification
- ❖ Pseudoarthrosis
- ❖ Quadriparesis
- ❖ Radiolucent areas with sclerotic margins
- ❖ Shortening
- ❖ Thin
- ❖ Thickening
- ❖ Wormian bones in the skull
- ❖ Zebra stripe sign—recovery lines in long bones during treatment.

### Differential Diagnosis

- ❖ *Battered baby syndrome:* The texture of bone will be normal
- ❖ *Hyperphosphatemia*: Osteoectasia (widening of bones) will be seen

* *Hypophosphatasia*: Deep cupping of end of diaphysis in long bones and widening of growth plate.

## Discussion

Hereditary familial disease is also known as brittle bone disease. This condition is associated with osteoporosis and excessive bone fragility.
* Incidence—1:20,000–1:50,000
* Structural or quantitative defect in type I collagen.

## Types

* Type I—mild type. This is associated with blue sclera, recurrent fractures during childhood, presenile hearing loss. There are two subtypes—A and B subtypes depending upon the absence or presence of dentigenous imperfecta respectively. Other connective tissue disorders:
  - Easy bruising
  - Joint laxity
  - Mild short stature
  - Fractures
  - Hearing loss begins in the early childhood.
* Type II—femur is shortened, broad, telescoped, or crumpled; tibia is short and bowed; fibula is thin.
* Type III—fractures and deformities of the limbs will develop in the first and second years of life femur is shortened but not crumbled.
* Type IV—more severe type that type I fracture occurs before puberty. Hearing loss is profound.

**What are the types of osteogenesis imperfecta?**

*Silence classification:*

*Types:* Common forms:
* Type I—mild type with triad of blue sclera, fragile bones, and deafness
* Type II—lethal type baby will be stillborn
* Type III—progressive disorder with progressive deformities
* Uncommon forms type IV to type VIII varies in severity
* Type IV—moderate bowing of legs, normal sclera, and moderate short stature
* Types II and III are severe types.

## Type I Osteogenesis Imperfecta

This type is mild and most common type.

**Complications:**
* Fractures even with mild trauma
* Deformities of bone
* Progressive kyphoscoliosis
* Hearing loss begins in the childhood.

**Investigations:**
X-ray.

**Management:**
* Prophylactic bracing of limbs and physical rehabilitation
* Administration of calcitonin, fluoride, and vitamin C.

**Prognosis:**
Presenile conductive hearing loss in adolescents and adults.

## Type II Osteogenesis Imperfecta

This is more rare. This type is lethal type, approximately 50% are stillborn and others will die soon after birth. The thighs will be broad and at right angles to the trunk.

## Type III Osteogenesis Imperfecta

This is associated with severe bone fragility, deformities, and fractures. They have normal birth weight and length.

X-ray will show multiple fractures and generalized osteopenia.

## Type IV Osteogenesis Imperfecta

This is inherited as autosomal dominant. This is more severe than type I and less severe than type III. Significant bowing of the lower limbs can be seen at birth fractures may occur at any age from birth to adult life. This type may show improvement with puberty, multiple fractures may be seen at birth, hearing impairment is less common, opalescent dentin can be present.

### Type V
Similar to type IV but with distinct histology.

### Type VI
Types VII, VIII clinically overlap types II and III.

### Treatment of Osteogenesis Imperfecta
- ❖ The babies should be nursed in a firm mattress
- ❖ Later splinting and correction deformities can be done
- ❖ Antenatal diagnosis—type II osteogenesis imperfecta can be diagnosed antenatally by ultrasonogram, X-ray, and biochemical studies.

### Prevention
Genetic counseling for primary prevention.

## QUESTION

**Q1. What are the extra skeletal manifestations of ontogenesis imperfecta?**
- ❏ Aortic valve disease—root dilatation or regurgitation or aortic dissection
- ❏ Bleeding
- ❏ Cardiovascular abnormalities—cardiac failure
- ❏ Cervical artery dissection
- ❏ Dentinogenesis imperfecta
- ❏ Early hypoacusis
- ❏ Fragility of skin increased
- ❏ Flat feet
- ❏ Gray teeth
- ❏ Hearing loss
- ❏ Hydrocephalus
- ❏ Hypermobility
- ❏ Infections—recurrent pneumonia
- ❏ Joint and ligament hyperlaxity due to ligament weakness and instability
- ❏ Kidney—renal calculi due to hypercalciuria
- ❏ Ligaments hyperlaxity
- ❏ Mitral valve prolapsed
- ❏ Malocclusion of teeth
- ❏ Macrocephaly
- ❏ Neurological manifestations—headache, lower cranial nerve palsy, quadriparesis, and ataxia due to basilar invagination.
- ❏ Ocular—blue sclera
- ❏ Pneumonia—recurrent pulmonary infections due to chest wall deformities.

## Osteopetrosis (Figs. 3.73A to C)
### Albers Schönberg Disease
**Radiological findings:**
- ❖ X-ray of any bone
  - Absent bone marrow
  - Bone within bone appearance
  - Cortical thickening
  - Corticomedullary distinction lost
  - Cortex not seen in the bones (the X-ray film will show white bones with almost no black shades inside the bones)
  - Dense bones
  - Diffuse sclerosis
  - Dentition defective
  - Dental caries
  - Enamel formation incomplete
  - Flaring of ends of bones
  - Fractures—multiple and healed
  - Generalized thickening of bones and marked increase in bone density including skull, long bones, pelvis, and vertebra
  - Height decreased
  - Hair-on-end appearance in areas of increased hematopoietic activity
  - Increased size and density of bones
  - Jaw—absence of normal trabecular pattern in both jaws, triangular opacity in the mandible due to calcification.
  - Knee—Erlenmeyer flask deformity at distal ends of femur (funnel

# Radiology—X-rays

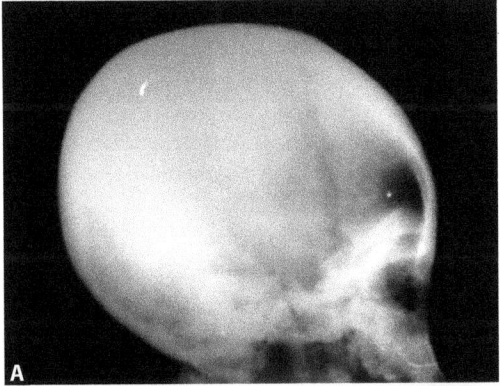

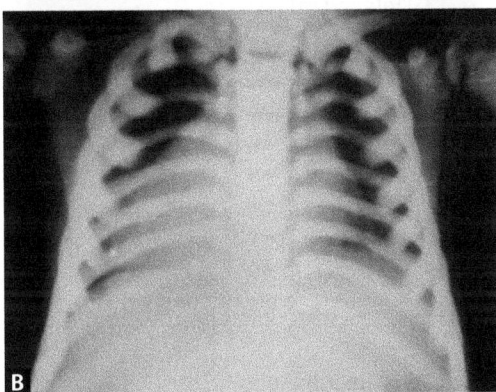

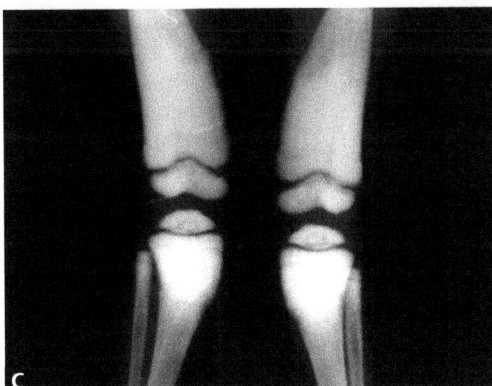

**Figs. 3.73A to C:** (A) Skull lateral view; (B) Osteopetrosis of ribs, vertebra is dense; (C) Osteopetrosis femur and tibia.

  like appearance) due to lack of tabularization and flaring of ends
- Longitudinal metaphyseal striations
- Minimal spur formation at the lower end of femur
- Nasal sinus architecture abnormalities, poorly pneumatized
- Osteosclerotic bone with alternate lucent bands due to abnormal bone
- Overgrowth of bones
- Phantom sign is due to increased density around the orbit
- Rugger jersey spine—sandwich appearance of vertebral bodies
- Splaying of metaphyses and rib ends
- Sandwich sign in vertebral body (cervical, thoracic, and lumbar regions) due to dense sclerotic end-plates alternating with central intervening portions, which is less dense bands
- Thickening of inner and outer table with widening of diploic space
- Trabeculations lost.

### Differential diagnosis:

❖ Hypervitaminosis D
❖ Lead poisoning
❖ Pyknodysostosis
❖ Fibrous dysplasia

### Discussion:

*Greek words:*
❖ Osteo—bone
❖ Petros—stone

### Types of osteopetrosis:

❖ Infantile autosomal recessive (malignant form more severe)
❖ Intermediate
❖ Adult autosomal dominant.

### Osteopetrosis—marble bone disease and Albers-Schönberg disease:

❖ Abnormal bone remodeling—osteopetrosis includes a group of inherited disorders caused by defect in bone resorption
❖ Albers-Schönberg, a German radiologist described osteopetrosis in 1904
❖ Age of onset—based of age and clinical features, three types are adult onset, infantile, and intermediate types are described

- ❖ Autosomal dominant—usually asymptomatic
- ❖ Autosomal recessive presents with severe symptoms like abnormal bone remodeling, deficient hematopoiesis, and neurological impairment in infancy. Prognosis is bad with reduced life span.

## QUESTIONS

**Q1. What is the pathogenesis of osteopetrosis?**
- ☐ Failure of osteoclasts to resorb the immature bone
- ☐ Bones will be sclerotic and thick but structurally weak.

**Q2. What is the age of presentation of osteopetrosis?**
- ☐ It usually presents by infancy. But the age of presentation will depend upon the severity of the gene mutation
- ☐ Antenatally—multiple fractures.

**Q3. What is the function of osteoclasts?**
To resorb and remodel the bone by secreting strong hydrochloric acid to dissolve the hard mineral part of the bone.

**Q4. What is malignant osteopetrosis?**
Osteopetrosis (autosomal recessive) with precocious manifestations—the onset is early with progressive course leading to death.

**Q5. What are the clinical features of osteopetrosis?**
- ☐ Anemia (severe anemia because of absence of bone cortex, which is the main site of formation of blood cells. Although blood is formed in other sites as liver, it will not be enough)
- ☐ Bleeding manifestations (due to marrow failure)
- ☐ Bone pain
- ☐ Cranial nerve paralysis:
- ☐ Callus-abundant
- ☐ Dental abnormalities
- ☐ Entrapment neuropathy.
- ☐ Failure to thrive
- ☐ Growth retardation
- ☐ Head—large
- ☐ Hepatosplenomegaly due to persistence of these organs as a site for formation of blood
- ☐ Increasing pallor
- ☐ Symptoms due to entrapment neuropathy
- ☐ Blindness
- ☐ Deafness
- ☐ Delayed mile stones
- ☐ Facial nerve palsy.

**Q6. What is the cause of hepatosplenomegaly in osteopetrosis?**
Extramedullary hematopoiesis or erythropoiesis.

**Q7. What is the cause of macrocephaly in osteopetrosis?**
Thickened calvaria.

**Q8. What are the complications of osteopetrosis?**
- ☐ Acute leukemia
- ☐ Anemia
- ☐ Bleeding
- ☐ Bone marrow failure—pancytopenia
- ☐ Cranial nerve compression (due to pressure by the bones, the adjacent structures will get compressed)
- ☐ Deafness
- ☐ Blindness
- ☐ Facial nerve palsy
- ☐ Dental caries
- ☐ Delayed union or nonunion of fractures
- ☐ Enamel problems
- ☐ Eye problems—failure to establish fixation, nystagmus, and strabismus
- ☐ Fractures
- ☐ Failure to thrive
- ☐ Growth retardation—short stature
- ☐ Hemorrhages (subarachnoid hemorrhage)

- Infections—increased susceptibility due to granulocytopenia mandible osteomyelitis
- Injuries—prone for trivial injury due to fragile bones
- Jaw fractures
- Joint degeneration problems.

**Q9. What are the dental problems in osteopetrosis?**
- Abscesses
- Ankylosis of teeth
- Bacterial infections
- Cysts
- Dental caries
- Eruption of teeth delayed
- Fistulas
- Fractures of jaw during extraction

**Q10. What is the cause of hypocalcemia in osteopetrosis?**
- Due to excessive deposition of immature bone leading to secondary hyperparathyroidism
- Serum acid phosphatase will be raised due to release from defective osteoclasts
- Bone specific creatinine kinase will be elevated.

**Q11. How will you treat osteopetrosis?**
Treatment of osteopetrosis is conservative
- Antibiotics (treatment of infections)
- Blood transfusion
- Bone marrow transplantation
- Calcitriol (oral)
- Corticosteroids—prednisolone
- Diet—low calcium diet
- Erythropoietin to correct anemia
- Fractures management
- Facial deformities correction by surgery
- Gamma interferon
- Genetic counseling should be given.

**Q12. What are the complications of osteopetrosis?**
Due to anemia secondary cardiac failure can occur.

**Q13. What is the differential diagnosis of osteopetrosis?**
Pyknodysostosis.

**Q14. What are the differentiating features between osteopetrosis and pyknodysostosis?**

| Features | Osteopetrosis | Pyknodysostosis |
|---|---|---|
| Angle of mandible | Acute | Obtuse |
| Terminal phalanges | Normal | Progressive acro-osteolysis |

## Achondroplasia

### Radiological Findings

❖ General:
  - Short stature
  - Bones are wide due to unaffected appositional growth.
❖ Skull:
  - Anteroposterior craniocervical diameter is 10 mm (normal 30–43 cm)
  - Brachycephaly
  - Base of skull small and shortened
  - Basilar impression
  - Calvarium large
  - Cervicomedullary kink
  - Communicating hydrocephalus due to narrow foramen magnum
  - Disproportionate craniofacial due to mid-face hypoplasia
  - Depressed nasal bridge
  - Enlarged skull vault and mandible
  - Elevation of brainstem resulting in large suprasellar cistern and vertically oriented straight sinus
  - Frontal bossing
  - Flat nasal bridge due to hypoplastic base of skull
  - Foramen of magnum small, narrow, and irregular.

- ❖ *Chest:*
  - Anterior flaring of ribs
  - Anteroposterior narrowing of chest and ribs.
- ❖ *Vertebra:*
  - Anterior wedging of vertebral bodies
  - Anteroposterior shortening of lumbar pedicles
  - Anterior beaking of vertebra in the upper lumbar spine (hurler)
  - Bullet nose (bullet shaped) thoracolumbar vertebra due to hypoplasia, anterior wedging
  - Canal stenosis
  - Concave scalloping of posterior surface of the vertebral bodies
  - Cuboid shaped vertebral bodies with L1 and L 2 anterior beaking
  - Decreased or narrowed interpedicular distance of lumbar vertebra from L1 to L5
  - Dorsal concavity of lumbar vertebra
  - Extension of elbow is limited—posterior bowing of distal humerus more than 20°(lateral radiograph)
  - Exaggerated lumbar or sacral lordosis
  - Foramen magnum at craniocervical junction (base of skull) and spinal canal are small
  - Gibbus in thoracolumbar region
  - Height of vertebral bodies decreased
  - Intervertebral disk bulging or herniation
  - Increased angle between sacrum and lumbar spine
  - Interpediculate narrowing
  - Kyphosis in thoracolumbar region
  - Laminar thickening.
- ❖ *Pelvis:*
  - Acetabular angle decreased and flattened causing tombstone appearance
  - Ball and socket arrangement of metaphysis with epiphysis
  - Broad iliac wings
  - Crescent-shaped iliac wing (paraglider-shaped pelvis) due to relatively well-ossified iliac wing
  - Deep and narrow sciatic notches
  - Elephant ear appearance of pelvis
  - Flat pelvis with round tomb stone like ileum
  - Glass (champagne glass) type of pelvic inlet due to squared iliac wings, narrow sacroiliac notch
  - Horizontal acetabular roofs
  - Iliac wings are vertical (flaring of iliac wings absent)
  - Mickey mouse ear pelvis
  - Short pelvis
  - Square-shaped iliac wings
  - Small sacrosciatic notch
  - Trident pelvis.
- ❖ *Limbs:*
  - Brachydactyly
  - Broad tubular bones
  - Ball in socket epiphysis
  - Bowing of legs
  - Caliber of shaft of tubular bone is normal
  - Cupping of metaphysis
  - Circumflex or chevron seat on the metaphysis (V-shaped growth plates)
  - Dysgenesis of upper femoral epiphysis, which will be small
  - Disproportionate metaphysical flaring—trumpet appearance of long bones
  - Extremities are short
  - Flaring of metaphysis
  - Femur—short, broad neck, and femoral head will be normally developed
  - Fibula long (compared to tibia) and bowed
  - Genu varum
  - Glenoid fossa incomplete
  - Humerus shortened
  - Rhizomelic shortening—proximal shortening more than distal shortening
  - Short stubby bones
  - Shortening of long bones with long distal fibula
  - Short distal ulna

- Trident hand with fingers widely opposed, equal length, separation of middle, and ring fingers`
- Trumpet bone appearance
- Thick and tubular bones of hand and feet
- Ulnar styloid longer than radius
- V-shaped growth plates
- Widening of shafts of long bones are the periosteal ossification proceeds normally.

## Discussion

Achondroplasia is inherited as autosomal dominant condition.

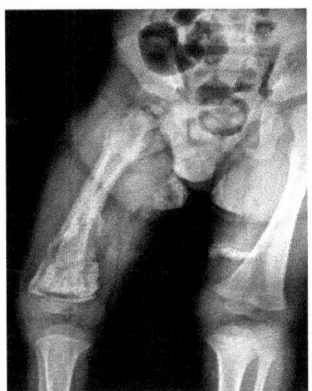

**Fig. 3.74:** Osteomyelitis.

## Clinical Features

- Head—large head with frontal bossing
- Hypotonia
- Dysmorphic facies—hypoplastic midface with cheekbones that lack prominence and a low nasal bridge with narrow nasal passages
- Genu varum
- Short fingers with trident hand (divergence between ring and middle finger)
- Hyperextensibility of the joints.

## Complications

- Acute otitis media
- Nerve root compression syndromes
- Hearing impairment
- Persistent kyphosis
- Hydrocephalus due to obstruction of foramen magnum.

## Osteomyelitis

Osteomyelitis is infection of bone and bone marrow (Fig. 3.74).

## Types

Acute, subacute, or chronic.

## Radiological Changes in Osteomyelitis

- Architecture of bone will be lost
- Areas of bone destruction
- Apposition of new bone
- Bone density decreased (osteopenia) in the affected region
- Bones will be thick and sclerotic with areas of bone destruction
- Bone formation—periosteal reaction with new bone formation or thickening
- Brodie's abscess is osteomyelitis consisting abscess in the bone
- Cortical destruction and irregularity
- Codman's triangle
- Deep soft tissue swelling
- Destruction of bone metaphysis results in patchy rarefaction of metaphysis
- Demineralization due to hyperemia and immobilization
- Endosteal scalloping
- Elevated periosteum
- Fat or fascial planes obliterated adjacent to metaphysis
- Focal bony lysis or cortical loss.

## Discussion

To produce radiological changes, osteomyelitis must extend at least 1 cm and compromise 30–50% of bone mineral content.

## Specific Features

- Chronic osteomyelitis will be associated with sequestrum surrounded by involucrum, which is new bone formed around the dead weakened sequestrum. Involucrum will be dense white
- Dactylitis osteomyelitis of short long bones of hand and feet

- Soft tissue swelling
- Sickle cell anemia will cause infarction of bone which will be associated with infection resulting in osteomyelitis
- Septic arthritis—the joint space will be widened later destruction of bone.

## QUESTIONS

**Q1. What are the features of acute osteomyelitis?**
- Initial X-ray will be normal up to about 10 days after infection
- Architecture loss
- New bone apposition
- Cortical loss
- Osteopenia
- Endosteal erosion
- Endosteal scalloping
- Extensive periosteal reaction or thickening
- Focal bony lysis in areas of metaphysis
- Intracortical fissuring
- Peripheral sclerosis.

**Q2. What are the features of subacute osteomyelitis?**
Brodie abscess—central area of radiolucency with surrounding rim of reactive bone sclerosis.

**Q3. What are the features of chronic osteomyelitis?**
- Air in the soft tissues
- Bone expansion (irregular, thick, and sclerotic) interspersed with radiolucencies
- Bone density loss
- Bone thickening
- Cloaca formation
- Cortical irregularities and thickening
- Draining sinuses
- Dead bone—sequestrum necrotic cortical bone (developed after 30 days)
- Elevated periosteum
- Involucrum—cloak of laminated or speculated periosteal reaction (developed after 20 days).

**Q4. What are the complications of osteomyelitis?**
- Abscess (subperiosteal)
- Brodie abscess
- Cloacae formation
- Deformities
- Disruption of intraosseous and periosteal blood supply causing osteonecrosis
- Dense, devitalized, dead bone surrounded by pus, not resorbed (sequestrum surrounded by pus), and granulation tissue
- Extension of infection into the adjacent structures or joint (septic arthritis)
- Fistula or sinus formation
- Fractures
- Growth disturbances, if epiphysis is involved
- Growth stimulation due to hyperemia results in premature maturation of adjacent epiphysis
- Height decreased as hyperemia stimulates growth resulting in premature maturation of adjacent epiphysis
- Hyperostosis
- Intraosseous abscess
- Involucrum—reactive shell of new bone formation
- Joint involvement.

**Q5. What are the early radiological changes seen in osteomyelitis?**
Soft tissue swelling and loss of fascial planes.

**Q6. What is the difference between soft tissue swelling?**
Muscle sign—soft tissue swelling in the muscle plane associated with osteomyelitis will extend along the whole length of the bone.

## SKULL

### Increased Intracranial Tension

*Radiological Features of Increased Intracranial Tension*

- Atrophy of bones at the inner wall of the skull due to pressure

- Beaten brass skull or copper beaten appearance or silver beaten appearance due to prominent convolutional markings which overlie the gyri.
❖ Cranial walls are thin:
  - Deep sella turcica due to enlargement due to pressure atrophy of base of skull
  - Depression of cribriform plate and os planum
  - Digital markings on the inner walls of the skull due to pressure by the pulsating vessels
  - Displacement of midline structure like pineal gland to one side
  - Diastasis of sutures
  - Widening of sutures
  - Enlargement of venous channels of the skull, diploic veins, venous sinuses, and emissary veins
  - Enlargement of skull
  - Erosion of posterior glenoids
  - Erosion of sella turcica.

## QUESTIONS

**Q1. How will you differentiate normal convolutional markings in the skull from those due to increased intracranial tension?**
In normal children, the convolutional markings may be confined to the posterior part of the skull.

**Q2. What is the duration of increased intracranial pressure (ICP) for changes in sella turcica?**
Alteration in sella turcica will be seen after about 6 weeks of increased ICP.

## NECK

### Cervical Rib
Accessory rib arises from seventh cervical vertebra (Fig. 3.75).

### Differential Diagnosis
❖ Elongation of transverse process of seventh cervical vertebra
❖ Hypoplastic first thoracic rib.

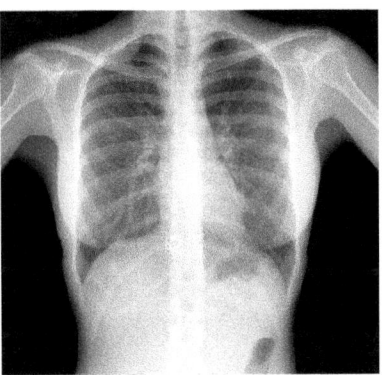

**Fig. 3.75:** X-ray of cervical rib.

### Discussion
❖ Usually bilateral
❖ Common in females

### Significance of Cervical Rib
It will reduce the space in the interscalene triangle through which roots and trunks of brachial plexus will traverse.

## QUESTIONS

**Q1. What are the clinical features of cervical rib?**
❑ Asymptomatic
❑ Neck pain radiating to the arms.

**Q2. What are the complications of cervical rib?**
❑ Aneurismal dilatation of subclavian artery
❑ Thoracic outlet syndrome by compression of brachial plexus and subclavian vessels.

**Q3. What are the anomalies associated with cervical rib?**
Klippel–Feil anomaly.

## PELVIS

### Developmental Dysplasia of Hip (Fig. 3.76)

### Radiological Findings
❖ Acetabular angle more than 30°
❖ Acetabular dysplasia

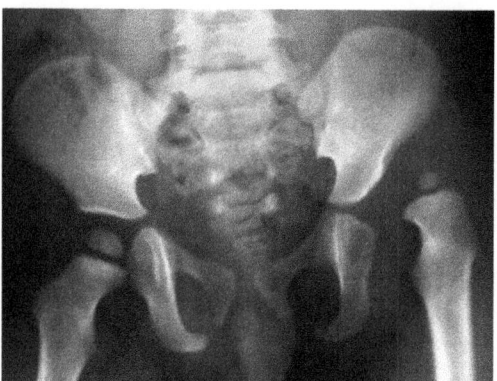

**Fig. 3.76:** Developmental dysplasia of hip left side.

- Acetabulum shallow
- Asymmetrical length—shortened limb on the side of developmental dysplasia of hip (DDH)
- Apex of metaphysis will be lateral to the edge of acetabulum
- Beaking of femoral metaphysis medially
- Center angle of Wiberg less than 25° (angle subtended by a first-line drawn from acetabular edge to the center of femoral head and second-line perpendicular to the line connecting centers of femoral heads)
- Deformity of acetabulum
- Delayed ossification of femoral epiphysis
- Eccentric position of proximal femoral epiphysis
- False acetabulum will be formed
- Flattening of femoral head
- Femoral shaft lies above the horizontal line drawn through Y-synchondrosis
- Femoral head lateral to Perkin's line
- Femoral head superior to Hilgenreiner's line
- Gender—girls are more commonly affected
- Hilgenreiner line (horizontal line connecting superolateral margins of triradiate cartilage) to femoral epiphysis length will be shortened
- Interrupted and discontinuous Shenton's line.

## Discussion

*Developmental dysplasia of hip*: The dysplastic hips may or may not be dislocated at birth. The dislocation can be partial or total. This will vary from mild acetabular dysplasia to total dislocation. It is more common in the first born babies. The incidence is less common in preterm babies.

Gender—females are more commonly affected. The left side is affected more than the right side.

## QUESTIONS

**Q1. What is the incidence of DDH?**
0.5–2% of live births.

**Q2. What is the incidence of true dislocation?**
1.5 in 1,000 live births.

**Q3. Describe Ortolani's test.**
This tests passive reduction—reentry of a dislocated femoral head. The hip and knee are kept in flexed position and gradually abducted.

**Q4. What is Galeazzi's sign?**
Compare the level of the knees with the infant in supine position and knee kept in flexed position and gradually abducted.

**Q5. Describe Burlow's test.**
This tests passive manipulation provoked dislocation. Hold the upper femur between the middle finger on the greater trochanter and the thumb on the groin by levering the femoral head in and out of the acetabulum the dislocation can be demonstrated.

**Q6. What are the factors associated with DDH?**
- ❏ Oligohydramnios
- ❏ Female babies
- ❏ First born infants
- ❏ Breech presentation.

Postnatal factors:
- ❏ Positioning of the infant with extended and abducted hips

- Muscle contractures associated with conditions like cerebral palsy.

**Q7. What are the types of DDH?**
There are two types:
1. Dislocatable at birth
2. Subluxated or dislocated at birth.
   The subluxation is a condition when the femoral head is present in the joint space but not concentric with the acetabulum at rest the dislocatable hip is a condition when the entire femoral head leaves the acetabulum with manipulation but will remain in the normal position at rest.

**Q8. What are the etiological features of DDH?**
- *Genetic predisposition*—Common in certain families
- *Environmental*—Common in certain geographical areas
- *Hormonal*—Relaxin is a hormone, which is specific for female tissues. This hormone may cross the placenta and act on the female tissues. Hence, this is more common in female babies
- *Mechanical factors*—Breech presentation (5-10 times more common), intrauterine manipulation. Oligohydramnios will predispose to hip dislocation
- *Structural defects*—Primary dysplasia of acetabulum
- Teratologic DDH will develop early in gestation and is associated with other serous malformations like arthrogryposis, lumbosacral agenesis, chromosomal disorders, and spina bifida. There will be significant contractures and displacement of femoral head. This condition is not reducible at birth
- Transplacental passage of maternal hormones especially relaxin, which results in ligamentous laxity.

**Q9. What is the treatment for DDH?**
- Pavlik harness
- Closed reduction
- Maintenance of the reduction
- The harness can be removed between 8 weeks to 12 weeks.

## NEWBORN

### General

*Pneumonia*

**Radiological findings in pneumonia:**
- The findings are variable and non-specific
- Strand-like opacities from the hilum
- Patchy infiltrates or diffuse reticulonodular densities
- Persistent focal or diffuse radiological changes associated with respiratory distress.

**Differential diagnosis:**
- Transient tachypnea of newborn
- Group B streptococcal (GBS) pneumonia
- Hyaline membrane disease (HMD).

In infants with transient tachypnea of newborn or atelectasis, the radiological changes will resolve within 48 hours.

Group B streptococcal pneumonia will resemble HMD.

In HMD, the lung volume will be less and in GBS, lung volume is normal.

## QUESTIONS

**Q1. What are the types of pneumonia in newborn?**
- Congenital pneumonia within 72 hours of life
- Acquired pneumonia after 72 hours of life, e.g. ventilator-associated pneumonia.

**Q2. What are the common causes of pneumonia in newborn?**
- *Gram-positive cocci*—Group A, Group B streptococci, and *Staphylococcus aureus*
- *Gram-negative bacilli*—*Escherichia coli*, *Klebsiella*, and *Proteus*.

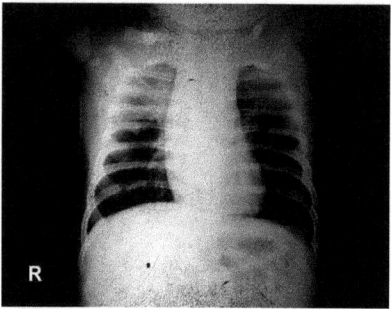

**Fig. 3.77:** Septicemia in newborn—narrowing of pedicle due to atrophy of thymus in sepsis, bow sign and right cardiac border resembles a bow), bilateral hyperventilation.

## Septicemia

**X-ray chest and abdomen findings in septicemia:**

*Chest:*
- Bilateral hyperventilation
- Tenting of diaphragm
- Narrowing of pedicle—due to atrophy of thymus
- *Bow sign*—The right border of heart will appear like a bow (Fig. 3.77).

*Abdomen:*
- Dilated bowel loops (due to stasis) causing abdominal distension.

**Differential diagnosis:** Neonatal pneumonia will present with persistent focal or diffuse radiological changes associated with respiratory distress. In infants with transient tachypnea of newborn of atelectasis, the radiological changes will resolve within 48 hours.

## QUESTIONS

**Q1.** What are the common organisms causing early sepsis in newborn?
- *Klebsiella*
- Group *B Streptococcus*
- *Escherichia coli.*

**Q2.** What is early neonatal sepsis?
Sepsis developing in the first 72 hours of life.

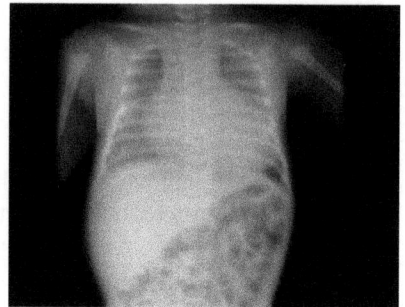

**Fig. 3.78:** Cardiomegaly.

**Q3.** What is late neonatal sepsis?
Sepsis developing after 72 hours of life.

**Q4.** What are the common organisms causing late sepsis in newborn?
- *Klebsiella*
- *Staphylococcus.*

## Cardiovascular System

### Cardiomegaly (Fig. 3.78)

Cardiothoracic ratio is more than 60% in newborn.

Cardiomegaly may be due to involvement of any of the following structures in the pericardial sac:
- *Cardiac chambers*—Ventricular dilatation
- *Cardiac wall*—Ventricular hypertrophy
- *Pericardial space*—Pericardial effusion
- *Additional structures*—Tumors.

## QUESTION

**Q.** What are the causes of cardiomegaly in newborn?
- Congenital heart disease with congestive cardiac failure (CCF)
- Myocarditis
- Dilated cardiomyopathy
- Pulmonary hypertension
- Hypertrophic cardiomyopathy
- Pericardial effusion
- Ebstein's anomaly
- Atrioventricular block
- Endocardial cushion defect.

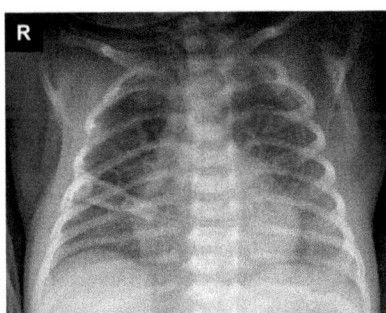

**Fig. 3.79:** Transient tachypnea of the newborn (TTN).

## Respiratory System

### Transient Tachypnea of the Newborn (Wet Lung)

Transient tachypnea in newborn (also known as retained fetal fluid or wet lung syndrome) (Fig. 3.79).

**Radiological findings:**

X-ray chest findings are:
- *Appearance*—Sunburst appearance is symmetric perihilar radiating congestion—streaky shadows emanating from hilum, parahilar, or perihilar radiating streaky densities (Figs. 3.80A and B)
- Bilaterally symmetrical opacities
- Cardiomegaly (mild) rarely
- Diaphragm flat
- *Effusion*—Minimal pleural fluid in the pleural space (small pleural effusion) or fissures
- Edema of interlobar septae
- Fissures thickened and prominent
- *Fluid in fissures*—Fluid in the interlobar fissure—prominent interlobar fissures
- Fine granular appearance due to interplay of air distended bronchioles and ducts in the background of atelectasis of alveoli
- Film-to-film variation, air disappears in expiration and small bubbles form with better aeration
- Ground-glass appearance
- Haziness in the perivascular region
- Hyperinflated or normal lungs
- *Hilum*—Prominent with prominent pulmonary vascular markings
- Interstitial edema
- Increased lung volume (over aeration)
- Interlobular septal thickening due to interstitial edema
- Kerley B lines
- Linear or strand-like opacities throughout the lungs (due to engorged lymphatics) and streaky shadows emanating from hilum—Linear streaky radiating densities at both hila due to dilated lymphatics
- Entire lung or lobe may be opaque (seen on the right side. This is rare).

Normal X-ray is after 48–72 hours. Radiological changes will resolve usually in 24–72 hours.

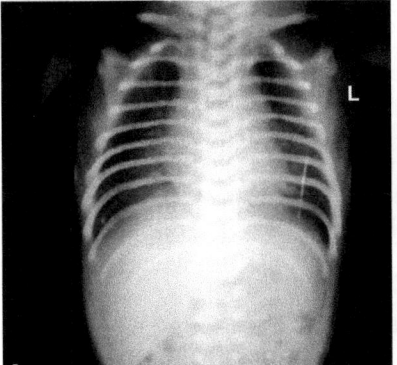
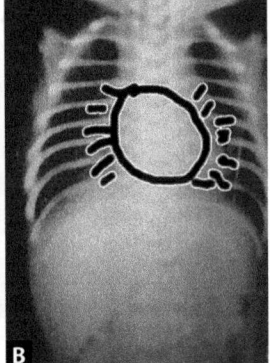

**Figs. 3.80A and B:** Transient tachypnea of the newborn (TTN) with sunburst appearance.

## QUESTIONS

**Q1. What is transient tachypnea of the newborn (TTN)?**
It is a mild, self-limited disorder. This is the most common cause of respiratory distress in newborn.

Usually affects near-term or term infants born by cesarean section.

**Q2. What is the pathogenesis of transient tachypnea of the newborn (TTN)?**
In TTN, basic pathogenesis is attributed to epithelial sodium channels (ENaC) which plays a major role in lung fluid resorption. In babies with channelopathy, fluid will get absorbed over a period of 24 hours through lymphatics and venous channels. These babies will present with tachypnea, failure of drainage of alveolar fluid will result in engorgement of lymphatics, decreased lung compliance.

**Q3. What is the pathophysiology of transient tachypnea of the newborn (TTN)?**
Transient tachypnea of the newborn is due to delayed resorption of the fetal lung fluid in the newborn period. It may be associated with abnormal epithelial ion transport. Catecholamines stimulate the lung fluid resorption. In babies delivered by cesarean, the levels are low in infants of diabetic mother. There is an interference by insulin on the β-adrenergic response of the lung.

The presence of unabsorbed lung fluid produces decreased lung compliance. The increased respiratory rate attempts to minimize the respiratory work. The incidence is more in babies delivered by cesarean section that the babies that are born by vaginal delivery. This is because the chest compression during the vaginal delivery expels the lung fluid.

**Q4. What are the predisposing factors for transient tachypnea of the newborn (TTN)?**
- Asthma in the mother
- Breech delivery
- Cesarean section delivery without preceding labor
- *Diabetes in the mother*—Infant of diabetic mother
- Excessive fluid administration to the mother
- Full-term babies
- *Gender*—Male babies
- *Hyporesponsiveness to beta-adrenergic stimuli*—Family history of asthma. Infants of asthmatic mothers will have beta-adrenergic hyporesponsiveness.
- *Increase birth weight*—Macrosomia
- Precipitous delivery.

**Q5. What are the clinical features of transient tachypnea of the newborn (TTN)?**
- Onset within 6 hours of life and peaks at first day of life
- Barrel chest
- Coarse breath sounds
- *Chest retractions*—Mild retractions/intercostal recessions
- Tachypnea (60–100 beats/min).

**Q6. What are the investigations in transient tachypnea of the newborn (TTN)?**
- X-ray chest
- Blood gas analysis will be normal.

**Q7. What are the differential diagnoses for transient tachypnea of the newborn (TTN)?**
- Alveolar phase of respiratory distress syndrome (RDS)
- *Aspiration*—Mild meconium aspiration syndrome (MAS)
- Bronchopneumonia/diffuse pneumonitis
- Cardiac failure (left heat failure)
- Drowned newborn syndrome and clear amniotic fluid aspiration

- Early-onset sepsis
- *Fetal circulation*—Persistent
- Fluid overload
- Group-B streptococcal pneumonia
- Hyaline membrane disease
- Hyperviscosity syndrome
- *Hemorrhage*—Pulmonary hemorrhage
- Immature lung syndrome
- Normal during first several hours of life.

**Q8. What is the treatment of transient tachypnea of the newborn (TTN)?**
No specific treatment is needed. Few babies may need oxygen/respiratory support to maintain oxygenation.

**Q9. What is the prognosis of transient tachypnea of the newborn (TTN)?**
This condition usually resolves spontaneously within 24–72 hours after birth—self-limited. Arterial pH and $PaCO_2$ are usually within normal limits. Overall prognosis is good.

## *Hyaline Membrane Disease*

### Radiological findings in hyaline membrane disease:

- Air bronchogram due to air-filled airways running to the periphery surrounded by dense lung tissue
- *Atelectasis of alveoli*—Expiratory film shows disappearance of air from the bronchioles and tubes
- Bilaterally symmetrical involvement
- Bell-shaped thorax
- Complete white-out of lungs (Fig. 3.81)
- Dense opacities
- Diffuse reticulogranular pattern
- Decreased lung volume
- Effacement of normal pulmonary vessels
- Fine granular appearance of the lungs
- *Ground-glass appearance*—Ground-glass mottling throughout both lung fields due to distended distal airway contrasted against the collapsed air spaces
- Hazy lungs
- Homogenous opacity (white lung)

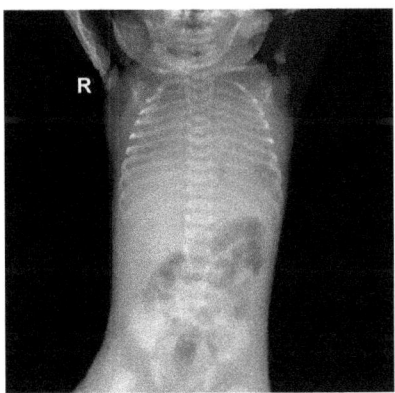

**Fig. 3.81:** White-out of lung in hyaline membrane disease (HMD).

- Hypoaeration of lungs (nonventilated lungs).

**Radiographic changes after intubation:**
Hyperinflation after intubation.

**Differential diagnosis:**

- Pneumonia
- Poor aeration or pulmonary hemorrhage may result in opaque lungs
- Sepsis
- Transient tachypnea of the newborn
- Pneumothorax
- Congenital heart disease
- Pulmonary hemorrhage
- Pulmonary venous congestion.

# QUESTIONS

**Q1. How will you classify hyaline membrane disease (HMD) according to the severity?**
- *Mild disease*—Reticulogranular pattern due to microatelectasis—in early and mild disease.
- *Moderate disease*—Air bronchogram due to atelectasis of lung tissue surrounding the airways—the contrast between the mottling and the air in the bronchi.

- *Severe disease*—Ground-glass opacity followed by white-out of the lungs with minimal distinction of pulmonary shadows. The lungs will appear opaque due to poor aeration or pulmonary hemorrhage.

**Q2. What are the clinical features of respiratory distress syndrome?**
- Apnea
- Breathing efforts will be more at birth
- *Chest wall retractions*—Intercostal and subcostal retractions
- Cyanosis
- Difficulty in breathing
- Expiratory grunt
- Flaring of nostrils
- *Fast breathing*—Increased respiratory rate (tachypnea).

**Q3. What are the four stages of hyaline membrane disease (HMD)?**
Four stages can be described as follows:

| Stages | Radiological features |
|---|---|
| I | Hazy lungs |
| II | Opacity more than stage I. Air bronchogram will overlap the heart shadow |
| III | Opacity more than stage II |
| IV | White lung (homogenous opacity) |

**Q4. What are the changes in pulmonary function tests in hyaline membrane disease (HMD)?**
Pulmonary function tests will show the following:
- Airway resistance decreased
- Compliance decreased
- Functional residual capacity decreased
- Residual volume decreased
- Tidal volume decreased
- Increased ventilation-perfusion (V/Q) mismatch.

**Q5. What are the risk factors for hyaline membrane disease (HMD)?**
- *Asphyxia*—Before, during, or after delivery
- *Aspirations*—Meconium aspiration syndrome (MAS)
- Babies with patent ductus arteriosus
- Caucasian babies
- Cesarean delivery
- Cold stress
- Diabetes in the mother
- Extreme preterm babies
- *Family history*—Sibling history of respiratory distress syndrome (RDS)
- *Gender*—Male baby
- *Gestational age*—Prematurity (less than 32 weeks)
- Hypoxia
- Infant of diabetic mother (IDM)
- Infection in the perinatal period
- Low birth weight less than 2.5 kg
- Lung development is poor
- Multiple pregnancy as the babies are premature.

**Q6. What are the factors that will impair surfactant production by type II pneumocytes?**
- Hypoxia
- $H^+$ increased (acidosis)
- Hypothermia
- Hypotension.

**Q7. Mention the clinical triad of symptoms in hyaline membrane disease (HMD).**
- Tachypnea
- Grunting (expiratory)
- Retractions

**Q8. How will you treat hyaline membrane disease (HMD)?**
Exogenous administration of surfactant by INSURE technique.
- Intubate
- Surfactant
- Extubate.

**Q9. What is the dose of surfactant?**
*Dose*: 100 mg/kg of phospholipids.

**Q10. What are the adverse effects of surfactant?**
- Hypotension
- Heart rate decreased (bradycardia)

- *Hemorrhage*—Pulmonary hemorrhage, intraventricular hemorrhage.

**Q11. How will you accelerate lung maturation in the fetus?**

Glucocorticoids act by accelerating lung maturation in the fetus. In infants delivered under 34 weeks of gestation, the mother should be given betamethasone/dexamethasone 24 hours before delivery. Steroids enhance the surfactant production and also improve the lung function.

**Q12. What are the steroids used for accelerating lung maturation in the fetus?**
- *Dexamethasone*: 6 mg intramuscular (IM), q 12 hours, and four doses
- *Betamethasone*: 12 mg IM, q 24 hours, and two doses.

**Q13. What are the complications of hyaline membrane disease (HMD)?**
- Apnea
- Atelectasis
- *Air leak syndromes*—Pneumothorax, pneumomediastinum, and pneumopericardium
- Alveolar collapse
- Bradycardia
- Bronchopulmonary dysplasia (extreme prematurity)
- Congestive cardiac failure. During recovery, the pulmonary vascular resistance will decrease which results in left to right shunt through patent ductus arteriosus (PDA). This will lead to congestive cardiac failure
- Disseminated intravascular coagulation
- *Emphysema*—Pulmonary interstitial emphysema
- Failure to thrive
- Gastrointestinal perforation
- *Hemorrhage*—Pulmonary, intracerebral, and intraventricular hemorrhage
- Interstitial emphysema
- Infection/septicemia
- *Jaundice*—Neonatal hyperbilirubinemia
- Kidney failure
- Localized interstitial pneumonia
- *Metabolic disturbances*—Hypocalcemia
- Neonatal necrotizing enterocolitis (NNEC)
- Oxygen toxicity
- Persistent PDA.

*Long-term complications*:
- Bronchopulmonary dysplasia
- Chronic lung disease
- Impaired hearing and vision
- Learning difficulties
- Movement problems
- Recurrent infections
- Subglottic stenosis due to intubation.

**Q14. How will you differentiate hyaline membrane disease (HMD) from pulmonary hemorrhage?**

Air bronchograms will be diminished during poor aeration whereas in pulmonary hemorrhage, it will not be diminished.

**Q15. What are the tests to evaluate for decreased surfactant during the antenatal period?**

Measure L:S ratio and desaturated phosphatidylcholine (DSPC) in the amniotic fluid.

**Q16. What is the course of the hyaline membrane disease?**

It is a progressive respiratory disease with the onset soon after delivery. The disease progresses up to 24–48 hours and may result in respiratory failure if untreated.

**Q17. What are the factors that will alter the course of hyaline membrane disease (HMD)?**

The course of the disease is altered by the following factors:
- Antenatal steroids
- Chronic hypoxia in utero

- ❏ Intervention with surfactant therapy
- ❏ Early continuous positive airway pressure (CPAP).

**Q18. What are the factors associated with accelerated maturation of lungs?**

Accelerated maturation is seen with the following:
- ❏ Aminophylline inhibits phosphodiesterase activity
- ❏ Beta-adrenergic agonists
- ❏ Betamethasone
- ❏ Cocaine abuse by mother
- ❏ Dexamethasone
- ❏ Estrogen
- ❏ *Factors for growth*—Epidermal growth factor
- ❏ Granulocyte-macrophage colony-stimulating factors (GMCSFs)
- ❏ *Hormones*—Thyroid hormones
- ❏ Heroin
- ❏ Insulin-like growth factors
- ❏ Prolactin.

**Q19. What are the factors associated with delayed maturation of lungs?**

Delayed maturation is seen with the following:
- ❏ Insulin
- ❏ Androgens
- ❏ Transforming growth factor-β.

## Meconium Aspiration Syndrome (Figs. 3.82A and B)

### Radiological findings:

X-ray of chest may show any of the following findings:
- ❖ Atelectasis, uneven aeration due to atelectasis and focal hyperaeration
- ❖ Areas of expansion
- ❖ *Air leak*—Pulmonary air leak, pneumothorax, and pneumomediastinum
- ❖ Bronchial tree obstruction
- ❖ Bilateral multifocal air space
- ❖ Bilateral asymmetrical nodular infiltrates
- ❖ *Consolidation*—Multifocal due to chemical pneumonitis
- ❖ Diffuse patchy, dense opacities

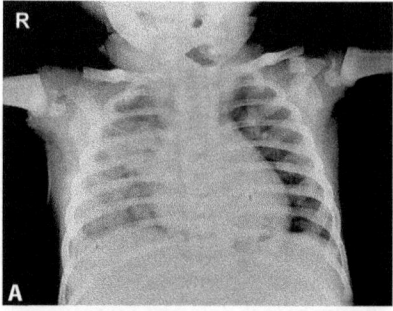
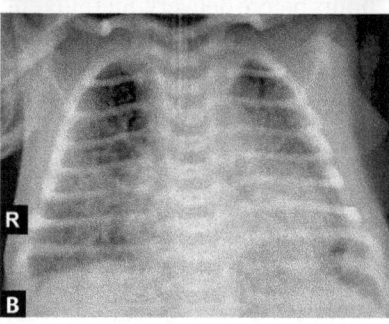

**Figs. 3.82A and B:** Meconium aspiration syndrome (MAS).

- ❖ *Densities*—Streaky, linear
- ❖ *Emphysema*—Obstructive emphysema
- ❖ *Effusion*—Mild pleural effusion
- ❖ Fluffy or nodular opacities
- ❖ Flattening of diaphragm
- ❖ Gas trapping secondary to distal small airway obstruction
- ❖ Hyperinflation of lungs (hypertranslucency, ribs horizontal, depressed diaphragm, and inflation or more than seven intercostal spaces can be seen)
- ❖ Resulting in heterogeneous opacities
- ❖ hypertranslucencies
- ❖ Infiltrates (patchy).

*Lateral view*—Increased anteroposterior diameter of chest

*Note*—There will be no air bronchogram.

## QUESTIONS

**Q1. What is meconium aspiration syndrome?**

It is the respiratory distress in an infant born through meconium-stained amniotic fluid whose symptoms cannot be otherwise explained.

**Q2. What are the clinical criteria for meconium aspiration syndrome?**

Persistent respiratory distress after 24 hours of life in babies born through meconium-stained amniotic fluid (MSAF).

**Q3. What are the features of meconium?**

The features of meconium are:

| Features | Features of meconium |
|---|---|
| Color | Black-green |
| Consistency | Thick, viscous, and sticky |
| Odor | Odorless |
| Weight | 28% |
| Carbohydrate | 80% |
| Protein | Nil |
| Lipid | Minimal |
| pH | 5.5–7 (acidic) |

*Quantity*—At birth, the newborn passes 60–200 grams of meconium.

**Q4. What is Miller's triad?**
- Meconium in the glottis
- Respiratory distress soon after birth or with 1 hour after birth
- Radiological evidence of aspiration pneumonitis (atelectasis and/or hyperinflation).

**Q5. What are the complications of meconium aspiration syndrome?**
- Airway obstruction
- Inactivation of the surfactant by the meconium
- Chemical pneumonitis.

## Agenesis of Lung/Pulmonary Agenesis

It refers to failure of development of primitive lung bud (Fig. 3.83).

### X-ray findings of pulmonary agenesis:

- Absence of lung parenchyma on the side of agenesis

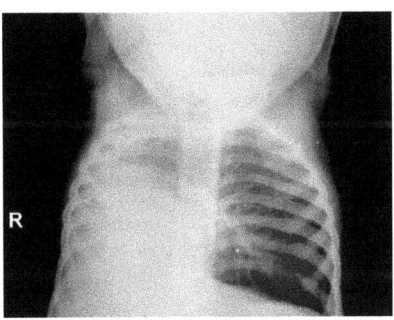

**Fig. 3.83:** Agenesis of right lung.

- Bilaterally symmetrical bone cage of thorax
- Bronchus rudimentary on the side of agenesis
- Cardiac borders will be indistinct on the side of agenesis
- Contralateral lung hyperinflation on the opposite side
- *Completely opaque hemithorax*—Homogeneous opacity on the side of agenesis
- Displacement of mediastinum to the side of agenesis
- Elevated hemidiaphragm on the side of agenesis
- Features of volume loss on the affected side
- Flattened hemidiaphragm on the side of agenesis
- *Hemithorax*—Opaque, white-out on the affected side
- Herniation of the opposite normal lung to the side of agenesis (this will be seen best in the lateral film)
- Intercostal spaces will be narrowed on the side of agenesis and widened on the opposite side
- Ipsilateral lung volume loss.

### Lateral view:

- Band-like opacity on the retrosternal area with variable width
- Herniation of the opposite normal lung to the side of agenesis (this will be seen best in the lateral film).

**Differential diagnosis:**

- *Atelectasis*—Total
- Aplasia of lungs (in aplasia, there will be short blind-ending bronchus)
- Bronchopneumonia
- Collapse lung
- Destroyed lung
- Diaphragmatic hernia
- Eventration of diaphragm
- Effusion (pleural)
- Pneumonectomy
- Pleural thickening
- *Pulmonary hypoplasia*—The lung tissue will be present but they are hypoplastic. It is usually bilateral and is associated with elevated diaphragm. The thoracic cage may be bell-shaped.

Unilateral pulmonary hypoplasia is associated with diaphragmatic hernia.

**Associated conditions:**

- Atrial septal defect
- *Bone abnormalities*—Absent ribs
- *Cardiac defects*—Ventricular septal defect (VSD), PDA, and coarctation of aorta
- Diaphragmatic defects
- Extrapulmonary sequestration
- Ear anomalies
- Fallot's tetralogy
- *Gastrointestinal anomalies*—Esophageal atresia
- *Genitourinary/renal anomalies*—Polycystic kidney
- Hemivertebra
- Imperforate anus
- VACTERL syndrome.

**Discussion:** This is due to arrest of lung development during embryonic period. This can be localized to a lobe or one lung and rarely both lungs.

Pulmonary angiogram will show absence of pulmonary artery.

Bronchogram will show absence of main bronchus.

Persistence of pleuroperitoneal canal will result in herniation of intestinal loops into the chest cavity.

# QUESTIONS

**Q1. How will you differentiate between agenesis and atelectasis?**
No respiratory distress in agenesis.
Respiratory distress in atelectasis.
Foreign body aspiration may lead to atelectasis and need flexible bronchoscopy.

**Q2. How will you group congenital developmental anomalies of lung?**
- *Group I*—Agenesis
- *Group II*—Aplasia
- *Group III*—Hypoplasia.

**Q3. What is the difference between agenesis, aplasia, and hypoplasia?**
Agenesis is complete absence of lung, bronchus with no blood supply on the affected side.

Aplasia is associated with rudimentary bronchus present with complete absence of parenchyma.

Hypoplasia is hypoplastic lung with presence of variable amounts of bronchial tree, pulmonary parenchyma, and its vasculature.

## Chronic Lung Disease (Fig. 3.84)
**Radiological findings:**

- *Atelectasis*—Lobar or segmental, shifting atelectasis
- Bronchopneumonia
- Coarse, irregular linear densities due to atelectasis or fibrosis
- Cardiomegaly in presence of pulmonary hypertension
- Cystic changes (bubbly lung)
- Diffuse involvement
- Emphysema
- Focal hyperexpanded areas of air trapping
- Generalized interstitial thickening

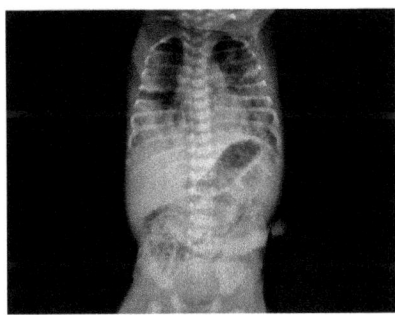

**Fig. 3.84:** Chronic lung disease (CLD).

* Granular pattern
* Hyperinflated lungs due to air trapping
* Heart borders obliterated
* Interspersed round lucent areas
* Ill-defined reticular markings.

**Lateral view:** Anteroposterior (AP) diameter will be normal, but in chronic cases decreased.

### Differential diagnosis:

* Bronchopulmonary dysplasia
* Congestive cardiac failure with pulmonary edema
* Hyaline membrane disease
* Infections
* *Pulmonary interstitial emphysema*—Pulmonary interstitial emphysema is associated with small air containing spaces (Fig. 3.85).

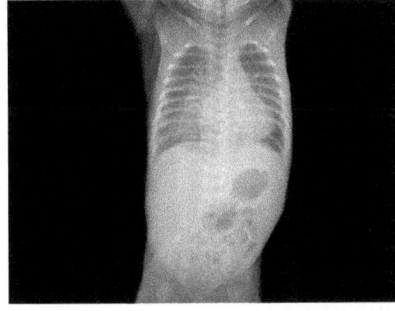

**Fig. 3.85:** Pulmonary interstitial emphysema.

**Discussion:** Chronic lung disease (CLD) is defined as continued oxygen need with chest X-ray abnormalities lasting for more than 28 days.

## QUESTIONS

**Q1. What are the predisposing factors for chronic lung disease?**
- *Artificial ventilation*—Prolonged mechanical ventilation
- *Infection*—Lung infection
- Immature, extreme premature lungs
- *Injury*—Lung injury.

**Q2. What are the complications of chronic lung disease (CLD)?**
- Asthma
- Pulmonary hypertension
- Sudden infant death
- Increased risk for pulmonary infection.

### Gastrointestinal System

#### Meconium Ileus

Bowel obstruction at the distal ileum by abnormally thick meconium.

### Radiological findings:

* Absence of air or minimal gas beyond the obstruction
* Bowel loop obstruction
* Bubbly bowel appearance of distal intestinal loops in the right lower quadrant
* *Calcifications*—Linear, curvilinear, and amorphous in the loops or in the abdomen
* Dilated gas filled proximal loops of varying caliber with relative lack of air-fluid levels due to thick meconium
* distension of small gut with no air and fluid level (X-ray of abdomen)
* Enema using water-soluble contrast medium, shows filling defects in the colon
* Filling defects in the ileum
* Functional microcolon
* Frothy or soap bubble sign due to mixture of air with meconium in the distal ileum or colon

- Ground-glass appearance due to small air bubbles mixed with meconium
- Mottled appearance of the affected loops (Neuhauser sign).

**Contrast enema findings:**
- Filling defects in the ileum
- Microcolon
- Distal ileum is packed with meconium and will be larger than microcolon.

**Differential diagnosis:**
- Meconium plug syndrome is functional colonic obstruction by a meconium plug. This usually affects the left colon known as small left colon syndrome. Contrast enema will show small left colon with multiple filling defects due to retained meconium. In meconium, ileus right colon is not dilated.
- *Hirschsprung's disease*—There will be reversed rectosigmoid ratio
- Small left colon syndrome
- Imperforate anus.

**Discussion:**

*Meconium ileus*: In babies with mucoviscidosis, the ileum may be obstructed by thick, putty-like meconium. This is the earliest manifestation of cystic fibrosis.

Meconium is not radiologically visible.

## QUESTIONS

**Q1. What are the clinical features of meconium ileus?**
- Abdominal distension
- Bilious vomiting
- Constipation (in older children)
- Doughy mass due to distended intestine
- Empty or relatively empty rectum
- Failure to pass meconium within 48 hours.

**Q2. What are the investigations in a patient with cystic fibrosis?**
- X-ray of abdomen
- Sweat chloride test.

**Q3. When meconium is produced?**
Meconium is produced after 13 weeks of gestation.
It accumulates in the distal colon and rectum by 20 weeks of gestation.

**Q4. When an X-ray should be taken in a baby with meconium ileus?**
X-ray should be taken after 6 hours after delivery of the child.

**Q5. What is the difference between meconium ileus and meconium plug syndrome?**
In meconium plug syndrome, the site of obstruction is at the distal portion of colon or in the rectum. Also, the severity of obstruction will be more in meconium plug syndrome.

**Q6. What is the treatment for meconium ileus?**
Hyperosmolar enema with gastrografin will draw fluid into the intestinal lumen.

**Q7. What are the complications of meconium ileus?**
- Ileal atresia
- Ileal stenosis
- Ischemic bowel
- Gangrene
- Perforation
- Meconium peritonitis
- Volvulus
- Pseudocyst.

**Q8. What are the conditions associated with meconium ileus?**
- Cystic fibrosis
- Pancreatic atresia
- Stenosis of pancreatic duct
- Gut immaturity.

### X-ray of Abdomen (Figs. 3.86A and B)

**Views:**
- Supine
- Decubitus views
- Prone cross table, translateral
- Supine translateral.

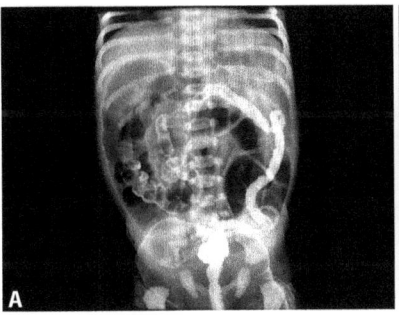
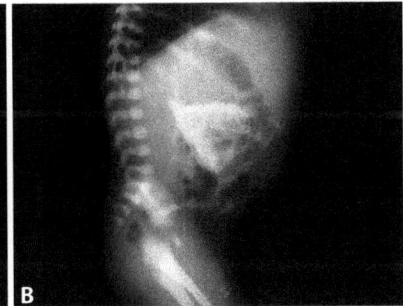

**Figs. 3.86A and B:** Meconium ileus with calcifications: (A) Anterioposterior view; (B) X-ray abdomen lateral view.

**Evaluation of X-ray of abdomen:** Evaluation of X-ray of abdomen in a newborn should be done in the following order:
- First focus on the relatively fixed structures like stomach and rectum.
- This should be followed by examination of solid organs like liver and spleen.
- Diaphragm
- Bony structures
- Soft tissues.

**Bowel gas pattern:** The gas may be abdominal intraluminal or abdominal extraluminal. The extraluminal may be intramural or extraintestinal.

The time required for the swallowed air to reach various parts of the gastrointestinal system is given here.

| Parts of the gastrointestinal tract (GIT) | The time required for the swallowed air |
|---|---|
| Stomach | 30–60 minutes |
| Duodenum | 30–60 minutes |
| Jejunum | 2–4 hours |
| Ileum | 4–6 hours |
| Colon | 12–18 hours |
| Rectum | 24 hours |

Decreased bowel gas will be seen in conditions in which swallowing is affected like central nervous system (CNS) depression, prematurity. Also in conditions like prolonged nasogastric aspiration or repeated vomiting, there will be diminished bowel gas.

Absent air shadow will be seen in conditions associated with anatomic discontinuity like esophageal atresia without fistula.

**Q1. When the abdomen is opaque, how will you differentiate whether it is due to airless abdomen or fluid-filled abdomen?**

In airless abdomen, the abdomen will not be distended. In fluid-filled abdomen, the abdomen will be distended.

Excessive bowel gas with abdominal distension.

Obstruction is functional or organic.

**Q2. How will you differentiate between the paralytic ileus and mechanical ileus?**

In paralytic ileus, the abdominal distension will be uniform.

In mechanical ileus, there will be differential distension of the gastrointestinal (GI) tract.

## Endocrine System

### Hypothyroidism

**Radiological feature:**

Absence of epiphysis at the lower end of femur (Fig. 3.87).

## QUESTION

Q. What are the epiphyses present at birth?
1. Cuboid
2. Lower end of femur
3. Upper end of tibia.

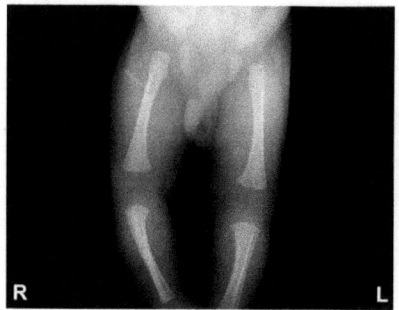

**Fig. 3.87:** X-ray showing absent epiphysis at the lower end of femur in hypothyroidism.

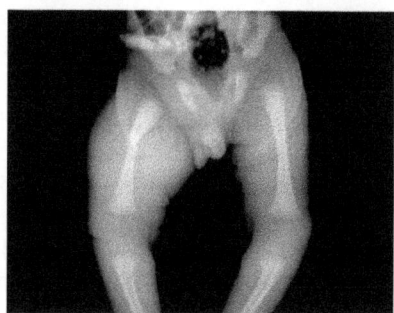

**Fig. 3.88:** Fracture of femur.

## Miscellaneous

### Birth Injuries—Fracture Shaft of Femur

Fracture shaft of femur is rare in newborns (Fig. 3.88).

#### Causes of fracture of femur in infants and children:

- Accidental injury
- Birth trauma
- Child abuse
- *Collagen disorder*—Osteogenesis imperfecta
- *Dietary deficiency*—Vitamin D deficiency (rickets).

## QUESTIONS

**Q1. What are the predisposing factors for fracture of femur in newborn?**
- *Accidents*—Sudden fall—precipitate deliveries
- *Breech presentation*—Malpresentation—internal podalic version
- *Birth weight*—Low/large for date baby
- *Collagen disorder*—Osteogenesis imperfecta
- Difficult deliveries
- *Density of bone decreased*—Osteopenia of prematurity, osteoporosis.

**Q2. What are the predisposing factors for fracture of femur in babies delivered by cesarean section?**
- Poor relaxation
- Small incision
- Wrong delivery techniques.

**Q3. What is the treatment of fracture of femur?**
- *Subtrochanteric fracture*—Strapping of the thigh to the abdomen
- *Fracture of shaft*—Toe groin cast.

**Q4. What are the complications of fracture of femur in newborn?**
- Limb length discrepancy
- Residual angulations.

# PEDIATRIC SURGERY

## CARDIOVASCULAR SYSTEM

### Pneumopericardium

Air will get accumulated in the pericardium.

### Radiological Findings of Pneumopericardium (Mnemonic A–E)

- **A**ir in the pericardium surrounds the heart. The air does not rise above the level of pericardial reflection at the root of the great vessels
- **A**ir limits to the anatomical limits of pericardium at the level of pulmonary artery and ascending aorta. The heart will be completely or partially surrounded by a rim of air appearing as lucent areas extending up to the pulmonary arteries
- **B**ase of the heart can be visualized. Lucent areas on the inferior border of the heart
- **C**ardiomegaly with relatively clear lung fields
- **D**iaphragm can be visualized below the heart—continuous diaphragm sign

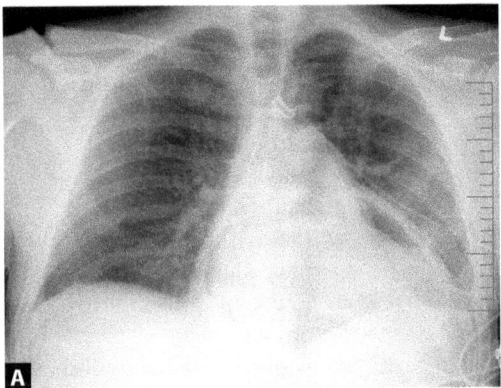
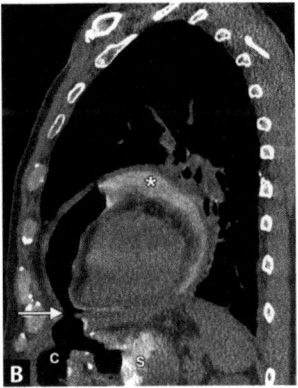

**Figs. 3.89 A and B:** (A) X-ray showing pneumopericardium; (B) CT scan showing pneumopericardium.

(continuous left hemidiaphragm sign in lateral view)
- **E**xtremely slender heart—(small heart sign) in tension pneumopericardium, the cardiothoracic ratio will be decreased
- **P**arietal pericardium will be visible as thin rim (Figs. 3.89A and B)
- Lateral decubitus—air in pericardial space shifts to nondependent site.

## Differential Diagnosis

- Pneumomediastinum—air will be outlining the aortic arch, superior vena cava above the azygos vein, and distal left pulmonary artery
- Gas does not surround the heart completely, will not be confined to heart and may extend to the superior mediastinum and neck
- The air in the pericardium will remain below the level of great vessels in pneumopericardium
- In lateral decubitus view the air is trapped in the mediastinal tissue and does not cross the midline to contralateral side.

## QUESTIONS

**Q1. What are the causes of pneumopericardium?**
- Assisted ventilation (positive pressure ventilation)
- Air leaks like pneumomediastinum, widespread pulmonary interstitial emphysema, and tension pneumothorax
- Barotrauma
- Blunt chest injury
- Bacterial infections
- *Clostridium perfringens* infection
- De novo by microorganism—*Klebsiella* infections
- Penetrating injuries
- Invasive procedures.

**Q2. What are the clinical features of pneumopericardium?**
- Hypoxia
- Heart rate decreased—bradycardia
- Hypotension
- Hamman's sign—continuous crunching synchronous with the heartbeat. This will be better heard in the left lateral position.
- Heart sounds will be muffled or absent.

**Q3. What are the complications of pneumopericardium?**
- Cardiac tamponade
- Pulsus paradoxus.

**Q4. What is the finding in jugular venous pulse?**
Rapid "x" descent.

**Q5. How will you differentiate between pneumomediastinum and pneumopericardium?**

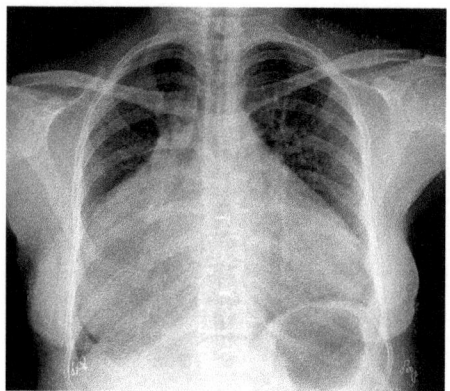

**Fig. 3.90:** Money bag appearance pericardial effusion.

- The air in the pericardium will change with change in position but in pneumomediastinum will not change
- The air surrounding the heart will not extend beyond the reflection of aorta or the pulmonary artery
- Transverse band of air sign air within the transverse sinus of the pericardium.

## Pericardial Effusion (Fig. 3.90)

Excess fluid collected in the pericardium.

### Radiological Features in X-ray Chest (Mnemonic A–G)

- *Anteroposterior view:*
  - Acute cardiophrenic angles will be more acute
  - Base of the heart will be widened in small effusions
  - Leather bottle appearance with pulmonary oligemia
  - Bilateral hilar overlay sign.
  - Cardiothoracic ratio increased
  - Cardiophrenic angles will be acute
  - Clear lung fields
  - Cardiomegaly—increased cardiothoracic ratio or rapidly increasing cardiothoracic ratio
  - Diminished vascular clarity
  - Distinct cardiac borders
  - Dimension of cardiomediastinal silhouette increased (water bottle sign)
  - Enlarged cardiac silhouette—obliteration of normal cardiac features
  - Epicardial fat pad sign
  - Elliptical stripe paralleling the left cardiac border
  - Flask shaped heart or water bottle shaped
  - Fields (lung) are clear due to pulmonary oligemia
  - Flask or water bottle configuration appearance
  - Globular or triangular or money bag appearance of cardiac silhouette without increasing pulmonary vascular markings
  - There will be widening of subcarinal angle without evidence of left atrial enlargement.
- *Lateral view*—filling of retrosternal space
- *Fluoroscopy* will show decreased or absent cardiac silhouette pulsations with normal aortic pulsations.

### Signs in Large Pericardial Effusion

- *Bilateral hilar over lay sign*
- *Epicardial fat–pad sign*—in small effusion, lateral view will show widened anterior pericardial stripe more than 2 mm thick.
- *Water bottle sign* is seen in very large pericardial effusion. *Water bottle sign*—the enlarged shape of cardiac silhouette on erect frontal view will show old fashioned water bottle sitting on a bench
- *Fat pad or Oreo Cookie sign*: In lateral view of X-ray chest the epicardial fat behind the sternum and pericardial fat will look as lucent line separated by vertical opaque line due to the pericardial fluid. Separation of retrosternal and inner epicardial fat stripe lines:
  - Normal pericardial sac will contain about 30–50 mL of pericardial fluid
  - Globular heart in large effusion
  - *Lateral view*—filling of retrosternal space.

## Differential Diagnosis

- Cardiomegaly
- Hemoperitoneum
- Dilated cardiomyopathy
- Constrictive pericarditis.

## Discussion—Pericardial Effusion

### Causes of pericardial effusion:

- Pericarditis—viral, tuberculosis, and bacterial
- Hydatid cyst
- Myocardial infarction
- Neoplasm
- Radiation pericarditis—more 40 Gy
- Systemic disease—uremia and collagen disorder.

### Classification according to type of fluid:

- Transudate—cardiac failure, uremia, myxedema, and collagen vascular disorders
- Exudate—inflammatory and neoplasm
- Hemorrhagic—traumatic, neoplastic, and aortic rupture
- Chylous—thoracic duct injury.

## QUESTIONS

**Q1. How will you differentiate cardiomegaly due to pericardial effusion and congestive cardiac failure (CCF)?**
- The pulmonary vascular markings will be increased in CCF whereas it will be decreased in pericardial effusion
- Pericardial effusion may be serous, purulent, or hemorrhagic.

**Q2. What are the ECG changes in pericardial effusion?**
Low voltage QRS complexes—electrical alternans will be seen in large effusion.

**Q3. What is Ewart's sign?**
Compression of left lower lobe of lung by pericardial effusion will produce bronchial breath sounds in the infrascapular area.

**Q4. What is the investigation of choice to diagnose pericardial effusion?**
Echocardiography.

**Q5. What is the investigation of choice to diagnose loculated or small pericardial effusion?**
Computed tomography (CT) scan or MRI.

**Q6. How much fluid can be accumulated in the pericardial sac without enlargement of its borders?**
About 200-250 mL.

**Q7. What is epicardial fat pad sign?**
In normal cases, the parietal pericardium will be separated from the epicardial fat by 1-2 mm. In pericardial effusion this distance will be increased. This will be seen best in lateral view.

**Q8. How will you treat pericardial effusion?**
Pericardiocentesis through subxiphoid approach with ECG monitoring will be useful.

**Q9. What is the amount of fluid accumulated in the pericardial cavity for any change in the cardiac silhouette to occur?**
About 250-300 mL should be accumulated in the pericardial cavity for any change in the cardiac silhouette to occur.

## RESPIRATORY SYSTEM

### Esophageal Atresia and Tracheoesophageal Fistula

#### Esophageal Atresia

- Abdomen should be included to find out if air is present in the abdomen. If there is a distal fistula there will be air in the abdomen
- X-ray will show coiled catheter in the upper esophageal pouch.
- Plain X-ray may show proximal blind pouch distended with air or esophagus dilated with air
- Roentgenography using contrast medium, which is water soluble and less than 1 mL can be used to outline the blind upper pouch
- Catheter cannot be passed into the stomach. Catheter will stop abruptly 10-11 cm

from the upper gum line. The tube cannot be passed beyond 11-12 cm
* Treatment—esophageal atresia is a surgical emergency
* Constant suction should be done to empty the esophageal pouch. The baby should be nursed prone to prevent aspiration
* Surgery should be done in stages.

## Tracheoesophageal Fistula

### Radiological Findings of Tracheoesophageal Fistula (Mnemonic A–G) (Figs. 3.91A and B)

The radiological findings depend upon the type of tracheoesophageal fistula (TEF).
* *Air bubble in the stomach* implies, there is a communication between the trachea and lower part of esophagus. This is seen in C type, which is the most common type.
  * In types A and B, there will be no air in the stomach and intestines.
* *Bowel gas* absent in type A with blind upper and blind lower segment without any fistula, bowel gas will be present in types C, E, and F. In types C and D air will be seen in the bowel loops
* *Coiled tube in the pouch*—X-ray (anteroposterior and lateral view) should be taken with a catheter having a radiopaque end in situ (nasogastric tube inserted in to the esophagus)
* Close proximity of trachea and esophagus (lateral view)
* Displacement of trace anteriorly (lateral view)
* *Esophageal pouch*, dilated, and air-fluid filled
* Fistula in the upper end of esophagus sloping toward the trachea (barium study)
* *Fluoroscopy*—H type of fistula can be demonstrated by injection water-soluble contrast (omnipaque) during cine fluoroscopy
* *Gasless abdomen* will be seen in TEF without fistula. In normal newborns, there will be air in the stomach 15 minutes after birth. Stomach air may be absent. This will indicate that the esophagus is obstructed and there is no communication between the trachea and the esophagus. Absence of stomach air indicates esophageal atresia without fistula connecting to the trachea.

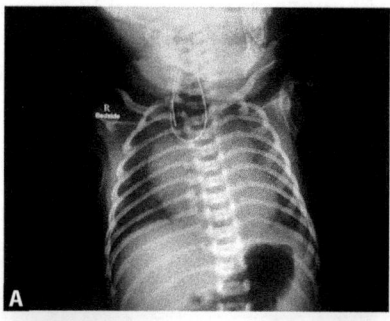
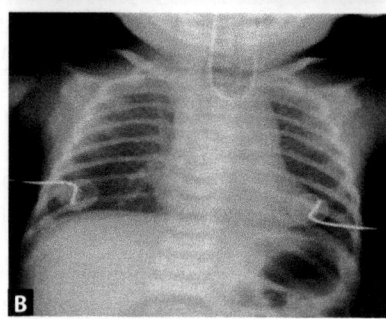

**Figs. 3.91A and B:** Tracheoesophageal fistula coiling of orogastric tube.

### Clinical Features
* Aspiration
* Breathing difficulties—respiratory distress
* Choking
* Copious secretions.
* Drooling
* Episodes of coughing and chocking cyanosis while feeding
* Fails to take first fed in the first day of life.
* Frothing
* Feeding difficulties.

### Complications
* Atelectasis—lungs may show atelectasis
* Bronchopneumonia—aspiration pneumonia right upper lobe
* *Consolidation* due to aspiration.

*Lateral view*—anterior displacement of trachea.

## Discussion

**Causes:**

- Congenital
- Acquired:
  - Malignancy
  - Traumatic—instrumentation
  - Infections—tuberculosis
  - Perforated diverticulum
  - Perforated cyst or sequestrated lung.

Inability to pass a nasogastric tube in to the stomach, in TEF large sized catheter size 8–10 should be passed. Nasogastric tube tends to coil in the blind upper esophageal pouch. The tube will be seen coiled in the pouch.

Insert a rubber catheter into the stomach. The length of the tube inserted can be measured by measuring the distance from the tip of the nose to the tragus and from tragus to the xiphisternum. The tube cannot be passed beyond the obstruction.

In a normal term, newborn air reaches rectum by 12 hours but in a babies with perinatal asphyxia, it will take longer. In preterm, it may take a longer time up to 36 hours depending upon the prematurity.

In TEF, except H type there will be an inability to pass a nasogastric tube into the esophagus.

## QUESTIONS

**Q1. What are the types of congenital tracheoesophageal fistula?**

*Types*: There are six types:
1. Type A—blind upper and blind lower segment without any fistula esophageal atresia without distal tracheoesophageal fistula. Upper end is blind with the lower end connected to the trachea
2. Type B—Fistula at the upper end esophageal atresia with fistula between trachea or main bronchus and proximal esophagus
3. Type C—esophageal atresia with fistula between trachea or main bronchus and the lower end of the esophagus. Upper end is blind with the lower end connected to the trachea
4. Type D—fistula at both upper and lower end of the esophagus. Esophageal atresia with fistula at both ends—proximal and distal tracheoesophageal fistula
5. Type E—H type fistula without atresia, H type will be seen high in the esophagus at the cervical level
6. Type F—congenital narrowing of the esophagus without atresia or fistula.

Of the above types, 'C' type is more common occurring in 82–86% of cases with TEF.

**Q2. Which is the most common type of tracheoesophageal fistula?**
- Upper end is blind with the lower end connected to the trachea (type C)
- Most common type is proximal esophageal atresia with distal tracheoesophageal fistula
- Also esophageal stenosis will be seen, which is a variant of esophageal atresia.

**Q3. What are the conditions associated conditions with TEF?**
- Maternal polyhydramnios
- Single umbilical artery
- VACTERAL (vertebral, anal atresia, cardiac, TEF, renal, and limb abnormalities).

**Q4. What are the anomalies associated with esophageal anomalies?**
- Major cardiac anomalies
- Gastrointestinal anomalies
- Genitourinary anomalies.

**Q5. What is the differentiating feature of esophageal stenosis and TEF?**
X-ray should be taken with the tube in situ. Air bubble will be seen in the stomach, if there is a communication between the lower segment and trachea or between upper and lower segments (esophageal stenosis).

**Q6. What are the complications of surgical repair of TEF?**
- ❑ Aspiration
- ❑ Asthma like symptoms
- ❑ Bacterial infections
- ❑ Chest infections
- ❑ Cough (persistent)
- ❑ Dysphagia
- ❑ Erosion of esophagus due to acid from stomach
- ❑ Fistula formation or recurrence
- ❑ Focal tracheomalacia
- ❑ Gastroesophageal reflux disease (GERD)
- ❑ Hiatus hernia due to shortening of esophagus
- ❑ Hypoplasia, if distal esophagus
- ❑ Impaired motility of esophagus
- ❑ Strictures.

## Congenital Lobar Emphysema or Congenital Lobar Overinflation

X-ray chest taken in both inspiration and expiration will show overdistension of one lobe, compression of the adjacent lung, herniation across the mediastinum, and depression of the diaphragm.

Most commonly affected part is left upper lobe followed by right middle lobe and right upper lobe. Radiological findings will depend upon the time in which the film is taken either before the fluid is expelled or after the fluid is expelled.

❖ Before the pulmonary fluid is expelled, the lungs will appear opaque
❖ After the fluid is expelled, a classical emphysematous picture will develop (mnemonic A-I):
  - Air-filled lobes of the lung
  - Atelectasis on the affected side
  - Collapse of adjacent lobes due to compression by the emphysematous lung
  - Diffuse reticular pattern due to distended lymphatic channels
  - Displacement of mediastinum to the opposite side
  - Downward displacement and flattening of hemidiaphragm

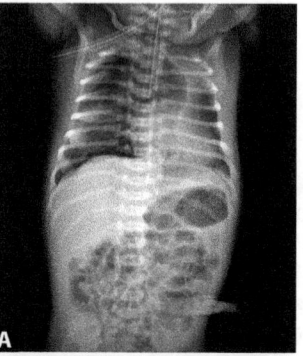
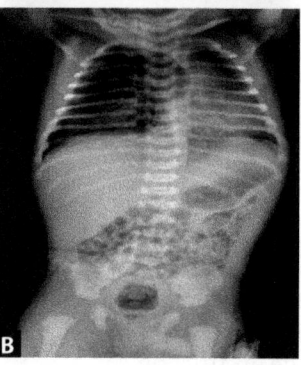

**Figs. 3.92A and B:** Congenital lobar emphysema with upper lobe herniation.

- Enlarged lobe of the lung
- Flat hemidiaphragm
- Fluid-filled lobe of the lung, which will become air-filled within few days
- Gas trapping in the lungs
- Herniation of the lobe across the midline and compressing the adjacent lobes
- Hazy mass like lesion immediately after birth
- Hyperlucency on the affected side after clearing of fluid extends to opposite side
- Increased space between the ribs (wide rib spaces)
- Increased space between widely spaced out thin pulmonary vessels will be seen on the lucent areas (Figs. 3.92A and B)
- *Lateral film*—posterior displacement of heart.

### Differential Diagnosis

❖ Pneumonia
❖ Lung cysts

- Mucus plug obstruction—vigorous suction and physical therapy should be done to exclude this condition
- Pneumothorax—the margins of the collapsed lung will be seen in pneumothorax.

## Discussion
- Congenital lobar emphysema (CLE) is due to hyperinflation of a lobe. There will be no emphysematous destruction of the lung tissue. This is a rare condition due to air trapping due to soft bronchus.
- Depending upon the number of alveoli, it can be hypoalveolar or polyalveolar.

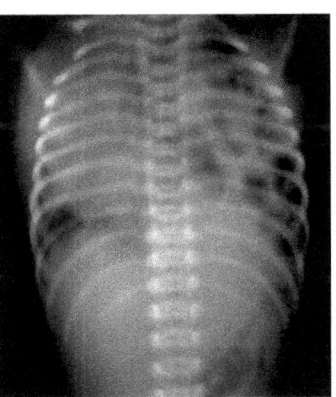

**Fig. 3.93:** Congenital pulmonary adenomatoid malformation.

## QUESTIONS

**Q1. What are the common sites of CLE?**
Common sites are left upper lobe, right middle lobe, and right upper lobes, are commonly affected.

**Q2. What is the treatment for CLE?**
- When the respiratory distress is mild and no oxygen is required the infant can be managed conservatively. The symptoms usually subside by the age of one year
- When associated with severe respiratory distress, treated by surgical excision of the affected lobe.

**Q3. What is the prognosis for CLE?**
Few cases will resolve spontaneously. Most of the cases will require surgery. The children treated medically or surgically may be associated with mild airway obstruction at the age of 10 years of age.

## Congenital Pulmonary Adenomatoid Malformation (Fig. 3.93)

### Radiological Findings in Congenital Pulmonary Adenomatoid Malformation of Lung

*(Mnemonic A–F)*
- **A**ir filled cysts—multiple
- **C**riss-cross septate markings in the hyperlucent lung
- **C**ystic lucencies in the hemithorax
- **C**ompression of lungs
- **C**yst formation
- **D**isplacement of the mediastinum to the opposite side by large cyst
- **D**epression of the diaphragm on the same side
- **E**nlargement of the affected lobe
- **F**luid filled cyst.

The findings will vary according to the types of congenital pulmonary adenomatoid malformation (CPAM):
- Type I and II will be seen as distinct, sharply outlined cysts
- Type III will be seen as opaque mass
- Type III will be associated with an opaque hemithorax.

### Differential Diagnosis

In diaphragmatic hernia, the abdominal gas shadow will be seen in the chest, but in CPAM, the abdominal gas shadow will be normal and the nasogastric tube can be passed in to the stomach. Magnetic resonance imaging (MRI) will be helpful in differentiating CPAM and diaphragmatic hernia. Pulmonary sequestration has a blood vessel supplying it.

### Discussion

*Congenital pulmonary adenomatoid malformation of the lung* is due to anomalous fetal development of terminal respiratory structures and adenomatous over growth of the terminal bronchioles. This will result in subsequent suppression of alveolar growth. The lung bud, during the development develops abnormally into multiple cysts of varying sizes. This is confined to one lobe or one lung.

### Pathology
- This is a type of hamartoma of terminal respiratory structures
- Anomalous fetal development of terminal respiratory structures
- Adenomatoid proliferation of bronchiolar elements
- Compression of lungs—the mass effect will result in lung compression
- Development of lung bud abnormally into multiple cysts of varying sizes
- Large CPAM will produce mediastinal shift
- Left-sided lesions are more common than the right. In few cases, they can be seen bilaterally.

### Anatomy
- This is confined to one lobe or one lung. Adenomatoid proliferation of bronchiolar elements and cyst formation results in enlargement of the affected lobe. This usually involves a single lobe. Involvement of an entire lung is very rare.
- The blood supply is from bronchial circulation.
- These have increased amount of elastic tissue and absent cartilage.

## QUESTIONS

**Q1. What are the types of CPAM?**
There are three types of cysts according to Stocker's classification:
1. Type I—macrocystic cysts larger than 2 cm in diameter or a single dominant cyst surround by smaller cysts. These become air-filled later. These become air-filled later. This the most common type
2. Type II—microcystic cysts about 1 cm. Multiple, evenly spaced cysts. Macroscopically solid lesion. A firm bulky mass containing tiny cysts less than 0.5 cm
3. Type III—macroscopically solid lesion.

**Q2. What are the clinical features of CPAM?**
- Before birth—hydrops fetalis and polyhydramnios
- After birth—mediastinal shift (this may be absent, if there is fibrosis due to recurrent infections)
- Respiratory distress.

**Q3. What is the differential diagnosis of CPAM?**
Pulmonary sequestration, bronchogenic cyst, congenital lobar emphysema, diaphragmatic hernia, and cystic bronchiectasis.

**Q4. What are the investigations of CPAM?**
- Antenatal—the lesions are seen as echogenic cystic masses in the lung.
- Prenatal diagnosis is by ultrasonogram.

**Q5. What is the treatment of CPAM?**
Surgical excision.

**Q6. What are the complications of CPAM?**
- Pulmonary hypoplasia
- Pulmonary hypertension
- Lung abscess.

**Q7. What is the prognosis of CPAM?**
- Macrocystic cysts have a better prognosis than the other two types.
- The prognosis is poor in larger lesions causing mediastinal shift or associated with hydrops.

**Q8. What is the differential diagnosis for radiological finding?**
Left-sided diaphragmatic hernia.

**Q9. What are the differentiating features between congenital diaphragmatic herniation and CPAM in X-ray?**
This can be differentiated from diaphragmatic hernia by the following features:

- ❏ The diaphragm will be well defined in CPAM
- ❏ Normal complement of bowel loops
- ❏ Gas in the stomach will be normal.

**Q10. How will you diagnose CPAM in the antenatal period?**

Prenatal diagnosis is by ultrasonogram. The lesions are seen as echogenic cystic masses in the lung.

## Congenital Diaphragmatic Hernia

### Radiological Findings in Congenital Diaphragmatic Hernia (Mnemonic A–I)

- ❖ Air-filled bowel loops in the thorax. Sometimes bowel loops may be airless
- ❖ Abdominal circumference decreased (scaphoid abdomen)
- ❖ Bowel loops absent in the abdomen
- ❖ Cyst like lucencies in the left side of the chest
- ❖ Cardiothymic shift to opposite side
- ❖ Displacement of mediastinum to opposite side
- ❖ Distension of stomach with air
- ❖ Endotracheal tube deviated to opposite side
- ❖ Fluid-filled loops at early stages before swallowing of air
- ❖ Gut in the thoracic cavity—X-ray with a feeding tube placed in the stomach shows the presence of the gut (signet ring radiolucencies) in the thoracic cavity. The stomach tube will be seen in the chest. Nasogastric tube will localize the stomach in the thorax
- ❖ Gasless abdomen or paucity of bowel gas in the abdomen. The abdomen will be devoid of gas patterns
- ❖ Herniation of liver or gut into the chest
- ❖ Indistinct diaphragm.

### Differential Diagnosis

- ❖ Eventration of diaphragm
- ❖ Congenital pulmonary adenomatoid malformation
- ❖ *Cystic bronchiectasis*: The abdominal gas shadow will be seen in the abdomen. There will be no mediastinal shift
- ❖ *Pulmonary sequestration*: This condition is due to an accessory lung bud, which originates in the lower down part of the primitive foregut. There may be associated polyhydramnios, mediastinal shift, or hydrops. Color Doppler will show a solid highly echogenic mass in the chest with systemic arterial supply. X-ray chest will show cystic lesions especially in the lower lobes. Triangular or oval shaped basal lung mass will be seen on one side of the lung contrast aortography, MRI or color Doppler study will delineate the feeding vessel to the sequestration.

### Diaphragm

*Development of diaphragm*: The diaphragm develops from the following structures (Figs. 3.94A and B):

- ❖ Septum transversum, from the mesoderm
- ❖ Pleuroperitoneal membranes
- ❖ Mesenchyme surrounding the esophagus
- ❖ Mesenchyme surrounding the aorta.

### Eventration of Diaphragm

- ❖ X-ray findings will resemble diaphragmatic hernia.
- ❖ X-ray chest will show a clear demarcation between the abdominal contents and the lung (Figs. 3.95A and B).

## QUESTIONS

**Q1. What is the cause of eventration of diaphragm?**

Eventration of diaphragm is due to insufficient muscle development or absence of phrenic nerves. The diaphragm will be replaced by a fibrous sheet, which may be localized or diffuse. In most cases, they are unilateral and are seen on the left side. The diaphragm is weak and it bulges in to the thoracic cavity. There is no opening in the diaphragm. This is seen usually in the left cupola of the diaphragm. The stomach is usually displaced upwards

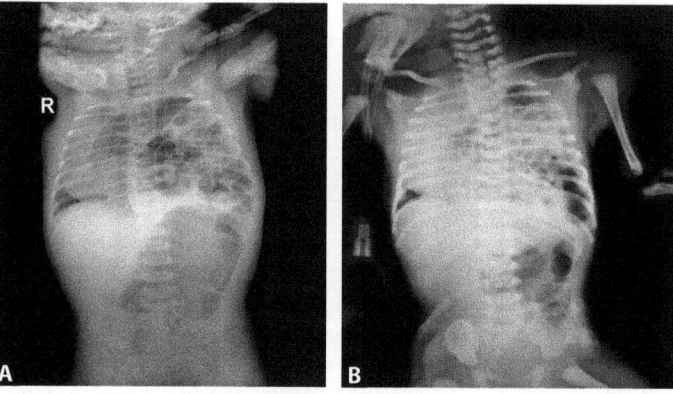

**Figs. 3.94A and B:** Left diaphragmatic hernia CDH.

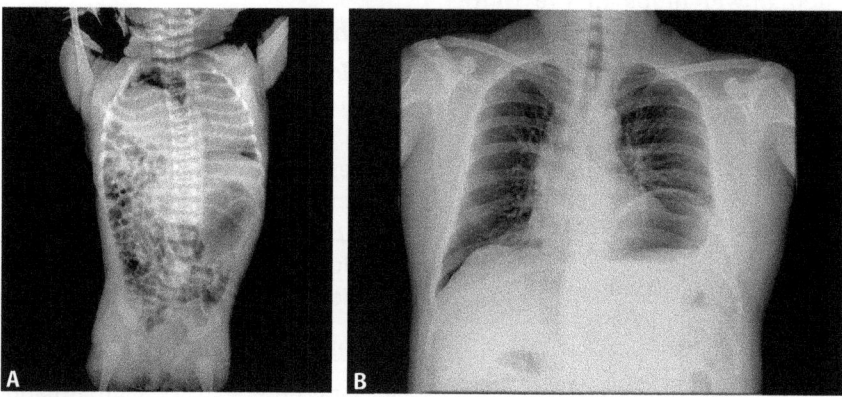

**Figs. 3.95A and B:** (A) Eventration of diaphragm right side; (B) Eventration of diaphragm left side.

with the esophagus and the cardia remaining in their normal positions.

**Q2. What are the clinical features of eventration of diaphragm?**
- Poor appetite, which results in slower growth.
- Respiratory distress will be seen, if the eventration is severe
- Inability to swallow more fluid, the esophagus may be kinked, which results in difficulty in swallowing.

**Q3. How will you differentiate between eventration and diaphragmatic hernia?**
In diaphragmatic hernia, there will be no clear demarcation between the abdominal contents and the lung.

In eventration, the movement may be paradoxical. During normal inspiration, the diaphragm will move down and move up during expiration, but in paradoxical respiration, the diaphragm moves up during inspiration and downwards during expiration.

**Q4. What is the treatment for eventration of diaphragm?**
Treatment is by plication of the diaphragm either by open or thoracoscopic approach.

**Q5. What are the radiological differences between diaphragmatic hernia and eventration of diaphragm?**
The intestinal shadows may reach the upper end of the lung in diaphragmatic hernia but in eventration of diaphragm the shadows will never reach upper end of the lung.

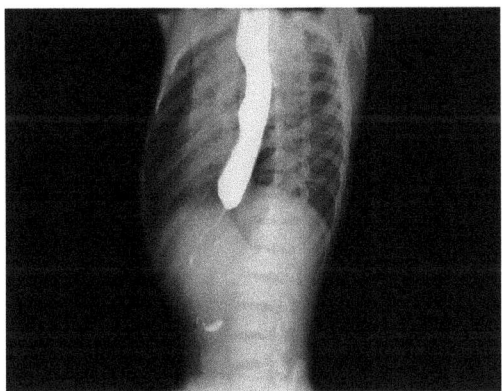

Fig. 3.96: Achalasia cardia.

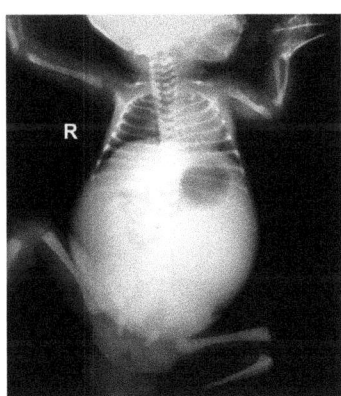

Fig. 3.97: Single bubble sign.

## GASTROINTESTINAL SYSTEM

### Achalasia Cardia (Fig. 3.96)

- Degeneration of nerve cells in the lower esophagus
- Failure of smooth muscles to relax results in incomplete lower esophageal sphincter relaxation.

### Barium Swallow

- Anteroposterior view and lateral views
- Air fluid level
- Bird's beak sign or rat tail sign—narrow region at the lower end of esophagus with dilatation of esophagus above
- Consolidation due to aspiration pneumonia
- Dilated esophagus
- Esophageal achalasia due to smooth eccentric narrowing at $D_{10}$ level
- Fixed narrowing at the lower end of esophagus.

## QUESTIONS

Q1. How will you differentiate between achalasia cardia, peptic stricture, and esophageal stenosis?
- In barium swallow the narrowing of the esophagus will be eccentric in achalasia cardia. In esophageal, stenosis will be in the center of the barium column. The narrowing will be smooth in both the conditions
- Peptic stricture will be seen in the lower end of the esophagus. The stricture will be irregular
- *Vascular anomalies*—posterior indentation at uppers thoracic esophagus.

Q2. What are the clinical features of achalasia cardia?
- Chest pain
- Dysphagia
- Fullness in the throat
- Heartburn
- Regurgitation.

Q3. What is the treatment for achalasia cardia?
- Esophageal balloon dilatation
- Heller myotomy.

### Idiopathic Hypertrophic Pyloric Stenosis—String Sign

#### Congenital Gastric Outlet Obstruction

- Single bubble sign due to distension of stomach by air or fluid (Fig. 3.97)
- No air shadow or minimal gas distal to the obstruction.

#### Hypertrophic Pyloric Stenosis

- *Radiological findings:*—Plain X-ray abdomen will show the following:
  - Bowel gas will be little
  - Distended single stomach bubble (diameter >7cm) with paucity of gas in the rest of the abdomen

- Distance between stomach and duodenal cap will be more
- Distension of both stomach and duodenal cap
- Distal gas pattern in the small and large bowel will be minimal
- Delayed gastric emptying due to obstruction to the outflow
- Elongation and narrowing of pyloric canal
- Fluid filled stomach after 2 hours of feeding
- Gastro-retroperistalsis and gastro-esophageal reflux can be observed.

❖ *Contrast studies*: Barium study will show narrow pyloric canal and retention of barium in the stomach

❖ *Antral beaking:* Streak of barium points toward the pyloric canal

❖ *Antral nipple sign in the lateral view*—seen in longitudinal ultrasonogram prolapse of redundant mucosa into the antrum

❖ *Beak sign:* The contrast medium will try to enter into the proximal portion of the pyloric canal causing beak sign. Beak sign in patients with hypertrophic pyloric stenosis, abrupt cut of the barium column in the pylorus

❖ *Cephalic orientation of pylorus Caterpillar sign*: Fluoroscopic study will show caterpillar sign due to vigorous active peristalsis that abruptly stops at the pyloric antrum

❖ *Diamond sign:* Transient triangular tent like cleft in the middle of the pyloric canal with apex pointing inferiorly. This is due to mucosal bulging between separated hypertrophied muscle bundles within the pyoric canal on the side of greater curvature

❖ *Double track sign or tram track sign*: Parallel mucosal folds in pyloric canals, contrast will remain in the redundant mucosa in the narrowed pyloric lumen, which separates barium column into two channels

❖ *Echogenicity* of pyloric muscle mass will be nonuniform

❖ Elongation and narrowing of pyloric canal 2-4 cm in length

❖ *Four millimeters* or more of pyloric mass thickness

❖ *Fifteen millimeters* or more of pyloric canal length

❖ *Failure of the channel to open* during 15 minutes of ultrasonogram scanning

❖ *Gastric emptying* delayed

❖ Gastric distension with fluid

❖ Hyperperistaltic contractions

❖ High intestinal obstruction

❖ *Kirklin sign or mushroom sign or umbrella sign:* The thickened muscle can indent the base of the duodenal bulb resulting in mushroom sign

❖ Olive pit sign—impression of the pyloric muscle on the antrum with a tiny barium seen on the orifice.

**Retrograde contractions:**

❖ *Shoulder sign:* The barium will outline the external thickened muscle, which bulges into the antrum and causes defect in the antrum

❖ *String sign or mouse tail*—typical elongation and narrowing of pyloric canal (length 2-4 cm). *String sign*, fine, narrowed, and elongated pyloric canal, is seen in hypertrophic pyloric stenosis. In barium meal study, the elongated pyloric canal will be seen as a single line of barium. Sometimes,

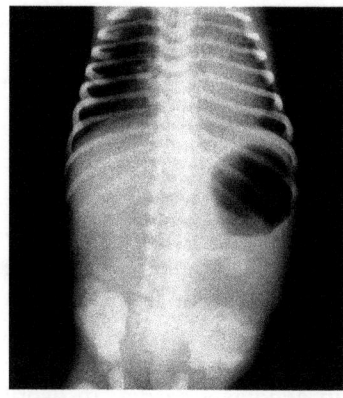

**Fig. 3.98:** Absence of air beyond stomach single bubble sign.

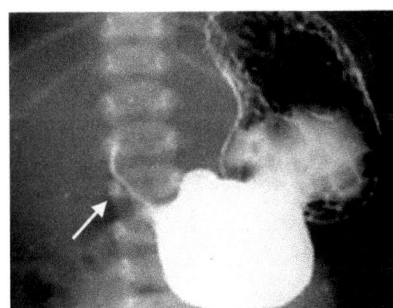

**Fig. 3.99:** Pyloric stenosis string sign.

it will be seen as a double line (Figs. 3.98 and 3.99)
* *Shoulder sign:* The hypertrophied pyloric muscle will cause an indentation of the barium-filled antrum in patients with hypertrophic pyloric stenosis
* *Target sign*—transverse ultrasonographic image and thick pylorus in the ultrasonogram in pyloric stenosis.

Abdominal ultrasonogram shows large thick pyloric mass with narrow pyloric canal. Longitudinal ultrasonogram of the pylorus will show thickened, circular mass, elongated pylorus, and narrowed pyloric channel. Transverse ultrasonographic image will show target sign and heterogeneous echo texture of the muscular layer. The sensitivity and specificity of ultrasonogram in diagnosing idiopathic hypertrophic pyloric stenosis (IHPS) is nearly 100%.

**Differential diagnosis:**

* Infantile pylorospasm
* Duodenal obstruction from midgut volvulus.

## QUESTIONS

**Q1. What are the risk factors associated with hypertrophic pyloric stenosis (HPS) (Mnemonic A-I)?**
- Age of mother—younger less than 20 years
- Boys
- Bottle fed babies
- Cesarean delivered babies
- Cigarette smoking by mother
- Caucasians of north European ancestry (less common in African-Americans and Asians)
- Drug abuse—alcohol addiction
- Drugs to antenatal mothers or babies—macrolide antibiotics erythromycin is a motilin agonist causing continuous contraction of pyloric muscle
- Environmental factors
- First born babies
- Genetic
- History of IHPS in family
- Infections—viral infections
- Immature or preterm baby.

**Q2. What is the typical finding of abdominal palpation?**
Palpable pyloric lump can be felt in the pyloric region just lateral to the rectus muscle (olive-shaped mass, smooth, and firm, when palpation is done in a baby with relaxed abdomen with empty stomach).

**Q3. What is the diagnostic triad of HPS (Mnemonic PPP)?**
- Peristalsis—visible gastric peristalsis
- Projectile vomiting
- Palpable pyloric mass.

**Q4. What are the features of HPS (Mnemonic PPPPP)?**
- Puny infant
- Projectile persistent vomiting
- Peristalsis visible
- Palpable pyloric mass
- Pyloric canal stenosis.

**Q5. What is the age of onset of IHPS and presentation?**
This is usually not present at birth. The symptoms usually appear in the early weeks of life, usually by 2–3 weeks of life.

It rarely presents in the first week of life. Its presentation in the preterm babies will be delayed.

**Q6. What are the features of IHPS? (Mnemonic A–P)**
- **A**ge of onset of symptoms after 2–3 weeks of life
- **A**lert
- **B**elching
- **C**onstipation
- **D**ehydrated
- **E**pigastric fullness
- **F**at will be lost
- **G**astric peristalsis will be visible
- **G**ain in weight will be poor
- **H**ungry
- **I**nterval between feed and emesis about 30 minutes
- **J**aundice may be present
- **K**$^+$ loss in urine due to hyperaldosteronism (hypokalemia)
- **L**ump in the pyloric region will be palpable
- **M**ass will be olive shaped, firm, and smooth
- **N**asogastric aspirate more than 10 mL with clear gastric contents
- **O**live-shaped mass
- **P**rojectile nonbilious and vomiting.

**Q7. What is the cause of jaundice in a child with HPS?**
Hyperbilirubinemia may be seen due to increased enterohepatic circulation.

**Q8. What is the surgical management for HPS?**
- Ramstedt's pyloromyotomy—treatment of choice
- An incision is made longitudinally over the entire length of the pylorus. Take care that only the muscles are incised and the mucosa should be left intact
- Balloon dilatation of the pyloric canal can be done
- Double-Y pyloromyotomy.

**Q9. What is the risk for the babies when the parents had this disorder?**
Father having this condition:

| Daughter | 1 in 10 |
|---|---|
| Son | 1 in 20 |

Mother having this condition during her infancy:

| Son | 1 in 5 |
|---|---|

**Q10. What are the complications of HPS (Mnemonic A–J)?**
- **A**lkalosis (metabolic) due to potassium depletion
- **B**leeding due to stomach irritation
- **C**hloride loss due to vomiting
- **D**ehydration
- **E**lectrolyte imbalance—hypokalemia
- **F**ailure to thrive—growth retardation
- **G**astritis
- **H**ypokalemic and hypochloremic metabolic alkalosis with compensatory respiratory acidosis
- **I**ntraoperative complications
- **J**aundice.

## Small Bowel Atresia

### Duodenal Atresia

- It usually occurs distal to the ampulla of Vater. This is the most common cause of congenital duodenal obstruction.
- *Double bubble sign*—two air-filled will be seen in the X-ray abdomen or abdominal ultrasound. First bubble is due to air in the distended stomach. The second bubble is due to air in the dilated proximal duodenum. There will be no gas distal to the obstruction.
- It is due to failure of recanalization of the duodenum, which occurs by 8–11 weeks of gestation.

**Differential diagnosis:**
- Duodenal atresia (Fig. 3.100)
- Duodenal web

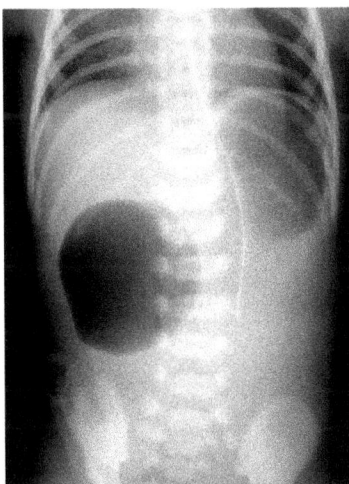

**Fig. 3.100:** Double bubble sign—duodenal atresia.

- Annular pancreas
- Midgut volvulus
- Ladd's bands are folds of peritoneum crossing anterior to the duodenum and obstructing it.

(1) Erect abdominal X-ray of a newborn infant showing obstructed upper small bowel loops with fluid levels. No air is visible in the distal bowel. (2) Contrast enema showing the unused or microcolon distal to a jejunoileal atresia. In addition, evidence of malrotation is present.

(a) Abdominal erect X-ray showing grossly distended stomach and duodenum with double bubble sign with no air beyond the duodenum. DB, (duodenal bubble); GB (gastric bubble). (b) Abdominal X-ray showing the double bubble sign. In this case, duodenal bulb is more prominent than the gastric bulb. At operation duodenal membrane was found and excised. DB, (duodenal bubble); GB (gastric bubble). (c) Duodenal atresia evident on upper gastrointestinal X-ray contrast study. D duodenum; S stomach.

Duodenal stenosis erect abdominal X-ray demonstrating.

A double bubble sign with air beyond the duodenum.

## QUESTIONS

**Q1. What are the conditions in which distal gas will be present?**

Distal gas will be seen in the following conditions:
- Duodenal web
- Annular pancreas
- Midgut volvulus.

**Q2. What are the radiological findings in duodenal atresia?**

Plain X-ray abdomen will show double bubble sign.

**Q3. What are the clinical features of duodenal atresia?**
- Vomiting
- Visible gastric peristalsis.

**Q4. What are the conditions associated with duodenal atresia?**

Increased incidence of the following:
- Anorectal anomalies (imperforate anus)
- Biliary atresia
- Bowel (small) atresia
- Cardiac anomalies
- Down syndrome 30–40%
- Esophageal atresia
- VACTERL anomalies

**Q5. What antenatal finding is seen in congenital duodenal atresia?**
- Antenatal—polyhydramnios
- Double bubble sign will be seen in the antenatal ultrasonogram.

**Q6. What is the treatment for duodenal atresia?**
- Kimura's duodenoduodenostomy
- Duodenojejunostomy.

### Jejunal Atresia

- Radiological findings:
- 2–3 dilated bowel loops
- Absence of gas in the lower part of the abdomen
- Triple bubble sign (Fig. 3.101)
- Barium enema may show microcolon (Fig. 3.102).

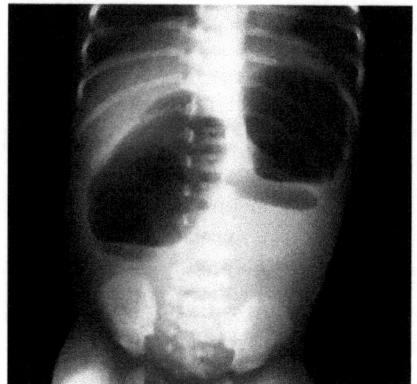

**Fig. 3.101:** X-ray jejunal atresia showing triple bubble sign.

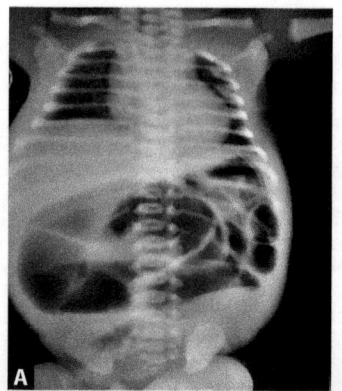

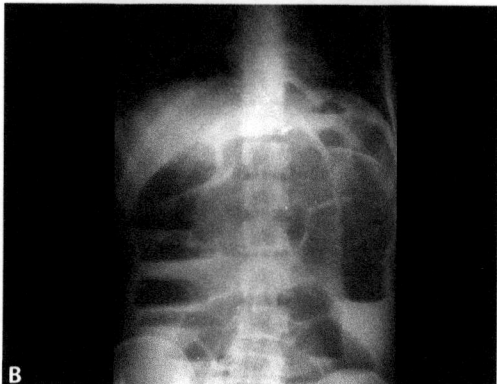

**Figs. 3.103A and B:** Intestinal atresia and intestinal obstruction (rectal gas absent).

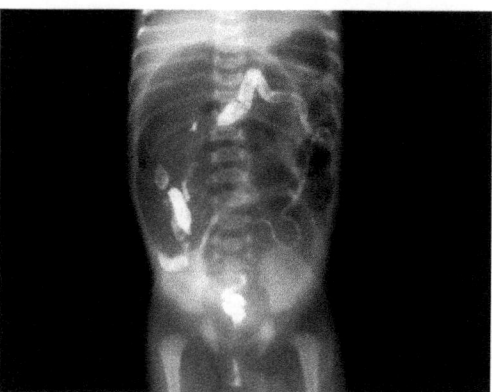

**Fig. 3.102:** X-ray barium enema showing microcolon.

## Intestinal Atresia

### Ileal atresia:

Radiological findings:
- Air fluid levels
- Air in the distended bowel loops proximal to the obstruction
- "Candy cane" appearance in erect position
- Disproportionate gaseous or fluid distension of small bowel in relation to colon
- Enema—microcolon due to lack of succus entericus from above
- Fluid-filled loops
- Gas fluid levels more than 2.5 cm wide, differing more than 2 cm in height from one another within the same bowel loop
- Hyperperistalsis or aperistalsis
- Absence of air beyond the level of obstruction (Figs. 3.103A and B).

## QUESTIONS

**Q1. What is the antenatal condition associated with ileal atresia?**
Polyhydramnios.

**Q2. What is the cause for string of beads appearance?**
String of beads appearance is due to peristalsis.

**Q3. What is the condition associated with stepladder pattern?**
Distal atresia will be associated with stepladder pattern.

**Q4. What is the radiological finding in intestinal atresia?**
Triple bubble sign.

## Intestinal Obstruction

- Plain X-ray in supine position dilated bowel with jejuna or ileal pattern proximal to the level of obstruction
- Prone translateral views will show absence of rectal gas shadow. However, in subacute obstruction, the rectal gas shadow may not be absent
- During the early stage of obstruction, the dilated bowel will try to overcome the obstruction and will produce pile of coins appearance of dilated jejunum
- Also a characterless tube like appearance of the dilated ileum can be seen. The bowel shadow distal to the obstruction will be present (Figs. 3.104A and B)
- Plain X-ray supine an prone translateral view before per rectal examination
- Presacral space is empty and devoid of any air shadow
- Distal jejunal or ileal obstruction would result in multiple, asymmetric centrally placed fluid levels often of different sizes
- The biggest shadow is just proximal to the site of obstruction
- Stepladder pattern may be seen.

## QUESTIONS

**Q1. How will you differentiate between intestinal obstruction and paralytic ileus?**
- In intestinal obstruction, prone translateral views will show absence of rectal gas shadow
- In paralytic ileus, there wail be uniform distension of abdomen
- X-ray abdomen in supine position will show uniformly dilated stomach and intestines
- X-ray prone translateral view will show presence of rectal gas shadow.

| Features | Intestinal obstruction | Paralytic ileus |
|---|---|---|
| X-ray abdomen supine view | Dilated stomach and intestines proximal to obstruction | Uniform distension of abdomen |
| X-ray prone translateral view | Rectal gas shadow | Rectal gas shadow |

**Q2. What are the clinical features of acute intestinal obstruction?**
- H/O bilious vomiting
- H/O obstipation.

Abdominal examination:
- Abdominal distension
- Visible intestinal peristalsis
- Per rectal examination—empty rectum.

**Q3. What are the radiological features of acute intestinal obstruction?**
- Plain X-ray in supine position will show dilated bowel with jejunal or

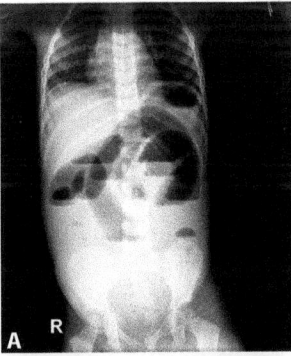

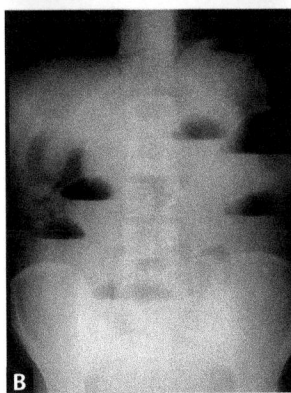

**Figs. 3.104A and B:** Intestinal obstruction multiple fluid levels.

ileal patterns proximal to the level of obstruction
- Prone translateral view will show absence of rectal gas shadow.

**Q4. How will you differentiate between acute and subacute intestinal obstruction?**

In acute intestinal obstruction, the bowel shadow distal to obstruction will be absent but in subacute intestinal obstruction, the bowel shadow distal to obstruction may be present.

**Q5. What are the clinical features of subacute intestinal obstruction?**
- Recurrent bilious vomiting
- Visible loops
- Visible intestinal peristalsis.

**Q6. What are the radiological features of subacute intestinal obstruction?**
- Plain X-ray in supine position—bowel shadow distal to the level of obstruction may not be absent.
- Prone translateral view—rectal gas shadow may not be present.

## Necrotizing Enterocolitis Pneumatosis Cystoides Intestinalis

### Radiological investigations in necrotizing enterocolitis (NEC):

*X-ray abdomen (Mnemonic A-I):* Supine (anteroposterior) or lateral decubitus view should be taken every 6 hours for babies with abdominal signs. The abdominal X-ray will show abnormal gas pattern and dilated bowel loops.
- Air shadows increased
- Ascites
- Air along the portal tracts (Fig. 3.105)
- Bowel wall edema
- Cystic bubbly pattern of intramural gas between mucosa and submucosa
- Curved linear radiolucent shadow in the walls of intestinal loops (pneumatosis intestinalis)
- Dilated bowel loops
- Edema bowel wall (thickening)
- Fixed loop sign—dilated fixed loops of intestine which do not change in size,

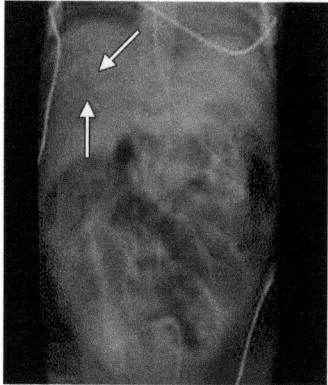

**Fig. 3.105:** Portal vein gas shadow.

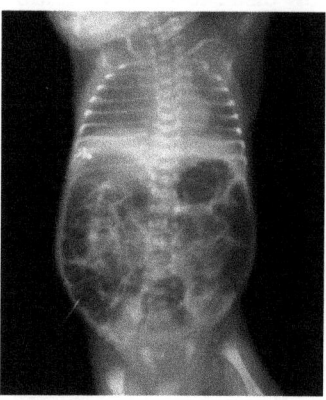

**Fig. 3.106:** Necrotizing enterocolitis with fixed ascending colon loop.

shape, and position on serial radiographs, which will indicate gangrenous part (Fig. 3.106)
- Football sign (Fig. 3.107)
- Falciparum ligament sign (Fig. 3.108)
- Gas pattern in the abdomen—abnormal
- Hypodense branching areas over the liver shadow. Gas in the portal venous system (portal gas)
- Intraperitoneal air (pneumoperitoneum) (Fig. 3.109)
- Ileus
- Intramural gas seen as train translucency and linear pattern (pneumatosis intestinalis) (Fig. 3.110)
- Intestinal perforation.

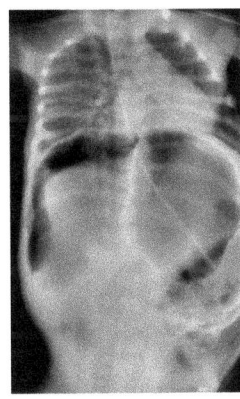

**Fig. 3.107:** X-ray of football sign.

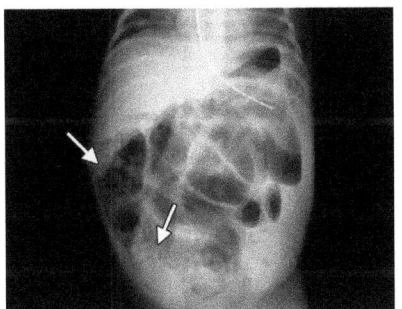

**Fig. 3.110:** X-ray of pneumatosis intestinalis.

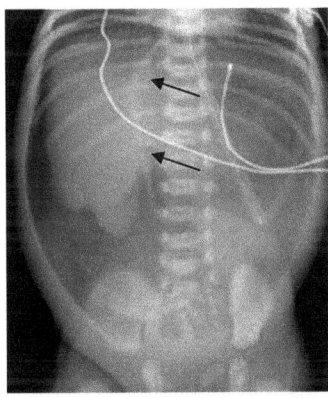

**Fig. 3.108:** X-ray of falciparum ligament sign.

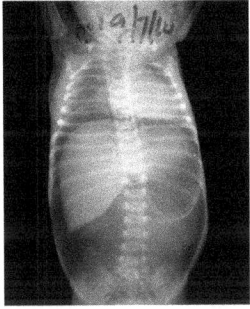

**Fig. 3.111:** X-ray of pneumoperitoneum.

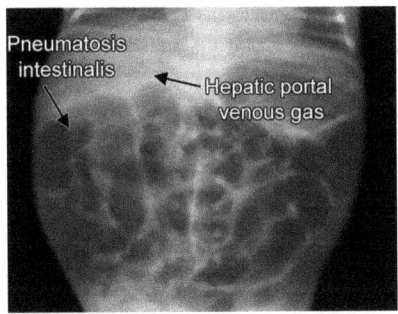

**Fig. 3.109:** X-ray of free gas in portal vein.

## Pneumoperitoneum (Fig. 3.111)

Terminal ileum is commonly affected.

- *Football sign:* If pneumoperitoneum is present. The free air over the liver with outlining of the falciform ligament. This is an indication of perforation and needs surgical treatment.
  - Air in the abdomen due to perforation—left lateral decubitus
  - Gas in the portal venous system.
- *Rigler's sign or double wall sign*—bowel wall is outlined by extra luminal air due to pneumoperitoneum and intraluminal air
- *Doge's cap sign*—presence of air in the Morrison's pouch, a potential space between right kidney and liver seen as triangular radiolucency with base down and apex facing upward.
- *Champagne flute sign*—due to portal air:
  - Dilated loops of intestine, fixed loops, and pneumoperitoneum
  - Pneumatosis cystoides intestinalis
  - Free gas in portal vein.
- *First sign:* Normal mosaic pattern will be lost followed by dilatation of some loops (Fig. 3.112).

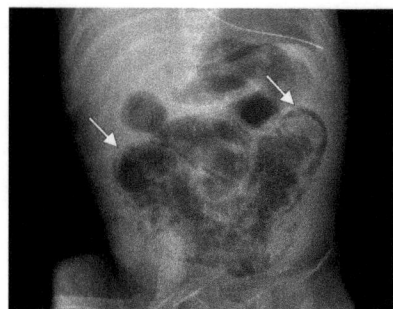

**Fig. 3.112:** Pneumatosis cystoides intestinalis.

Cross table abdominal X-ray intestinal bowel occlusion with air fluid levels in the distended loops.

**Discussion:**

- Age of onset rarely before 3 days of life
- Preterm 28–32 weeks will develop between 28 weeks to 32 weeks of life
- Lower the gestational age later will be the onset of NEC
- *Abdominal ultrasonogram*—ascites will be seen in the later stages in babies with perforation
- *Barium meal study* can be done to rule out volvulus and Hirschsprung's disease
- *Doppler study* may show an increased peak flow velocity in the celiac and superior mesenteric arteries
- *Magnetic resonance imaging* can be used, if available. This will pick up the intestinal necrosis.

# QUESTIONS

**Q1. What is the age of onset of NEC?**
The age of onset of NEC is related to the postconceptional age. The age of onset varies inversely with age of gestation. Term babies may develop NEC on the first day of life and the extreme preterm babies develop NEC few weeks after birth. Thus, the preterm babies develop NEC several weeks after birth.

**Q2. What is diving reflex?**
In birth asphyxia, the blood supply will be diverted toward the vital organs like brain. This will result in decreased blood supply to the gastrointestinal tract, which will predispose to NEC.

**Q3. What are the risk factors for NEC?**
Risk factors for NEC are:
- Anemia
- Apgar low (5-minute APGAR below 7)
- Birth asphyxia
- Birth weight—babies less than 1,000 g are at highest risk for NEC
- Catheterization (umbilical artery or vein)
- Cyanotic heart disease
- Congenital cardiac disorders—patent ductus arteriosus
- Drugs—infants exposed to cocaine
- Early feeds or prelacteal feeds
- Formula feeds
- Gut ischemia
- Gestational age—babies less than 28 weeks are at highest risk for NEC
- Hyperosmolar feeds
- Hypotension
- Hypoxia
- Hyaline membrane disease
- Infections or sepsis
- Polycythemia
- Prematurity
- Rapid advancement of feeds
- Shock
- Thrombocytosis
- Thrombocytopenia
- Antenatal period:
  - Antenatal hemorrhage
  - Prolonged rupture of membranes beyond 36 hours.

**Q4. When to suspect NEC?**
The NEC should be suspected in the presence of any of the following particularly in high-risk babies:
- Apnea
- Activity decreased or sluggish
- Bowel sounds absent or decreased
- Blood in stools
- Color—pallor
- Distension of abdomen
- Emesis (bilious)

- Erythema over the abdominal wall, especially around the umbilicus
- Fever
- Gastric residual increased
- Heart rate decreased
- Localized mass in the abdomen.

**Q5. What are the complications of NEC?**
- Fistula formation
- Failure to thrive
- Gangrene of Bowel
- Short bowel syndrome
- Intestinal Perforation
- Malabsorption syndrome
- Pneumoperitoneum
- Stricture formation.

**Q6. What are the preventive steps for NEC?**
- Antenatal steroids
  - Aminoglycosides (oral)
- Acidic pH in the stomach (avoid H1 blockers):
  - Breast milk feeding
  - Avoid preterm deliveries
  - Avoid hyperosmolar feeds.
- Advancement of feeds should be slow about 10 mL/kg/day:
  - *Advance of feeds*: Stimulation of gut with minimal or trophic feeding to prime the gastrointestinal tract has decreased the incidence of NEC.

**Q7. What are the patterns of intramural gas?**
There are two patterns of intramural gas:
1. Cystic or bubbly pattern due to presence of air in the mucosal or submucosal areas
2. Liner or curvilinear thin radiolucent lines due to presence of air between tunica mucosa and subserosa.

**Q8. What is circle sign in ultrasonogram?**
Presence of intramural gas seen in ultrasonogram.

**Q9. What is the modified Bell's staging?**
*Modified Bell's staging criteria for NEC:*

| Stage | Clinical diagnosis | | Abdominal signs | Systemic signs | Radiological signs |
|---|---|---|---|---|---|
| I | Suspected NEC | A | Abdominal distension, vomiting, and blood in stools | Apnea, bradycardia, and temperature instability | Normal or dilatation of intestines, mild ileus, and mild abdominal distension |
| | | B | Abdominal distension and frank or gross blood in the stools | Apnea, bradycardia, and temperature instability | Normal or dilatation of intestines, ileus, and mild abdominal distension |
| II | Proven or definite NEC | A—mildly ill | IIB features plus: Absent bowel sound and intestinal dilatation | IIB features plus: Temperature instability | Ileus or pneumatosis intestinalis or ascites |
| | | B—moderately ill | IIA features plus: Absent bowel sound, definite abdominal tenderness, abdominal cellulitis, and right lower quadrant mass | IIA features plus: Metabolic acidosis and temperature instability, thrombocytopenia | Portal vein gas with or without ascites |
| III | Advanced NEC | A—Severely ill Bowel intact | IIB features plus: Generalized peritonitis abdominal distension and erythema + tenderness | IIB features plus: Hypotension and acidosis | Same as II plus portal vein gas with or without Ascites + free air |
| | | B—Severely ill bowel perforated | IIIA features plus | IIIA features plus | |
| IV | Severely ill | | Peritonitis + tenderness | Disseminated intravascular coagulation | Portal venous gas plus pneumoperitoneum |

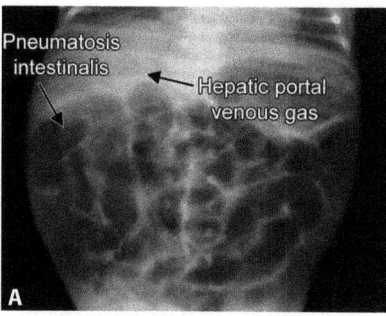 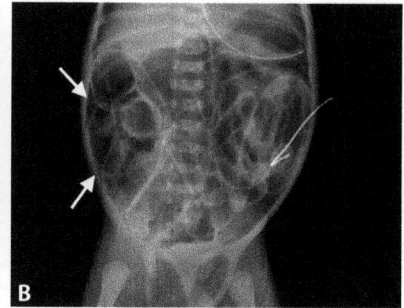

**Figs. 3.113A and B:** Free gas in portal vein and triangular sign.

## *Intestinal Perforation (Figs. 3.113A and B)*

### Radiological findings:
- X-ray will show pneumoperitoneum
- Air under the diaphragm.
- Crescent under the diaphragm (in erect X-ray abdomen).

### Discussion
- The clinical features of perforation will depend upon the location of perforation
- The perforation in the upper GIT will be associated with severe generalized pain whereas the lower GIT will be associated with gradual and localized pain.

## QUESTIONS

**Q1. What are the clinical features of intestinal perforation?**
- ❏ Abdominal distension
- ❏ Clinical features of pneumoperitoneum
- ❏ Obliteration of liver dullness
- ❏ Hematemesis
- ❏ Bilious vomiting.

**Q2. What is the treatment of intestinal perforation?**
Early surgery should be done.

## *Pneumoperitoneum*
- Gas within the peritoneal cavity
- Subdiaphragmatic gas
- Triangular collection of air in the Morison pouch.

The liver shadow will be more lucent than the cardiac shadow. In few cases, opacification of the falciparum ligament will be seen as a bright, thin, and vertical line over the spine. This is football sign.

### Signs of pneumoperitoneum:
- *Continuous diaphragm sign*—due to presence of air, the whole diaphragm is visible as thin radiopaque strip. In massive pneumoperitoneum, the entire diaphragm will be visible as thin radiopaque strip due to air above in the lungs and below (Fig. 3.114)
- *Sign of dome*—due to presence of air, which is radiolucent in correspondence to the tendon at the center of the diaphragm, which is raised and appears like a dome (Fig. 3.115)
- *Doge's cap sign* is due to presence of free air in Morrison's pouch a potential space between right kidney and the liver. The air shadow will be triangular with the base down and apex upward like the hat of an ancient Venetian Doge.

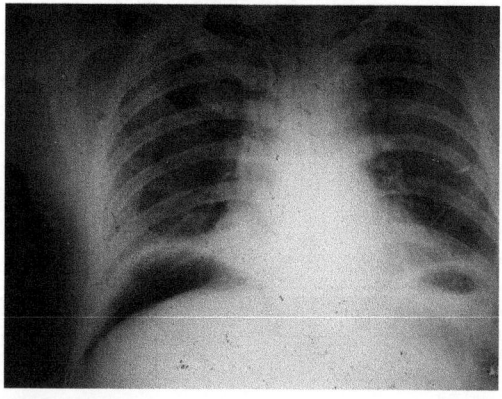

**Fig. 3.114:** Pneumoperitoneum air under diaphragm.

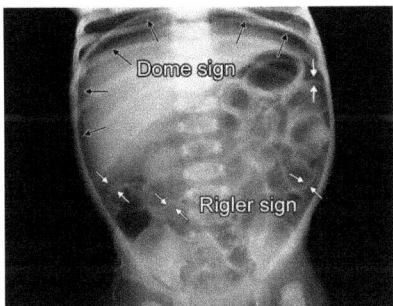

**Fig. 3.115:** X-ray of sign of dome.

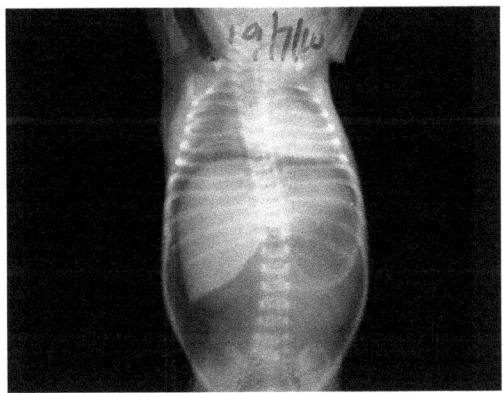

**Fig. 3.117:** Free gas in peritoneum.

- ❖ *Rigler's sign or double-wall sign*—on supine radiograph air can be visualized in the peritoneal cavity. The bowel wall will be outlined by intraluminal and extraluminal air. Both sides of the bowel wall will be visualized (Figs. 3.116A to C).
- ❖ *Radiological signs:* Gas present inside the lumen of the bowel and pneumoperitoneum. Free air presents outside the lumen will result in various signs, which will be helpful in diagnosis of pneumoperitoneum.
- ❖ *Bowel related signs*
  - *Double wall sign or Rigler sign or Gas relief sign*: Gas outlines both sides of the bowel wall with bowel gas lining inside and free gas outlining the outer surface of the bowel (Fig. 3.117)
    - *Triangle sign*—radiolucent triangle of gas is formed in between three loops of bowel or between two loops of bowel and the abdominal wall (*See* Fig. 3.114).
- ❖ *Peritoneal ligament related signs* (falciparum ligament will connect anterior abdominal wall to the liver) (Figs. 3.118A and B):
  - *Football sign* is seen in massive pneumoperitoneum. Abdominal cavity is outlined by gas with air surrounding the falciparum ligament, which looks like laces of football. *Football sign (See* Fig. 3.107)—oval radiolucent shadow running superior—inferiorly. The oval edges are formed by the diaphragm above and pelvic floor below. This is due to distension of peritoneal cavity by air in large pneumoperitoneum (Figs. 3.119A and B).
  - *Falciparum ligament sign or Silver sign,* the falciparum will be outlined by gas (*See* Fig. 3.108)
  - *Lateral umbilical ligament sign or Inverted V sign*—free gas outlines the lateral umbilical ligament seen as inverted V shaped in the pelvis and extends from internal iliac arteries to the umbilicus inverted V shaped (Fig. 3.120)

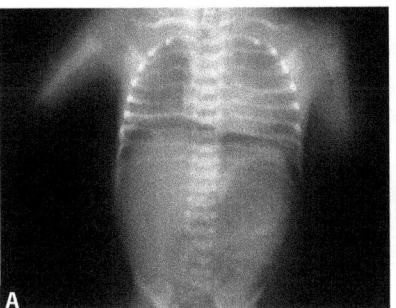
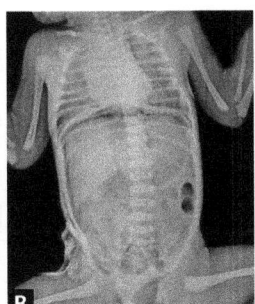
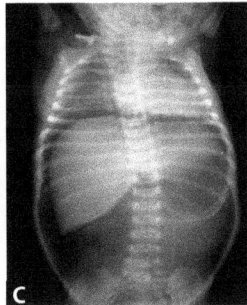

**Figs. 3.116A to C:** X-ray of pneumoperitoneum.

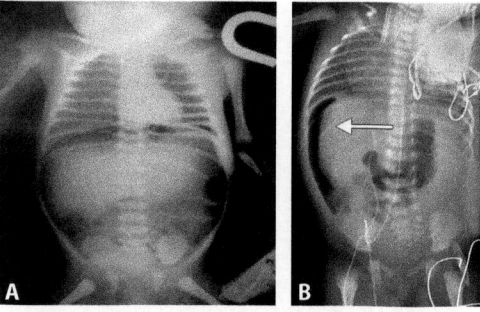

**Figs. 3.118A and B:** Saddle bag sign and decubitus film.

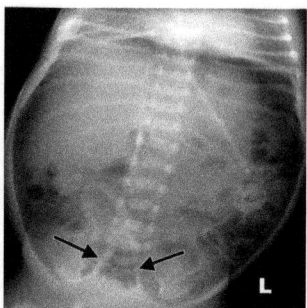

**Fig. 3.120:** X-ray of inverted V sign.

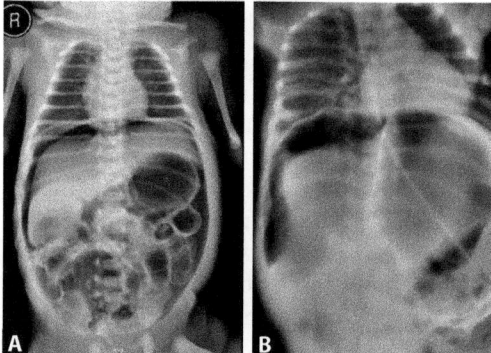

**Figs. 119A and B:** Pneumoperitoneum football sign.

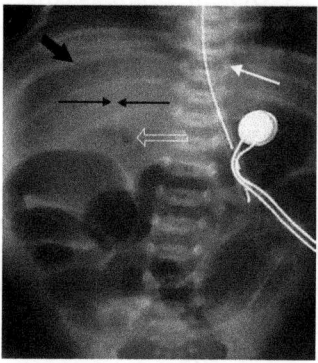

**Fig. 3.121:** X-ray of cupola sign.

- *Urachus sign* median umbilical cord extends from the urinary bladder to the umbilicus.
- ❖ *Right upper quadrant sings:*
  - *Cupola sign:* Cupola sign will be seen on supine film gas accumulates under the diaphragm in the midline. Lucency will be seen overlying the lower thoracic vertebral bodies. Superior border will be well defined and the inferior margin is not well defined (Fig. 3.121).

## Discussion

The following conditions will be associated with pneumoperitoneum:
- ❖ Interruption of walls of hollow viscus
  - Trauma
  - Iatrogenic
  - Perforation of gastric or duodenal ulcer
  - Perforation of appendix
  - Ruptured diverticulum (Meckel or sigmoid or jejunal diverticulum)
  - Necrotizing enterocolitis with perforation
  - Inflammatory bowel disease (toxic megacolon).
- ❖ Through peritoneal surface
  - Transperitoneal manipulation
  - Endoscopic procedures
  - Penetration abdominal injuries.
- ❖ Intraperitoneal
  - Peritonitis with gas forming organisms
  - Ruptured abscess.
- ❖ Genital problems in females
  - Iatrogenic—culdocentesis and perforation of vagina or uterus
  - Spontaneous—Knee chest exercise and sports.

## QUESTIONS

**Q1. What is pseudopneumoperitoneum?**
Gas in the chest or fat may mimic pneumoperitoneum.

## Q2. What are the causes of spontaneous pneumoperitoneum?
- ❑ Perforation of peptic ulcer
- ❑ Bowel obstruction
- ❑ Bowel ischemia
- ❑ Toxic megacolon
- ❑ Inflammation (appendicitis, NNEC, and tuberculosis).

## Intussusception
### Radiological features of intussusception:
X-ray abdomen will show a soft tissue mass with bowel obstruction (Mnemonic A—G)
- ❖ Air fluid levels (multiple) due to bowel obstruction
- ❖ Bowel dilatation—distension of small bowel
- ❖ Collapsed bowel (absence of gas) distal to intussusception
- ❖ Distal bowel pseudoobstruction
- ❖ Elongated soft tissue mass
- ❖ Fluid levels in upright view
- ❖ Gas under diaphragm (if perforation occurs). X-ray abdomen may show signs of intestinal obstruction.

### Radiological signs of intussusception (Fig. 3.122):
- ❖ *Absent liver edge sign*—absence of subhepatic angle
- ❖ *"Bowel in bowel sign" or "sandwich sign"* (in CT scan or ultrasound)—in longitudinal scan inner and outer hypoechoic shadows will be seen
- ❖ *Bull's eye of coiled-spring sign*: Bull's eye of coiled-spring lesion in barium contrast enema
- ❖ *Claw sign or spring sign*—concave filling defect in barium enema barium will outline the rounded head of the leading end
- ❖ *Colon cut off sign*—abrupt cut off of intestinal or colonic gas with a convex shadow inside the transverse colon seen in barium enema
- ❖ *Crescent sign*—plain X-ray shows the lead point of intussusceptum will protrude into the gas-filed pocket.
- ❖ *Dance sign*—clinical examination shows an abdominal mass in right upper quadrant of abdomen and empty right lower quadrant
- ❖ *Doughnut sign or target sign (plain X-ray abdomen or ultrasonogram):* Target sign of tissue mass in right upper quadrant of abdomen causing concentric circular lucency due to mesenteric fat of the intussusceptions
- ❖ *Meniscus sign*—crescent gas within the colonic lumen that outlines the intussusceptions
- ❖ *Pseudokidney sign* (on ultrasonogram)
- ❖ *Barium enema:*
  - Pitch fork sign in barium enema
  - Coiled spring deformity
  - Colon cut off sign—with a convex shadow inside the transverse colon
  - Barium enema will be diagnostic and therapeutic in early stages.

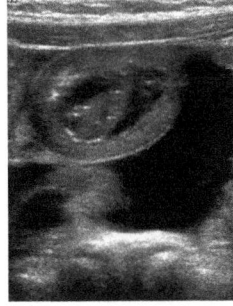

**Fig. 3.122:** Ultrasound finding in intussusception.

## QUESTIONS

**Q1. What is intussusception?**
- ❑ Intussusception is telescoping of one part of the intestine into the other distal to it
- ❑ This is usually seen in healthy infants less than 1 year of age but it is rare in neonates
- ❑ Males are affected more than females.

**Q2. What is the most common site for intussusception?**

The most common site is ileocecal region just proximal to the ileocecal valve.

**Q3. What is the pathogenesis of intussusception?**
The Peyer's patch may get hypertrophied due to a change in bacterial flora accompanied by weaning of feeds or introduction of other feeds. The hypertrophied Peyer's patch may predispose to a loop of intestine invaginating in to the distal loop of intestine. The hypertrophied Peyer's patch will act as a leading point the part of the intestine that is invaginating into the distal loop is known as intussusception. The part of intestine into which invagination occurs is known as intussuscipiens there will be venous congestion resulting in bloody mucus secretion. In some cases, there will be vascular compromise resulting in gangrene.

**Q4. What are the clinical features of intussusception?**
Mnemonic A B C D E
- Abdominal pain
- Banana-shaped mass can be palpated.
- Colicky pain and paroxysmal pain
- Currant jelly stools (red)
- Distension of abdomen
- Emesis—bilious vomiting.
- Infant awakes from sleep due to violent abdominal colic, flexes the thigh, vomits, and then passes stools
- Initially, the infant passes normal stools and the passes blood and mucus.

**Q5. What is the finding in abdominal examination in a child with intussusception?**
Typical banana-shaped mass can be palpated. The concavity will be toward the umbilicus.

**Q6. What are the investigations to be done in intussusception?**
- Ultrasonogram
- X-ray abdomen—X-ray abdomen may show signs of intestinal obstruction.

**Q7. What is the classical triad of intussusception?**
- Abdominal colicky pain
- Bilious vomiting
- Currant jelly stools—passing of blood and mucus (red currant jelly) without stool.

**Q8. How will you treat intussusception?**
- Pneumatic reduction—pushing air will push back the invaginated mass of intestine
- Hydrostatic reduction—pushing water per rectally will push back the invaginated mass of intestine
- Barium enema will push back the invaginated mass of intestine. If the barium fills freely, it is an indication of complete reduction. Reduction using barium or saline is indicated in the following cases:
  - Early stages
  - Within 24 hours of the onset
  - No signs of intestinal obstruction.
- Surgical correction—if the intussusception is not reduced by conservative methods, surgical reduction should be done.
  - If there is no evidence of gangrene manual reduction can be done
  - If there is gangrene resection of the entire intussuscepted mass should be done.

**Q9. What are the indications for surgery?**
- Irreducible—intussusception
- Ischemic—intussusception
- To remove the lead points for intussusception like polyps, duplications, and Meckel's diverticulum.

**Q10. What is the prognosis of intussusception?**
- Prenatal intussusception may be a cause for intestinal atresia:
  - 10% recurrence after barium enema reduction
  - 2-5% recurrence after surgical reduction.

- Mortality is seen in delayed diagnosis, septic shock, perforation, and recurrence.

## Peritonitis—Paralytic Ileus

### Radiological findings in paralytic ileus:
- Plain X-ray abdomen—uniformly dilated stomach and intestines
- Prone translateral view will show presence of rectal air shadow.

## QUESTIONS

**Q1. What are the types of peritonitis?**
Primary and perforative peritonitis.

**Q2. What are the radiological findings in perforative peritonitis?**
- Air under the diaphragm
- Ground glass appearance.

**Q3. What are the radiological findings in perforative peritonitis in plain X-ray supine view?**
- Gas under the diaphragm
- Football sign.

**Q4. What are the clinical features of peritonitis?**
*History of:*
- Abdominal pain
- Vomiting

*Examination:*
- Poor general condition
- Tenderness
- Guarding or rigidity
- Shifting dullness
- Positive peritoneal tap.

**Q5. What is the diagnostic test?**
Peritoneal tap will be positive for bile.

**Q6. What are the predisposing factors for primary peritonitis?**
- Nephrotic syndrome
- Ventriculoperitoneal shunt.

**Q7. What are the clinical features of paralytic ileus?**

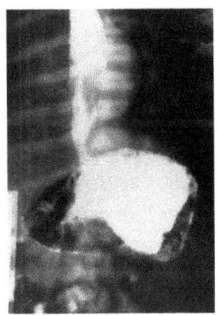

**Fig. 3.123:** Barium study confirming mesenteroaxial gastric volvulus.

The features of the causes of paralytic ileus like septicemia:
- Vomiting
- Abdominal distension
- Absent bowel sounds
- Empty rectum.

### Volvulus
- Bowel twists around its mesentery
- Torsion will result in narrowing of lumen at the point of rotation. Also the vessels will get obstructed resulting in compromise of blood supply to the gut.
  - Plain abdominal X-ray showing a distended stomach but only a single fluid level in this neonate with mesenteroaxial gastric volvulus
  - Barium study confirming mesenteroaxial gastric volvulus (Fig. 3.123).

## QUESTIONS

**Q1. What are the clinical features of volvulus (Mnemonic A-G)?**
- Abdominal pain
- Bloating
- Bloody stools
- Constipation
- Distension of abdomen
- Emesis—bilious vomiting
- Flatus not passed
- Fever (during ischemia)
- Gastrointestinal features—nausea.

*Radiological signs of volvulus:*
- *Coffee bean sign or Kidney bean sign* distinct midline crease corresponding to the mesenteric root in a largely distended loop
  - Tyre tube appearance.
- *Bent inner tube sign* air-filled closed loop of colon forming the volvulus
  - Ace of spades.

*Types of volvulus:*
- Gastric volvulus—stomach twists on its mesentery more than 180°
- Midgut volvulus
- Cecal volvulus
- Sigmoid volvulus (most common about 60%).

*Radiological signs of volvulus depend upon the type of volvulus:*
- *Gastric volvulus:*
  - Stomach upside down due to inversion of stomach, extending into the thorax (Fig. 3.124)
  - Large distended stomach (Fig. 3.125)
  - Small bowel collapsed
  - Double air fluid level (Figs. 3.126A to D).
- *Midgut volvulus:*
  - Signs of bowel obstruction
  - Occasionally double bubble sign.

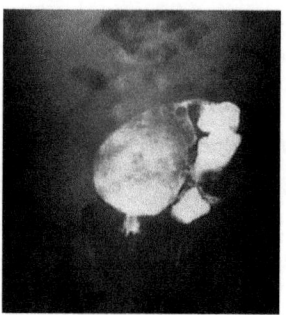

**Fig. 3.124:** Upside down or mirror image stomach indicates gastric volvulus.

- *Cecal volvulus:*
  - Distension of loop of large bowel with its long axis extending from the right lower quadrant to the epigastrium
  - If the obstruction is complete, the distal colon will be empty.
- *Sigmoid volvulus:*
  - Coffee bean sign
  - Absent rectal gas
  - Frimann-Dahl sign—three dense lines will converge toward the site of obstruction.

**Q2. What are the signs of volvulus? Mnemonic—COW.**
- **C**offee bean sign
- **O**mega sign
- **W**hirlpool sign.

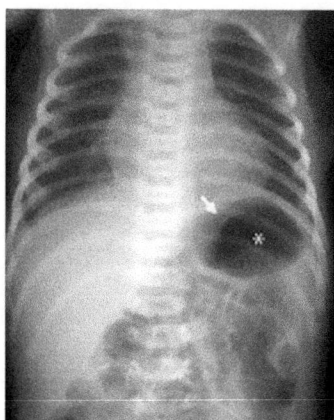 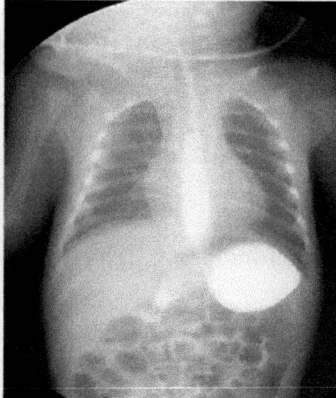 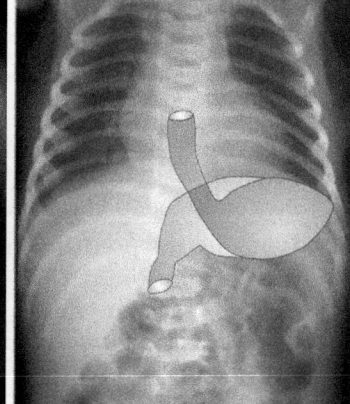

**Fig. 3.125:** Distended stomach with mesenteroaxial volvulus.

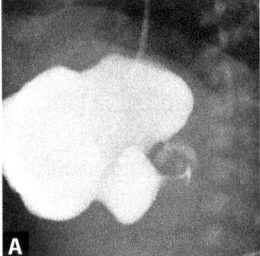 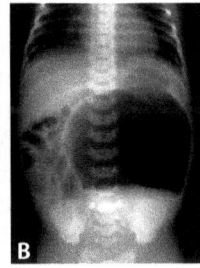 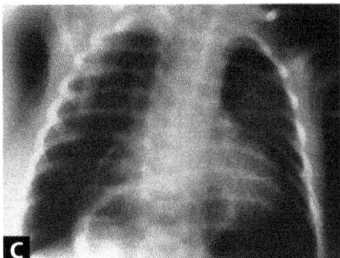 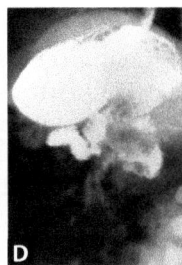

**Figs. 3.126A to D:** (A) Upside down or mirror image stomach indicates gastric volvulus; (B) Distended stomach in lateral view; (C) Air filled viscus in the chest barium study shows stomach in the chest with greater curvature lying uppermost; (D) Oblique view showing organoaxial volvulus gastric.

*Barium enema signs:*
- *Omega sign* in Barium enema—singly grossly dilated loop of colon arising out of pelvis.

## CT Scan Signs
- *Bird beak sign* is a sign of sigmoid volvulus in water-soluble contrast enema. Gradual narrowing/or tapering of sigmoid colon up to the level of obstruction tapered hook like end of barium colon at the point where the segment of proximal and distal bowel rotate. The tapering will look like a bird beak
- *Whirlpool sign* twisting of mesentery and mesenteric vessels
- *Split wall sign*—mesenteric fat will be seen indenting or invaginating the wall of the bowel.

*Gastric volvulus:*
- *Midgut volvulus*: If the mesenteric attachments do not develop properly, the mid gut will be line freely with only two attachments to the posterior abdominal wall at the duodenum and at the proximal colon. The gut can twist in either direction. The volvulus usually occurs in the clockwise direction.
  - Clinical features—the newborn may present with features of high intestinal obstruction often during the first week of life.
  - Sudden bilious vomiting with abdominal distension in a previously well newborn.
  - Complications—mesenteric vascular compromise of midgut, rapidly progressive peritonitis, sepsis, and shock
  - Investigations—X-ray abdomen—high intestinal obstruction
  - *Treatment*—laparotomy should be done and the volvulus is rotated anticlockwise. The viability of the intestines should be carefully evaluated.
  - Ladd's procedure including lysis of the peritoneal bands, appendectomy, and replacement of the bowel in a malrotated position may prevent recurrence of volvulus.

## Intestinal Malrotation
- Congenital anatomical anomaly due to abnormal rotation of the gut as the intestines return into the abdominal cavity
- Normal rotation will be for 270° counterclockwise. The mesenteric attachment will be broad
- In malrotation, the rotation will be only to 180°. The mesentery will be narrow, which predisposes to midgut volvulus
- Normally duodenum will pass from right to left and the transverse colon will overlap the duodenum
- The mesentery will run obliquely from left to right.

## Radiological findings:

- *Contrast enema findings:*
  - Abnormal position of cecum
  - Barium filled small bowel on the right side
  - Cecum will be displaced from usual right iliac fossa to right hypochondrium or epigastrium
  - Duodenojejunal flexure does not cross to the left of the midline
  - Duodenal junction lied inferior to the duodenal bulb
  - Entire duodenum lies to the right side of spine
  - Right sided jejunum.
  - 20% can have normal cecum
  - Absence of stool filled colon in the right lower quadrant of abdomen (Fig. 3.127)
  - Barium meal may show absence of "C" loop of duodenum.
- *Ultrasonogram findings:*
  - Inversion of superior mesenteric artery (SMA) or superior mesenteric vein (SMV) relationship—normally, the SMV is located on the right and anterior to the SMA. In intestinal rotation, it will be reversal of this relationship between SMA and SMV (in 60% of cases)
  - Small intestine found predominantly on the right side of the abdomen
  - Ligament of Treitz will be displaced to the right side and inferiorly
  - Whirlpool sign of mesenteric artery.

## QUESTIONS

Q1. What are the clinical features of malrotation?
- ❑ Asymptomatic throughout the life
- ❑ Abdominal mass
- ❑ Abdominal pain
- ❑ Bleeding per rectum
- ❑ Emesis—vomiting
- ❑ Gastric peristalsis visible.

Q2. What are the complications of intestinal malrotation?

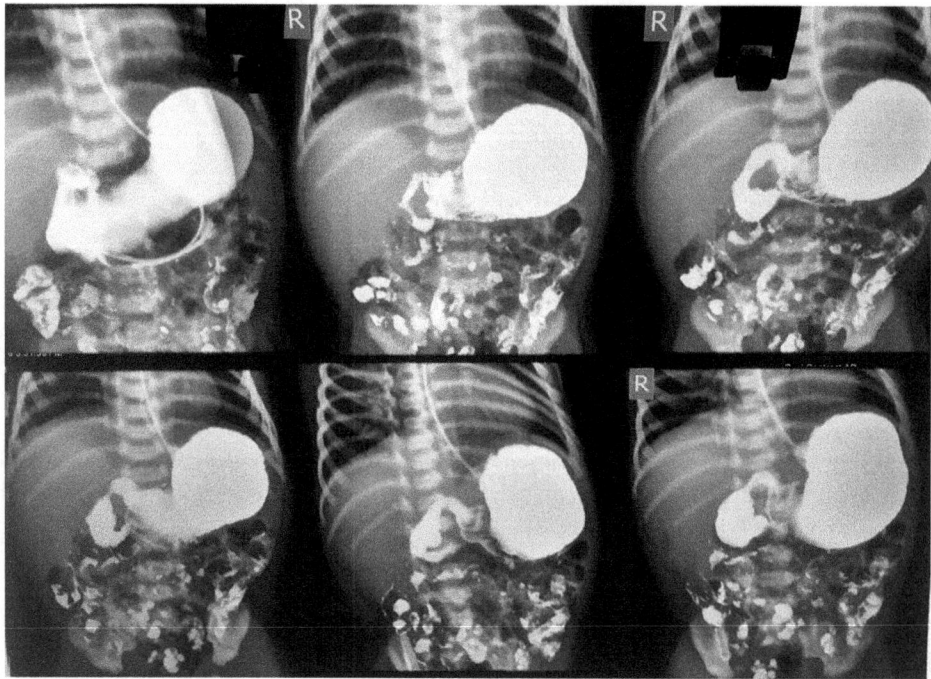

**Fig. 3.127:** X-ray of malrotation.

- Duodenal obstruction by Ladd bands
- Intestinal ischemia due to twisting of mesenteric vessels
- Volvulus—midgut volvulus acute or chronic
- Superior mesenteric artery syndrome
- Internal hernias
- Obstruction—intestinal obstruction by fibrous band of Ladd, which course over the vertical portion of duodenum.

**Q3. What are the conditions associated with intestinal malrotation?**
- Absence of kidney
- Biliary atresia
- Congenital diaphragmatic hernia (Bochdalek)
- Congenital short bowel
- Duodenal web
- Esophageal atresia
- Fistula—tracheoesophageal fistula
- Gut atresia
- Gastroschisis
- Hirschsprung disease
- Imperforate anus
- Intestinal pseudo obstruction
- Omphalocele
- Pyloric stenosis.

**Q4. What are the syndromes associated with intestinal malrotation?**
- Cornelia de Lange syndrome
- Cat eye syndrome
- Familial intestinal malrotation
- Heterotaxy (asplenia and polysplenia)
- Marfan syndrome
- Trisomy 13, 18, and 21.

## Hirschsprung's Disease (Colonic Aganglionosis or Congenital Megacolon)

- Arrest of craniocaudal migration of neural crest cells—this results in relaxation failure of aganglionic segment. Absent ganglionic cells from both the myenteric and the submucosal plexus
- Mostly involves rectosigmoid region
- Myenteric plexus (Auerbach plexus between smooth muscle layers of gastrointestinal tract
- Submucosal plexus (Meissner plexus).

**Radiological signs of Hirschsprung's disease:**
- X-ray abdomen.
- *Plain X-ray abdomen will show (mnemonic A–G):*
  - Absence of air in the rectum (gasless rectum)
  - Bowel obstruction
  - Cut off sign—in the rectosigmoid region with absence of air distally:
    - Dilatation of colon loops, large and small intestine abnormally from the transitional zone
    - Empty aganglionic segment.
  - Feces filled, enlarged sigmoid:
    - Fluid—filled loops of intestine.
  - Gas filled loops of intestine
  - Gasless colon in the newborn babies as the colon is empty (Fig. 3.128).

**Barium enema:**
- Abrupt change in caliber between the ganglionic and aganglionic segments of the bowel at the rectosigmoid's junction (visualization of rectosigmoid zone)
- Air fluid levels
- Barium evacuation delayed—marked retention of barium on delayed films.

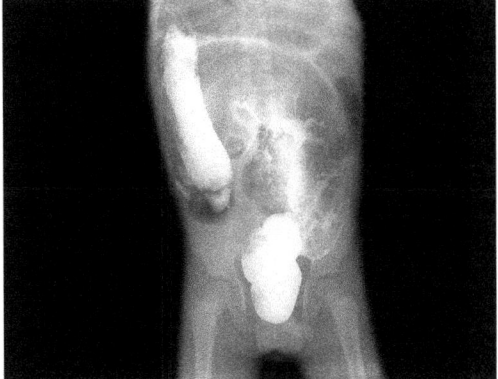

**Fig. 3.128:** Hirschsprung's disease Barium enema.

Persistence of the contrast in the rectosigmoid for more than 24 hours after the examination can occur. However, when the total colon is affected barium enema is not useful
- Cobble stone appearance
- *Cone-shaped colon or pig tail deformity* consists of a narrowed rectosigmoid segment distal to a dilated portion of the colon at the junction of the ganglionic and aganglionic segments. The typical transition zone may not become apparent until the infant is aged 3-4 weeks.
- Corrugated rectum
- Dilated sigmoid with narrow rectal segment
- Dilated descending colon
- *Duck neck sign*—narrowing of the rectosigmoid region
- Empty rectum with no gas in the rectum
- Diameter of rectum decreased and sigmoid increased
- Failure to evacuate the barium
- Ganglionic segment will be dilated
- Hypertrophy of proximal colon
- Irregular saw tooth contractions *(saw tooth appearance)* of the aganglionic bowel segment
- Inverted cone shaped at the transition zone between normal and abnormal usually at the rectosigmoid
- Jejunization of the mucosa and irregularity of mucosa
- Rectosigmoid ratio will be less than 1 (Fig. 3.129)

- *Contrast enema*, mixed barium, stool pattern of delayed radiographs.
  - Transition zone is absent in the long segment variety
  - Postevacuation films after 24 hours will show persistence of contrast in the left colon
  - Parallel transfolds in the dilated proximal colon.

Depending upon the finding of barium enema three types of findings are:
1. Compatible—cone shaped transition zone seen
2. Suggestive—questionable transition zone
3. Unremarkable—no transition zone seen.

### Differential diagnosis:
- Hypoganglionosis intestinal pseudo-obstruction
- Necrotizing enterocolitis
- Microcolon.

### Discussion—Hirschsprung's disease:
- It is also known as congenital aganglionic megacolon. Males are more commonly affected than females
- Male to female ratio is 4:1
- Relatives will be affected and the risk is more when the length of the affected segment is more
- Incidence—1 in 5,000-7,000 births
- Age of onset—the babies may present with symptoms at birth or later. The newborns may pass meconium beyond 48 hours of life. In 15 % of cases, the condition can be diagnoses in the first month of life. In majority of cases, the condition is diagnosed by 4 months of life.

### Grading of Hirschsprung's disease:
- Short segment—most common, 70-80% transitional zone at rectosigmoid region, rectum, and sigmoid colon only
- Long segment transitional zone above descending colon extends to splenic flexure or transverse colon

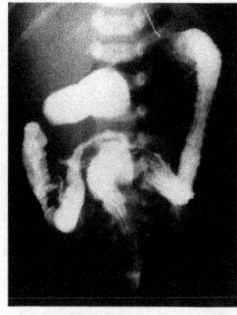

**Fig. 3.129:** Enterocolitis complicating Hirschsprung's disease.

- Ultrashort-segment disease—transitional zone anorectal region 3-4 cm of internal sphincter only
- Total colonic aganglionosis transitional zone at distal ileus 1-4%.
- Total intestinal aganglionosis is rare.

## QUESTIONS

**Q1. What is the cause of Hirschsprung's disease?**

Hirschsprung's disease is caused by failure of migration of ganglion cell from neural crest to the colon. The most common site is rectosigmoid region.

**Q2. What are the conditions associated with Hirschsprung's disease?**
- Aarskog syndrome
- Bardet–Biedl syndrome
- Congenital central hypoventilation syndrome
- Down syndrome
- Fryns syndrome
- Multiple endocrine neoplasia (MEN) type 2
- Smith–Lemli–Opitz syndrome
- Waardenburg syndrome.

**Q3. What are the types of Hirschsprung's disease?**

Two types:
1. Aganglionosis involves the distal sigmoid and rectum—more common type, common in males
2. Long segment variety—common in both males and females.

**Q4. What is the pathogenesis of Hirschsprung's disease?**

Hirschsprung's disease is caused by failure of migration of ganglion cell from neural crest to the colon. The most common site is rectosigmoid region. It extends proximally from the anorectal junction. Anus will be always involved. In most cases, the involvement does not extend more proximally than the sigmoid colon. In about 8–10% of cases entire colon may be involved.

Absent ganglionic cells from both the myenteric Auerbach's and the submucosal, Meissner's plexus is a feature of this condition. This will result in absence of parasympathetic innervation of the internal anal sphincter and varying portions of the colon and terminal ileum. Parasympathetic ganglia are absent from Meissner's plexus and Auerbach's plexus. This will result in absence of peristalsis in this segment, which will be spastic and contracted. There will be increased nerve fibers in the affected segment. The proximal colon will dilate.

**Q5. What are the clinical features of Hirschsprung's disease?**
- Hirschsprung's disease will present with a range of symptoms like acute intestinal obstruction in the newborn to constipation in older infants and children:
  - Abdominal distension (due to intestinal obstruction)
  - Bloated abdomen
  - Brown vomit
  - Bilious vomiting
  - Blood in stools
  - Constipation
  - Delayed passage of meconium
  - Diarrhea
  - Explosive stools after per rectal examination
  - Emesis—vomiting
  - Failure to thrive (in older children)
  - Fatigue (in older children)
  - Functional obstruction
  - Fecal retention
  - Gaseous distension of bowel loops with absence of rectal gas shadow
  - Growth retardation
  - Height decreased
  - Infrequent stooling or intermittent constipation
  - Obstipation (no gas or stools passed)
- Few infants may present with frank enterocolitis with diarrhea, dehydration, and shock

- Per rectal examination will show a normal anal sphincter and empty rectum. Explosive passage of stools will follow rectal examination.

**Q6. How will you confirm the diagnosis of Hirschsprung's disease?**
- Rectal biopsy—full thickness biopsy. Anorectal manometry
- Anal tonometry reveals the absence of normal reflex relaxation of the internal anal sphincter when the rectum is dilated.

**Q7. What is the definitive test for Hirschsprung's disease?**
*Rectal biopsy*—full thickness biopsy is the definitive test. There will be absence of intrinsic innervations of the distal colon with both myenteric and submucosal plexuses are absent. In contrast, the extrinsic innervations containing sympathetic and parasympathetic nerves obtained from the spinal cord may be increased as a result of lack of feedback from the intrinsic nerves.

**Q8. What are the biopsy findings in Hirschsprung's disease?**
Absent ganglionic cells from both the myenteric and the submucosal plexus.

**Q9. What is the use of anal manometry in Hirschsprung's disease?**
- Anorectal manometery measures the contraction and relaxation of internal sphincter in response to rectal distension. Anal tonometry reveals the absence of normal reflex relaxation of the internal anal sphincter when the rectum is dilated
- Rectal biopsy will confirm the diagnosis—full thickness biopsy shows absence of ganglionic cells.

**Q10. What is the treatment of Hirschsprung's disease?**
- Periodic obstruction can be relieved by digital rectal stimulation, enema, and laxative
- The treatment depends upon the length of the segment involved:
  - Ultrasegment disease—rectal suction biopsy will be both diagnostic and therapeutic
  - Diversion colostomy followed by anorectal pull through should be done.

**Q11. What is the aim of the surgery in Hirschsprung's disease?**
The aim of surgery is to remove the aganglionic segment and bring down the ganglionic segment to the anus surgical removal of the affected segment and anastomosis of the ganglionic segment to the rectum. This can be done as a single stage or in two stages.

**Q12. What is the difference between congenital and acquired megacolon?**
In congenital megacolon, there will be normal anal sphincter and empty rectum. In acquired megacolon, the rectum will be full. There will be explosive passage of feces and flatus immediately after the finger is removed after per rectal examination.

**Q13. Why rectal examination, enema or bowel preparation should not be done before radiological examination?**
Air will enter the rectum and the diagnosis will be missed.

**Q14. What are the complications of Hirschsprung's disease?**
- Enterocolitis
- Bowel obstruction
- Intestinal perforation
- Intestinal obstruction
- Volvulus
- Toxic megacolon
- Pelvic abscess
- Short bowel syndrome.

*Surgical complications:*
- Abscess:
  - Anastomosis leakage
  - Bleeding per rectum

- Bowel obstruction
- Constipation
- Diarrhea
- Enterocolitis.
- ❏ Fistula formation
- ❏ Stenosis
- ❏ Incontinence—damage to sphincter.

**Q15. What is the single most reliable sign of Hirschsprung's disease?**
Visualization of rectosigmoid zone.

## Anorectal Anomalies

### Prone cross table translateral view:

*Prone cross table view or prone translateral view* should be taken. The baby should be in genupectoral position. At this position, the anorectal fistula becomes the lowest point and the rectum is better distended with air.

### Discussion:

- High anorectal anomaly or low depends upon whether the defect is above or below the levator ani muscle (Fig. 3.130)
- *M line* is a horizontal line running through the lower third and upper two-thirds of the ischium. The M line will be the level of puborectal sling. This is used to classify the anorectal anomalies as high, intermediate or low
- *Embryology*—the cloaca is divided into the rectum and urogenital sinus. The development of perineum is associated with posterior displacement of the lower part of rectum and anal orifice. Anorectal anomalies are associated with failure of the urorectal septum to divide the cloaca completely or failure of the posterior migration of the rectum in the perineum Persistence of the anal membrane results in imperforate anus. Persistence of communication between cloacal membranes will result in rectovaginal or rectovesical fistulae
- *X-ray—invertogram:* Place a radio-opaque material like coin at the anal site. A plain X-ray is taken with the child held upside down about 24 hours after births. Air from the gut will reach the anal ends of the gut by this time. The type of anorectal anomaly can be assessed by looking at the distance between the coin and the air in the intestine. Invertogram is not routinely done now (Figs. 3.131A and B)
- Also a lateral view of the pelvis should be taken. A line should be drawn from the pubis to the coccyx (pubococcygeal line). Look if the gut ends above or below this line. Ultrasonogram, intravenous pyelogram, and micturating cystourethrogram should be done to diagnose associated urinary tract abnormalities. Fistulogram by injecting a contrast in to the fistula can be done
- *Invertogram:* This should be taken 24 hours after birth so that the swallowed air reaches the rectum. A radiopaque coin is

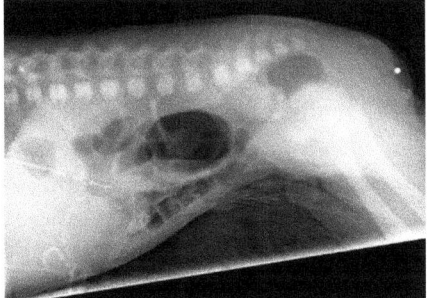

**Fig. 3.130:** X-ray normal—in prone translateral view.

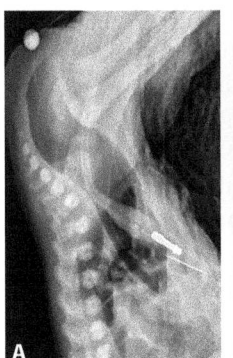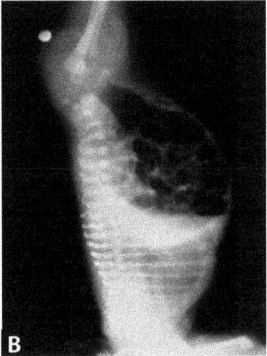

**Figs. 3.131A and B:** X-ray invertogram.

placed at the anal dimple. The distance between the coin and the air shadow should be noted.

- ❖ If the distance between the coin and the air shadow is <2 cms it is high anorectal anomaly. If the distance is <2 cms it is low anomaly.
- ❖ X-ray should be taken 12-24 hours after birth as air takes 12-24 hours to reach the distal part of the colon.

## QUESTIONS

**Q1. What are the types of anorectal anomalies?**
- ❏ High—the bowel ends above the levator sling—anorectal agenesis
- ❏ Intermediate—rectobulbar fistula, rectourethral fistula, rectovaginal fistula, and rectovestibular fistula
- ❏ Low—sling the colon and rectum will be patent distal to levator sling
   - ➢ Anocutaneous fistula, imperforate anus, anal stenosis, anal membrane, and anovestibular fistula in females
   - ➢ Associated conditions are more common in high lesions. The anomalies are esophageal, cardiac, renal, and skeletal anomalies.
   - ➢ High and middle types are supralevator and low type is translevator.

**Q2. What are the clinical features of anorectal anomalies?**
- ❏ Vary from fistula to complete obstruction
- ❏ Flat bottom without a dimple
- ❏ Presence of meconium in the urine
- ❏ Impulse on crying
- ❏ Failure to pass meconium.

**Q3. What are the conditions associated with anorectal anomalies?**
- ❏ VACTERL
- ❏ Renal anomalies
- ❏ Sacral agenesis
- ❏ Vascular abnormalities
- ❏ Ventricular septal defect (VSD)
- ❏ Single umbilical artery.

**Q4. What is the investigation done instead of invertogram for anorectal anomalies? What are the advantages?**
- ❏ X-ray abdomen prone cross table translateral view is used now
- ❏ The advantages of prone cross table view in comparison to invertogram are *(Mnemonic A-G)*:
   - ➢ **A**ccuracy for diagnosis good
   - ➢ **B**etter information than invertogram for level of rectal atresia
   - ➢ **C**ooperation of the patient will be better
   - ➢ **C**omfortable to the baby
   - ➢ **D**elineation of the rectal gas shadow will be better
   - ➢ **E**asy positioning
   - ➢ **F**indings more precise in prone cross table translateral view
   - ➢ **G**ravity effect will be eliminated.

**Q5. Why it is important to know the type of anomaly?**
Surgical treatment to correct the anomalies depends on the type of anomaly. A single stage correction can be done to correct the low anomalies. Perineal anoplasty (cruciate incision) on the membrane will be enough in simple cases. A two stage correction is needed to treat the high anomalies. A colostomy is done, which can be followed by a pull through operation later.

**Q6. What is the prognosis for anorectal anomalies?**
The prognosis will be good for low anomalies and no associated anomalies. High defects are difficult to correct and may lead to incontinence if perineal musculature is ill developed.

**Q7. What is pouch-perineal distance?**
- ❏ It is the distance between the distal rectal pouch and the perineum. It is useful for differentiating between low and high and intermediate anomalies. The cut off distance is 15 mm

❏ It can be measured by transperineal sonography.

## Meconium Ileus (Fig. 3.132)

Radiological findings:
- Air-filled loops—Air fluid levels are absent
- Bubbly appearance of distended intestinal loops
- Calcification
- Contrast enema will be helpful in diagnosis
- Cylindrical filling defect in the colon
- Dilated intestinal loops—proximal to obstruction
- Enema (water-soluble contrast or Gastrografin) shows microcolon
- Filling defects in the distal ileum and colon
- Functional microcolon
- Associated with cystic fibrosis
- Normal meconium may not be visible in X-rays
- Mottled appearance may be seen in.

Discussion:
- Age of onset in the neonatal period
- Abdominal distension
- Bilious vomiting
- Bubbly appearance of intestinal contents
- Cystic fibrosis
- Desiccated meconium pellets get impacted causing small intestinal obstruction
- Earliest clinical manifestation of cystic fibrosis
- Failure to pass meconium within 48 h of life.

## QUESTIONS

**Q1. What is the difference between meconium ileus and meconium plug syndrome?**
The consistency of meconium will be thick in meconium ileus.

**Q2. What are the predisposing factors for meconium ileus?**
Cystic fibrosis.

**Q3. What are the complications of meconium ileus?**
- Ileal atresia
- Ileal stenosis
- Ileal perforation
- Meconium peritonitis
- Volvulus with or without pseudocyst formation.

## Genitourinary System

### Normal Micturating Cystourethrogram (Fig. 3.133)

Micturating cystourethrogram (MCUG) is used to image the lower urinary tract especially urethra using iodinated contrast media. Contrast dye is injected into the catheter inserted into the urethra and bladder. The X-rays are taken while the child is micturating and before and after micturition.

Various X-ray films should be taken:
- Scout film—to evaluate the spine and pelvis
- Filling phase

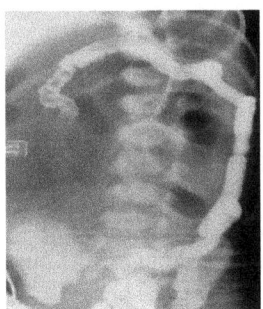

**Fig. 3.132:** Distal microcolon.

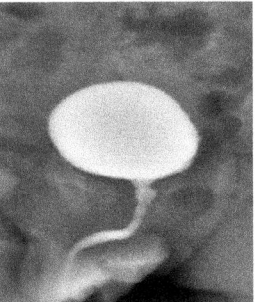

**Fig. 3.133:** Normal micturating cystourethrogram.

- ❖ Voiding phase
- ❖ Postvoid film.

X-rays should be taken in the following views:
- ❖ Right anterior oblique with left leg abducted and knee flexed
- ❖ Left anterior oblique view with right leg abducted and knee flexed
- ❖ Supine posteroanterior view
- ❖ Anterior oblique view will be useful in viewing bilateral vesicoureteric junctions
- ❖ Postvoid X-rays will be helpful in diagnosis of ureterocele
- ❖ Retrograde urethrogram.

Indications:
- ❖ Urinary tract infections (under antibiotic cover)
- ❖ Trauma to urethra
- ❖ Strictures of urethra
- ❖ To check the integrity of urethra
- ❖ Urethral tears
- ❖ Fistula
- ❖ Diverticula of urethra
- ❖ Urethral obstructions
- ❖ Dysfunctional voiding
- ❖ Reflux nephropathy

Contraindications:
Acute urinary tract infections.

### Normal Micturating Cystourethrogram

The following structures are seen in MCUG:
- ❖ Bladder
- ❖ Urethra
- ❖ Flow of the urine can be seen
- ❖ Vesicoureteral reflux
- ❖ Posterior urethral valve
- ❖ X-ray posterior urethral valve

## QUESTION

**Q1. What are the complications of MCUG?**
- ❑ The complications may be due to contrast medium or due to techniques
- ❑ Complications due to contrast medium:
  - ➢ Contrast medium induced cystitis
- ❑ Complications due to techniques:
  - ➢ Urethral trauma
  - ➢ Urinary tract infections
  - ➢ Retention of Foley catheter
  - ➢ Hematuria
  - ➢ Urinary retention
  - ➢ Perforation of bladder
  - ➢ Injury to vagina or ectopic urethral orifice

### Posterior Urethral Valve (Figs. 3.134A and B)

*Present only in boys:*
- ❖ These are small folds in the normal urethra arising from the lower end of verumontanum, which passes downwards toward the external urethral sphincter
- ❖ Common in boys
- ❖ Incidence—1 in 5,000–8,000 male births.
- ❖ Cricket ball bladder palpable in the suprapubic area.
- ❖ *Embryology*—by about 6 weeks after conception, the formation of urethra begins. The mesonephric ducts open into the cloaca at the Mullers tubercle, which is at the midpoint between the cranial and caudal portions of the urogenital sinus. The persistence of the urethrovaginal folds to the urogenital sinus and results in posterior urethral valve
- ❖ *Types:* There are three types:
  1. *Type I:* This is the most common type. This arises from the lower end of the verumontanum and passes toward the anterolateral walls of the bladder
  2. *Type II:* This arises from the lower end of the verumontanum and passes toward the bladder neck. Here, it divides into a fin like membrane. This is usually nonobstructive
  3. *Type III:* Diaphragm with a central perforation. This arises proximal to the bladder.
- ❖ *Clinical features:*
  - ▪ Antenatal—oligohydramnios
  - ▪ In the neonatal period:
    - ♦ Features of renal failure and acidosis
    - ♦ Palpable bladder.

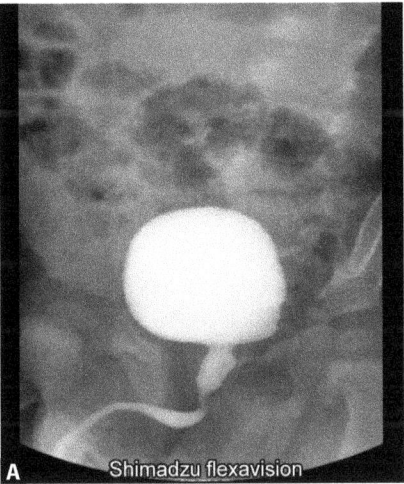 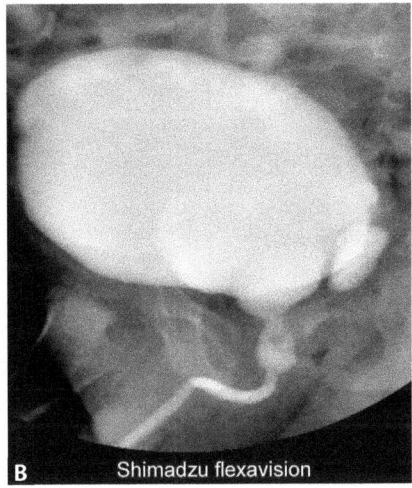

**Figs. 3.134A and B:** Posterior urethral valve.

- Nonurinary—abdominal distension and bladder with kidney will be palpable
- Urinary—straining, poor stream, dribbling thin stream of urine, straining, and crying while voiding urine.
  - *Urinary ascites:* Urinary ascites in neonates is usually due to intraperitoneal bladder or ureteric or upper tract perforation as a result of distal obstruction.
- ❖ *Investigations:*
  - Antenatal diagnosis by ultrasonogram-hydroureteronephrosis
  - Micturating cystourethrogram (MCU)
  - Radioisotopic
  - Renography.
- ❖ *Micturating cystourethrogram:*
  - Dilated posterior urethra
  - Trabeculated bladder
  - Thin anterior urethral
  - Stream
- ❖ *Treatment:*
  - Cystoscopic ablation
  - Electrocauterization, or laser fulguration
  - Transurethral fulguration
  - Ablation of valves
    - Upper tract diversion
    - Vesicostomy.

- ❖ *Prognosis:* If not identified and treated early the following can occur:
  - An UTI, renal failure, metabolic acidosis, and death (due to septicemia, metabolic acidosis, and end-stage renal diseases)
  - Obstructive lesions—may manifest as:
    - Infection
    - Sepsis
    - Acute febrile UTI
    - Failure to thrive
    - Vomiting or diarrhea
    - Prenatal diagnosis—ultrasound.

## QUESTIONS

**Q1. What are the clinical features of posterior urethral valve in newborn infants?**
- ☐ Distended bladder with dribbling of urine
- ☐ Vomiting
- ☐ Diarrhea
- ☐ Abdominal distension
- ☐ Nonspecific symptoms
- ☐ Obstructive symptoms may be absent.

**Q2. What are the obstructive symptoms in posterior urethral valve?**

- Weak stream
- Dribbling
- Straining
- Crying on voiding urine.

### Vesicoureteric Reflux

- It can be demonstrated by micturating cystourethrogram
- The ureterovesical valve mechanism is defective and result in urine flowing from the bladder to the ureter.

**Discussion:** Reflux may be unilateral or bilateral.

## QUESTION

**Q1. What are the complications of vesicoureteric reflux?**
- Stasis of urine will predispose to infections
- Recurrent pyelonephritis
- Posterior urethral valve
- Mucosal fold arising from the distal most part of the verumontanum
    - Can be demonstrated by micturating cystourethrogram

*Vesicoureteral Reflux:*
It is the retrograde propulsion of urine in to the upper urinary tract during bladder contraction. It is due to the insertion of the ureter into the bladder wall. This results in shorter intravesicular ureter, this acts as an incompetent valve during urination.

In normal babies, urine will enter the bladder through vesicoureteric junction. This junction will act as a one-way valve and will not allow the urine to reflux up the ureters. Ureter will be not dilated.

The reflux does not occur due to the distensibility of the bladder, which can hold much urine by distension and maintain allow pressure. Also the anatomy at the vesicoureteric junction will prevent reflux of urine back to the ureters. When the vesicoureteric junction is defective in function or faulty insertion of ureter will allow urine to reflux back in to the ureter.

Vesicoureteral reflux may be familial.
- *Primary—congenital anomaly:*
    - Trigone underdeveloped
    - Short or absent intravesical ureter
    - Absence of adequate detrusor backing
    - Lateral displacement of the ureteral orifice
    - Paraureteral (Hutch) diverticulum
    - Posterior urethral valve
    - Duplication of ureters
- *Secondary causes:*
    - Cystitis or UTI
    - Bladder outlet obstruction
    - Neurogenic bladder
    - Detrusor instability
    - *Ureterocele*: An ureterocele is a swelling at the bottom of one of the tubes (ureters) that carry urine from the kidney to the bladder. The swollen area can block urine flow. But not the reflux.
    - Diverticulum

*Grade (Figs. 3.135A to C):*
- I—reflux into a nondilated distal ureter
- II—reflux in to the upper collecting system without dilatation
- III—reflux with blunting of calyceal fornices dilated ureter
- IV—reflux into a grossly dilated ureter
- V—massive reflux.

I and II—in 80% of cases spontaneous cessation with maturation of child.

Obstructive lesions—may manifest as:
- Infection
- Sepsis
- Acute febrile UTI
- Failure to thrive
- Vomiting or diarrhea

*Evaluation:*
- Urine culture
- Voiding urethrography (yearly)

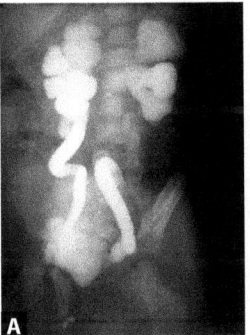 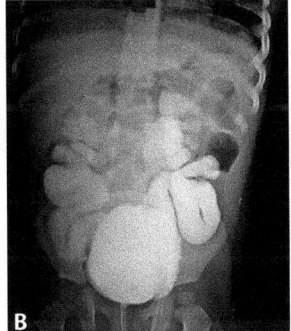 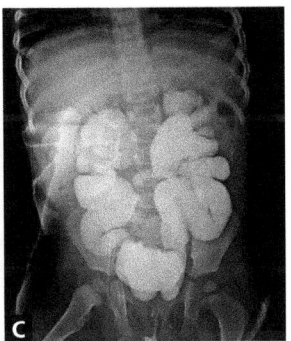

**Figs. 3.135A to C:** Bilateral vesicoureteric reflux with hydronephrosis.

Urodynamic studies will show functional abnormalities in the lower urinary tract.
- Ultrasound
- Endoscopic injection of polytef (polytetrafluoroethylene)
- Effective short-term radioisotopic
- Renography
- Technetium labeled—diethylenetriaminepentaacetic acid (DTPA) with furosemide in (less reliable in the 1st year of life)
- Iodine-labeled Hippuran (with obstructive lesions radiation hazard is more)
- Accuracy safety is more – MAG 3 (Tc mercaptoacetylglycine)
- Circumcaval ureter invariably on the right side (anomalous development of vena cava).

*Outcome*:
The ureter elongates with growth and most of the mild grades get corrected spontaneously. Most of the cases with grades I to III will resolve spontaneously.

*Management*:
- UTI prophylaxis is indicated to prevent infection.
- Surgical repair is indicated in cases with urinary tract infections or high grade reflux.
- Endoscopic treatment—dextranometer hyaluronic acid is injected through a cystoscope near the ureteric orifice.

*Complications:*
- Hypertension
- Renal scarring
- Chronic renal failure.

### Hydronephrosis (Figs. 3.136A and B)
- Most common cause of hydronephrosis in childhood is congenital narrowing of pelvic ureteric junction
- Pyeloplasty can be done
- The obstruction should be removed and the size of the pelvis should be reduced
- In nonfunctioning hydronephrosis and gross pyonephrosis nephrectomy can be done.

## MISCELLANEOUS

### Thrombocytopenia absent Radius Syndrome (Fig. 3.137)
- TAR syndrome
- X-ray showing absent radius
- Genetically determined condition
- Bilateral radial aplasia
- Absence or hypoplasia of megakaryocytes
- Presents in early infancy
- Prognosis—remits over the first few years of life.

### Radiological Features
- Bilateral absence of radius in the forearm with radial deviation of hand

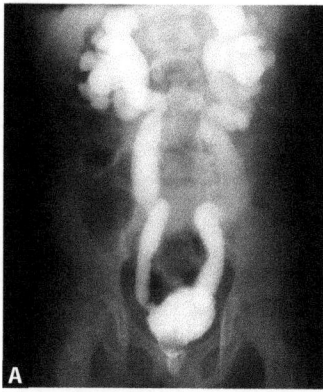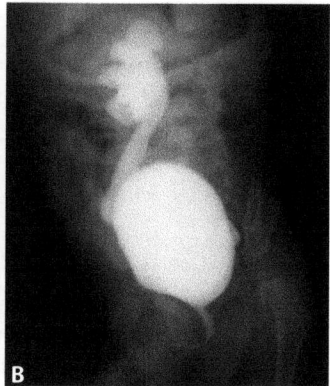

**Figs. 3.136A and B:** (A) Bilateral hydroureteronephrosis; (B) Right hydroureteronephrosis.

- ❖ The legs will be normal in most of the cases, but can be associated with dislocation of hip, femoral torsion, tibial torsion, varus or valgus deformities, etc.
- ❖ Thumbs will be normal:
  - Asymmetrical limb shortening
  - Bilateral abnormalities
  - Clavicle abnormal
  - Digits hypoplastic
  - Extremities abnormal
  - Five fingered hand will arise from the shoulder (in humeral aplasia)
  - Glenoid fossa hypoplastic
  - Humerus may be abnormal or absent

## Discussion

- ❖ It is a rare condition with autosomal recessive inheritance.

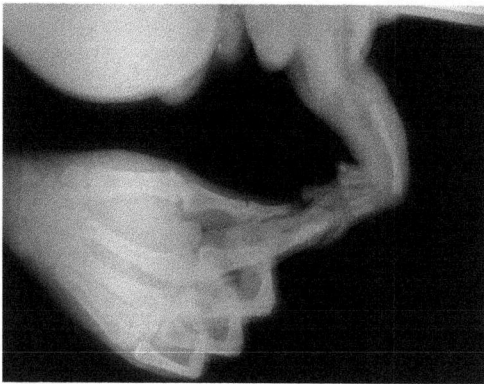

**Fig. 3.137:** TAR syndrome.

- ❖ Platelet count will be decreased. The count will be decreased in infancy and will improve as the age advances. The count can be normal in some cases.

## QUESTIONS

**Q1. What is the bone marrow finding in thrombocytopenia absent radius (TAR) syndrome?**
Hypoamegakaryocytic thrombocytopenia.

**Q2. What are the complications seen in TAR syndrome**
Intracranial hemorrhage in the first year of life.

**Q3. What are the congenital cardiac defects associated with TAR syndrome?**
Atrial septal defect and tetralogy.

**Q4. What is the prognosis in TAR syndrome?**
Death due to hemorrhage in 50% of cases in early infancy.

**Q5. What is the problem of feeding in infants with TAR syndrome?**
Intolerance to Cow's milk is common.

## Habitual Constipation (Fig. 3.138)

### Radiological Features

The part with fecal matter will be equal or greater diameter than the normal part of the colon.

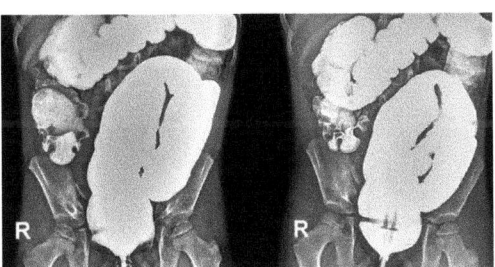

**Fig. 3.138:** Habitual constipation: Note that the size of rectum will be more than that of the colon.

## Discussion

- Defecation because of prolonged retention of stool in the colon
- Less than three times per week
- Rule out organic causes of constipation.

*Differential Diagnosis*

Hirschprung disease.

## QUESTIONS

**Q1. What are the predisposing factors for habitual constipation?**
- Motion devoid of poorly digestible ingredients
- Lack of physical activities.

**Q2. Describe the management of habitual constipation.**
- Conservative
- Diet rich in digestible ingredients
- Regular pattern of eating and defecation
- Hydrophilic colloid laxative.

# CHAPTER 4

# Drugs

## CHAPTER OUTLINE

- Antibiotics
- Antivirals
- Antifungals
- Antiprotozoal
- Anthelmintics
- Antihistaminics
- Cholinergic Drugs
- Sympathomimetic/Inotropic Drugs
- Antihypertensives
- Antiasthmatics
- Sedatives Hypnotics
- Opioids
- Anticonvulsants
- Corticosteroids (Glucocorticoids)
- Hormones
- Diuretics
- Cardiac Glycosides
- Chelating Agents
- H2-receptor Blockers
- Miscellaneous

## INTRODUCTION

Almost all drugs are associated with one or more complications. Some complications may be mild and some may be severe. Some complications may be reversible and some may be irreversible. Combining drugs may be associated with more complications.

The benefits and the risks should be analyzed before providing them and decision should be taken whether to administer them or not. The medicines given as injections will enter the body directly and can result in damage, which is inevitable. All the medical professional and patients should be aware of the complications of the drugs before using them. The beneficial effects of the drugs and the adverse effects should be analyzed and a wise decision should be taken whether to use the drug or not. The adverse effects and contraindications are discussed in this chapter. Always explain the possible adverse effects to the patients or to their caretakers. This can prevent unnecessary apprehension to the patients and wasting of time and money for consulting for the new symptoms due to adverse effects. For example, the stools may be black colored in those who are taking iron tablets. If they are not warned of this, they may fear that they are passing blood in stools. They may go for consulting doctors and performing unnecessary investigations. Drugs like ampicillin may cause diarrhea. If the patient is not aware of this, they will fear about this and will come to the doctor who had prescribed the drug and blame them that the wrong treatment was given which was the cause for diarrhea. Some others may go to other doctors for consultations.

Before administering any drug to the patient, it is the duty of the medical professionals to know the indications, contraindications, side effects, and complications of the drugs. The patients or caretakers also should be explained about the possible adverse effects.

The patients also can develop complications that are not listed in this book. In that case the patients have to report about those adverse effects to their doctor and it should be intimated to the concerned authorities. Any new adverse effect that had occurred after taking a drug should be considered as the adverse effect of that drug unless proved otherwise.

Do not take any medicine or vaccine without knowing the adverse effects that it can cause. If the adverse effect is irreversible then it is going to be a lifelong problem for the patient and the family.

Both the medical professional and patients should observe for complications and adverse effects that are not listed. Many adverse effects not identified during phase III trials of drugs were identified later during postmarketing surveillance. If any such adverse effects are noted it should be intimated to appropriate health authorities who in turn should take effort to notify to appropriate authorities.

# ANTIBIOTICS

## Antibacterials

### Sulfonamides

**Mechanism of action:** Sulfonamides are bacteriostatic by inhibiting folic acid synthesis. They are competitive inhibitors of dihydropteroate synthetase an enzyme needed for folate synthesis.

**Woods fields theory:** Sulfonamides have a structural similarity to para-aminobenzoic acid (PABA) and compete with paba for incorporation into folic acid.

**Pharmacological actions:** Sulfonamides are bacteriostatic which will inhibit the growth and multiplication of bacteria and do not kill the bacteria. Sulfonamides will inhibit the growth of gram-positive and gram-negative bacteria, *Actinomyces*, *Nocardia*, and chlamydia organisms.

**The spectrum of action of sulfonamides:** Bacteriostatic against many gram-positive and gram-negative organisms.

**Dosage:** 6/kg/day in two divided doses.

**Indications:**
- Urinary tract infections
- Respiratory tract infections
- Typhoid
- Bacterial diarrhea and dysentery
- Chancroid
- Granuloma inguinale
- *Pneumocystis carinii*
- Trachoma
- Inclusion conjunctivitis
- Lymphogranuloma venereum
- Toxoplasmosis
- Nocardiosis
- Bacillary dysentery
- Prophylaxis of streptococcal pharyngitis
- Shigellosis.

**Contraindications:**
- Children below 2 years of age
- Allergy to any sulfonamide, thiazide diuretics, and sulfonylureas
- Porphyria
- Pregnancy
- Renal insufficiency
- Hepatic disorders
- Pyruvate kinase deficiency
- Glucose-6-phosphate dehydrogenase (G6PD) deficiency.

**Precautions:** Should be used cautiously in kidney stones and renal disease.

**Effects on pregnancy:** Teratogenic and should be avoided during pregnancy.

**The effects of sulfonamides (long acting) on the fetus and newborn:** Kernicterus can occur at low serum bilirubin levels by displacing bilirubin from albumin, can cause hemolytic anemia in G6PD deficient babies.

**Side effects:**

- *General*: Dizziness
- Headache
- Lethargy
- Gastrointestinal disorders:
  - Nausea
  - Anorexia
  - Vomiting
  - Diarrhea
  - Epigastric pain
- Urinary tract disorders:
  - Crystalluria
  - Albuminuria
  - Hematuria
- Hematopoietic disorders: Hemolysis in G6PD deficiency patients
- Allergic reactions: Skin rash
- Hypersensitivity reactions (rashes and hives):
  - Stevenson–Johnson syndrome
  - Toxic epidermal necrolysis (Lyell syndrome)
  - Agranulocytosis
  - Hemolytic anemia
  - Thrombocytopenia
  - Fulminant hepatic necrosis
  - Acute pancreatitis
- Urticaria
- Drug rash with eosinophilia and systemic symptoms (DRESS) syndrome
- Severe cutaneous adverse reactions (SCARs)
- Precipitation of kernicterus in newborn as sulfonamides will replace bilirubin from albumin.
- Photosensitivity
- Porphyria
- Hepatitis.

**Drug interactions:** Will intensify the effects of warfarin, phenytoin, oral hypoglycemic, hence will require reduction in dosage.

## QUESTIONS

**Q1. What are the sulfonamides that can cause allergy?**
Sulfonamides that contain arylamine group at N4 are associated with hypersensitivity, sulfamethoxazole, sulfasalazine, sulfadiazine, antiretrovirals amprenavir, and fosamprenavir.

**Q2. What is the sulfonamide used in the treatment of inflammatory bowel disease?**
Sulfasalazine.

**Q3. As sulfonamides inhibit folate synthesis, will it affects human cells?**
Humans will acquire folate from food.

**Q4. What are the sulfonamides used as anticonvulsants?**
- Ethoxzolamide
- Sultiame
- Zonisamide.

**Q5. What are the sulfonamides used in skin conditions?**
Mafenide.

**Q6. What are the sulfonamides used as antiretrovirals?**
- Amprenavir
- Darunavir
- Delavirdine
- Fosamprenavir
- Tipranavir.

**Q7. Why sulfonamides are preferred in treating urinary tract infections?**
Bactericidal concentrations are achieved in urine.

**Q8. What are the sulfonamides used for gastrointestinal infections?**
Sulfaguanidine.

**Q9. How will you classify sulfonamides?**
Classification of sulfonamides:
- Short-acting sulfonamides (4–8 hours)—sulfadiazine, sulfadimidine, and sulfafurazole

- Intermediate-acting sulfonamides (12 hours)—sulfadoxine and sulfamethoxazole
- Long-acting sulfonamides (7 days)—sulfadimethoxine and sulfamethoxypyridazine
- Ultra long-acting—sulfadoxine and sulfametopyrazine.

## Co-trimoxazole

- It is a fixed dose combination of trimethoprim and sulfamethoxazole
- Available as tablet and syrup:
  Pediatric and adult tablets are available.

**Mechanism of action:** It has synergistic bactericidal action.

**Dosage:** Dose of 6 mg/kg in two divided doses.

**Indications:**
- Urinary tract infections
- Respiratory infections
- Bacterial diarrhea
- Gonorrhea
- Typhoid fever
- Prophylaxis and treatment of *Pneumocystis carinii*.

**Contraindications:**
- Newborn
- Infants early infancy
- Blood dyscrasias
- Severe renal failure.

**Precautions:** Patients with urinary obstruction.

**Effects on pregnancy:** Not recommended because of teratogenic effect. Co-trimoxazole should be avoided during pregnancy and in patients with G6PD deficiency as hemolysis will be precipitated.

**Side effects:**
- Nauseas
- Vomiting
- Folic acid deficiency
- Blood dyscrasia
- Skin rashes
- Anemia
- Leukopenia
- Thrombocytopenia
- Stomatitis
- Glossitis
- Crystalluria
- Stevenson-Johnson syndrome.

**Drug interactions:** When combined with pyrimethamine cause megaloblastic anemia.

## QUESTIONS

**Q1. What is co-trimoxazole?**
Co-trimoxazole is a fixed dose combination of trimethoprim and sulfamethoxazole.

**Q2. Why sulfamethoxazole is used in combination with trimethoprim?**
- It is because the half life of both is about 10 hours
- Both are given in a ratio of 5:1 trimethoprim will enter many tissues and has a high volume of distribution.

## Diaminopyrimidines

**Trimethoprim:**
- It is a pyrimidine derivative
- Oral availability (F) (%) 100
- Half-life (h) 11.

**Trimethoprim–sulfamethoxazole:** Available in double strength with 160 mg trimethoprim and 800 mg of sulfamethoxazole and 80 mg trimethoprim/400 mg of sulfamethoxazole.

**Mechanism of action:** It is bacteriostatic. This inhibits the enzyme dihydrofolate reductase by binding to it, which results in inhibition of conversion of dihydrofolic acid to tetrahydrofolic acid.

The affinity of trimethoprim for bacterial dihydrofolate reductase is thousand times more that that for human dihydrofolate reductase.

**Pharmacological actions:** Effective against:
- Streptococci
- *Staphylococcus aureus*

- *Escherichia coli*
- *Salmonella*
- *Shigella*
- *Proteus.*

**Dosage:**
- *Oral dose*: 15–20 mg/kg in divided doses
- *Intravenous dose*: 8–12 mg/kg/day
- *Adult dose*: One tablet bd for 10 days.

**Indications:**
- Urinary tract infections
- Prostatitis
- Prophylaxis against *Pneumocystis pneumonia*
- Whipple disease
- Disulfiram like reaction with alcohol
- Traveler's diarrhea.

**Contraindications:**
- Age less than 2 months
- Creatinine clearance less than 15 mL/minute
- Hypersensitivity to sulfonamides
- Megaloblastic anemia due to folate deficiency.

**Precautions:**
- Use cautiously in patients with anemia, kidney disease, liver diseases, bone marrow suppression, and G6PD deficiency
- Hyperkalemia
- Hyponatremia
- Do not take any vaccines with this drug. The effect of typhoid vaccine will be affected
- Decrease the dose if the creatinine clearance is 15–30 mL/minute.

**Effects on pregnancy:** Can cross the placenta and affect metabolism of folate. Contraindicated in the first trimester of pregnancy. This will lower folic acid levels and cause spinal cord defects. Displaces bilirubin from proteins in the blood in infants if used to pregnant mothers near term.

**Side effects:**
- Appetite loss
- Bone marrow toxicity
- Cyanosis
- Diarrhea
- Emesis
- Fever and chills
- Gustatory—change in taste
- Headache
- Hypersensitivity
- Itching
- Jaundice
- Joint aches
- $K^+$ excess (hyperkalemia)
- Lyell syndrome (toxic epidermal necrolysis)
- Mouth sores
- Muscle pain
- Nausea
- Photosensitivity
- Phototoxic skin eruptions
- Rash
- Stevens-Johnson syndrome
- Thrombocytopenia.

**Drug interactions:** Trimethoprim may inhibit hepatic metabolism of phenytoin.

## QUESTION

Q1. What are the advantages of using trimethoprim and sulfamethoxazole in combination?
- ☐ Synergistic action
- ☐ Reduces the development of drug resistance as compared to use of either drug alone
- ☐ Competes with creatinine for secretion in to the renal tubule.

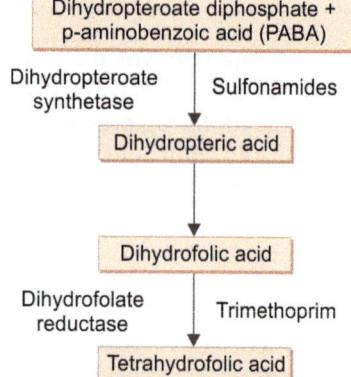

## Quinolones

### Ciprofloxacin:

- It is a second generation fluoroquinolones
- Oral availability (F) (%) 60
- Half-life (h) 4.1

**Mechanism of action:** Quinolones will block bacterial deoxyribonucleic acid (DNA) synthesis by inhibiting bacterial topoisomerase II DNA gyrase and topoisomerase IV.

**Dosage:** 15 mg/kg in two divided doses.

**Indications:**
- Urinary tract infections
- Respiratory infections
- Ear, nose, and throat (ENT) infections
- Intra-abdominal infections
- Soft tissue infections—cellulitis
- Gynecological infections
- Systemic infections
- Infections of bone and joints
- Anthrax
- Chancroid.

**Contraindications:**
- Hypersensitivity to ciprofloxacin
- Myasthenia gravis

**Precautions:**
- Renal impairment, cerebral atherosclerosis, and epilepsy
- Adequate hydration should be maintained to prevent crystalluria.

**Effects on pregnancy:**
- Contraindicated
- Category C
- No study in humans, but animal studies have suggested potential harm to the fetus.

**Side effects:**
- Arthralgia
- Burning sensation
- Bloody/black tarry stools
- Chest pain/discomfort
- Central nervous system (CNS) effects
- Diarrhea
- Dizziness
- Emesis (vomiting)
- Exacerbation of muscle weakness in myasthenia gravis
- Fainting
- Gastrointestinal tract (GIT) symptoms
- Headache
- Insomnia
- Jaundice
- Joint stiffness
- Kidney problems
- Light headedness
- Muscle weakness
- Numbness
- Peripheral neuropathy
- Restlessness
- Skin rash
- Tendinitis
- Unsteadiness.

**Drug interactions:** The following drugs will decrease absorption of ciprofloxacin:
- Magnesium
- Aluminum hydroxide
- Calcium
- Iron
- Zinc
- Rifampicin will decrease the serum concentration of ciprofloxacin
- Ciprofloxacin will potentiate oral anticoagulants.

## QUESTIONS

Q1. What are the other fluoroquinolones?
- ❏ Norfloxacin
- ❏ Gatifloxacin
- ❏ Genifloxacin
- ❏ Moxifloxacin.

Q2. Fluoroquinolones are not routinely recommended in patients under 18 years?
- ❏ Damage growing cartilage
- ❏ Arthropathy which is reversible.

### Norfloxacin:

- Fluoroquinolone
- Fluorinated 4—quinolone.

**Mechanism of action:** Bactericidal, inhibits subunit A of DNA gyrase (topoisomerase) that is essential for bacterial DNA replication. It is a powerful broad spectrum antibacterial agent.

**Dosage:**
- Oral 5–6 mg/kg/day maintenance
- 10 mg/kg/day up to a maximum of 15 mg/kg/day.

**Indications:**
- Urinary tract infections
- Typhoid fever
- Gonorrhea
- Bacterial gastroenteritis.

**Contraindications:**
- Hypersensitivity to quinolones
- Convulsions
- Blood dyscrasias
- Pregnancy
- Lactation.

**Precautions:**
- Renal impairment
- Convulsions
- Pregnancy
- Maintain adequate hydration and urine output.

**Effects on pregnancy:** Contraindicated.

**Side effects:**
- Arthralgia
- Bronchospasm
- Bone marrow depression
- Dry mouth
- Eosinophilia
- Edema of larynx
- Facial edema
- Gastrointestinal problems—abdominal pain
- Hypersensitivity reactions
- Hypotension
- Insomnia
- Jaundice
- Kidney problems.

**Drug interactions:**
- Theophyine will cause disulfiram like reactions when used with alcohol
- Cyclosporine levels will be increased
- Effects of oral contraceptives will be increased
- The effects of caffeine will last longer.

The following drugs will decrease the levels of norfloxacin:
- Multivitamin containing zinc and iron
- Antacids
- Sucralfate
- Probenecid will decrease the urinary excretion of norfloxacin.

## QUESTION

Q1. What is the cause of diarrhea in child taking norfloxacin?
 Infection with *Clostridium difficile*.

### Beta-lactam Antibiotics

**Amoxycillin:** Amoxycillin is semi-synthetic penicillin an analogue of ampicillin beta-lactam antibiotic.

**Mechanism of action:** Inhibits biosynthesis of cell wall mucopeptide and also inhibits the cross linkage between linear peptidoglycan polymer chains in both gram-positive and gram-negative organisms.

**Pharmacological actions:** Broad spectrum bactericidal activity against gram-positive and gram-negative organisms.

**Dosage of amoxycillin:** Dose—100 mg/kg/day in three to four divided doses.

**Indications:**
- Typhoid fever
- Urinary tract infections
- Respiratory infections—acute sinusitis, acute otitis media, and pharyngitis
- ENT infections
- *Haemophilus influenzae*
- *Neisseria gonorrhea*
- Prophylaxis against infective endocarditis.

**Contraindications:** Allergic to penicillin.

**Precautions:**
- Assessment of renal and hepatic functions
- Super infections with mycotic infections may occur.

**Effects on pregnancy:** No risk.

**Side Effects:**
- Nausea
- Vomiting
- Diarrhea
- Indigestion
- Serum sickness
- Rise in serum glutamate-oxaloacetate transaminase (SGOT)
- Nonallergic rash
- Allergic reactions—hives
- Anaphylaxis
- Increased risk for yeast infections.

**Rare side effects:**
- Drowsiness
- Hallucinations
- Coma
- Neutropenia
- Thrombocytopenic purpura
- Antibiotic associated colitis
- *Clostridium difficile* infection.

**Drug interactions:**
- Amoxycillin will reduce the absorption of oral contraceptives
- Uricosuric drugs
- Typhoid vaccine
- Anticoagulants
- Allopurinol.

# QUESTIONS

**Q1. What is the use of combining clavulanic acid along with amoxycillin?**
Clavulanic acid is a potent inhibitor of beta-lactamase. Thus, it will prevent the effect of beta-lactamase on beta-lactamase susceptible antibiotics.

**Q2. What is the advantage of combining clavulanic acid with amoxicillin?**
- Amoxycillin is susceptible to beta-lactam producing organisms.
- Clavulanic acid is a beta-lactamase inhibitor. Hence, the combination reduces the susceptibility to beta-lactamase resistance, *Staphylococcus aureus*, *Bacteroides fragilis*, and beta-lactamase producing *E. coli* and *H. influenzae*.

**Q3. What are the differences between ampicillin and amoxycillin?**
- Amoxycillin will be absorbed better and food does not interfere with absorption of amoxycillin.
- The blood levels will be more sustained.
- Amoxycillin is less active against *Shigella* and *H. influenzae*.
- The incidence of diarrhea will be less.

**Q4. Why amoxycillin is better than ampicillin?**
Amoxycillin is superior to ampicillin because it is absorbed better in the GIT.

**Ampicillin:**
- Ampicillin is a semi-synthetic penicillin
- It is inactivated by penicillinase producing organisms
- Beta-lactam antibiotic
- Ampicillin injection: 100, 250, and 500 mg powder in vials
- *Drops*: 100 mg/mL
- Acid resistant.

**Mechanism of action:** Inhibits cell wall synthesis by binding to specific penicillin binding proteins.

**Pharmacological properties:**
- Excreted largely unchanged in the urine
- The spectrum of action of ampicillin:
  - Ampicillin acts against gram-positive organisms
  - *H. influenzae, E. coli, Proteus, Salmonella,* and *Shigella.*

**Dosage:**
- Gram-positive organisms—dose: 50–100 mg/kg/day for 10–14 days
- Meningitis dose: 100–200 mg/kg/day every 6–8 hourly.

**Indications:**
- Urinary tract infections
- Respiratory infections
- Meningitis

- Gonorrhea
- Typhoid fever
- Bacillary dysentery
- Cholecystitis
- Subacute bacterial endocarditis
- Septicemia.

**Contraindications:** Hypersensitivity to penicillin.

**Precautions:**
- Rash will occur in patients with infectious mononucleosis
- Allergic and anaphylactic reactions
- Use of allopurinol
- Periodic assessments of renal and hepatic functions are needed.

**Effects on pregnancy:** Can be given during pregnancy safely.

**Side effects**
- Rash (maculopapular)
- Pruritis
- Gastrointestinal upset
- Diarrhea.

**Drug interactions:**
- Drug interactions with ampicillin
- Hydrocortisone will inactivate ampicillin
- Oral contraceptives by inhibiting intestinal flora, deconjugation and enterohepatic circulation will be decreased. This results in failure of oral contraception
- Probenecid will retard and increase the blood levels
- Oral contraceptives will cause breakthrough bleeding.

## QUESTIONS

Q1. What are the conditions which increase the incidence of rashes?
- Acquired immune deficiency syndrome (AIDS)
- Epstein-Barr (EB) virus infections
- Lymphatic leukemia
- Allopurinol.

Q2. What is the cause of diarrhea in patients taking oral ampicillin?
Ampicillin is incompletely absorbed and causes irritation of lower intestines. Also this drug will cause marked alteration of bacterial flora.

Q3. What are the derivatives of ampicillin?
Acylureidopenicillins like mezlocillin, azlocillin, and piperacillin. These have broad spectrum of action than ampicillin. Like ampicillin they are susceptible to beta-lactamases.

Q4. What are the fluids compatible with ampicillin?
- Compatible with normal saline and ringer lactate
- Incompatible with dextrose solutions and sodium bicarbonate.

**Penicillin:**
- Bactericidal drugs
- Penicillins are beta-lactam antibiotics.

## QUESTIONS

Q1. What are the types of penicillin?
- Short-acting: Benzyl penicillin given every 6 hourly
- Intermediate-acting: Procaine penicillin given once daily
- Long-acting: Benzathine penicillin rheumatic prophylaxis is give once in 21 days after test dose.

Q2. What are the types of preparations of penicillin?
- Oral penicillin
- Parenteral preparations (aqueous penicillin G, procaine penicillin, and benzathine penicillin).

Q3. What are repository preparations?
Penicillins are rapidly eliminated through urine and have to be given in a interval of 4-6 hours. To prevent this risk relatively insoluble penicillins are prepared. These should be given deep by intramuscular route. This should not given by intravenous route.

The following are some of the repository preparations:
- Procaine benzyl penicillin
- Benzathine penicillin
- Penicillin with probenecid.

**Q4. What are the routes of administration of penicillin?**
- Benzyl penicillin by intravenous route
- Phenoxymethyl penicillin (penicillin V) by mouth
- Procaine penicillin by intramuscular route
- Benzathine penicillin through intramuscular route.

**Q5. What is semisynthetic penicillin?**
- Acid-resistant penicillin
- Potassium phenoxy methyl penicillin
- Potassium phenoxy ethyl penicillin.

**Q6. What is penicillinase-resistant penicillin?**
Penicillinase-resistant penicillins are:
- Methicillin
- Cloxacillin
- Nafcillin.

**Q7. What is broad spectrum penicillin?**
Broad spectrum penicillins are:
- Ampicillin
- Amoxycillin.

**Q8. What are the penicillinase-resistant penicillins?**
- Methicillin
- Cloxacillin

**Q9. What is the spectrum of action of penicillins?**
Highly sensitive against the following organisms:
- Acts against gram-positive organisms
- Both gram-positive and gram-negative organisms are sensitive to penicillins
- Streptococcal infections except enterococci
- Pneumococcal infections
- Meningococcal infections
- Gonococci—gonorrhea
- *Neisseria*
- *Treponema pallidum* (syphilis)
- Diphtheria
- Anaerobes
- Tetanus gas gangrene
- Leptospirosis
- Rat bite fever.

**Q10. What are the conditions in penicillin used for prophylaxis?**
- Rheumatic fever
- Gonorrhea
- Bacterial endocarditis
- Patients with agranulocytosis.

**Q11. What are the adverse effects of penicillin?**
- Allergy to penicillin
- Acute anaphylactic reaction and angioedema
- Breathing problems–fast and irregular breathing
- Convulsions and coma
- Diarrhea
- Dermatitis
- Encephalopathy—accumulation in patients with renal failure may lead to encephalopathy
- Erythema
- Emesis
- Fever
- Mental confusion and muscular twitching
- Gastrointestinal problems—abdominal tenderness, abdominal cramps, and nausea
- Glossitis
- Gustatory problems—abnormal taste perception
- Genitourinary problems—vulvovaginitis
- Headache
- Hypersensitivity—rash, itching, urticaria, and pyrexia
- Infections—superinfections, e.g. candidiasis
- Itching
- Jarisch-Herxheimer reaction
- Joint pain

- Kidney problems—interstitial nephritis (with high doses of parenteral penicillin)
- Light headedness
- Lymphadenopathy
- Mental depression
- Myoclonus
- Neuropathy (paresthesia) (with high doses of parenteral penicillin)
- Edema—larynx and angioedema
- Pruritis
- Pancytopenia—anemia, thrombocytopenia, neutropenia, and agranulocytosis.

**Q12. What are the doses of different types of penicillins?**
- *Benzyl penicillin (penicillin G)*: 100,000–150,000 units/kg/24 hours in two divided doses
- *Procaine penicillin*: 25,000–50,000 units/kg/24 hours, single dose, intramuscularly
- *Benzathine penicillin*: Less than 27 kg, 60,000 units intramuscular
- *1.2 million units (mega units) once in 3 weeks*: This injection will be painful.

**Q13. What is the duration of action of different types of penicillin?**
- Benzyl penicillin is most active penicillin and should be given by injection. Duration of action will be for 6–8 hours. The duration of its action can be prolonged by combining with procaine or benzathine
- Phenoxymethylpenicillin is acid-resistant penicillin and can be given by mouth as it is absorbed through gastrointestinal tract
- Procaine penicillin duration of action will be for 24 hours
- Benzathine penicillin duration of action will be for 3–4 weeks.

**Q14. What is Jarisch-Herxheimer reaction?**
When penicillin is injected into a syphilitic patient particularly secondary syphilis the following features will develop:
- Shivering
- Fever
- Myalgia
- Exacerbation of lesions
- Vascular collapse.

**Q15. What are the predisposing factors to development of toxicity?**
- Renal insufficiency
- Dose more than 20 MU.

**Q16. What are the contraindications to penicillin treatment?**
Allergy to penicillin.

**Q17. What are the shortcomings of penicillin?**
- Poor oral efficacy
- Susceptibility to penicillinase
- Narrow spectrum of activity
- Hypersensitivity.

**Q18. Why penicillin should not be applied locally?**
Skin sensitization can occur when penicillin is applied locally.

**Q19. What is the problem of giving penicillin in patients with renal failure?**
Accumulation of penicillin in renal failure can predispose to encephalopathy. The injectable preparations of penicillin are formulated as sodium or potassium salts. This will predispose to hypernatremia or hyperkalemia is patients with renal failure.

**Q20. What is the problem of giving penicillin intrathecally?**
Excessive dose may predispose to fatal encephalopathy.

**Q21. What is the problem of giving procaine penicillin intravenously?**
Very severe reaction can occur which may be fatal. The patient may have sensation of impending death, paresthesia, and confusion which may last up to 1 hour followed by exhaustion and anxiety.

**Modified penicillins:**
- Ampicillin
- Carbenicillin
- Amoxicillin
- Amoxicillin with clavulanic acid
- Piperacillin
- Mezlocillin
- Azlocillin.

**Q. What are the penicillinase resistant penicillins?**
- ☐ Methicillin
- ☐ Cloxacillin
- ☐ Nafcillin

**Mechanism of action of penicillins:** Beta-lactam antibiotics will interfere with the synthesis of bacterial cell wall. They inhibit the penicillin binding proteins, which catalyze the cross-linking of bacterial cell wall.

**Pharmacology:** Metabolized in the liver and excreted through the kidneys.

**Precautions:**
- Serious fatal anaphylaxis can occur
- Always epinephrine, oxygen, steroids, and equipment for airway management should be kept ready to use if needed.

**Phenoxymethylpenicillin—potassium phenoxymethylpenicillin (penicillin V)**
- 250 = 4 lacs units
- Acid-resistant penicillin
- Acid stable and can be given orally
- As compared to benzyl penicillin, phenoxymethylpenicillin (penicillin V) is less active against gram-negative organisms.

**Mechanism of action:** Not inactivated by gastric acid. Food does interfere with the absorption.

**Pharmacological actions:** Are similar to benzyl penicillin.

**Dosage:**
- Dose for children:
  - 25-75 mg/kg/day in three to four divided doses
  - 125-250 mg orally every 6-8 hours
- Adult dose: 125-500 mg orally every 6-8 hours.

**Indications:** Gram-positive infections.

**Contraindications:** Allergy to penicillin.

**Precautions:** Should be given 1 hour before or 2 hours after food.

**Effects on pregnancy:**
- Category A
- The drug crosses placenta, but no adverse effects were noted. The drug is excreted in breast milk, but no adverse effects were noted.

**Side effects:**
- Allergy
- Abdominal pain
- Bloody diarrhea
- Convulsions
- Depression
- Emesis
- Fever
- Gastrointestinal problems
- Headache
- Icterus
- Join pain.

**Drug interactions:** Penicillin V can make oral contraceptives ineffective.

## QUESTIONS

**Q1. What are the conditions in which phenoxymethylpenicillin is useful?**
- ☐ Streptococcal pharyngitis
- ☐ Sinusitis
- ☐ Otitis media
- ☐ Rheumatic fever prophylaxis.

**Q2. What is the advantage of penicillin V (phenoxymethylpenicillin)?**
This penicillin is acid stable and dissolves only after reaching duodenum. This results in achievement of high serum levels of penicillin.

**Benzyl penicillin (penicillin G):**
- 100,000–150,000 units/kg/24 hours in two divided doses

- Spectrum of activity: Narrow spectrum with activity limited to gram-positive organisms and few other infections.

**Dosage:** 100,000–150,000 units/kg/24 hours in two divided doses.

**Indications:**
- Organisms:
  - Streptococcal infections
  - Pneumococcal infections
  - Meningococcal infections
  - Staphylococcal infections
  - Syphilis
  - *Gonococcus*
- Diseases:
  - Diphtheria
  - Tetanus
  - Pharyngitis
  - Otitis media
  - Scarlet fever
  - Rheumatic fever
  - Gas gangrene
  - Rheumatic prophylaxis
  - Infective bacterial endocarditis
  - Rat bite fever

**Contraindications:**
- Hypersensitivity
- Allergic reactions
- Wheezing
- Angioneurotic edema

**Precautions:** A test dose should be given intradermally or a scratch test should be done before the administration of this drug.

**Effects on pregnancy:** Can be used in pregnancy.

**Side effects:**
- Nontoxic drug
- Pain at the site of injection
- Intolerance—allergic or anaphylactic reactions.

**Drug interactions:**
- The drug levels will be increased and prolonged by probenecid
- The effects will be decreased by the following drugs:
  - Chloramphenicol
  - Tetracycline.

## QUESTION

**Q1. What are the disadvantages of benzyl penicillin?**
- ❑ Gets inactivated by gastric acid
- ❑ Gets inactivated by penicillinases produced by organisms resistant to penicillin
- ❑ Narrow spectrum of activity
- ❑ Duration of action will be short
- ❑ Anaphylaxis.

### Procaine penicillin:

**Dosage:** 25,000–50,000 units/kg/25 hours single dose intramuscularly.

**Indications:**
- Treatment of impetigo and streptococcal infection
- Rheumatic prophylaxis
- Treatment of syphilis—gonorrhea
- Meningococcal meningitis—penicillin 4-5 lacs units/kg/day 4 hourly
- Syphilis.

**Contraindications:** Allergy to penicillin.

**Precautions:** Serious fatal anaphylaxis can occur.

**Effects on pregnancy:**
- Category B
- Procaine penicillin will be excreted in breast milk.

**Side effects:** Intravenous injection of procaine penicillin may result in:
- Anxiety
- Agitation
- Behavior—abnormal
- Central nervous system stimulation, confusion, and convulsions
- Depression
- Emesis
- Fear of impending death

- Hallucinations
- Because it is insoluble it may cause micro-embolism.

### Benzathine penicillin:
**Dosage:**
- Less than 27 kg, 60,000 units intramuscular
- 1.2 million units (mega units) once in 3 weeks
- This injection will be painful.

**Indications:** Used in secondary rheumatic prophylaxis.

**Contraindications:** Allergy to penicillin.

**Precautions:** Anaphylaxis and death had occurred.

**Effects on pregnancy:** No adverse fetal defects were noted.

**Side effects:**
- Local effects—pain and erythema
- Hypersensitivity
- Hypotension
- Neurovascular reactions—warmth pallor and numbness.

**Drug interactions:**
- Methotrexate
- Tetracycline
- Probenecid.

## Cephalosporins

These are semisynthetic substances derived from a fungus *Cephalosporium gramineum*.
- *First-generation cephalosporins*:
  - Cefazolin
  - Cephalexin, cephradine, and cefadroxil
- *Second-generation cephalosporins*:
  - Cefuroxime and cefoxitin
  - Cefaclor and cefuroxime
- *Third-generation cephalosporins*: These will achieve higher concentration in all body tissues and fluids including blood, urine, and bile.
  - Cefotaxime: 100 mg/kg/day in four divided doses
  - Ceftriaxone: 100 mg/kg/day in single dose or two divided doses. This is the preferred drug in multidrug resistant typhoid
  - Cefoperazone: 100 mg/kg/day in two divided doses. This will achieve better concentration in the bile than in the blood. The safety studies for use in children are not adequate.
  - Cefixime (Orally active 3rd generation cephalosporin)
- *Fourth-generation cephalosporins*:
  - Cefepime
  - Cefpriome.

## QUESTIONS

**Q1. What are the conditions in which cephalosporins are useful?**
- ❑ Respiratory tract infections
- ❑ Urinary tract infections
- ❑ Soft tissue infections
- ❑ Septicemia
- ❑ Gonorrhea
- ❑ Syphilis
- ❑ *H. influenzae* meningitis.

**Q2. What are the adverse effects of cephalosporins?**
- ❑ Pain
- ❑ Diarrhea
- ❑ Electrolyte imbalance
- ❑ Hypersensitivity reactions
- ❑ Renal toxicity
- ❑ Neutropenia
- ❑ Thrombocytopenia
- ❑ Cefoperazone will be associated with disulfiram like reaction with alcohol.

### Cephalexin:
- First-generation cephalosporin
- Oral availability (F) (%) 90
- Half-life (h) 0.9.

**Mechanism of action:**
- Inhibits bacterial cell wall synthesis
- Binds to specific penicillin binding proteins in the cell wall of bacteria
- Cell lysis will occur, which is mediated by bacterial cell wall autolytic enzymes.

**Pharmacological aspects:** 90% of the drug is excreted in the urine.

**Dosage:**
- 25–100 mg/kg/day
- Oral route.

**Indications:**
- Superficial infections
- Respiratory infections
- Gynecological and obstetric infections
- Ear infections
- Urinary tract infections.

**Contraindications:** Hypersensitivity to cephalosporins.

**Precautions:** It can be given to patients allergic to penicillin, but rarely cross-reactions can occur.

**Effects on pregnancy:**
Category B

**Side effects:**
- Allergy—rashes
- Breathing difficulty
- Behavior changes—agitation and confusion
- Cramps
- Diarrhea—*Clostridium difficile*-associated diarrhea
- Emesis—vomiting
- Fever
- Fatigue
- Gastrointestinal upset and nausea
- Hypersensitivity
- Hallucinations
- Itching
- Joint pain
- Neutropenia (reversible).

**Drug interactions:**
- Combination with aminoglycosides or potent diuretics like furosemide and ethacrynic acid may affect renal function
- Probenecid
- Metformin.

**Cefotaxime:**
- Third-generation cephalosporin
- Available as injectable solutions and powder forms.

**Mechanism of action:**
- Binds to penicillin binding proteins
- Inhibits transpeptidation of peptidoglycan synthesis which results in death of cell wall
- Resistant to beta-lactamase.

**Pharmacological:** Metabolized in liver and excreted in urine.

**Dosage:** Dosing depends on the condition for which it is used.
- 50–100 mg/kg/day in two divided doses
- 100–150 mg/kg/day in two to three divided doses.

**Indications:**
- Respiratory tract infections
- Urinary tract infections
- Soft tissue infections
- Gonorrhea
- Urethritis.

**Contraindications:**
- Hypersensitivity to cephalosporins
- Renal failure.

**Precautions:**
- Pseudomembranous colitis may develop
- Injection sites should be changed frequently to minimize inflammation
- Bacterial or fungal overgrowth can occur when used for along time
- The dose should be adjusted in patients with renal failure.

**Effects on pregnancy:** Category B; animal studies showed mild risk and human studies showed no risk.

**Side effects:**
- Arrhythmia
- Allergy—rash
- Blood urea nitrogen (BUN) elevated
- Colitis
- Diarrhea
- Emesis
- Eosinophilia
- Fever
- Gastrointestinal—nausea
- Granulocytopenia

- Hepatic enzymes—elevated
- Itching/pruritis.

**Drug interactions:** Cefotaxime will potentiate the nephrotoxic effect of nephrotoxic drugs [aminoglycosides, nonsteroidal anti-inflammatory drugs (NSAIDS), and furosemide].

## QUESTION

**Q1. What are the fluids used for diluting cefotaxime?**
Diluted with normal saline or D5W.

### Ceftriaxone
- Longer duration of action
- Good cerebrospinal fluid (CSF) penetration
- Available as solution and powder.

**Mechanism of action:** Bactericidal action inhibits cell wall synthesis.

**Pharmacological aspects:** Excreted through bile and renal excretion.

**Dosage:** 50–100 mg/kg.

**Indications:**
- Bacterial meningitis
- Multidrug resistant typhoid
- Otitis media
- Urinary tract infections
- Septicemia
- Gonorrhea.

**Contraindications:**
- Newborn with high bilirubin
- Preterm.

**Precautions:**
- Avoid if the patient is allergic to penicillin or other cephalosporins
- May affect immunity developed by typhoid vaccines
- Should be used cautiously in patients with colitis.

**Effects on pregnancy:**
Category B.

**Side effects:**
- Allergic reactions
- Breathing problems
- Bleeding
- *Clostridium difficile*-associated diarrhea
- Candidiasis—oral thrush (with prolonged use)
- Dizziness
- Easy bruising
- Emesis
- Frequent urination
- Flushing
- Gallbladder disease
- Hypoprothrobinemia
- Hemolytic anemia
- Involuntary and incontrollable movements
- Jaundice
- Kidney problems
- Mental/mood changes.

**Drug interactions:**
- Use of calcium containing solution with ceftriaxone intravenously will precipitation in lungs
- Calcium containing ringer lactate and Harman solutions also should be avoided
- Should not be used in total parenteral nutrition/peripheral parenteral nutrition (TPN/PPN)
- Antagonizes action of chloramphenicol.

### *Aminoglycosides*

**Gentamycin:** 20 mg/2 mL.

**Q. What is the therapeutic concentration levels of gentamycin?**
5–10 µg/mL 30 minutes after intravenous administration and 60 minutes after intramuscular injection.

**Mechanism of action—bactericidal:**
- The aminoglycosides acts by binding to ribosomes and inhibiting protein synthesis
- Streptomycin binds to 30S ribosomes where as other aminoglycosides bind to 50S subunit as well as to 30-50S interface.

**Dosage:** Dose depends upon age, weight, and renal function of the patient.
- Depending upon the weight: 2.5 mg/kg/dose

- Depending upon the age of the patient:
  - Less than 7 days every 12 hourly
  - More than 7 days every 8 hourly
- Depending upon the renal function:

  | Creatinine clearance | Dose interval |
  |---|---|
  | 30–70 mL/minute | 12 hours |
  | 10–30 mL/minute | 24 hours |
  | Less than 10 mL/minute | 48 hours |

- Depending upon the organism:
  - *E. coli*: 3–5 mg/kg/day in two divided doses
  - 7.5 mg/kg/day for 10–14 days for *Salmonella*.

**Indications:**
- Acts mainly on gram-negative organisms
- Urinary tract infections
- Osteomyelitis
- Middle ear infection
- Meningitis caused by gram-negative organisms.

**Spectrum of action:**
- Acts against gram-negative bacteria
- More potent against *Pseudomonas aeruginosa*, most of the strains of *Proteus, E. coli, Klebsiella, Enterobacter* and *Serratia*.

**Contraindications:**
- Allergic to gentamycin
- Uremia
- Decreased renal function.

**Precautions:** Monitor serum creatinine levels for those who require the drug for more than 72 hours. Dose should be decreased if serum creatinine is elevated. Other ototoxic or nephrotoxic drugs should be avoided.

**Effects on pregnancy:**
- Category D
- Contraindicated as it can cause ototoxicity
- Can be safely given during breastfeeding.

**Side effects/adverse reactions of gentamycin:**
- Ototoxicity—vestibular and auditory is associated with high peak and trough levels and is usually reversible. Loss of hearing.
- Nephrotoxicity—kidney failure
- Neurotoxicity
- Thrombocytopenia
- Itching
- Joint pain
- Allergy—rashes
- Breathing problems
- Confusion
- Depression
- Dizziness
- Emesis
- Fever
- Generalized burning sensation
- Hoarseness.

**Drug interactions:**
- Along with ethacrynic acid will potentiate ototoxicity and nephrotoxicity
- Potentiates neuromuscular blocking agents
- Compatible with 5% dextrose and normal saline
- Compatible with heparin and chloramphenicol.

Q. What are the drugs that will potentiate nephrotoxicity?
- ❑ Cephalosporins
- ❑ Hydrocortisone
- ❑ Indomethacin.

## QUESTIONS

Q1. What are the adverse effects of aminoglycosides?
- ❑ Ototoxicity
- ❑ Nephrotoxicity.

Q2. What are the precautions for aminoglycosides?
Aminoglycosides should be used with caution in elderly and those with kidney problems.

Q3. What are the drug interactions for aminoglycosides?
- ❑ Concurrent use of ototoxic (high ceiling diuretics) or nephrotoxic

drugs (amphotericin B, vancomycin, cyclosporine, and cisplatin) should be avoided
- Neuromuscular blockage.

**Q4. What are the fluids compatible with gentamycin?**
Compatible with 5% dextrose and normal saline.

## Amikacin:
- It is a semisynthetic aminoglycoside
- Dose 15 mg/kg in two divided doses. Single daily dose is also given.

**Mechanism of action:** Inhibits protein synthesis by irreversibly binding to specific 30S subunit proteins.

**Pharmacological aspects:**
- Absorbed by intramuscular route
- Excreted in urine by glomerular filtration
- Highly active against *Pseudomonas*.

**Dosage:** 15 mg/kg/day in two divided doses.

**Indications:**
- Bacterial infections resistant to penicillin
- *E. coli*.

**Contraindications:** Hypersensitivity to aminoglycosides.

**Precautions:** Adequate hydration should be maintained. Impaired renal function.

**Effects on pregnancy:** Contraindicated.

**Side effects:**
- Headache
- Nausea
- Vomiting
- Ototoxicity
- Nephrotoxicity
- Skin rash
- Neuromuscular blockade
- Tremor
- Eosinophilia.

**Drug interactions:**
- Neuromuscular blocking drugs and ethacrynic acid will increase the nephrotoxicity
- Potentiates action of penicillin, cephalosporins, and beta-lactam antibiotics.

## QUESTIONS

**Q1. What are the advantages of amikacin?**
- Wide spectrum of activity
- Resistance to bacterial aminoglycoside inactivating enzymes
- In higher doses, it is useful against *Pseudomonas* and *Proteus*.

**Q2. What are the disadvantages of amikacin?**
- More toxic both ototoxic (more hearing loss than vestibular toxicity) and nephrotoxic
- Lacks activity against *Pseudomonas*.

## Streptomycin:

**Mechanism of action:**
- Protein synthesis inhibitor
- Blocks the ability of 30S ribosomal subunits to make proteins.

**Pharmacological aspects:**
- Poorly absorbed orally
- It is not metabolized and excreted in the urine.

**Dosage:**
- 20–30 mg/kg in divided doses
- Route of administration–intramuscular.

**Indications:** It has a narrow spectrum of activity.
- Bacterial spectrum:
  - *H. ducreyi*
  - Brucella
  - *Yersinia pestis*
  - *Nocardia*
  - *Mycobacterium tuberculosis*
  - Plague
  - Tuberculous meningitis
- Treatment of tuberculosis—first-line of drug.

**Contraindications:**
- Pregnancy
- Myasthenia gravis
- Labyrinthine disorders
- Old age
- After live bacterial vaccination like Bacillus Calmette-Guérin (BCG) and typhoid

- Hypersensitivity to streptomycin or aminoglycosides.

**Precautions:**
- Development of resistance is more common on prolonged use
- In renal impairment decrease the dose
- In neuromuscular disorders use cautiously
- Do not mix with any other drug in the same syringe or infusion
- May affect response to immunization with BCG and typhoid.

**Effects on pregnancy:**
- Category D
- Should not be given in pregnancy as it is ototoxic and may cause permanent deafness in the baby.

**Side effects**
- Allergy—skin rash
- Anaphylactic shock
- Angioneurotic edema
- Aplastic anemia
- Agranulocytosis
- Blood dyscrasias
- Clumsiness
- Cochlear problems
- Dizziness
- Dermatitis
- Emesis
- Eosinophilia
- Fever
- Gastrointestinal upset
- Hemolytic anemia
- Hypotension
- Nephrotoxicity—proteinuria and oliguria
- Neurotoxicity—optic nerve dysfunction and neuromuscular blockade
- Ototoxicity—deafness (transient or permanent)
- Vestibular disturbances (tinnitus, vertigo, ataxia, and disequilibrium).

**Drug interactions:**
- Ototoxicity will be potentiated by other ototoxic drugs like high ceiling diuretics, ethacrynic acid, furosemide, mannitol, and minocycline
- Nephrotoxicity will be potentiated by other nephrotoxic drugs like amphotericin B, vancomycin, cephalothin, cyclosporine, and cisplatin
- Muscle relaxants should be used cautiously in a patient who is on streptomycin.
- Potentiates the nephrotoxicity of other aminoglycosides, vancomycin, and cephalosporins
- Plasma levels will be increased by indomethacin and H2 receptor blockers
- May potentiate neuromuscular blockade and respiratory paralysis when used along with muscle relaxants or anesthetics
- Intravenous diuretics will increase aminoglycoside concentration and toxicity.

## QUESTIONS

**Q1. What are the disadvantages of streptomycin?**
- Development of resistance is common
- Cross resistance may occur between other aminoglycosides
- Streptomycin dependence
- It is not absorbed from the gut
- Attains low concentrations in the serous fluids
- Streptomycin is excreted by glomerular filtration, in conditions associated with low glomerular filtration, the dose should be decreased.

**Q2. Why streptomycin should not be given intravenously?**
Sudden rise in high levels will increase the risk of toxicity.

**Q3. What is the problem of ototoxicity caused by streptomycin?**
Ototoxicity is irreversible, unlike nephrotoxicity which is reversible.

## *Macrolides*

**Erythromycin:**
- Acid labile
- Poorly absorbed

- Erythromycin estolate will be absorbed well
- Erythromycin base is acid labile, hence should be given as enteric coated tablets
- It is a macrolide antibiotic.

**Mechanism of action:** It is bacteriostatic in low concentrations and bacteriocidal in high concentrations. Erythromycin acts by inhibiting bacterial protein synthesis by binding to ribosomes. Erythromycin combines with 50S ribosome subunits and will interfere with translocation.

**Dosage:**
- 250–500 mg every 6 hourly by oral route
  - 30–60 mg/kg/day
- *Adults*: 250–500 mg/day up to a maximum of 8 g/day
  - Three divided doses
  - Give after food.

**Indications:** Gram-positive organism including streptococci and staphylococci.
- *First line of drug*:
  - Streptococcal pharyngitis
  - Atypical pneumonia by *Mycoplasma pneumoniae*
  - *Bordetella pertussis*—whooping cough
  - Legionnaires disease
- *Second line of drug*:
  - *Campylobacter enteritis*
  - Chancroid
  - Chlamydia trachomatis
  - Diphtheria
  - Endocarditis
  - Prophylaxis against rheumatic fever and subacute bacterial endocarditis
  - Treatment of infections resistant to penicillin
  - Useful for gram-positive organisms in penicillin sensitive patients
- *Spectrum of action*:
  - Useful for gram-positive organisms in penicillin sensitive patients
  - Erythromycin is bacteriostatic at low concentrations against most gram-positive organisms, mycoplasma pneumonia, and spirochetes.

**Contraindications:**
- Allergy
- Liver disorders
- Myasthenia gravis
- Deafness.

**Precautions:** Erythromycin is not excreted in urine. So the dose need not be altered in renal failure.

**Effects on pregnancy:**
- Category B
- Erythromycin estolate may cause hepatotoxicity during pregnancy
- Erythromycin can be given during breast-feeding.

**Side effects:**
- Allergic reactions—fever, urticaria, and dermatitis
- Breathing problems
- Cholestasis
- Diarrhea, promotes intestinal motility (stimulates motilin receptors in the gut and increases gut motility and hastens gastric emptying)
- Epigastric pain
- Emesis—vomiting
- Fainting
- Gastrointestinal problems—gastritis and nausea
- Hepatic dysfunction
- Hepatitis with cholestatic jaundice
- Hypersensitivity
- Itching
- Cholestatic jaundice in adults
- Very high doses can cause reversible hearing impairment.

**Drug interactions:**
- Erythromycin will inhibit hepatic oxidation of many drugs resulting in rise in level of theophylline, carbamazepine, valproate, warfarin, terfenadine, astemizole, and cisapride
- Erythromycin will inhibit hepatic oxidation of many drugs.

## QUESTIONS

**Q1. What is the antibacterial spectrum of erythromycin?**
Most gram-positive and few gram-negative organism.

**Q2. What are the newer macrolides?**
- Roxithromycin
- Clarithromycin
- Azithromycin.

**Q3. What is the disadvantage of erythromycin?**
Most of the cocci develop resistance to erythromycin.

**Azithromycin:**

**Mechanism of action:** Bacteriostatic drug acts by inhibiting protein synthesis by binding irreversibly to 50S ribosomal subunits of the microorganism.

**Pharmacological aspects:** Acid stable and can be given orally. The drug is excreted unchanged in the bile. About 6% will be excreted in the urine.

**Dosage:** 12 mg/kg.

**Indications:**
- Pharyngitis
- Tonsillitis
- Sinusitis
- Otitis media
- Pneumonia
- Respiratory infections
- *H. influenzae*
- Chlamydial infections.

**Contraindications:** Age less than 6 months.

**Precautions:**
- Azithromycin can cause severe allergic reactions
- Myasthenia gravis patients will become worse.

**Effects on pregnancy:**
Category B

**Side effects:**
- Abdominal pain
- Breathing problems
- *Clostridium difficile* (antibiotic associated) diarrhea
- Dizziness
- Emesis
- Fainting
- Gastric upset
- Headache.

**Serious side effects:**
- Allergic reactions
- QT prolongation
- Liver problems
- Acute generalized exanthematous pustulosis
- Toxic epidermal necrolysis
- Stevens–Johnson syndrome.

**Drug interactions:**
Combination with warfarin will increase the risk for bleeding.

## QUESTION

**Q. Can the child get vaccinated along with azithromycin?**
The vaccine effect may get affected.

**Clarithromycin:**

**Mechanism of action:** Bacteriostatic drug acts by inhibiting protein synthesis by binding irreversibly to 50S ribosomal subunits of the microorganism.

**Pharmacological aspects:**
- Well absorbed orally
- Excreted through liver and kidneys.

**Dosage:**
- Children:
  - 125 mg 12 hourly
  - 250 mg 12 hourly
- Adult dose: 500 mg 12 hourly
- Extended dose: 1,000 mg once a day.

**Indications:**
- *Mycobacterium*
- Upper and lower respiratory tract infections
- Sinusitis
- Otitis media
- *Helicobacter pylori* infection.

**Contraindications:**
- Allergy/hypersensitivity to drug or its components
- Arrhythmias
- Coronary artery disease
- *Clostridium difficile* infection
- Myasthenia gravis
- Hepatic dysfunction
- Kidney dysfunction
- Concomitant use of statins.

**Precautions:**
- If creatinine clearance is less than 30 mL/min, decrease the dose of clarithromycin by 50%
- When combined with ritonavir, decrease the dose of clarithromycin by 50–75%.

**Effects on pregnancy:**
- Adverse effects are observed during pregnancy
- Should not be given during pregnancy unless no other options available.

**Side effects:**
- Allergy
- Arrhythmias and QT prolongation
- Bradycardia
- Breathing problems
- Cholestasis
- Diarrhea—*Clostridium* associated diarrhea (pseudomembranous enterocolitis)
- Emesis
- Fainting
- Gustatory problems—abnormal taste in mouth
- Hypersensitivity
- Hepatic dysfunction
- Itching.

**Drug interactions:**
- When combined with atazanavir, decrease the dose of clarithromycin by 50–75%.
- Calcium channel blockers are metabolized by cytochrome p450 which will be inhibited by clarithromycin resulting in increased blood levels to harmful levels.
- Combination of clarithromycin and cyp3a4 substrates should be avoided.
- Drugs like verapamil, amlodipine, nifedipine, and diltiazem that are metabolized by cytochrome cyp3a4 like calcium channel blockers will result in acute kidney injury.
- Combination of clarithromycin and colchicine can result in fatal reactions. The dose of colchicine should be reduced.
- Combination of clarithromycin and midazolam or triazolam will cause increased sedation or prolonged sedation.
- Combination of clarithromycin and oral hypoglycemic agents or insulin will result in profound hypoglycemia.
- Combination of clarithromycin and warfarin will increase INR and prothrombin time.

## QUESTION

Q. What are the indications for extended release clarithromycin?
- ❏ Acute maxillary sinusitis
- ❏ Acute bacterial exacerbation of chronic bronchitis
- ❏ Community acquired pneumonia.

### Nitrofuran Derivatives

**Furazolidone:** A nitrofuran compound.

**Mechanism of action:** Acts by cross-linking with DNA.

**Dosage:** 5 mg/kg/day.

**Indications:**
- Gram-negative bacilli
- *Salmonella*
- *Shigella*
- *Giardia*
- *Trichomonas*
- Diarrhea due to protozoa
- Giardiasis
- Bacterial diarrhea.

**Contraindications:**
- Intolerance to alcohol
- Primaquine sensitivity

- Infants below 1 month (increased risk for hemolytic anemia).

**Precautions:** The urine color will be orange when this drug is taken.

**Effects on pregnancy:** Must be administered with caution.

**Side effects:**
- Arthralgia
- Allergy—rash
- Blood pressure—decreased
- Chest tightness
- Dyspnea
- Dizziness
- Emesis
- Flushing
- Gastrointestinal tract—nausea
- Headache
- Hemolysis.

**Drug interactions:**
- Monoamine oxidase inhibitors (MAOIs) will cause hypertensive crisis
- Orthostatic hypotension can occur with the following drugs:
  - Sedatives
  - Antihistamines
  - Tranquilizers
  - Narcotics.

## Glycopeptides

### Vancomycin:
- Capsules: 125 mg and 250 mg
- Injectable: 3 mg/mL.

**Mechanism of action:**
- Bactericidal drug acts by inhibiting cell wall biosynthesis
- Blocks glycopeptides polymerization
- Induce platelet reactive antibodies predisposing to thrombocytopenia.

**Dosage:**
- 40 mg/kg in three to four divided doses
- 10 mg/kg every 6 hourly
- Should be given slowly by intravenous route over 1 hour or more and should not exceed 10 mg/minute.

**Indications:**
- Acts against *Staphylococcus aureus* and methicillin-resistant *Staphylococcus aureus* (MRSA).
- *Indications for parenteral administration*:
  - Antibiotic-induced colitis
  - Bacterial meningitis
  - *Staphylococcus septicemia*
  - Endocarditis
  - Peritonitis
  - Preoperative prophylaxis like implantation of prosthesis with increased risk for MRSA or methicillin-resistant *Staphylococcus epidermidis* (MRSE)
- *Indications for oral administration*:
  - Colitis caused by MRSA
  - *Clostridium difficile*-associated diarrhea
  - Pseudomembranous colitis
  - Oral administration is useful for antibiotic associated pseudomembranous enterocolitis.

**Contraindications:**
- Allergy
- Hypersensitivity to the drug.

**Precautions:**
- If frozen liquid is used, thawing by microwave or water bath should be avoided
- Should be given very slowly by intravenous route. Rapid infusion may cause erythema, flushing, hypotension, pruritus, and urticaria
- Dose should be modified in patients with impaired renal functions, elderly to about 15 mg/kg
- Extravasation may cause necrosis
- Reconstituted solution should be stored at 2–8°C and discarded after 14 days
- Should be used with caution in newborn babies.

**Effects on pregnancy:**
- Category C
- Not recommended in lactating mothers.

**Side effects:** Local pain and thrombophlebitis are more common.

- Anaphylaxis
- Bitter taste
- Bleeding/ecchymoses/hemorrhage/wet purpura
- Blood dyscrasias
- Chills
- *Clostridium difficile*-associated diarrhea
- Dizziness
- Drug fever
- Drug rash with eosinophilia and systemic symptoms (DRESS) syndrome
- Emesis
- Eosinophilia
- Erythema multiforme
- Fatigue
- Hypersensitivity
- Interstitial nephritis
- Kidney damage
- Nephrotoxicity
- Nerve deafness
- Ototoxicity
- Phlebitis
- Red man syndrome
- Reversible neutropenia
- Stevens–Johnson syndrome
- Super infections
- Thrombocytopenia
- Tinnitus
- Toxic epidermal necrolysis

**Drug interactions:**
- With other nephrotoxic drugs like aminoglycosides, cisplatin can cause renal toxicity.
- Increased nephrotoxicity and ototoxicity when used along with other nephrotoxic and ototoxic drugs.

# QUESTIONS

**Q1. What is red man syndrome?**
- Rapid injection of vancomycin will be associated with chills, fever, urticaria, and intense flushing.
- This is erythematous rash on face and upper part of the body after rapid infusion of vancomycin.

**Q2. What is the disadvantage of vancomycin?**
Systemic toxicity is very high.

## Tetracycline

Class of antibiotics having a nucleus of four cyclic rings.

**Mechanism of action:** Tetracyclines are bacteriostatic. They inhibit protein synthesis by binding to 30S subunit of ribosomes in susceptible organism. This inhibition is reversible on withdrawal of the drug.

**Pharmacological aspects:**
- Absorbed in the gut and serum level are achieved by 1–2 hours.
- Excreted in the urine.

**Dosage:** 20–40 mg/kg/day.

**Indications:**
- Gram-negative bacilli like *H. ducreyi*, *Campylobacter*, and *Helicobacter pylori*
- All *Rickettsia* species
- *Mycoplasma*
- *Actinomyces*.

**Contraindications:**
- Allergy to tetracycline
- Age below 8 years
- Liver problems
- Kidney problems
- Breastfeeding mothers
- Pregnancy
- Porphyria
- *Clostridium difficile* infection.

**Precautions:**
- To be taken before administering tetracyclines
- Rule out renal or hepatic failure
- Tetracyclines should be avoided during pregnancy, lactation, and in children
- Not recommended before 8 years of age
- Outdated tetracyclines can cause many complications like pesudotumor cerebri

- Tetracyclines should not be injected intrathecally
- Tetracyclines will worsen symptoms of myasthenia gravis.

### Effects on pregnancy:
- Teratogenic effects of tetracycline
- Staining of teeth in children results in discolored and deformed teeth, if given after 5 months of gestation, enamel hypoplasia, and intrauterine growth restriction (IUGR). To prevent this doxycycline can be given.

### Side effects:
- Antianabolic effect—reduces the protein synthesis
- Benign intracranial hypertension (Pseudotumor cerebri caused by outdated tetracyclines)
- Brown discoloration of tooth
- Chelating property—in children between 3 months and 5 years of age will affect permanent anterior dentition
- *Clostridium difficile*-associated diarrhea
- Diabetes insipidus—demeclocycline will antagonize antidiuretic hormone (ADH) action and cause diabetes insipidus
- Ear problems—vestibular toxicity
- Fanconi syndrome (caused by outdated tetracyclines)
- Gastrointestinal disturbances
- Infections—oral thrush
- Liver and kidney damage
- Phototoxicity.

### Drug interactions:
- Tetracycline and penicillin should not be mixed which will result in inactivation
- Tetracycline and isotretinoin should not used concomitantly as it may cause pseudotumor cerebri
- Avoid in patients on diuretics
- Will enhance the action of warfarin.

**Doxycycline:** Doxycycline is available as tablets.

**Mechanism of action:** It binds with ribosomes and inhibits bacterial protein synthesis.

### Pharmacological aspects:
- Well absorbed from the gut even after food
- Excreted in the bile
- More potent.

### Dosage:
- Children more than 8 years: 4.4 mg/kg in two divided doses
- Adults:
    - 100–200 mg
    - 100 mg/day 12 hourly followed by 100/day.

### Indications:
- Respiratory tract infections
- Genitourinary tract infections
- Eye infections
- Ear, nose and throat infections
- Gynecological infections
- Venereal infections
- Chlamydia infections
- Mycoplasma infections
- Falciparum malaria resistant to chloroquine
- Rocky Mountain spotted fever
- Prophylaxis against malaria and leptospirosis.

### Contraindications:
- Age less than 8 years
- Hypersensitivity
- Liver dysfunction
- Pregnancy
- Lactating mothers
- Porphyria.

### Precautions:
- Impaired hepatic function
- Blood dyscrasias
- Not recommended before 8 years of age
- Doxycycline should be taken with a glass of water to prevent injury to esophagus.

**Effects on pregnancy:** Contraindicated.

### Side effects:
- Antibiotic associated diarrhea
- Anorexia
- Blurring of vision

- Bone problems—reduced fibular growth rate
- Brown discoloration of tooth
- Congestion of nose
- Dry mouth
- Diarrhea
- Emesis
- Enamel hypoplasia
- Fever
- Gastrointestinal tract—nausea
- Hives
- Increased intracranial hypertension (outdated tetracyclines)
- Photosensitization.

**Drug interactions:**
- Isotretinoin intake will increase the risk for increased intracranial tension
- Warfarin—dose of warfarin should be decreased as tetracycline will inhibit bacterial flora and there by decreased vitamin K production
- The substances that will reduce absorption of doxycycline are:
  - Antacids
  - Bismuth subsalicylate
  - Barbiturates
  - Carbamazepine
  - Calcium
  - Eptoin
  - Ferrous sulfate/iron
  - Milk
  - Magnesium.
- The following will enhance the metabolism of doxycycline:
  - Phenytoin
  - Phenobarbitone
  - Carbamazepine
  - Rifampicin.

## Antituberculous Drugs

Isoniazid (INH) interferes with pyridoxine metabolism and predisposes to pyridoxine deficiency. It is more effective than streptomycin and para-aminosalicylic acid (PAS).

**Mechanism of action:**
- Inhibition of synthesis of mycolic acids, which are components of cell wall.
- Bactericidal in actively growing bacteria and bacteriostatic in slow growing bacteria.
- Isoniazid is metabolized in the liver.

**Dosage:** 5-10 mg/kg (maximum 300 mg/day) orally, once daily.

**Indications:** Treatment of tuberculosis.

**Contraindications:**
- Hepatic dysfunction
- Severe renal impairment
- Gout
- Alcoholism
- Allergy.

**Precautions:** Chronic alcoholism, epilepsy, and hepatitis.

**Effects on pregnancy:** Pyridoxine should be given along with INH.

**Side effects:**
- Peripheral neuritis
- Hepatitis
- Rashes
- Fever
- Arthralgia
- Anemia
- Pellagra.

Q. What are the neurological adverse effects of INH?
- ❑ Peripheral neuritis:
  - ➢ Paresthesia
  - ➢ Numbness
- ❑ Mental disturbances:
  - ➢ Convulsions (rarely)
  - ➢ Incoordination
  - ➢ Encephalopathy.

**Drug interactions:**
- Isoniazid along with acetaminophen will increase acetaminophen toxicity
- Alcohol intolerance with alcohol cause hyperpyrexia, tremor, and death
- Para-aminosalicylic acid will inhibit INH metabolism and increase the efficacy of INH

- Aluminum hydroxide will inhibit INH absorption
- Increases the effect of phenytoin
- Isoniazid will antagonize the hypoglycemic action of insulin
- Prednisolone will decrease the INH level
- Isoniazid will decrease the metabolism of carbamazepine
- Isoniazid will increase the phenytoin, theophylline, and valproate levels in the body.

## QUESTIONS

**Q1. What is the drug used for prophylaxis against INH induced neurotoxicity?**
Pyridoxine 10 mg/day.

**Q2. How will you treat INH neurotoxicity?**
Pyridoxine 100 mg/day.

**Pyrazinamide (PYZ):** Pyrazine analog of nicotinamide.

**Mechanism of action:** It diffuses into *Mycobacterium tuberculosis*. The enzyme pyrazinamidase will convert PYZ into pyrazinoic acid which is the active form. Pyrazinoic acid will accumulate inside the cell and inhibit fatty acid synthase. Pyrazinoic acid also will inhibit RpsA ribosomal protein S1 and inhibit trans-translation.

**Pharmacological aspects:** 70% of oral dose will be excreted in urine.

**Dosage:**
- 20–35 mg/kg in three to four divided doses
- With a maximum of 3 g/day.

**Indications:**
- Treatment of tuberculosis.

**Contraindications:**
- Hepatic dysfunction
- Gouty arthritis.

**Precautions:**
- Liver function tests and uric acid levels should be done
- Pyrazinamide should be discontinued if these tests are abnormal.

**Effects on pregnancy:**
- Contraindicated
- Category C
- Pyrazinamide is excreted in breast milk.

**Side effects:**
- Nausea
- Vomiting
- Hepatotoxicity
- Hyperuricemia, gout due to inhibition of uric acid secretion in the kidney
- Arthralgia
- Flushing
- Rashes
- Fever
- Loss of diabetic control
- Anorexia
- Sideroblastic anemia.

**Drug interactions:**
- Reduces serum INH concentration
- Affects control of diabetes.

## QUESTIONS

**Q1. What are the advantages of pyrazinamide?**
- More active in acidic medium
- Good penetration in CSF
- Highly effective during first 2 months of therapy when inflammatory changes are present.

**Q2. What are the disadvantages of pyrazinamide?**
- When used alone tuberculous bacilli will develop resistance
- When given along with INH the sensitivity will be present.

**Rifampicin (RFM):**
- 10 mg/kg (maximum 600 mg/day)
- Once daily in empty stomach.

**Mechanism of action:**
- Inhibits production of ribonucleic acid (RNA) by bacteria by inhibiting DNA dependent RNA synthesis
- Inhibits DNA dependent RNA polymerase.

**Pharmacological aspects:**
- Absorbed from the GIT
- The drug is deacetylated and excreted
- Highly bactericidal.

**Dosage:** 10 mg/kg.

**Indications:**
- Tuberculosis
- Leprosy
- Meningococcal prophylaxis
- *H. influenzae* prophylaxis
- *Brucellosis* (along with doxycycline)
- Legionnaires disease.

**Contraindications:**
- Diabetes
- Porphyria
- Hepatic problems
- Abnormal liver function tests
- Jaundice.

**Precautions:** Orange red discoloration of secretions, urine will occur.

**Effects on pregnancy:**
- Fetal hemorrhage can occur if given during late pregnancy
- Should be given only if indicated.

**Side effects:**
- Nausea
- Vomiting
- Skin rash
- Hepatitis
- Respiratory syndrome (shock and collapse with breathlessness)
- Purpura
- Hemolysis
- Cutaneous syndrome (flushing and pruritus)
- Flu like syndrome (fever, headache, malaise, and bone pain)
- Peripheral neuropathy
- Abdominal syndrome.

**Drug interactions:**
- Amino salicylic acid may delay the absorption of rifampicin
- Avoid concurrent administration of anticoagulants or oral contraceptives
- The following drugs will lower the blood levels:
  - Phenobarbitone
  - Phentoin
- Probenecid will increase the blood levels
- When combined with INH, severe hepatitis may occur
- Will reduce the efficacy of oral contraceptive pills.

## Ethambutol (EMB)

**Mechanism of action:**
- Bacteriostatic drug
- Interfere with the metabolism of bacteria and affecting formation of cell wall.

**Pharmacological aspects:** Well absorbed from the gut excreted unchanged in the urine.

**Dosage:** 15–25 mg/kg.

**Indications:**
- Treatment of tuberculosis
- *Mycobacterium species*; *M. avium* and *M. kansasii*
- It is given along with other antituberculous drugs.

**Contraindications:**
- Age below 6 years
- Hypersensitivity
- Kidney problems
- Liver damage
- Optic neuritis
- Susceptibility to epilepsy.

**Precautions:**
- Not given to children below 6 years of age
- Assess the visual function before and during the drug administration
- Toxic effects will be more in patients with impaired renal function
- Antacids should not be given with ethambutol.

**Effects on pregnancy:** Not recommended during pregnancy and breastfeeding.

**Side effects:**
- Anorexia
- Blurred vision

- Color blindness
- Dark urine
- Dizziness
- Disorientation
- Eye—retrobulbar neuritis
- Field defects in vision
- Gout
- Hepatotoxicity
- Hallucinations
- Itching
- Joint pain
- Kidney problems
- Lichenoid eruptions
- Mental confusion
- Nausea
- Neurotoxicity—numbness, paresthesia, and neuropathy.

**Drug interactions:** Aluminum hydroxide will reduce the absorption.

## Miscellaneous

**Meropenem:** It is a broad spectrum carbapenem antibiotic.

### Mechanism of action:
- Inhibits cell wall synthesis
- This drug will penetrate bacterial cells and interfere with synthesis of vital cell wall components.

### Pharmacological aspects:
- This drug will be excreted unchanged in the urine
- Active against both gram-positive and gram-negative organisms
- Bactericidal drug.

### Dosage:
- *For skin infections*:
  - 10 mg/kg every 12 hours
  - Maximum dose of 1 g/dose
- *For intra-abdominal infections*:
  - Preterm less than 32 weeks of gestation—20 mg/kg every 12 hours
  - More than 3 months of age—20 mg/kg intravenously every 8 hours
  - Maximum dose of 1 g/dose
- *Meningitic dose*:
  - More than 3 months of age—3 mg/kg intravenously every 8 hours
  - Maximum dose of 2 g/dose.

**Indications:** Complicated skin infections, intra-abdominal infections, bacterial meningitis, and bacterial infections.

**Contraindications:**
- Kidney disease
- Seizures
- Allergy.

**Precautions:** Dose should be reduced in patients with renal failure.

**Effects on pregnancy:** Category B.

**Side effects:**
- Diarrhea
- Nausea
- Vomiting
- Rash
- Thrombophlebitis.

**Toxicity:**
- Ataxia
- Convulsions
- Dyspnea.

**Drug interactions:**
- When used along with BCG vaccine, the efficacy of BCG vaccine will be decreased
- When combined with probenecid, the serum concentration of meropenem will be increased
- When combined with valproic acid, the serum concentration of meropenem will be decreased.

## Linezolid:

Available in the form of Tablet.

**Mechanism of action:** Inhibits protein synthesis by binding 23S fraction of 50S ribosome.

**Dosage:**
- 10 mg/kg intravenously or orally
- More than 12 years: 600 mg every 12 hourly

- The drugs can be given in 0.9% sodium chloride solution, 5% dextrose or ringer lactate.

**Route:** Oral or intravenous.

**Indications:**
- Nosocomial pneumonia
- Vancomycin resistant enterococcal infections
- Skin infections
- Methicillin-resistant *Staphylococcus aureus*
- Infections caused by gram-positive organisms that are resistant to other antibiotics.

**Contraindications and cautions:**
- Allergy
- Adrenocortical tumor—pheochromocytoma
- Bone marrow suppression
- *Clostridium difficile* infection
- Carcinoid syndrome
- Decreased blood cells—anemia, leukopenia, and thrombocytopenia
- Endocrine problems—thyrotoxicosis
- Eye problems
- Fits/convulsions
- Hypertension—uncontrolled
- Hypersensitivity to drug.

**Precautions:**
- Food containing high amounts of tyramine like cheese, bananas, and yeast extracts should be avoided
- Should not be used for more than 28 days.

**Effects on pregnancy:**
- Category C
- Should be used only if benefit outweighs risk for the fetus.

**Side effects:**
- Allergy
- Agitation
- Bleeding
- Confusion
- Constipation
- Discoloration tongue
- Diarrhea
- Emesis (vomiting)
- Eye problems—change in color vision, blurred vision
- Fever
- Forgetfulness
- Gastrointestinal problems—abdominal pain and nausea
- Gustatory problems—altered taste
- Hoarseness
- Headache
- Hallucinations
- Hypertension
- Itching.

**Serious adverse effects:**
- Anemia
- Allergic reactions
- Blurring of vision
- Bone marrow suppressions—anemia, leukopenia, and thrombocytopenia
- *Clostridium* associated diarrhea
- Colitis
- Diarrhea
- Eye problems—optic neuritis causing blindness (if used for >28 days)
- Fungal infections—oral/vaginal candidiasis
- Gastrointestinal upset
- Hypoglycemia
- Irreversible peripheral neuropathy
- Serotonin syndrome
- Rarely pseudomembranous colitis.

**Drug interactions:**
- Linezolid is a weak MAOI and should not be used with other MAOIs or with in 2 weeks after taking those drugs
- Should not be given to patients on treatment with vasopressors like epinephrine, norepinephrine, or dopaminergic agents like dopamine and dobutamine.

**Piptaz:** It is a combination of piperacillin and tazobactam.

**Mechanism of action:**
- Prevents formation of cell wall
- Tazobactam is a beta-lactamase inhibitor.

**Dosage:**
- 250 mg/kg/day in divided doses
- Should be given intravenously.

**Indications:**
- Pelvic inflammatory disease
- Pneumonia
- Intra-abdominal infections
- Cellulitis
- Sepsis
- Both gram-positive and gram-negative bacteria
- *Pseudomonas aeruginosa*.

**Contraindications:**
- Allergy to penicillin and beta-lactam
- Bleeding disorders
- *Clostridium difficile* infection
- Hypokalemia
- Neutropenia
- Kidney dysfunction.

**Precautions:** It should be used with caution in patients with renal insufficiency.

**Effects on pregnancy:**
- Can be used during pregnancy
- Not secreted in the breast milk.

**Side effects:**
- Common side effects:
    - Nausea
    - Vomiting
    - Diarrhea
    - Rash
    - Sleep problems
- Serious side effects:
    - Allergy
    - Anaphylaxis
    - Agranulocytosis
    - Bleeding
    - Convulsions
    - Diarrhea—*Clostridium difficile*-associated diarrhea
    - Erythema multiforme
    - Stevens–Johnson syndrome
    - Toxic epidermal necrolysis.

**Drug interactions:**
- Methotrexate
- Piptaz will interfere with lab results like urine glucose tests.

# ANTIVIRALS

## Acyclovir (Acycloguanosine)

It is a deoxyguanosine compound and requires a virus-specific enzyme, which will convert it into the active metabolite.

### Mechanism of Action

Acts by inhibiting the viral DNA synthesis. This will interfere with nucleic acid synthesis and thereby inhibit viral multiplication.

### Dosage

- Dose of acyclovir for children:
    - *Genital herpes simplex*: 5% ointment should be applied locally six times a day for 10 days
    - Recurrent herpes zoster: Parenteral acyclovir 5 mg/kg infusion over 1 hour every 8 hourly for 10 days
    - Intravenous: 30–40 mg/kg/day 6 hourly for 10–14 days
    - Oral: 20 mg/kg/day 6 hourly for 10–14 days. This drug is absorbed partially when given orally
    - Should not be given below the age of 2 years
- Dose for adults:
    - For herpes simplex: 200 mg give times a day for 5 days
    - For herpes zoster: 600 mg five times a day for 5 days
    - Herpes simplex encephalitis: Acyclovir 10 mg/kg/8 hour intravenously for 10 days
    - Herpes simplex keratitis: Acyclovir ointment should be applied daily till 3 days after healing
    - Herpes zoster: 5–10 mg/kg/8 hourly intravenously for 7 days

- The infected mother can be given varicella zoster immunoglobulin
- Treatment: Acyclovir can be given for treating the infection. Dose—10 mg/kg orally every 8 hours for 7 days
- Herpes simplex: Acyclovir 10-15 mg/kg/dose. Infusion with normal saline, intravenously for 10-14 days. The dose should be given for 21 days in babies with disseminated infection or if CNS is involved.

## Indications
- Herpes simplex infections
- Herpes simplex (genital, mucocutaneous, encephalitis, and keratitis)
- Chicken pox
- Varicella zoster
- Can be topically applied for genital herpes, herpes labialis, and herpetic corneal ulcer
- Herpes simplex encephalitis.

## Contraindications
- Hypersensitivity to acyclovir
- Glaucoma
- Psychiatric problems like depression
- Contraindicated during pregnancy.

## Contraindications for Topical Acyclovir Treatment
Hypersensitivity to acyclovir.

## Precautions
- To be taken during the treatment with acyclovir
- One should maintain adequate hydration during the treatment with acyclovir
- Decrease the dose in patients with renal impairment.

## Effects on Pregnancy
- *First trimester*: Fetal loss and abortion
- Gastrointestinal tract anomalies and neural tube defects.

## Side Effects
- *Oral*: Headache, nausea, malaise, vomiting, and CNS effects
- *Intravenously*: Sweating, emesis, hypotension, dose dependent decrease in glomerular filtration rate (GFR), reversible neurological manifestations like tremors, disorientation, hallucinations, convulsions, and coma
- *Topical acyclovir*: May cause local irritation and transient burning sensation after application.

## Complications
- Thrombophlebitis
- Elevation of blood urea and plasma creatinine.

## Drug Interactions
Probenecid will increase and prolong the half-life and plasma level.

# QUESTIONS

**Q1. What is the indication for reducing the dose?**
Renal failure.

**Q2. Mention a natural antiviral compound?**
Interferon.

**Q3. Does acyclovir cross the blood brain barrier?**
Yes, acyclovir will cross the blood brain barrier. The concentration achieved will be about 50% of the level in the plasma.

## Interferon
- Interferon alpha, beta, and gamma are produced by body cells in response to viral infections.
- Type I interferons are produced by cells like fibroblasts, epithelial cells, and hepatocytes.
- Type II interferons are produced by macrophages, natural killer cells, and T lymphocytes.

## Mechanism of Action
- Interferons will bind to the specific cell surface receptors and affect cell multiplication. They will also affect viral protein synthesis.

- Interferons will inhibit both RNA and DNA viruses.

### Dosage
5 mu/m$^2$/dose subcutaneously three times a week for 6 months.

### Indications
- Chronic hepatitis B and C
- Herpes simplex
- Herpes zoster
- Interferons are useful in multiple sclerosis and autoimmune disorders. Certain malignancies like hairy cell leukemia and chronic myeloid leukemia.

### Contraindications for the Use of Interferon in Chronic Hepatitis B Infection
- Allergy to drug or ribavirin
- Advanced renal, neurological, and cardiac disease
- Autoimmune diseases—polyarteritis nodosa and rheumatic arthritis
- Blood cell disorders—thalassemia and sickle cell anemia
- Coinfection with human immunodeficiency virus (HIV) infection
- Depression
- Decompensated liver disease with normal or near normal transaminases
- Encephalopathy (hepatic)
- Epilepsy
- Febrile seizures
- Granulocytopenia
- Hepatic decompensation
- Hypothyroidism
- Pregnancy
- Thrombocytopenia
- If the female partner is pregnant the male partner should not use this drug.

### Precautions
Factors to be monitored during the treatment with interferon:
- Liver function tests and hemogram
- Hepatitis B serology, especially hepatitis B virus (HBV) DNA, should be checked every 2–3 months.

### Effects on Pregnancy
Can harm the fetus, birth defects, and can result in miscarriage.

### Side Effects
- Allergy—rash
- Body aches
- Cough
- Dizziness
- Diarrhea
- Dry mouth
- Emesis
- Erythema
- Flu-like symptoms
- Fever with chills and rigors
- Fatigue
- Granulocytopenia
- Headaches
- Hearing loss
- Hypothyroidism
- Itching
- Jaundice
- Myalgia
- Pancreatitis
- Thrombocytopenia.

**Serious side effects:**
- Aggressive behavior
- Bleeding
- Convulsions
- Depression (severe).

### Drug Interactions
- Interferons will increase the blood levels of zidovudine resulting in liver toxicity.
- Interferons will affect excretion of theophylline and require reduction in dose of theophylline.

## Nevirapine

### Mechanism of Action
Non-nucleoside reverse transcriptase inhibitor, blocks function of reverse transcriptase. Nevirapine is a non-nucleoside reverse transcriptase inhibitor (NNRTI), which controls intrapartum and postpartum transmission of

HIV. It acts on the cell-free HIV-1 virions and viruses with in the cell.

## Pharmacological Aspects
- Rapid development of resistance is seen
- Readily absorbed from the gut
- Biotransformed by cytochrome P450 isoenzymes into several hydroxylated metabolites.

## Dosage
Dose will depend upon the body surface area.

## Indications
HIV-1 infected cases with decreased CD4 count.

## Contraindications
- Hypersensitivity
- Hepatitis.

## Precautions
- Monotherapy will be associated with increased risk for development of resistance.
- Nevirapine extended release tablets should not be used in children below the age of 6 years.

## Effects on Pregnancy
Safe during pregnancy.

## Side Effects
- Allergy: Skin rash
- Liver problems
- Severe life-threatening
- Hepatotoxicity
- Stevens–Johnson syndrome
- Toxic epidermal necrolysis
- Hypersensitivity
- Immune reconstitution inflammatory syndrome (IRIS).

## Drug Interactions
- Rifampicin which will induce CYP3A and CYP2B6 enzymes will lower serum levels of nevirapine.
- Fluconazole and ritonavir are inhibitors of the above enzymes and will increase the serum levels of nevirapine.

## QUESTION

**Q1. What is nevirapine prophylaxis?**
Given to antenatal mother within 6 hours before delivery in a single dose of 200 mg. The newborn should be given nevirapine in a single dose of 2 mg/kg. This will prevent mother-to-child transmission of HIV.

## Zidovudine
### Mechanism of Action
Inhibits the activity of HIV-1 reverse transcriptase. This will compete with thymidine trophosphate for incorporation into the newly synthesized viral DNA.

### Dosage
- Zidovudine 400 mg/day (100 mg four times a day) for at least 6 weeks before delivery for the mother.
- Zidovudine 24 mg/kg/day in four divided doses (8 mg/kg/dose) to the infant for 4–6 weeks. This should be started within 2 hours of delivery.

### Indications
Asymptomatic and symptomatic HIV can be treated with combination therapy, which includes this drug.

### Contraindications
- Anemia
- Bone marrow suppression.

### Precautions
- Measure the serum levels during treatment
- Hepatic impairment
- Renal impairment
- Dose adjustment should be done if needed in conditions like development of anemia and myelo depression.

### Effects on Pregnancy
- Effect on fetus and newborn
- *First trimester*: Fetal bone marrow depression, anemia, IUGR, and prematurity.

### Side Effects
- Anorexia
- Allergy: Skin rash
- Bone marrow suppression: Anemia, neutropenia, and leukopenia
- Dizziness
- Emesis
- Fever
- Gastrointestinal tract symptoms: Nausea
- Headache
- Hepatotoxicity
- Insomnia
- Inflammation of muscles: Myalgia.

### Drug Interactions
The following drugs will inhibit the metabolism of zidovudine:
- Aspirin
- Codeine
- Cimetidine
- Clofibrate
- Dapsone
- Indomethacin
- Lorazepam
- Morphine
- Probenecid will decrease renal excretion
- Ribavirin will antagonize zidovudine.

## ANTIFUNGALS

### Amphotericin B

### Mechanism of Action
This is polyene with conjugated double bonds on one side which is highly hydrophilic and OH groups on the other side which is highly lipophilic. This polyene will bind to cholesterol in the cell membranes and predispose to rapid leakage of monovalent ions like $K^+$, $Na^+$, $H^+$, and $Cl^-$. This will cause death of the fungus.

### Pharmacological Aspects
Orally not absorbed from gut.

### Dosage
- *Oral*: 50–100 mg QID
- Intravenous infusion at a rate of 0.3 mg/kg
- Intrathecal route for fungal meningitis: 0.5 mg twice daily.

### Indications
- Systemic mycosis
- Oral, vaginal, cutaneous, and systemic candidiasis infection
- Vaginitis
- Otomycosis
- Fungal meningitis.

### Contraindications
- Hypersensitivity
- Renal impairment.

### Precautions
Aminoglycosides, cyclosporine, and other nephrotoxic drugs will enhance the renal impairment.

### Effects on Pregnancy
Category B.

### Side Effects
This is a highly toxic drug.
- *Acute reactions*:
  - Aches
  - Bone marrow depression (anemia)
  - Chills
  - Dyspnea for 2–5 hours due to release of cytokines
  - Emesis
  - Fever
  - Gastrointestinal features: Nausea
  - Hypotension
  - Thrombophlebitis
- *Long-term toxicity*:
  - Nephrotoxicity (azotemia, acidosis, blood in the urine, concentrating ability

of kidneys lost, decreased urine output, edema, flank pain, Fanconi syndrome, GFR reduced, and hyperkalemia)
- Anemia due to bone marrow suppression
- Neurotoxicity following intrathecal injection for fungal meningitis. Intrathecal injections is associated with following adverse effects:
  - Headache
  - Emesis
  - Nerve palsy.

## Drug Interactions
- Rifampicin will potentiate the action of amphotericin B.
- Flucytosine will have a additive effect.
- Other nephrotoxic drugs like aminoglycosides, cyclosporine, and diuretics will enhance the nephrotoxicity.

## Clotrimazole Cream

### Mechanism of Action
Alters the permeability of fungal cell wall by binding to the phospholipids in the fungal cell wall. It inhibits biosynthesis of sterols required for cell membrane production.

### Dosage
- Topical application twice a day
- Dosage and duration will depend upon the type of infections
- Five times a day for 14 days for oral thrush
- Twice daily for 2-8 days for skin infections
- Once daily for 3-7 days for vaginal infections.

### Indications
- Skin fungal infections
- Pityriasis caused by tinea versicolor
- Vulvovaginal candidiasis.

### Contraindications
Allergy/hypersensitivity to clotrimazole.

### Precautions
Avoid application into the eyes, nose, and mouth.

### Effects on Pregnancy
Should be used only if clearly indicated.

### Side Effects
- Burning sensation
- Irritation
- Tenderness
- Itching
- Flaking of skin
- Allergic reactions rare.

### Drug Interactions
- CYP450 enzyme inhibitors
- Any drug metabolized by CYP3A4 will be elevated when used along with clotrimazole.

## Fluconazole
Has wider range of activity than ketoconazole.

### Mechanism of Action
Prevents formation of ergosterol, which is required for growth of cell membrane.

### Dosage
- Depends upon the type and site of fungal infections
- Fluconazole 200 mg for 2 weeks
- Can be given orally or intravenously.

### Indications
- Candidiasis
- Tinea infections
- Cryptococcal meningitis
- Systemic fungal infections.

### Contraindications
- Allergy to fluconazole
- Liver problems
- Pregnancy

- Abnormal electrocardiogram (ECG) like QT changes and prolonged QT interval
- Renal impairment.

## Precautions

Ventricular arrhythmias can occur when given along with cisapride. Do not administer with other drugs which will prolong QT interval like cisapride, erythromycin, astemizole, and quinidine.

## Effects on Pregnancy

- Category D
- Contraindicated in pregnant and lactating women.
- It can cause birth defects and is secreted in milk.

## Side Effects

- Abdominal pain
- Allergy: Rashes
- Anorexia
- Breathing problems
- Constipation
- Dizziness
- Delirium
- Emesis: Vomiting
- Fatigue
- Gynecomastia
- Headache
- Hepatotoxic: Mild with elevation of transaminases
- Itching
- Insomnia
- Jaundice
- Joint pain
- Kidney problems: Polyuria and renal pain
- Loss of hair
- Loss of libido
- Menstrual irregularities
- Nausea
- Neurotoxicity
- Oligozoospermia
- Oliguria
- Paresthesia
- Prolongation of QT interval
- Psychiatric disturbances.

**Severe:**
- Anaphylaxis
- Blood dyscrasias—thrombocytopenia
- Convulsions/seizures
- Stevens–Johnson syndrome
- Hepatotoxicity.

## Drug Interactions

Increases the serum levels of the following drugs by affecting the hepatic drug metabolism.
- Phenytoin
- Warfarin
- Sulfonylureas
- Zidovudine.

## Ketoconazole

- Broad spectrum antifungal drug
- Orally effective.

## Mechanism of Action

- Inhibits ergosterol synthesis and increases fungal cellular permeability.
- Ketoconazole will interact with demethylase, a cytochrome P450, which is necessary for conversion of lanosterol to ergosterol.

## Pharmacological Aspects

- Metabolized in the liver and excreted in the urine
- Replaces testosterone from protein binding sites
- Decreases androgen production form the testes
- Suppression of estradiol production will predispose to menstrual irregularities.

## Dosage

- Depends upon the type and site of fungal infections.
- 200–400 mg once daily.

## Indications
- Oral thrush
- Mucocutaneous candidiasis
- Dermatophytosis
- Deep mycosis.

## Contraindications
- Allergy
- Achlorhydria
- Abnormal ECG: QT changes and prolonged QT interval
- Abnormal heart rate: Tachycardia
- Adrenal dysfunction
- Abnormal liver function tests: Hepatitis.

## Precautions
In high doses it can affect adrenals and decrease testosterone levels and decrease in sperm production.

## Effects on Pregnancy
Category C.

## Side Effects
- Allergic reactions
- Breathing problems
- Cardiotoxicity: Prolonged QT interval
- Diarrhea
- Dizziness
- Enlarged tender breasts in men
- Loss of libido and sexual ability
- Menstrual changes
- Less toxic than amphotericin B.

## Drug Interactions
Rifampicin and phenytoin will reduce the efficacy by inducing the metabolism of ketoconazole. Following drugs will reduce the gastric acidity and absorption of ketoconazole.
- $H_2$ blockers
- Proton pump inhibitors
- Antacids.

# ANTIPROTOZOAL

## Artemether
It is an artemisinin derivative.

## Mechanism of Action
- Acts at the late stage of ring parasites and trophozoites.
- Erythrocytic stages of *Plasmodium* species.
- In the body it is metabolized into the active form dihydroartemisinin. In this it will inhibit the nucleic acid and protein synthesis.
- Interaction of peroxide containing drug with heme forming potentially toxic oxygen and carbon-centered radicals.

## Pharmacological Actions
- Acts against all malarial parasites resistant to other antimalarials.
- Rapidly metabolized into active form dihydroartemisinin.

## Dosage
Artemether (20 mg)–lumefantrine (120 mg) can be used as six dose regimen (1 bd × 3 days).

## Indications
- Falciparum malaria infection
- Resistant malaria.

## Contraindications
- Pregnancy
- Hyperkalemia
- Hypermagnesemia
- Prolonged QT interval
- Brady/tachycardia
- Allergy.

## Precautions
- Dose should be reduced in elderly people.
- Avoid using with drugs that will prolong the QT interval.

## Effects on Pregnancy
Contraindicated.

## Side Effects
- Abdominal pain
- Anorexia
- Allergy
- Breathing problems
- Bradycardia

- Bleeding
- Cough
- Chills
- Emesis
- Fever
- Headache
- Heart blocks: QT interval prolongation and first-degree atrioventricular (AV) block
- Insomnia
- Itching
- Joint pain
- Myalgia
- Rise in alanine amino transferase (ALAT)
- Rise in aspartate amino transferase (ASAT)
- Decreased reticulocyte count.

### Drug Interactions
- Lumefantrine can be combined with artemether to treat nonsevere malaria.
- Artemether should be combined with lumefantrine for improved efficacy.
- Should not be used along with drugs that inhibit CYP3A4.
- Will decrease the effectiveness of hormonal contraceptives.

## Artesunate
It is derived from artemisinin.

### Mechanism of Action
It is a prodrug which will be converted to active form dihydroartemisinin. This inhibits DNA replication and transcription.

### Dosage
- Intravenous route for severe malaria
- Intramuscular route
- Oral doses can be given for less severe cases; uncomplicated falciparum malaria
- Rectal route can be given.

### Indications
- Severe malaria
- Uncomplicated falciparum malaria
- Preferred for quinine in treating cerebral malaria
- Schistosomia hematobium.

### Contraindications and Cautions
- Previous allergic reactions to the drug
- Should be avoided in liver or kidney impairment.

### Precautions
- Not used for prevention of malaria.
- The powder should be mixed in 5% sodium bicarbonate. The powder will not get mixed easily. It should be verified if the powder is completely dissolved.

### Effects on Pregnancy
- Considered as safe during pregnancy, but not established
- Should not be used in the first trimester of pregnancy.

### Side Effects
- Allergic reactions—skin rash
- Bradycardia
- Cardiotoxicity (with high doses)
- Counts decreased (WBC count, platelet, reversible reduction of neutrophil, and reticulocyte)
- Dizziness
- Emesis
- Fever
- Gastrointestinal tract problems—abdominal pain, diarrhea, nausea, and constipation
- Headache
- Hemolysis delayed (by around 2 weeks after initiating treatment)
- Injection site pain.

### Drug Interactions
- Should not be used along with mefloquine, which results in increased clearance of mefloquine
- Interactions with drugs that inhibit:
  - CVP246
  - Amiodarone
  - Isoniazid
  - Ketoconazole.

## QUESTION

**Q1. What is combination therapy?**
- ❏ Artesunate + sulfadoxine/pyrimethamine
- ❏ In vivax, this combination therapy is associated with development of resistance
- ❏ This combination should be avoided in newborns as the effects on bilirubin.

## Chloroquine

### Mechanism of Action

Rapidly acting erythrocytic schizonticide against all species of plasmodia. Chloroquine enters the red blood cell and inhibit the parasite cell and digestive vacuole by simple diffusion. In the acidic pH chloroquine becomes protonated and cannot leave the cell by diffusion. This prevents biocrystallization of heme resulting in accumulation of heme. Conversion of toxic heme to nontoxic hemozoin by the parasite will be prevented. Chloroquine will bind to the heme forming FP-chloroquine complex, which causes cell lysis by disrupting the cell membrane. The parasites will get autodigested, but the parasites that do not form hemozoin are resistant to chloroquine.

In rheumatoid arthritis, chloroquine acts by inhibiting lymphocyte proliferation, production of interleukin 1 (IL-1), and release of enzymes form lysosomes.

### Pharmacological Aspects

- ❖ 4-aminoquinolines
- ❖ Rapidly absorbed from the gut
- ❖ Partially metabolized in the liver and more than 50% excreted in the urine unchanged.

### Dosage

- ❖ Dose 600 mg stratum followed by 300 mg after 6 hours and 300 mg daily for next 2 days
- ❖ 10 mg/kg stratum followed by 5 mg/kg after 8 hours
- ❖ 5 mg/kg once daily for next 2 days.
- ❖ Dose—10 mg (base)/kg followed by 5 mg/kg after 6 hours. The dose of 5 mg/kg should be repeated for 2 days.

### Indications

- ❖ Suppressive prophylaxis of all types of malaria
- ❖ Extraintestinal amoebiasis
- ❖ Rheumatic arthritis
- ❖ Discoid lupus erythematosus
- ❖ Lepra reactions
- ❖ Photogenic reactions
- ❖ Symptomatic relief in infectious mononucleosis
- ❖ *Entamoeba histolytica*
- ❖ Giardiasis.

### Contraindications

- ❖ Pregnancy
- ❖ Liver damage
- ❖ Eye impairment
- ❖ Gastrointestinal diseases
- ❖ Hematological diseases.

### Precautions

- ❖ Tablet should not be chewed
- ❖ Cumulative toxicity can occur in long-term use
- ❖ Can cause acute hemolysis in patients with G6PD deficiency.

### Effects on Pregnancy

No teratogenic effects or abortifacient effects are observed.

**Effect on fetus and newborn:** Deafness and retinal pigmentation.

### Side Effects/Adverse Effects of Oral Chloroquine

- ❖ Allergy: Rash
- ❖ Abdominal pain/cramps
- ❖ Anorexia
- ❖ Bone marrow suppression: Pancytopenia and aplastic anemia
- ❖ Central nervous system toxicity: Convulsions
- ❖ Deafness

- ❖ Difficulty in accommodation
- ❖ Emesis
- ❖ Eye problems: Corneal deposits and chloroquine retinopathy
- ❖ Gastrointestinal: Nausea
- ❖ Gustatory problems: Unpleasant metallic taste
- ❖ Headache
- ❖ Hypotension
- ❖ Itching (uncontrollable).

Parenteral administration can be associated with the following:
- ❖ Arrhythmias
- ❖ Blood pressure: Decreased (hypotension)
- ❖ Cardiac depression
- ❖ Central nervous system toxicity: Convulsions.

Long-term use can be associated with the following:
- ❖ Deafness
- ❖ Photoallergy
- ❖ Mental disturbances
- ❖ Myopathy
- ❖ Graying of hair
- ❖ Attacks of porphyria and psoriasis may be precipitated.

**Q. What are the adverse effects of parenteral administration of chloroquine?**
- ❏ Hypotension, cardiac depression, arrhythmias, CNS toxicity, and convulsions
- ❏ Corneal deposits which may affect vision and is reversible on discontinuation
- ❏ Rashes
- ❏ Loss of hearing
- ❏ Rashes, photoallergy, mental disturbances, myopathy, and graying of hair on long-term use
- ❏ May precipitate porphyria and psoriasis
- ❏ Chloroquine given parenterally may cause seizures in the newborn.

### Drug Interactions

The following drugs will decrease the absorption of chloroquine:
- ❖ Antacids
- ❖ Kaolin
- ❖ Combination with mefloquine will increase the risk of convulsions
- ❖ Chloroquine will reduce the levels of ampicillin.

## QUESTIONS

**Q1. What is the disadvantage of treating *Plasmodium falciparum* with chloroquine?**
*Plasmodium falciparum* acquires resistance with chloroquine.

**Q2. What are the features of chloroquine overdose?**
CNS toxicity can cause convulsions
- ❏ Abdominal cramps
- ❏ Accommodation problems
- ❏ Allergy/rashes
- ❏ Blurred vision
- ❏ Cardiorespiratory arrest
- ❏ Cardiovascular collapse
- ❏ Deafness
- ❏ Drowsiness
- ❏ Emesis
- ❏ Epigastric pain
- ❏ Eye problems: Visual disturbances
- ❏ Fits
- ❏ Gastrointestinal problems: Nausea
- ❏ Headache
- ❏ Hypotension
- ❏ Itching (uncontrollable)

Radical therapy is not indicated as this is a form of transfusion malaria, which is not associated with exoerythrocytic phase.

**Q3. What is the treatment for chloroquine resistant malaria?**
Quinine sulfate 25 mg/kg/day for 3–5 days (for chloroquine resistant cases).

### Metronidazole
- ❖ Available as 200 mg and 400 mg tablets
- ❖ *Injection*: 100 mL vial, dose of 5 mg/mL
- ❖ Preparation for intravenous infusion is available.

### Mechanism of Action
- ❖ Metronidazole enters the microorganism by diffusion, its nitro group is reduced to

intermediate compounds which will be cytotoxic and cause damage to DNA.
- Inhibit cell mediated immunity.

## Dosage
- 20–30 mg/kg in three divided doses
- Anaerobic organisms: 15 mg/kg loading dose.

## Indications
- Anaerobic organisms
- Amoebiasis (*Entamoeba histolytica*)
- Anaerobic organisms
- Anaerobic cocci
- Bacteroides species: *Bacteroides fragilis*
- *Clostridium perfringens*
- *Fusobacterium*
- Giardiasis
- Guinea worm infestation
- *Helicobacter pylori*
- Pseudomembranous enterocolitis
- *Trichomonas vaginalis*
- Ulcerative gingivitis

## Contraindications
- Neurological disease
- Blood dyscrasias
- First trimester of pregnancy
- Chronic alcoholism.

## Precautions
- If the patient is on disulfiram within last 2 weeks do not give metronidazole
- Avoid alcohol intake or other alcohol containing preparations
- Cytotoxic may cause damage to DNA.
- This drug will not be active against aerobic organisms.

## Effects on Pregnancy
This drug should not be given during first trimester of pregnancy because fetal abnormalities are reported in animals.

## Side Effects/Adverse Effects
- Anorexia and nausea
- Allergy: Rashes
- Abdominal cramps
- Brain problems: Mental/mood changes
- Coordination problems
- Dryness of mouth
- Dizziness
- Emesis
- Fever
- Gait problems
- Glossitis
- Gustatory problems: Metallic taste
- Headache
- Transient neutropenia
- Peripheral neuropathy and CNS effects after prolonged administration
- Seizures with high doses.

## Drug Interactions
- Alcohol should not be given when the patient is on metronidazole as metronidazole has similar action like disulfiram. Acute psychosis can occur.
- Enzyme inducing drugs like phenobarbitone and rifampin will reduce the therapeutic effect
- Cimetidine will reduce the metabolism of metronidazole
- Metronidazole will decrease the renal excretion of lithium.

# ANTHELMINTICS

## Albendazole
Broad-spectrum anthelmintic.

## Mechanism of Action
Causes degenerative alterations in the worm, especially in the tegument and intestinal cells. They prevent polymerization or assembly of tubulin by binding to the colchine sensitive site of tubulin.

## Dosage
- Dose of albendazole for hookworms, *Enterobius*, and trichuris:
  - Single dose
  - 400 mg for more than 2 years of age
  - 200 mg for 1–2 years of age

- Dose of albendazole for tapeworms and strongyloidiasis: 400 mg daily for 3 consecutive days
- Dose of albendazole for neurocysticercosis: 15 mg/kg for 1 month
- Dose of albendazole for trichinosis: Albendazole for 3 days, steroids may be given if systemic manifestations are severe
- Dose for hydatid diseases: 400 mg twice a day for 28 days. If needed, the dose can be repeated after 2 weeks up to three courses.

### Indications
- Ascariasis
- Hookworm
- *Enterobius vermicularis*
- *Trichuris trichiura*
- Tape worms
- Trichinosis
- Strongyloidosis
- Neurocysticercosis
- Hydatid disease
- Cutaneous larva migrans

### Contraindications
- Hypersensitivity
- Pregnancy
- Lactating mothers
- Albendazole is contraindicated below 1 year of age.

### Precautions
The drug should be taken along with food.

### Effects on Pregnancy
- Category C
- Contraindicated
- As it has caused embryotoxicity in animals, the drug should not be used in pregnancy and lactating mothers.

### Side Effects
- Abdominal pain
- Bone marrow suppression: Aplastic anemia, leucopenia, thrombocytopenia, and granulocytopenia
- Central nervous system: Meningeal signs
- Dizziness
- Emesis
- Fever
- Gastrointestinal disturbances
- Hair loss
- Increased intracranial pressure.

### Drug Interactions
- Antidiabetics will potentiate the action of albendazole
- $H_2$ antagonists will increase the serum level of albendazole
- Cimetidine, corticosteroids, praziquantel, and levamisole will increase serum levels of albendazole.

## QUESTION

Q. What are the advantages of albendazole?
- ❑ Broad-spectrum activity
- ❑ Single-dose administration.

## Ivermectin

### Mechanism of Action
Paralyses and kills patients.

### Dosage—Single Dose
- 150–200 µg/kg of body weight
- Applied to skin or taken by mouth
- Orally with about 250 mL of water on a empty stomach.

### Indications
- Scabies
- Round worm infestations
- River blindness (onchocerciasis)
- Strongyloidiasis
- Filariasis.

### Contraindications
- Allergic reactions
- Asthmatic patients
- Liver disorders.

## Precautions

- The drug should be taken in an empty stomach with about 240 mL of water. The tablet should not be cut or crushed.
- May cause dizziness avoid driving or working in machinery.
- Dizziness may be prevented by getting up slowly from bed or sitting position.
- Safety is not established in children weighing under 15 kg.

## Effects on Pregnancy

- Category C
- In animal studies adverse effects are noted on the fetus. In humans no enough studies.
- Ivermectin is secreted in breast milk and may cause side effects in the breastfed babies.

## Side Effects

- Allergic reactions
- Breathing problems
- Chest pain
- Convulsions
- Dizziness
- Diarrhea
- Edema
- Eye swelling, redness, pain, and loss of vision
- Facial swelling
- Fever
- Gastrointestinal problems: Nausea
- Headache
- Itching
- Joint pain
- Jaundice
- Knee swelling
- Lymphadenopathy
- Muscle pain
- Neurotoxicity: Depression and ataxia.

## Drug Interactions

- Barbiturates
- Benzodiazepines
- Valproic acid
- Along with warfarin can cause bleeding.

# Mebendazole

- 100 mg tablets
- Broad anthelmintic.

## Mechanism of Action

- Acts by blocking glucose uptake in the parasite and depletion of its glycogen stores inhibits polymerization of microtubules.
- Interferes with carbohydrate metabolism.

## Dosage

Q. What is the dose of mebendazole for children aged more than and equal to 2 years?
- Hookworm, roundworm, and trichuris whipworms: 100 mg twice a day for 3 consecutive days. Can be repeated after 3 weeks if not cured.
- *Enterobius*: 100 mg single dose, repeat after 2–3 weeks
- Pinworms: 100 mg once, repeat the dose after 2 weeks
- Tapeworm: 0.2 g 12 hourly for 3 days
- Hydatid disease: 200–400 mg 12 hourly for 3–4 weeks.

## Indications

- Pinworms (*Enterobius vermicularis*)
- Guinea worms
- Hydatid
- Giardiasis
- Roundworms (*Ascariasis lumbricoides*)
- Hookworms (*Necator americanus*) (*Ancylostoma duodenale*)
- Whipworm (*Trichuris trichiura*).

## Contraindications

- Hypersensitivity
- Age below 2 years.

## Precautions

Periodic assessment of hematopoietic and liver functions during long-term therapy should be done.

### Effects on Pregnancy
Contraindicated.

### Side Effects
- Abdominal pain
- Anaphylaxis
- Allergy: Rashes
- Agranulocytosis
- Angioedema
- Bone marrow suppression (thrombocytopenia and neutropenia)
- Convulsions
- Diarrhea
- Dizziness
- Elevated liver enzymes
- Expulsion of worms
- Fever
- Glomerulonephritis
- Granulocytopenia
- Gastrointestinal tract symptoms: Nausea
- Headache
- Hair loss
- Hepatitis
- Joint pain
- Urticaria
- Stevens-Johnson syndrome
- Toxic epidermal necrolysis.

### Drug Interactions
Mebendazole combined with metronidazole can cause Stevens-Johnson syndrome and toxic epidermal necrolysis (TEN).

The following drugs will lower serum levels of mebendazole:
- Carbamazepine
- Phenytoin
- Cimetidine will inhibit mebendazole metabolism.

## ANTIHISTAMINICS

- Chlorpheniramine: 2-5 mg
- Diphenhydramine: 15-25 mg
- Promethazine: 15-25 mg.

## Chlorpheniramine Maleate
### Mechanism of Action
- Antihistamines will act by competing for $H_1$ histamine receptors in the tissues.
- Suppresses the cough center in medulla
- Serotonin reuptake inhibitor.

### Pharmacological Actions
- Sedation
- Antiemetic
- Antidyskinetic
- Autonomic nervous system: Weak anticholinergic
- Dryness of mouth
- Local anesthetic effect.

### Dosage
- *Pediatric dose*:
  - 3-5 months: 0.5 mg orally every 12 hourly
  - 18 months—6 years: 2 mg
  - 6-11 years: 2 mg every 6 hours
  - More than 12 years: 4 mg every 4-6 hours
- *Adult dose*: 4 mg every 4-6 hours.

### Indications
- *Allergy*: Symptomatic treatment of allergic disorders
- Catarrh
- Rhinitis
- Hay fever
- Urticaria
- Prevent allergic reactions during blood transfusion
- Treatment of motion sickness.

### Contraindications and Cautions
### (Mnemonic A-I)
- Allergy to antihistaminics
- Bronchial asthma
- Bladder neck (urinary) obstruction and prostatic hypertrophy
- Closed-angle glaucoma
- Chronic idiopathic constipation

- Chronic obstructive pulmonary disease (COPD)
- Duodenal peptic ulcer (stenosing)
- Enlarged prostate
- Elderly patients
- Fits: Epilepsy/seizure disorder
- Gastric/gastrointestinal obstruction
- Hyperthyroidism
- Hypertension
- Intestinal obstruction
- Increased intraocular pressure.

## Precautions
Use with caution in asthma.

## Effects on Pregnancy
- Category B
- Breastfeeding: Not excreted in milk.

## Side Effects
**(Mnemonic A-H)**
- *Appetite altered*: Increased/anorexia
- *Blood dyscrasias*: Agranulocytosis, leucopenia, and hemolytic anemia
- *Cardiovascular system*: Hypotension and palpitation
- Dryness of mouth
- Dysuria/urinary retention
- *Drowsiness*: Moderate sedation
- *Eyes*: Dry
- Respiratory failure
- *Gastrointestinal disturbances*: Nausea, anorexia, and epigastric pain
- Hypotension.

## Drug Interactions
The following drugs will decrease the effectiveness of chlorpheniramine:
- Monoamine oxidase inhibitors
- Iodide
- Anticholinergics.

# QUESTIONS—PHENIRAMINE MALEATE (AVIL)

**Q1. What is the dose of pheniramine maleate?**
Oral adult dose—25–75 mg.

**Q2. What are the uses of pheniramine maleate?**
- Allergic disorders
- $H_1$ receptor antagonists will block the actions of histamine on the skin, mucous membranes, and plain muscles but do not antagonize the histamine induced gastric secretions.

# Cetirizine
A metabolite of hydroxyzine.

## Mechanism of Action
Antihistaminic with marked affinity for $H_1$ receptors.

## Pharmacological Actions
Mild-sedative action.

## Dosage
More than 6 years of age 10 mg/dose/day.

## Indications
- Allergic conditions
- Itching
- Sneezing
- Running nose.

## Contraindications and Cautions
- Allergy to cetirizine
- Age less than 2 years or more than 65 years
- Blood pressure increased (hypertension)
- Cardiovascular problems
- Diabetes
- Endocrine disorders: Thyroid diseases
- Enlarged prostate with inability to empty bladder
- Kidney failure
- Glaucoma
- Hepatic disease
- Should not be used with other antihistaminics like hydroxyzine or levocetirizine as they are similar to cetirizine.

## Precautions
- The dose should not exceed 10 mg/day
- Not useful in treatment of anaphylaxis

- This drug can cause drowsiness, so avoid driving and working at machinery
- Consuming alcohol will be dangerous.

### Effects on Pregnancy
Should not be used during pregnancy and breastfeeding.

### Side Effects
- Abdominal pain
- Blurred vision
- Convulsions
- Drowsiness
- Dry mouth
- Diarrhea
- Emesis
- Fatigue
- Gustatory problems: Dysgeusia
- Gastritis
- Headache
- Irritability
- Insomnia (when cetirizine hydrochloride is combined with pseudoephedrine hydrochloride)
- Tiredness.

### Drug Interactions
- Other drugs that cause drowsiness like opioids and codeine should be avoided.
- Theophylline will prolong excretion of cetirizine.

## CHOLINERGIC DRUGS

### Atropine
Well absorbed on oral and parenteral administration.

### Mechanism of Action
Atropine will block the muscarinic effects of endogenous as well as exogenously administered acetylcholine by competitive blockage of muscarinic receptors. This will compete with acetylcholine for muscarinic receptors. Atropine will produce mild stimulation of medullary vagal nuclei producing bradycardia and increase in rate and depth of respiration.

### Pharmacological Actions
- *General*: Increase in body temperature due to inhibition of sweating and stimulation of temperature regulating center on the hypothalamus
- *Eyes*:
  - Mydriasis by blocking the cholinergic nerves supplying the smooth muscles of the sphincters of the eye ciliary smooth muscle will be paralyzed
  - Cycloplegia with eye fixed for distant vision
  - Increases intraocular tension
  - Mild local anesthesia on the cornea
- *Heart*:
  - Sino atrial (SA) node-increases firing at SA node by blocking the actions of vagus nerve
  - Blocks the parasympathetic influences on the heart
  - Increases conduction at atrioventricular (AV) node
- *Respiratory tract*: Relaxes smooth muscles causing bronchodilatation and reduces airway resistance in asthma patients.
- *Gastrointestinal*: Reduces both the tone and motility of all parts of GIT and salivary secretion.
- *Biliary tract*: Antispasmodic action.
- *Genitourinary*: Reduces urethral peristalsis.
- *Urinary bladder*: Reduce the tone of the fundus of the bladder and enhance the tone of the trigonal sphincter. This will result in urinary retention.
- *Central nervous system*:
  - Atropine will stimulate medullar centers like vagal, respiratory, and vasomotor centers
  - Depresses vestibular excitation
  - Blocks relative cholinergic overactivity in basal ganglia
  - Toxic doses will result in central cortical excitation causing restlessness, irritability, hallucinations, and delirium
  - Peripheral vagal paralysis.

- *Smooth muscles*: Smooth muscles of gastrointestinal tract, eye, and heart receiving parasympathetic supply are relaxed by atropine due to blockade of M2 receptors.
- *Skin*: In high doses atropine will cause vasodilatation of cutaneous vessels.
- *Glands*: Decreases sweat, lacrimal, salivary, and tracheobronchial secretions.

## Dosage

- 0.01 mg/kg intravenously
- Minimum dose 0.1 mg/kg
- Maximum single dose 0.5 mg for child and 1 mg for adolescents.

## Indications

- *Eyes*: Mydriatic and cycloplegic
- *Cardiac*:
  - AV block in block caused by excess vagal activity
  - Symptomatic bradycardia
  - Heart block
- *Gastrointestinal system*:
  - Antispasmodic in gastrointestinal colic
  - Peptic ulcer
  - Biliary antispasmodic
- *Genitourinary*: Renal colic
- *Poisoning*:
  - Organophosphorus poisoning
  - Anticholinesterase poisoning
  - Snake bite
- *Anesthesia*: Preanesthetic medication reduces respiratory secretions
- *Nervous system*: Parkinsonism controls the tremor and rigidity
- *Miscellaneous*: Motion sickness.

## Contraindications

- Narrow iridocorneal angle
- Atropine will aggravate the obstruction and precipitate acute congestive glaucoma.

## Precautions

- Belladonna poisoning can occur on consuming datura or belladonna
- In patients with prostrate hypertrophy, acute urinary retention can occur.

## Effects on Pregnancy

- Crosses placental barrier
- Secreted in the milk.

## Side Effects and Toxicity

- Ataxia
- Behavior changes: Restlessness and psychotic behavior
- Blurring of near vision
- Convulsions
- Coma
- Delirium
- Dryness of mouth
- Difficulty in swallowing
- Difficulty in micturition: Urinary urgency
- Difficulty in speech
- Dry skin
- Dilatation of pupils: Mydriasis
- Excitement
- Fever
- Flushed skin
- Hot skin
- Hallucinations
- Hypotension
- Increased pulse rate
- Incoordination: Motor incoordination
- Cardiovascular collapse with depression of respiration can occur in severe poisoning.

## Drug Interactions

- Atropine will slow the gastric emptying and thereby slow the absorption of most of the drugs
- The absorption of digoxin and tetracycline will be increased
- Antacids will interfere with the absorption of anticholinergics.

## QUESTIONS

**Q1. How the competitive type of antagonism can be overcome?**

The competitive type of antagonism can be overcome by increasing the agonist concentration at the receptor site. The acetylcholine levels can be increased by administration of anticholinesterase.

**Q2. What are the indications of atropine application in the eyes?**
Mydriatic, cycloplegic, and during refraction.

**Q3. What are the effects of topical application of atropine?**
Mydriasis, abolition of light reflex and cycloplegia, photophobia, blurring of vision, and palpitation.

**Q4. What is cycloplegia?**
Paralysis of accommodation.

**Q5. What is atropine flush?**
In high doses, atropine will cause vasodilatation of cutaneous vessels.

**Q6. How does atropine cause hypotension?**
Atropine produces hypotension by depression of vasomotor center or peripheral vasomotor paralysis.

**Q7. What are the sites in which muscarinic receptors are found?**
- Heart
- Sweat gland cells
- Glands of gastrointestinal, respiratory and urinary tracts
- Smooth muscles
- Nervous system
- Eyes
- Blood vessels
- Autonomic ganglia.

**Q8. What are the muscarinic actions of acetylcholine?**
- Accommodation for near vision
- Blood vessels are dilated
- Bladder–detrussor contraction, sphincter relaxation, voiding of urine
- Contraction of smooth muscles
- Constriction of bronchus
- Diarrhea
- Emesis
- Eyes: Miosis, lacrimation increased
- Flushing
- Fall in blood pressure
- Gastrointestinal secretions increased
- Heart rate is decreased
- Increased salivation, sweating, tracheobronchial gastric secretions
- Intraocular tension is decreased.

**Q9. What is the meaning of belladonna?**
Pretty lady.

**Q10. The secretion of which exocrine gland is not affected by atropine?**
- Secretion of milk
- Salivary secretion is extremely sensitive to atropine blockade
- The antagonism between atropine and acetylcholine is of competitive type which can be reversed by increase in the concentration of acetylcholine.

**Q11. What is the action of atropine on the central nervous system?**
Atropine is a central nervous system stimulant. Mild stimulation of medullary vagal nuclei in therapeutic doses. This results in bradycardia and increase in rate and depth of respiratory center.

**Q12. How will you differentiate the mydriasis caused by atropine and a sympathomimetic amines?**
Sympathomimetic amines will not produce cycloplegia.

**Q13. What are the clinical features of acute belladonna poisoning?**
- The atropine is associated with wide margin of safety
- Dryness of mouth
- Difficulty in swallowing
- Difficulty in speech
- Tachycardia
- Dilatation of pupils, blurred near vision, mydriasis, and paralysis of accommodation
- Photophobia
- Dry flushed and hot skin
- Difficulty in micturition
- Hyperpyrexia due to inhibition of sweating
- Intense thirst

- ❏ Urinary urgency
- ❏ In severe poisoning convulsions and coma can occur.

**Q14. What is the test used to diagnose belladonna poisoning?**
Methacholine 5 mg or neostigmine 1 mg given subcutaneously will not induce any muscarinic effects.

**Q15. What is the treatment of acute belladonna poisoning?**
- ❏ Gastric lavage with tannic acid
- ❏ Physostigmine intravenously 2–5 mg subcutaneously will antagonize both central and peripheral effects. This drug can be repeated at intervals of 4–6 hours till satisfactory control over muscarinic blockade occurs. Neostigmine will be less satisfactory.

**Q16. What is the supportive treatment of acute belladonna poisoning?**
- ❏ Diazepam for restlessness and tremors
- ❏ Dark room for photophobia
- ❏ Urinary catheterization for urinary retention
- ❏ Tepid sponging for pyrexia
- ❏ Artificial respiration for respiratory depression
- ❏ Maintain the blood volume.

**Q17. What are the clinical features of chronic belladonna poisoning?**
- ❏ Dryness of mouth
- ❏ Skin eruptions
- ❏ Tremors
- ❏ Speech disturbances.

**Q18. What is the lethal dose of atropine?**
- ❏ 10–20 mg in children
- ❏ 80–130 mg in adults.

**Q19. What is the effect of atropine on uterus?**
There is no effect on the tone or motility of uterus.

**Q20. What are the indications of atropine application in the eyes?**
Mydriatic, cycloplegic, and during refraction.

## Neostigmine

Inhibits anticholinesterase which is responsible for degradation of acetylcholine there by indirectly stimulates nicotinic and muscarinic receptors.

### Mechanism of Action

Anticholinesterase will improve contraction ach, will be released from the prejunctional endings ach, and will accumulate and act on receptors over a larger area. It will directly depolarize the end plate. It does not cross blood brain barrier.

### Pharmacological Actions

- ❖ *Eyes*: Decreases intraocular tension
- ❖ *Gastrointestinal tract*: Increase in gastrointestinal motility and secretions
- ❖ *Skeletal muscle*: Stimulation followed by depression
- ❖ *Secretions*: Increases bronchial, lacrimal, salivary, gastric, and pancreatic secretions
- ❖ *Smooth muscles*: Constriction of bronchioles and ureters.

### Indications

- ❖ Glaucoma
- ❖ Diagnose and treat myasthenia gravis
- ❖ Treatment of atropine poisoning
- ❖ Treatment of curare poisoning
- ❖ Postoperative paralytic ileus
- ❖ Paroxysmal atrial tachycardia and supraventricular tachycardia
- ❖ Postoperative urinary retention
- ❖ Postoperative paralytic ileus
- ❖ Postoperative decurarization
- ❖ *Snake bite*: Cobra bite
- ❖ Belladonna poisoning
- ❖ Over doses of tricyclic antidepressants, phenothiazines, and antihistaminics.

### Dosage

0.3–0.5 mg/kg.

### Indications

- ❖ Diagnostic tests for myasthenia gravis
- ❖ Postoperative paralytic ileus

- Postoperative urinary retention
- Belladonna poisoning
- Reverse the nondepolarizing effects of muscle relaxants neuromuscular blocking agents tubocurarine, rocuronium, and vecuronium
- Snake bite.

## Contraindications
- Asthma
- Bradycardia (sinus)
- Blockage of urinary tract
- Convulsions
- Coronary artery disease
- Dysrhythmias
- Elderly patients
- Fits/seizures
- Gastric ulcer
- Gastrointestinal obstruction
- Genitourinary tract obstruction
- Hypersensitivity to the drug
- Hyperthyroidism
- Intestinal obstruction
- Peritonitis
- Megacolon.

## Precautions
- The dose should be adjusted according to the response and duration
- Muscarinic actions can be blocked by using atropine
- The dose requirement may increase as the disease progresses
- Overdosage may cause cholinergic crisis increasing muscle weakness and respiratory paralysis.

## Effects on Pregnancy
- Intravenous use will predispose to premature labor
- Use only if clearly indicated.

## Side Effects and Toxicity
- Anaphylaxis
- Atrioventricular block
- Bronchospasm
- Cardiac arrhythmias, atrioventricular block, and cardiac arrest
- Central nervous system: Respiratory depression
- Dermatologic: Diaphoresis, flushing, rash, pruritus, and urticaria
- Emesis
- Fasciculation
- *Gastrointestinal*: Dry mouth and flatulence
- *Genitourinary*: Increased urinary frequency
- Hypotension

## Features of Anticholinesterase Poisoning
- Anorexia
- Bradycardia
- Abdominal cramps
- Diarrhea
- *Eye problems*:
  - Allergic reactions
  - Blurred vision
  - Congestive iritis
  - Detachment of retina
  - Increased lacrimation
  - Pericorneal congestion
  - Phacodonesis
- Flatulence
- Headache
- Insomnia
- Muscle cramps
- *Neurological*: Syncope, weakness, convulsions, dysarthria, miosis, and visual changes.

## Drug Interactions
- Neostigmine will prolong the block of depolarizing muscle relaxants like succinylcholine and decamethonium so it should not be used along with suxamethonium
- Neomycin and kanamycin will accentuate neuromuscular block.

# QUESTIONS

Q1. What is the feature of neostigmine overdose?
Cholinergic crisis.

## Q2. What are the features of cholinergic crisis?
- Nausea
- Diarrhea
- Emesis
- Excess salivation
- Rapidly progressive paralysis.

# SYMPATHOMIMETIC/INOTROPIC DRUGS

## Introduction
The drugs that produce effects similar to stimulation of postganglionic sympathetic nerves.

## Catecholamines
Some catecholamines are:
- Adrenaline
- Noradrenaline
- Dopamine
- Isoprenaline.

### Q1. What are the types of catecholamines?
- Endogenous and synthetic catecholamine
- Endogenous catecholamines are epinephrine, norepinephrine and dopamine
- Synthetic catecholamines are isoprenaline, dobutamine and dopexamine.

## Epinephrine (Adrenaline)
Epinephrine is a potent alpha- and beta-agonist. Adrenaline is synthesized in adrenal medulla.

## Mechanism of Action
It has both alpha- and beta-adrenergic stimulating effects. In cardiac arrest, it is the alpha-adrenergic stimulating effect will be more important which causes vasoconstriction. The vasoconstriction will elevate the perfusion pressure during chest compression thereby enhancing the delivery of oxygen to the heart and the brain. Also this drug will enhance the myocardial contractility, stimulates spontaneous contractions and increases the heart rate.

### Q. Mechanism of action of epinephrine at various doses?
- Low-dose epinephrine 0.01–0.03 µg/kg/minute will provide predominant beta-adrenergic agonistic effect.
- At higher dose of 0.1 µg/kg/minute, alpha effect will predominate resulting in vasoconstriction.
- Epinephrine will mediate renal artery vasoconstriction.

## Pharmacological Actions
- *Heart*: It is potent inotropic. Increase in force of contraction, increases stroke volume/cardiac output, increases the heart rate and coronary blood flow.
- Respiratory tract—adrenaline will cause bronchodilatation.
- Gastrointestinal tract—relaxation of smooth muscles of the gut, decreases the motility.
- Bronchi—relaxation of bronchial smooth muscles.
- Uterus—contraction in nonpregnant through alpha receptors and relaxation in term uterus through beta receptors
- Spleen—contraction of capsule releases erythrocytes into the circulation.
- Hair follicle—erection of hair follicle contraction of pilomotor muscle of the hair follicle.
- Eyes—mydriasis.
- Skeletal muscles—improves neuromuscular transmission.
- Metabolic effects—increases blood sugar level.
- Smooth muscles—intravenous administration will cause vasoconstriction, particularly skin and kidneys. The vessels supplying skeletal muscles will dilate.
- Blood vessels—constriction of blood vessels in skin and mucous membrane.
- Blood pressure—biphasic effect on blood pressure will be seen on intravenous administration.

Stimulation of alpha-receptors will cause rise in blood pressure initially. Later there will be a fall in blood pressure due to stimulation of beta-receptors. The blood pressure will increase in a dose-dependent manner.

Last choice when other inotropes fail.

## Dosage

The dosage will depend upon the age and weight of the patient.

**Q1. What is the dose of epinephrine?**
1:10,000 concentration of adrenaline is recommended.
Dose: 0.1-0.3 mL/kg of 1:10,000 solution (0.01-0.03 mg/kg). Repeated every three to five minutes as indicated should be given as a bolus very rapidly.
Doses of 1 in 1,000 adrenaline are:
- <6 month—0.01
- 6 months—6 years—0.15
- 6-12 years—0.3
- >12 years—0.5.

**Q2. What is the dose of adrenaline in asthma?**
- Adrenaline should be given subcutaneously in a dose of 0.2-0.5 mL of 1 in 1,000 aqueous solution.
- Dose greater than 2.0 µg/kg will cause renal vascular ischemia.

**Q3. What are the routes of administration of adrenaline?**
- Route of administration can be intravenous or through other veins like umbilical vein.
- Or through endotracheal tubes, subcutaneous or pulmonary routes.

**Q4. How will you administer the drug through endotracheal route?**
The drug is directly injected into the endotracheal tube and pushed inside using positive pressure ventilation.

**Q5. What is the disadvantage of administering adrenaline into the endotracheal tube?**
Small amount of drug is injected into a large endotracheal tube.

A 5-F feeding tube may be inserted into the endotracheal tube and the drug can be injected through this tube.

0.01 mL/kg subcutaneously.
Concentration to administer—1:1,000.

| Weight | Total mL |
|--------|----------|
| 1 kg   | 0.1–0.3  |
| 2 kg   | 0.2–0.6  |
| 3 kg   | 0.3–0.9  |
| 4 kg   | 0.4–1.2  |

Precautions—give rapidly as quickly as possible.
Monitor heart rate and blood pressure
Higher doses will be associated with hypertension
Route of administration:
- Endotracheal.
- Intravenous
- Umbilical vein.

**Q6. When can the next dose of adrenaline be repeated?**
- If the heart rate is less than 60 after 30 seconds after administration of adrenaline, the dose can be repeated every three to five minutes. If there is no response.
- An assessment regarding hypovolemia, acidosis should be done and corrected.

## Indications

- Anaphylactic shock
- Allergic reactions—anaphylaxis
- Advanced cardiac life support
- Angioedema
- Asystole
- Bronchial asthma—acute exacerbation
- Bronchospasm during anesthesia
- Bleeding control from local site, mucosal membranes
- Cardiac arrest
- Control of hemorrhage—nasal packs of gauze or cotton soaked in adrenaline will control
- Croup
- Drug allergy
- Epistaxis
- Fibrillation (ventricular) not responding to defibrillation

- Glaucoma—open angle glaucoma
- Hypotension—arterial/low cardiac output—shock

**Q1. What are the indications of epinephrine?**
- If the heart rate is less than 60 beats/minute, after a minimum of 30 seconds of adequate positive pressure ventilation and coordinated, synchronized chest compressions.
- Asystole.

**Q2. What are the conditions of bolus dose is used?**
Bolus dose is used in treating acute exacerbation of bronchial asthma and anaphylactic reaction.

**Q3. What are the routes of administration of epinephrine?**
- Intravenous route
- Subcutaneous routes
- Pulmonary route—epinephrine can be administered through endotracheal tube or intravenously.

## Contraindications
- Arrhythmias
- Adrenocortical pheochromocytoma
- Blood pressure elevated—arterial hypertension
- Cardiac asthma
- Cerebrovascular disease—myocardial disease, coronary insufficiency
- Diabetics
- Elderly/Older patients with intrinsic asthma
- Fibrillation (ventricular)
- Glaucoma (closed angle)
- Hypovolemic shock
- Hypersensitivity to sympathomimetics
- Hyperthyroidism
- Hypoxic patients with status asthmatics
- Hypertrophic obstructive cardiomyopathy
- Ischemic heart disease.

## Precautions
- Adrenaline resistance can develop with prolonged use in asthmatics
- Should not be injected into the digits, hands, feet as it may cause vasoconstriction and loss of blood flow
- Should be used cautiously with halogenated hydrocarbon general anesthetics, cyclopropane
- Epinephrine will mediate renal vasoconstriction, so it should be given carefully in patients with renal failure.

**Q1. What are the parameters to be monitored during administration of adrenaline?**
Heart rate, blood pressure, electrocardiography (ECG).

**Q2. What is the precaution to be taken during infusion?**
The drug should be infused through a large peripheral vein or through a central vein.

**Q3. Why epinephrine should be used with caution in patients with renal failure?**
It is because this drug can mediate renal artery constriction.
Epinephrine will mediate renal vasoconstriction, so it should be given carefully in patients with renal failure.
Last choice when other inotropes fail.

**Q4. What is the danger in administering adrenaline soon after isoprenaline inhalation?**
Administering adrenaline soon after isoprenaline inhalation can result in sudden death.

**Q5. How adrenaline acts in asthmatic patients?**
- Adrenaline relieves bronchospasm by stimulating beta-receptors
- It inhibits antigen-induced release of histamine form mast cells
- Adrenaline relives pulmonary congestion by constricting the pulmonary arteries.

**Q6. What are the preconditions in using sodium bicarbonate for neonatal resuscitation?**

The baby should be adequately ventilated and oxygenated before administering sodium bicarbonate during neonatal resuscitation.

**Q7. What is the dose of adrenaline in neonatal resuscitation?**
0.1–0.3 mL/kg of 1 in 10,000

## Effects on Pregnancy

- Category C
- Crosses placenta and may cause congenital anomalies, anoxia, fetal tachycardia, extrasystoles, etc.
- During second stage of pregnancy, adrenaline can cause anoxia to the fetus
- Adrenaline is secreted in the breast milk and breastfeeding should be avoided.

## Side Effects

- Anxiety
- Angina pectoris
- Arrhythmias—ventricular arrhythmias
- Blood pressure elevation (hypertension)
- Cerebral hemorrhage
- Dizziness
- Extravasations may produce skin necrosis
- Fear
- Fatigue
- Gastrointestinal—nausea, vomiting
- Headache
- Ischemia
- Palpitations
- Tremor
- Diabetics may have a transient increase in glucose level.

## Drug Interactions

- Additive effect with other sympathomimetic drugs
- Potentiation of pressor effects with tricyclic antidepressants—monoamine oxidase inhibitors (MAOIs), levothyroxine
- Antagonized by alpha-blockers, beta-blockers
- Beta-blockers—severe hypertension
- Spironolactone will diminish the vasoconstriction effects.

# QUESTIONS

**Q1. What is Dale's vasomotor reversal?**
When adrenaline is given after administration of ergotoxine an alpha-blocking drug, there will be a fall in blood pressure.

**Q2. Why injection of adrenaline should be avoided into the buttocks?**
Injection of adrenaline into the buttocks is associated with gas gangrene.

**Q3. What are the preconditions that must be fulfilled before administering epinephrine?**
The baby should have been adequate ventilated and oxygenated because epinephrine will increase the oxygen consumption by the cardiac muscles. If hypoxia is present, there is a risk of myocardial ischemia.
Precautions—give rapidly as quickly as possible.
*Acidosis* will be corrected spontaneously, with resuscitation and adequate circulation.

## Norepinephrine

- Noradrenaline is a sympathomimetic amine.
- A neurotransmitter in the brain, sympathetic nervous system.

## Mechanism of Action

- It acts on both alpha-1 and alpha-2 receptors.
- Predominantly stimulates alpha-adrenergic causing peripheral vasoconstriction.
- Stimulation of beta-1 adrenergic is also seen which results inotropic action on heart and dilatation of coronary arteries.

## Pharmacological Actions

- Blood vessels—constricts blood vessels of skin and mucous membranes.
- Blood pressure: Intravenous administration of norepinephrine will increase the blood

pressure due to increased systemic vascular resistance. It increases blood pressure due to severe vasoconstriction. This decreases renal blood flow with splanchnic vasoconstriction.
- Heart: Norepinephrine will increase the heart rate.
- Bronchus—no bronchodilator effect.
- Gastrointestinal system—relaxation of smooth muscle of intestines.
- Eyes—increases production of tears.

## Dosage of Noradrenaline
Intravenous infusion in a dose of 0.3–2 µg/kg/minute.

## Indications
- Shock especially septic shock when systemic vascular resistance is low
- Acute hypotension.

## Contraindications and Cautions
- Hypertension
- Hypersensitivity
- Hypovolemic shock without blood volume replacement

This drug should be used cautiously in patients with the following conditions:
- Angina pectoris (Prinzmetal's angina)
- Blood clot in arteries—peripheral vessels, mesenteric artery
- Coronary thrombus
- Diabetes
- Elderly people
- Fluid loss hypotension without fluid replacement
- Gastrointestinal tract thrombosis—mesenteric artery thrombosis
- Hypotension following heart attack
- Hyperthyroidism
- Hypoxia.

## Precautions
Appropriate volume replacement should be given during administration of this drug. If not, hypotension will recur after discontinuation of the drug.

## Effects on Pregnancy
Noradrenaline can reduce the blood supply to the placenta. It can cause fetal bradycardia. Contraction of uterus may cause fetal asphyxia especially late in pregnancy. It should be used only if indicated.

There will be no effect to the baby as it is not absorbed from the intestines. But it can lead to decreased milk production.

## Side Effects of Noradrenaline
- Appetite decreased
- Anxiety
- Arrhythmias
- Blood pressure elevated (hypertension)
- Confusion
- Dyspnea
- Emesis
- Extravasations may produce skin necrosis at the site of injection
- Feeling sick
- Gangrene of extremities
- Glaucoma (closed angle glaucoma)
- Hypoxia
- Heart rate increased or decreased
- Hypovolemia
- Insomnia
- Ischemia
- Increased myocardial oxygen demand
- Increased pulmonary vascular resistance
- Palpitations.

## Drug Interactions
- Noradrenaline is compatible with 5% glucose, sodium chloride solutions.
- Noradrenaline should not be used with anesthetic agents, cyclopropane and halothane as it will increase cardiac autonomic irritability.
- The following drugs may cause prolonged hypertension or arrhythmias:
  - Adrenergic drugs
  - Linezolid
  - Halogenated anesthetic agents
  - Monoamine oxidase inhibitors
  - Serotonergic drugs
  - Tricyclic antidepressants.

- Noradrenaline is incompatible and should not be mixed with the following drugs:
  - Barbiturates
  - Sodium bicarbonate
  - Chlorthiazide
  - Chlorpheniramine

## QUESTIONS

**Q1. What is the role of noradrenaline in tetralogy of Fallot (TOF) after Blalock-Taussig (BT) shunt?**
Noradrenaline will be used to increase the blood pressure to facilitate blood flow through BT shunt.

**Q2. What are the differences between epinephrine and norepinephrine?**

| Features | Epinephrine | Norepinephrine |
| --- | --- | --- |
| Receptors | Potent alpha- and beta-adrenergic receptors agonist in lower doses | Stimulates predominantly alpha-adrenergic receptors |
| Stroke volume | Increase | |
| Blood pressure | Increases stroke volume | Increase in blood pressure due to increase in SVR |
| Cardiac output and coronary blood flow | | No change in cardiac output or mild increase in stroke volume and coronary blood flow |
| Renal blood flow | Vasoconstriction in kidneys | Decreases renal blood flow with splanchnic vasoconstriction and reduced hepatic blood flow |
| Respiratory tract | Bronchodilatation | No bronchodilator effect |
| Metabolic effects | Raises blood sugar | Does not raise the blood sugar |
| Routes of administration | • Intravenous route<br>• Subcutaneous route<br>• Pulmonary route | |

*Contd...*

*Contd...*

| Features | Epinephrine | Norepinephrine |
| --- | --- | --- |
| Uses | • Asthma<br>• Shock<br>• Heart failure<br>• Advanced cardiac life support | |

## Dopamine

- Injection 200 mg/5 mL ampoules
- 200 mg/5 mL that is 40 mg/mL
- Add 15 mg to 50 cc of 5% dextrose
- Dopamine-mediated positive inotropic action depends on conversion of dopamine to norepinephrine
- Inotropic support by dopamine 5–10 µg/kg/minute by continuous infusion (To give a dose of 10 µg/kg/minute, 30 mg/kg of the drug is added to 50 mL of normal saline and infused at 1 mL/hour).

### Mechanism of Action

- This is a neurotransmitter and precursor of epinephrine and norepinephrine.
- It acts on dopaminergic (D1 and D2) receptors and adrenergic (alpha and beta-1) receptors.
- It acts on dopaminergic receptors (D1) present in the renal and splanchnic vasculature and produces vasodilatation in low doses by raising cyclic adenosine monophosphate (cAMP). This will increase glomerular filtration rate (GFR) and $Na^+$ excretion.
- It acts on alpha- and beta-adrenergics in the myocardium.
- Stimulation of beta-adrenergic receptors will result in positive chronotropy, inotropy and dromotropy.
- Indirect effects—inhibitions of norepinephrine reuptake at the nerve terminal, release of norepinephrine at the nerve terminal and synthesis of norepinephrine.
- Reversible suppression of prolactin and thyrotropin secretion.

**Q. What is the mechanism of action of dopamine?**

Dose-related stimulation of dopaminergic beta- and alpha-receptors with dose-related inotropic and vasopressor effects. Dopamine acts in part by releasing norepinephrine from the nerve endings of the heart.

  a. *Low dose (renal dose)*: At relatively low doses, 1–5 µg/kg/minute, dopamine stimulates dopaminergic receptors increasing the blood flow due to its effect on dopaminergic receptors. It will cause renal, mesenteric and cerebral vasodilatation.

  1–5 µg/kg/minute increases renal and mesenteric blood flow, less effect on heart rate and cardiac output. The dopaminergic receptors are affected. The urine output will be increased.

  b. *Intermediate dose (cardiotonic dose)*: 5–15 µg/kg/minute. At moderate doses, it predominantly acts on beta-adrenergic receptors positive inotropic effect due to direct beta-1 action and that due to NA release with less chronotropic effect on heart. This will cause increased myocardial contractility, increase in heart rate and cardiac output. This will be an advantage in treating shock.

  It increases renal blood flow, heart rate and cardiac output. This will be increased myocardial contractility. Beta-1 receptors are affected.

  With a dose above 10 µg/kg/minute beta-receptor action will predominate.

  c. *High dose (pressor dose)*: Greater than 20 µg/kg/minute. At higher doses, alpha-adrenergic (alpha-1) stimulation will be predominate causing severe vasoconstriction, marked cardiac effect and decrease in renal blood flow.

  *Large doses* greater than 20 mg/kg/minute will produce vasoconstriction. It increases the heart rate and increases renal blood flow. There will be peripheral vasoconstriction. Alpha-1 and beta-1 receptors are affected. The risk of tachyarrhythmia is increased.

| Dose of dopamine (µg/kg/minute) | Mechanism of action |
|---|---|
| 2–5 µg/kg/minute | Increases renal perfusion and urinary output |
| 5–15 µg/kg/minute | Beta-1 receptor stimulation causes increased myocardial contractility, cardiac output, heart rate |
| >20 µg/kg/minute | Alpha-receptor stimulation causes vasoconstriction and increase blood pressure |

*Pharmacological Actions*

- Chronotropic
- Arrhythmogenic
- Selective renal vasodilation
- Increases cardiac output and urinary outflow
- Improves blood pressure.

**Q1. What are the blood pressure changes in a patient receiving dopamine?**

Dopamine acts by a positive inotropic effect on the cardiac muscle resulting in increased blood pressure.

*Dosage*

Dosage of dopamine will depend upon the condition treated. The alpha, beta or dopaminergic effects depends upon the dose.

**Q1. How will you calculate the amount of dopamine to be infused?**

Milligram of dopamine/100 mL solution =

$$\frac{6 \times \text{weight (kg)} \times \text{Desired dose (µg/kg/minute)}}{\text{Desired fluid (mL/hour)}}$$

- Monitor heart rate and blood pressure
- Begin as 5 µg/kg/minute (if necessary increase up to 20 (µg/kg/minute)

- Available as 40 mg/mL, 5 mL ampoules are available
- 0.3 mL/kg of dopamine should be added to 20 mL of 5% dextrose and should be run at a rate of 0.55 mL/hour. This will provide 5 µg/kg/minute of dopamine.

## Indications

- Adjunctive therapy for shock refractory to adequate volume replacement
- Bradycardia
- Bactremic shock even after adequate volume expansion
- Cardiogenic shock
- Cardiac output low
- Decompensated congestive cardiac failure (CCF) (severe)
- Hypotension even after adequate volume expansion.

## Contraindications

- Pheochromocytoma, tachyarrhythmias, hypovolemia
- Hyperthyroidism
- Primary pulmonary hypertension (PPHN)
- Asthma
- Buerger's disease
- Coronary artery disease
- Circulation problems like Raynaud's syndrome
- Diabetes
- Frostbite.

## Precautions

Precautions that should be taken before dopamine administration:
- Correct hypovolemia before administering dopamine
- Extravasations can cause tissue necrosis and gangrene
- Monitor vital signs constantly
- Give as an infusion using an infusion pump.

## Effects on Pregnancy

Category C.

## Side Effects/Adverse Reactions of Dopamine

- Arrhythmias, tachycardia, widened QRS complex, bradycardia
- Angina pain
- Azotemia
- Blood pressure elevated (hypertension)
- Chest pain
- Diuresis (excessive diuresis)
- Ectopic beats
- Fast heart beats
- Gangrene of extremities (high does over prolonged periods)
- Hypotension due to vasodilatation
- Higher doses will cause vasoconstriction
- Subcutaneous infiltration may predispose to subcutaneous necrosis
- High doses will cause tachycardia, ectopic heart beats
- Worsen pulmonary hypertension and thereby worsening of ventilation perfusion mismatch.

## Drug Interactions

- Monoamine oxidase inhibitors (MAOIs)
- Hypotension (the risk is more when phenytoin is administered along with this).

## QUESTIONS

Q1. What are the indications of dopamine toxicity? How will you treat?
Decreased urine output, tachycardia and arrhythmias. It can be treated with alpha-blocker phentolamine.

Q2. What is the danger of infusing large doses for a long time?
It may cause ischemia and gangrene of limbs.

Q3. Can dopamine be given with phenytoin?
No, bradycardia and hypotension may be exacerbated.

Q4. What is the effect of intravenously administered dopamine on CNS?
The intravenously administered dopamine will not cross the blood-brain barrier.

**Q5. How will you prepare dopamine for infusion?**
First calculate the amount of dopamine needed by following formula.
  Milligram of dopamine to be added in 100 mL of solution = 6 × infants weight in kg.
  Flow rate of 1 ml/per hour will deliver 1 µg/kg/minute.
  (To give a dose of 10 µg/kg/minute, 30 mg/kg of the drug is added to 50 mL of normal saline and infused at 1 mL/hour.)
  The drug is started with a dose of 2 µg/kg/minute and then slowly increased until the desired effect is achieved at low doses of 5 µg/kg/minute. This causes renal vasodilatation. In high doses of 10 µg/kg/minute, the drug causes increased total peripheral resistance and increased heart rate.
  Dopamine-mediated positive inotropic action depends on conversion of dopamine to norepinephrine.
  Inotropic support by dopamine 5–10 µg/kg/minute by continuous infusion.

**Q6. What is the action of dopamine on CNS?**
As this does not cross blood-brain barrier, there is no action on CNS.

**Q7. What is the precaution to be taken before infusing dopamine?**
Give as an infusion using an infusion pump.

## Dobutamine

- It is a derivative of dopamine.
- Dopamine-mediated positive inotropic action depends on conversion of dopamine to norepinephrine.
- Dobutamine dose 0.5 mL/hour of this preparation will provide 5 µg/kg/minute.
- Available as 12.5 mg/mL, 15 mg/mL and 50 mg/mL. This will not bind to dopamine receptors and will not increase renal blood flow.

## Mechanism of Action

- Selective beta-1 agonist.
- Dobutamine is a derivative of dopamine with selective inotropic effect and negligible chronotropic effect and peripheral vascular actions. This has a selective inotropic effect in patients with low cardiac output with little change in heart rate and no change in systemic vascular resistance or blood pressure. Unlike dopamine this drug does not cause renal vasodilatation. Dobutamine primarily a direct-acting beta-adrenergic agonist selectively acting on beta-adrenergic 1 receptor. This drug acts weakly on beta-2 receptors causing vasodilatation.
- Dobutamine is used as an adjunct to dopamine therapy in a dose of 5–8 µg/kg/minute. It has direct inotropic effects with a moderate reduction in peripheral vascular resistance.

**Q1. What will be the action of dobutamine in low and high doses?**
In doses less than 10 µg/kg/minute, beta-1 receptors are affected. This will cause increased myocardial contractility.
  In doses greater than 10 µg/kg/minute, alpha-1 and beta-1 receptors are affected. This will cause increased myocardial contractility. In high doses of 10 µg/kg/minute, the drug causes increased total peripheral resistance and increased heart rate.

## Dosage

- 5–8 µg/kg/minute.
- The drug is started with a dose of 2 µg/kg/minute and then slowly increased until the desired effect is achieved at low doses of 5 µg/kg/minute. This causes renal vasodilatation.
- Inotropic support by dopamine 5–10 µg/kg/minute by continuous infusion (To give a dose of 10 µg/kg/minute, 30 mg/kg of the drug is added to 50 mL of normal saline and infused at 1 mL/hour).

## Indications

*Dobutamine* is used as an adjunct to dopamine therapy in a dose of 5-8 µg/kg/minute. It has direct inotropic effects with a moderate reduction in peripheral vascular resistance.
* Refractory cardiac failure not responding to digitalis
* Cardiac pump failure associated with myocardial infarction
* Bacteremic shock—beneficial hemodynamic changes in bacteremic shock.

## Contraindications

* Obstructive lesions in the heart like idiopathic hypertrophic subaortic stenosis
* Arrhythmias
* Hypersensitivity to dobutamine.

## Precautions

* During dobutamine infusion, blood pressure and ECG should be monitored. Cardiac output and pulmonary wedge pressure monitoring should be done if possible.
* Hypovolemia should be corrected before infusion of dobutamine.
* Mechanical obstruction like severe valvular aortic stenosis should be ruled out.
* Serum potassium levels should be monitored as dobutamine can lower serum potassium.

## Effects on Pregnancy

Category B.

## Side Effects/Adverse Reactions of Dobutamine

* Arrhythmias
* Bronchospasm
* Cutaneous vasoconstriction
* Dyspnea
* Ectopics—increase AV conduction and may precipitate ventricular ectopy
* Fever
* Hypertension
* Hypotension—high infusion will predispose to hypotension due to vasodilatation
* Hypersensitivity—skin rash
* Increased heart rate (tachycardia).

## Drug Interactions

Cardiac output will be increased if use along with nitroprusside and low pulmonary wedge pressure.

## QUESTIONS

**Q1. How will you prepare the dobutamine solution for use?**
Add 2.4 mL of 12.5 mg preparation or 1.2 mL of 25 mg preparation or 0.6 mL of 50 mg preparation in 50 mL of 5% dextrose 0.5 mL/hour of this solution will provided 5 µg/kg/minute of dobutamine.

**Q2. What is the rate of infusion of dobutamine?**
Rate of infusion of dobutamine is 2.5-15 µg/kg/minute. Maximum dose is 20 µg/kg/minute.

**Q3. Can dobutamine be infused in an alkaline medium?**
In alkaline medium, dobutamine will lose it potency like other catecholamines.

**Q4. What is the advantage of dobutamine over dopamine?**
Dobutamine will reduce the systemic resistance with only modest increase in the heart rate. Also the blood pressure is not much affected. As it does not bind with dopamine receptors, it will not cause increase in renal blood flow. It is less arrhythmogenic than adrenaline.

**Q5. What is the contraindication for dobutamine?**
  ❑ Obstructive lesions in the heart like idiopathic hypertrophic subaortic stenosis
  ❑ Arrhythmias

**Q6. What is rule for dopamine?**

| Dopamine | 0.6 × body weight = mg to be added to 100 mL, 1 mL/hour will deliver 1 µg/kg/minute |
|---|---|

By reducing the ventricular filling pressure, it will tend to reduce the myocardial oxygen demand and improve the myocardial perfusion and coronary oxygen reserve. Dobutamine infusion 5–20 µg/kg/minute will improve the heart function and tissue oxygenation.

**Q7. Can you use dobutamine along with dopamine?**
Yes. Dobutamine will be helpful to prevent vasoconstriction caused by dopamine.

**Q8. How will dobutamine differ from dopamine?**
Dobutamine will not cause renal vasodilatation like dopamine. This will be useful in refractory chronic cardiac failure not responding to dopamine.

Dobutamine will lose its effect in alkaline medium like other catecholamines.

In low output cardiac failure, dobutamine will increase the cardiac output without increasing the heart rate.

**Q9. How does dobutamine differ from other catecholamines?**
Unlike other catecholamines, dobutamine will not increase the blood pressure due to increasing vasoconstriction.

**Q10. What are the advantages of combining dopamine and dobutamine?**
Use of dopamine and dobutamine will offset the adverse effect of each other.

**Q11. What is the precaution to be taken before infusing dobutamine?**
Hypovolemia should be corrected.

**Q12. What are the parameters you will monitor in a patient on dobutamine?**
Continuous monitoring of heart rate and blood pressure is needed.

# ANTIHYPERTENSIVES

Antihypertensive drugs include many drugs acting at various site and are used to control, prevent or treat hypertension.

## Alpha-blockers—Prazosin

- Alpha-adrenergic blockers/antiadrenergic drugs
- It is a quinazoline derivative
- Effect of single dose will last up to 6–8 hours.

### Mechanism of Action

Prazosin, a postsynaptic alpha-1 receptor blocker, will reduce preload and left ventricular impedance without causing tachycardia. It should be given only after improving blood pressure in hypotensive patients.

Prazosin is a selective alpha-1 receptor blocker which causes dilatation of both resistance and capacitance vessels (arterial and venous vessels).

This drug causes both arterial and venous dilatation by causing only slight reduction in venous return and cardiac output. This drug causes more arterial dilatation than venous dilatation.

Prazosin also inhibits phosphodiesterase which will degrade cyclic adenosine monophosphate (cAMP). This results in increased smooth muscle cAMP which causes vasodilatation.

It is helpful in left ventricular failure by reducing preload and afterload.

Prazosin will relax smooth muscles in the prostate by blocking alpha-1 receptors.

### Pharmacological Actions

- Prazosin is metabolized in the liver and excreted in the bile
- Moderately potent antihypertensive that blocks sympathetically-mediated vasoconstriction
- It is a peripheral vasodilator that dilates arterioles more than the veins.

## Dosage
- Effective orally
- Metabolized in the liver and excreted in the bile.

## Indications
Prazosin is used in the treatment of following conditions:
- Essential hypertension
- Scorpion sting
- Left ventricular failure not controlled by digitalis and diuretics
- Raynaud's disease
- Prostatic hypertrophy—by blocking alpha receptors in the trigone of the bladder and prostate improves the urinary flow. Reduces residual urine in the bladder
- Pheochromocytoma.

## Contraindications
Congestive cardiac failure due to mechanical outflow obstruction.

## Precautions
- Hepatic impairment
- Pregnancy
- Lactation
- Pheochromocytoma
- Children below 12 years
- Abrupt withdrawal
- About 90% of prazosin will be metabolized in the liver and only 10% will be available. Hence in liver impairment, the dose should be decreased
- As a first dose effect, dizziness and fainting can occur which can be minimized by starting the low dose at bed time.

## Effects on Pregnancy
It should be used only if benefits outweigh the risk for fetus.

## Side Effects/Adverse Effects of Prazosin
- Allergy—rash
- Blurred vision
- Constipation
- Consciousness lost (in large dose)
- Dry mouth
- Dizziness
- Drowsiness
- Dreaming
- Emesis
- Fainting
- Gastrointestinal tract (GIT) symptoms—nausea
- Headache
- Postural hypotension
- Weakness
- Palpitation
- Nasal blockade.

In higher doses, ejaculation in males will be impaired.

## Drug Interactions
It enhances effects of antihypertensives and diuretics.

## QUESTIONS

**Q1. Why there is no relative tachycardia as compared to phentolamine and phenoxybenzamine?**
Prazosin is a selective alpha-1 receptor blocker. It is less potent on alpha-2 receptor blockers.

**Q2. Why prazosin is not used as first line of drug in treating hypertension?**
Prazosin is not used as first line of drug in treating hypertension due to development of tolerance with monotherapy.

**Q3. What are the advantages of prazosin?**
This drug will not affect the renal function, cardiac output, or renin-angiotensin axis.

**Q4. What is the duration of action of prazosin?**
The duration of action of prazosin is about 10 hours.

**Q5. What is first dose effect? How can it be prevented?**
Prazosin can cause postural hypotension which can follow first dose causing

dizziness and fainting. This can be prevented by starting at a low dose and starting the drug at bed time.

Effect of single dose will last up to 6–8 hours.

## Beta-blockers—Propranolol

Beta blockers act by blocking the beta adrenergic effects of adrenaline (epinephrine)

### Mechanism of Action

This drug will block the action of catecholamines mediated through β-receptor stimulation. It inhibits the activity of the membrane enzyme adenylyl cyclase resulting in decreased production of cAMP.

It prevents adrenaline-induced glycogenolysis.

It inhibits release of free-fatty acids from the adipose tissue.

### Pharmacological Actions

- Antihypertensive
- Antianginal
- Decreases the heart rate and force of contraction
- Decreases cardiac output
- Increases bronchial resistance by blocking β2-receptors
- Reduces intraocular pressure
- Modifies carbohydrate and lipid metabolism.

**Q1.** What are the effects of β-receptor stimulation on the heart?
- ❑ Increases automaticity enhances atrioventricular (AV) conduction
- ❑ Shortens the refractory period in the supraventricular tissues.

**Q2.** What is the pharmacological action of propranolol on the normal heart?
There is no marked effect on the normal heart at rest.

**Q3.** What are the pharmacological actions of propranolol on the heart in conditions with increased sympathetic tone?

Prevents increase in heart rate, cardiac output, and stroke work.

### Dosage

0.1–0.2 mg/kg/day.

### Indications

Propranolol is useful in the treatment of following conditions:
- Angina pectoris
- Adrenocortical pheochromocytoma
- Anxiety states—propranolol will reduce the palpitations, tachycardia, sweating, and diarrhea
- Blood pressure increased—hypertension
- Cyanotic spell in tetralogy of Fallot (TOF)
- Dysrhythmias/cardiac arrhythmias
- Endocrine problems—thyrotoxicosis
- Esophageal variceal bleeding in portal hypertension
- Familial (essential) tremors
- Fibrillation—atrial fibrillation
- Glaucoma—chronic open angle glaucoma
- Hypertrophic obstructive cardiomyopathy
- Infarction—postmyocardial infarction
- Migraine.

### Contraindications

- Acute myocardial infarction
- Acute decompensated cardiac failure
- Atrioventricular (AV) block second or third degree
- Bronchial asthma (can precipitate life-threatening asthma)
- Bradycardia less than 60 beats/min
- Cardiogenic shock
- Chronic obstructive pulmonary disease (COPD)/chronic obstructive lung disease
- Diabetes (insulin dependent)—hypoglycemia symptoms will be masked
- Endocrine—hypothyroidism
- Failure (cardiac failure)
- Gestational period—pregnancy
- Heart block—partial or complete heart block
- Heart—myocardial insufficiency

- Inadequate/reduced cardiac reserve
- Myasthenia gravis.

**Relative contraindication for use of propranolol:**
- Active airway disease
- Bradycardia
- Cardiogenic shock
- Moderate or severe left ventricular failure
- Hypotension.

## Precautions
- Impaired hepatic and renal functions
- Reduced cardiac reserve.

### Effects on Pregnancy—Category C
Contraindicated, the drug will cross the placenta and slow the heart rate, lower the blood sugar and blood pressure.

The drug will be secreted in the breast milk and lower the blood pressure in the babies.

**Effect on fetus and newborn:** Growth retardation [intrauterine growth restriction (IUGR) due to decrease in placental blood flow], thrombocytopenia, birth asphyxia, depression, hyperbilirubinemia, bradycardia, hypotension, hypoglycemia, and polycythemia.

### Side Effects/The Adverse Effects of Propranolol
- Aggravation of AV conduction defects
- Bradycardia may be pronounced resulting in cardiac asystole
- Bronchospasm in patients with asthma and other forms of airway obstruction
- Cold hands and feet
- Carbohydrate tolerance will be impaired
- Cardiac failure—myocardial failure due to direct depression of myocardium
- Congestive cardiac failure (CCF)—it can precipitate CCF in cases of myocardial insufficiency by blocking sympathetic support to the heart
- Central nervous system (CNS)—sedation, sleep disturbances, depression, and loss of concentration
- Dysphoria
- Dizziness
- Dreams (unpleasant)
- Depression
- Drowsiness
- Erectile dysfunction
- Exacerbates of peripheral vascular disease—Raynaud's syndrome
- Exacerbation of angina—prinzmetal angina (variant angina) due to unopposed action of alpha-mediated coronary constriction
- Fatigue
- Fever
- Forgetfulness
- Gastrointestinal problems—constipation/diarrhea, nausea, and vomiting
- Hypotension (sudden)
- Hallucinations
- Hypoglycemia
- Insomnia
- Intermittent claudication
- Lack of drive
- Muscle fatigue
- Nightmares
- Psychotic reactions—Rarely
- Plasma lipid profile will be altered
- Peripheral neuropathy
- Raynaud's phenomenon
- Reduced exercise capacity
- Rash
- Sick sinus syndrome
- Tiredness.
- Will worsen chronic obstructive lung disease

### Drug Interactions
- Adrenaline with propranolol will result in hypotension and bradycardia
- Beta blockers will potentiate the negative inotropic action of antiarrhythmic drugs like verapamil, a calcium channel blocker which can result in bradycardia or even asystole
- Cimetidine will inhibit propranolol metabolism and increase the plasma level of propranolol.

- Digitalis and beta blockers may cause severe bradycardia due to depression of sinus node and sinoatrial (SA) node
- Enhances the hypotensive effects of angiotensin-converting enzyme (ACE) inhibitors—propranolol
- Indomethacin may cause hypotension
- Propranolol will be the plasma level of chlorpromazine and increase bioavailability of chlorpromazine by decreasing the first-pass metabolism
- Propranolol will elevate the serum levels of cimetidine
- Propranolol will increase the cardiotoxicity of tricyclic antidepressants.

## QUESTIONS

Q1. **What are the pharmacological actions of propranolol?**
- Decreases the heart rate and force of contraction
- Decreases cardiac output and results in decrease in blood pressure
- Increases bronchial resistance by blocking β2-receptors
- Reduces intraocular pressure
- Modifies carbohydrate and lipid metabolism.

Q2. **What are the effects of β receptor stimulation on the heart?**
- Increases automaticity that enhances atrioventricular (AV) conduction
- Shortens the refractory period in the supraventricular tissues.

Q3. **What are the indications of propranolol in cyanotic heart diseases?**
Treatment of cyanotic spells.

Q4. **What are the causes of propranolol toxicity?**
Blockage of cardiac, vascular, and bronchial β receptors.

Q5. **What is hypoglycemia unresponsiveness?**
Propranolol will prevent correction of hypoglycemia by adrenergic body mechanism.

Q6. **What is the danger of abrupt withdrawal of propranolol in angina?**
Abrupt withdrawal of propranolol in angina may precipitate myocardial infarction. To prevent this, propranolol should be withdrawn gradually.

Q7. **What are the withdrawal symptoms of propranolol after prolonged use?**
- Withdrawal symptoms like nervousness, tachycardia, increased intensity of angina, and increase in blood pressure
- Myocardial infarction may occur.

Q8. **What are the complications of prolonged administration of propranolol?**
- Fatigue, cramps, lethargy, mental depression and hallucinations, and peripheral neuropathy
- Allergic reaction, thrombocytopenia, and agranulocytosis.

Q9. **Why propranolol should be withdrawn gradually after chronic use?**
Abrupt withdrawal will result in rebound hypertension, worsening of angina, or sudden death.

Q10. **What is the danger of combining propranolol and calcium antagonist verapamil?**
- Severe hypotension
- Bradycardia
- Heart failure
- Cardiac conduction abnormalities.

Q11. **Why beta-blockers are dangerous in bronchial asthma?**
Blockage of beta receptors in the bronchi and bronchioles will result in increase in airway resistance.

## Calcium Channel Blockers

### Nifedipine

**Mechanism of action:** This directly acts on the smooth muscle by inhibiting calcium influx.

Nifedipine will cause peripheral arteriolar dilatation and fall in peripheral vascular resistance resulting in fall in blood pressure.

**Pharmacological actions:**
- It has a relaxing effect on bladder
- Absorbed well after oral administration. Nifedipine is metabolized into inactive metabolites and excreted in the urine.

**Dosage:**
- 0.25–0.5 mg/kg in divided doses to maximum of 10 mg/dose
- One dose orally in empty stomach.

**Indication:** Hypertension.

**Contraindications:**
- Hypersensitivity
- Hypotension
- Acute myocardial infarction.

**Precautions:**
- Decrease the dose in elderly
- The tablet should not be bitten and should be swallowed as a whole
- While withdrawing the drug, it should be slowly withdrawn under supervision.

**Effects on pregnancy:** Category C

Not contraindicated during lactation.

**Side effects:**
- Ankle edema
- Allergy—skin rashes
- Breathing problems
- Constipation
- Cramps—leg cramps
- Cough
- Chest pain
- Dizziness
- Drowsiness
- Flushing
- Fatigue
- Gastrointestinal blocks
- Gastrointestinal symptoms—nausea
- Headache
- Hypotension (orthostatic)
- Hematuria
- Increased heart rate—tachycardia
- Palpitation.

**Drug interactions:** Makes diabetic control difficult by decreasing insulin resistance.

Metabolized by cytochrome P450 3A4 system and the drugs affecting this will alter the clearance of nifedipine.

## *Verapamil*

**Mechanism of action:** Calcium channel blocker.

**Dosage:** Oral three to four times a day.

**Indications:**
- Hypertension
- Angina
- Antiarrhythmic
- Migraine
- Cluster headache.

**Contraindications:**
- Allergy/hypersensitivity
- Blood pressure less than 90 mm of Hg/hypotension
- Cardiogenic shock
- Left ventricular dysfunction/failure.

**Precautions:**
- Sick sinus syndrome
- Wolff-Parkinson-White (WPW) syndrome
- Muscular dystrophy
- Myasthenia gravis
- Liver and kidney disorders
- Neurological disorders
- Heart rhythm problems
- Third-degree heart block.

**Effects on pregnancy:**
- During pregnancy use only if indicated
- Passed into breast milk.

**Side effects:**
- Allergic reaction
- Block—atrioventricular block
- Constipation
- Congestive cardiac failure
- Depression
- Dizziness
- Edema

- Flushing
- Gingival hyperplasia
- Headache
- Hypotension
- Nausea.

**Drug interactions:**
- Erythrocin, rifampicin will affect excretion of verapamil from the body
- Verapamil will slow the excretion of midazolam, triazolam, and colchicine.

## *Flunarizine*

Oral tablet/capsule.

**Mechanism of action:**
- Nonselective calcium antagonist
- Weak calcium channel blocker
- Blocks serotonin receptors
- Antihistaminic
- Blocks dopamine $D_2$ activity
- Inhibits sodium channels.

**Pharmacological aspects:** It is effective as propranolol.
- Well absorbed from gut
- Crosses the blood–brain barrier
- Metabolized in the liver.

**Dosage:** 5 mg/day in the evening for 4–8 weeks.

**Indications:**
- Migraine
- Peripheral vascular disease
- Vertigo.

**Contraindications and cautions:**
- Depression
- Stroke
- Parkinson's disease
- Hypotension
- Heart failure
- Arrhythmias.

**Precautions:**
- Liver disorders
- Movement disorders
- History of depression
- Allergy
- Avoid work requiring alertness
- Alcohol intake can predispose to excessive drowsiness
- Glaucoma
- Elderly
- Children
- Liver
- Heart problems
- Avoid excess dose.

**Effects on pregnancy:**
Category C.

**Side effects:**
- Common:
  - Allergy—skin rash
  - Blood pressure decreased
  - Central nervous system—anxiety, vertigo, and dizziness
  - Constipation
  - Depression
  - Drowsiness
  - Dry mouth
  - Extrapyramidal effects
  - Gastrointestinal tract—nausea, vomiting, and heart burn
  - Gain in weight
  - Heart burn
  - Involuntary movements
  - Sedation
  - Weakness
  - Muscle aches
  - Tremor.

**Drug interactions:** The effects of sedatives, antihypertensives will be increased.

## *Amlodipine*

Long-acting calcium channel blocker.

**Mechanism of action:** Angioselective calcium channel blockers inhibit calcium ions influx across the cell membranes.

**Pharmacological actions:**
- Dilatation of blood vessels
- Negative inotropic effect by inhibiting contraction of cardiac muscle cells

- Decreases peripheral vascular resistance by inhibiting vascular smooth muscle cells causing vasodilatation.

### Dosage:
- Children more than 6 years—2.5–5 mg/day
- Maintenance—5–10 mg/day
- Adults—5 mg/day orally once a day not to exceed 10 mg/day
- Maximum dose—10 mg/day.

### Indications:
- Angina (stable and variant)
- Blood pressure elevated (hypertension)
- Coronary artery disease.

### Contraindications:
- Allergy to drug
- Cardiogenic shock
- Children less than 6 years of age.

### Precautions:
- The safety of drugs is not established below the age of 6 years
- It can cause hypotension in patients with aortic stenosis, liver disease.

### Effects on pregnancy:
- Category C
- Safety is not known in use, there is a possible hazard to the fetus. Only if needed. The drug is secreted through the breast milk. The breastfeeding women should not use this drug.
- It is contraindicated during lactation.

### Side effects:
- Allergy
- Abdominal pain
- Breathing problem—bronchospasm
- Cholestasis
- Convulsions
- Dizziness
- Edema of feet—ankle/legs
- Flushing
- Fatigue
- Gastrointestinal symptoms
- Gingival enlargement
- Hepatitis
- Hypotension
- Insomnia
- Itching
- Jaundice
- Joint pain
- Lightheadedness
- Muscle pain
- Palpitation.

### Severe side effects:
- Fainting
- Chest pain.

### Drug interactions:
The following drugs will increase the serum levels of amlodipine:
- Ketoconazole
- Clarithromycin
- Sildenafil will be associated with hypotension
- Simvastatin will be associated with myopathy
- Calcium channel blockers.

## Alpha Methyldopa

Alpha methyl analog of Dopa is the precursor of dopamine and noradrenaline (NA).

Alpha methyl NA is a selective alpha-2 agonist formed in the brain from methyldopa that will act on alpha-2 receptors that will decrease efferent sympathetic activity.

Alpha methyl dopa has both central and peripheral action. Dopa decarboxylase in the brain and periphery.

### Mechanism of Action

Alpha methyl dopa has both central and peripheral action. This drug will be metabolized into alpha-methyl NA which will act at the alpha-adrenergic receptors in the vasomotor center and decrease the adrenergic neuronal outflow from the brainstem.

This will also inhibit secretion of renin from kidney.

## Pharmacological Actions

**Q1. How does methyldopa decrease the blood pressure?**

By reducing the peripheral vascular resistance, decreasing the heart rate, and cardiac output.

Acts centrally and decreases the sympathetic outflow.

## Dosage

- 10 mg/kg/day in two to four divided doses
- It can be administered orally or intravenously.

## Indications

Antihypertensive in mild to moderate hypertension.

## Contraindications

- Pheochromocytoma
- Hepatic impairment
- Jaundice
- Hypersensitivity.

## Precautions

- Pregnancy
- Renal impairment
- Cardiac disease
- Acquired hemolytic anemia.

## Effects on Pregnancy

May develop a positive direct Coombs test.

## Side Effects of Methyldopa

- Altered sleep rhythm
- Bone marrow depression
- Central nervous system—decreased intellectual drive, impaired mental concentration, nightmares, mental depression, vertigo, extrapyramidal signs, reduced mental capacity, lethargy, and sedation
- Cognitive impairment
- Dryness of mouth
- Drugs
- Electrolyte imbalance—sodium retention
- Fever
- Fluid retention
- Gain in weight
- Gynecomastia
- Postural hypotension
- Headache
- Hypersensitivity
- Hepatitis
- Hemolytic anemia
- Mild rebound hypertension on sudden withdrawal of methyldopa
- Impotence
- Jaundice
- Lactation in females due to increased prolactin secretion
- Nasal stuffiness
- Tolerance
- Toxic epidermal necrolysis.

Toxicity is probably due to inhibition of dopaminergic mechanism in the hypothalamus.

## Drug Interactions

- Tricyclic antidepressants will reverse the actions of methyldopa by blocking its active transport into the adrenergic neurons
- Reserpine and haloperidol will accentuate the mental symptoms.

# QUESTIONS

**Q1. How does methyldopa decrease the blood pressure?**

By reducing the peripheral vascular resistance, decreasing the heart rate, and cardiac output.

**Q2. Why cross-matching of blood is difficult in patients receiving methyldopa?**

About 10-20% of patients receiving methyldopa for longer than 12 months will develop positive Coombs test. This will make cross-matching of blood that is difficult in patients receiving methyldopa.

**Q3. Why methyldopa should not be used in pheochromocytoma?**

Injected methyldopa may release catecholamines (CAs).

## Angiotensin-converting Enzyme Inhibitor

### Captopril

Angiotensin-converting enzyme inhibitor.

**Mechanism of action:** It will interfere with calcium entry into the myocardial and smooth muscles. The contractility of cardiac and smooth muscles will depend upon the levels of extracellular calcium.

**Pharmacological actions:**
- Antihypertensive
- Antianginal.

**Dosage:**
- *Children*—0.3–0.5 mg/kg/dose up to a maximum of 6 mg/kg/day, not to exceed 450 mg/day
- *Adults*—12.5–25 mg orally two to three times per day.

**Indications:**
- Hypertension
- Cardiac failure.

**Contraindications:**
- Allergy to other ACE inhibitors
- Aortic stenosis
- Bilateral renal artery stenosis
- Congestive cardiac failure
- Dialysis with high flux membranes
- Elderly patients
- Failures—renal failure, bone marrow failure
- Gestational period—pregnancy
- Hypotension
- Hyperkalemia
- Hyponatremia
- Idiopathic angioedema.

**Precautions:** As this drug can cause hyperkalemia, avoid taking potassium salts or potassium-sparing diuretics.
The drug should not be given during pregnancy.

**Effects on pregnancy:**
- Category D
- It can cause fetal growth retardation, fetal death when given during later half of pregnancy
- Secreted in breast milk and is not recommended during breastfeeding.

**Side effects:**
- Angioedema
- Abdominal pain
- Bowel upset
- Cough
- Dizziness
- Emesis
- Electrolyte imbalances—hyperkalemia, hyponatremia
- Fainting
- Fatigue
- Gustatory—loss of taste, dysgeusia
- Gastrointestinal—constipation, diarrhea
- Headache
- Hypotension
- Itching
- Jaundice/liver failure
- Kidney failure.

**Drug interactions:**
- Potassium-sparing diuretics will result in hyperkalemia
- Potassium supplements should be avoided
- Will increase the lithium levels
- Nonsteroidal anti-inflammatory drugs (NSAIDs), indomethacin will reduce the hypotensive effects of ACE inhibitors
- Antacids will reduce the effects of captopril.

### Enalapril

Angiotensin-converting enzyme inhibitor.

**Mechanism of action:** Enalapril will inhibit ACE which converts angiotensin I to angiotensin II. The levels of angiotensin which constricts the blood vessels will be decreased.

**Pharmacological actions:** Onset of action will be by 1 hour with a peak effect by 4-6 hours. The action will last for 12-24 hours.

**Dosage:** 1 month to 17 years—0.05-0.1 mg/kg/day up to 1.25 mg/dose.

### Indications:
- Hypertension
- Cardiac failure.

### Contraindications and cautions:
- Age less than 1 month (newborn)
- Preterm babies less than 44 weeks
- Renal failure or glomerular filtration rate (GFR) less than 30 mL/min
- Liver failure.

### Precautions:
- If GFR is less than 30 mL/min, the dose should be reduced
- If the blood pressure is not reduced by enalapril alone, a diuretic should be added.

**Effects on pregnancy:** Contraindicated during pregnancy. It can affect the fetus.

### Side effects:
- Angioedema
- Breathing problems
- Cough—dry cough
- Dizziness
- Emesis
- Face swelling
- Gastrointestinal tract—nausea
- Hives
- Hypotension
- Itching
- Jaundice
- Syncope.

### Drug interactions:
- Along with diuretics can cause hypotension
- Potassium-sparing diuretics may increase the risk for hyperkalemia
- Lithium toxicity is common.

# ANTIASTHMATICS
## Bronchodilators
### Aminophylline
- Injection 250 mg in 10 mL ampoules
- It is a combination of theophylline and ethylenediamine
- It is safer than adrenaline and isoprenaline in hypoxic patients and patients with concomitant heart disease. When it is doubtful whether the patient is suffering from cardiac or bronchial asthma aminophylline can be used
- In adrenaline resistant cases aminophylline infusion can be given.

### Mechanism of action:
- Aminophylline acts directly on the smooth muscle. This also improves the contractility of diaphragm.
- Aminophylline will inhibit the enzyme phosphodiesterase.
- Aminophylline will increase the local concentration of cyclic adenosine monophosphate (AMP) resulting in bronchodilatation.
- Aminophylline will increase the contractility of diaphragm and renders it less susceptible to fatigue.

**Pharmacological actions:** Adenosine antagonist, mucociliary stimulation, spasmolytic action, respiratory center stimulation, and respiratory muscle stimulation.

### Dosage:
- 3-6 mg/kg in 20 mL of normal saline to be run in 20 minutes
- Three times a day. The drug can be repeated after 4 hours
- Oral dose: 4 mg/kg/dose every 6 hourly
- Loading dose: 7.0-8.0 mg/kg intravenously
- Maintenance: 2 mg/kg/dose every 8 hourly intravenously
- Dilute 1 mL of aminophylline with 9 mL of water. This will give 2.5 mg/mL. This is administered intravenously over 20 minutes.
- Intravenous infusion at a rate of 0.5-1 mg/kg/hour

❖ 5 mg/kg intravenously followed by maintenance of 1.2-1.

### Indications:
❖ Treatment of asthma: It is useful when the asthmatic is not responding to adrenaline or resistant to adrenaline
❖ Apnea of prematurity in newborn
❖ In adrenaline resistant cases, aminophylline infusion can be given.

### Contraindications:
❖ Allergy
❖ Hyperthyroidism
❖ Hypothyroidism
❖ Diabetes
❖ Angina
❖ Seizures.

**Precautions:** Rapid administration especially in presence of cardiac damage may result in nausea, vomiting, and collapse. Convulsions can occur even death had occurred.

### Effects on pregnancy:
❖ Category C
❖ Contraindicated in third trimester of pregnancy
❖ Aminophylline is excreted in the breast milk and cause irritability in the infants.

### Side effects:
❖ Gastrointestinal upset and gastroesophageal reflux
❖ Given rapidly can cause nausea
❖ Cardiovascular system: Arrhythmias, tachycardia and palpitations
❖ Central nervous system stimulation: Cerebral irritation, seizures (when given rapidly). Watch for twitching of mouth or the facial muscles or for severe hyperventilation.
❖ Insomnia.

**Drug interactions:** Aminophylline should not be mixed with ascorbic acid, chlorpromazine, promethazine, morphine, pethidine, phenytoin, phenobarbitone, insulin, tetracyclines, erythromycin, and penicillin G.

## QUESTIONS

**Q1. What is the drug of choice when one cannot decide if the child is suffering from cardiac asthma or bronchial asthma?**
Aminophylline is the drug of choice when one cannot decide if the child is suffering from cardiac asthma or bronchial asthma.

**Q2. What is the problem of giving aminophylline rapidly?**
❑ The drug can cause nausea, vomiting or collapse
❑ It is safer than adrenaline and isoprenaline is hypoxic patients and patients with concomitant heart disease. When doubtful cardiac or bronchial asthma it is used.

**Q3. What are the solutions with aminophylline is compatible and not compatible?**
❑ Compatible with 5% dextrose normal saline and ringer lactate
❑ Incompatible with alkaline solutions.

**Q4. Why aminophylline should not be given intramuscularly?**
Do not give intramuscularly as it will cause severe pain and sloughing.

**Q5. What are the things that should be monitored while administering aminophylline?**
Heart rate and blood glucose.

## Salbutamol
❖ Salbutamol is a highly selective β2-agonist
❖ Available as tablet 2-4 mg, 8 mg SR
❖ 2 mg/5 mL syrup
❖ 100 μg metered dose inhaler.

### Mechanism of action:
❖ β2 stimulation, ↑ cyclic AMP
❖ Salbutamol is a highly selective β2-agonist
❖ β2 adrenergic stimulant, which has prominent bronchodilator action (β2-receptor action). Stimulation of β2-receptors will activate the enzyme adenylyl

cyclase resulting in forming cyclic AMP from ATP. The cyclic AMP will cause bronchodilatation
- This has a poor β1 action, hence cardiac side effects are less prominent. It also has poor cardiac β2 action.

## Dosage:
- Oral dose: 0.2–0.3 mg/kg/day in three divided doses
- Nebulization: 0.02 mL/kg with 2 mL of normal saline for 5 minutes
- 100–200 µg by inhalation
- 0.25–0.5 mg intramuscular/subcutaneously.

**Q1. What is the duration of action of salbutamol?**
4–6 hours.

**Indications:** Bronchial asthma.

## Contraindications:
- Hypersensitivity
- Cardiac tachyarrhythmias.

**Precautions:** Should be used cautiously in the following conditions:
- Arrhythmias
- Blood pressure elevated: Hypertension
- Convulsive disorders
- Diabetes
- Endocrine problems: Hyperthyroidism.

## Effects on pregnancy:
- Category C
- Salbutamol is excreted in breast milk, but no adverse effects are noted.

## Side effects:
- Arrhythmias
- Anxiety
- Allergic reactions: Urticaria
- Bronchospasm (paradoxical)
- Cramps
- Collapse
- Dry mouth
- Edema (ankle edema)
- Flushing of skin
- Fine tremor
- Hypotension
- Headache
- Irritation of throat
- Palpitation
- Restlessness
- Nervousness.

## Drug interactions:
- This may interact with tricyclic antidepressants, monoamine oxidase inhibitors, loop diuretics, and thiazide diuretics
- Beta-blockers should be avoided.

# QUESTIONS

**Q1. Why salbutamol is better in cardiac patients?**
Because of its poor cardiac stimulant action it is safer that adrenaline and isoprenaline in presence of cardiac disease and hypoxia in status asthmaticus.

**Q2. Salbutamol is more effective by oral route or by inhalation?**
Salbutamol is more effective by inhalation (100 µg) than by oral route (2–4 mg).

**Q3. What are the advantages of salbutamol inhalation?**
- Salbutamol is more effective in low doses by inhalation
- Onset of action is rapid
- Less side effects.

**Q4. Why salbutamol is better than adrenaline and isoprenaline?**
It is because of its poor cardiac stimulant action.

**Q5. What are the causes of adverse effects of salbutamol?**
Adverse effects of salbutamol is due to stimulation of extrapulmonary β2-receptors.

**Q6. What are the advantages of salbutamol?**
- Cardiac side effects are less prominent
- May not produce palpitations or rise in blood pressure in therapeutic doses

❑ Resistant to inactivation by catechol-O-methyltransferase (COMT), resulting in longer duration of action.

## Theophylline

- ❖ Naturally occurring methyl xanthine
- ❖ Well absorbed orally.

### Mechanism of action:

- ❖ Has adrenergic effects and stimulate endogenous catecholamine release
- ❖ Phosphodiesterase inhibition preventing breakdown of cyclic AMP in smooth muscles
- ❖ Adenosine antagonist prevents adenosine mediated bronchospasm, mucociliary stimulation, spasmolytic action, respiratory center stimulation, and respiratory muscle stimulation.

### Pharmacological actions:

- ❖ It is a potent bronchodilator
- ❖ Theophylline will cross the blood brain barrier and stimulate the central nervous center
- ❖ The sensitivity of the central nervous center to carbon dioxide will be increased
- ❖ Theophylline will cross the blood brain barrier and stimulate the central nervous center
- ❖ The sensitivity of the central nervous center to carbon dioxide will be increased
- ❖ Central nervous system:
  - Stimulant especially the higher centers
  - Theophylline will antagonize the narcotic induced CNS depression and regularize the breathing pattern
- ❖ Cardiovascular system:
  - Directly stimulate the heart and will increase the rate and force of contractions there by increasing the cardiac output
  - Dilatation of blood vessels and coronary arteries
  - Smooth muscles: Relaxation of smooth muscles
  - Mast cells: Theophylline will inhibit release of histamine
  - Improves mucociliary clearance
  - Augments diaphragmatic contractility
  - Decreases the release of inflammatory mediators
  - The peripheral actions of theophylline
- ❖ Increases the cardiac output, vital capacity, and diaphragmatic contractility.

### Dosage:

- ❖ Loading dose:
  - 5–7 mg/kg; orally
  - Dose interval: 6–8 hourly
  - Maintenance dose: 2–5 mg/kg/day
  - Plasma concentration: 7–12 µg/mL
- ❖ Dose: 12–15 mg/kg/day in three divided doses.

### Indications:

- ❖ Bronchial asthma
- ❖ Apnea of prematurity.

### Contraindications and cautions:

- ❖ Angina
- ❖ Alcoholics
- ❖ Blood pressure elevated
- ❖ Cystic fibrosis
- ❖ Cor pulmonale
- ❖ Diabetes
- ❖ Endocrine problems: Hyperthyroidism/hypothyroidism
- ❖ Fits
- ❖ Gastric ulcer/peptic ulcer disease
- ❖ Hepatic problems
- ❖ Hypersensitivity to drug.

### Precautions:

- ❖ This is not a first line of drug for treatment of asthma.
- ❖ It has a narrow therapeutic window. The therapeutic levels should be maintained between 10 µg/mL and 20 µg/mL. Clearance of this drug will vary in children and the serum levels should be measured frequently. The serum levels can be measured by 1 hour after an intravenous dose and 2–6 hours after oral dose.

**Effects on pregnancy:**
- Contraindicated during third trimester of pregnancy
- Theophylline crosses placenta and secreted in milk.

**Side effects:**
- *Gastrointestinal tract*: Gastrointestinal irritation, gastric irritation, nausea, vomiting, gastrointestinal bleeding, hematemesis, dyspepsia, gastric irritation, and abdomen pain
- *Central nervous system*: Convulsions, jitteriness, tremors, irritability, poor sleep, poor concentration, headache, nervousness, insomnia, restlessness, tremors, agitation, tachypnea, flushing, increased muscle tone, and delirium
- *Cardiovascular system*: Cardiac stimulation, tachycardia, palpitation, diuresis, hypotension, extrasystoles, worsening cardiovascular status, shock, and arrhythmias
- *Metabolic*: Hyperglycemia and increased insulin levels.

**Q1. What are the plasma concentrations associated with adverse reactions?**
- 15 mg/L: Headache, nervousness, and insomnia
- 20 mg/L: Palpitation, diuresis, restlessness, and tremors
- More than 40 mg/L: Shock, arrhythmias, seizures, and arrhythmias.

**Drug interactions:**
- Doxapram and theophylline should not be given simultaneously as both are incompatible
- Theophylline will decrease the effects of phenytoin and lithium.

**Q1. What are the agents which will induce theophylline metabolism?**
- Smoking
- Phenytoin
- Rifampicin
- Phenobarbitone.

**Q2. What agents will inhibit theophylline metabolism and thereby increase the plasma level?**
When the following drugs are given along with theophylline the dose should be reduced to two-thirds.
- Erythromycin
- Ciprofloxacin
- Cimetidine
- Oral contraceptives
- Allopurinol.

**Q3. What are the agents whose effects will be enhanced by theophylline?**
- Furosemide
- Sympathomimetics
- Digitalis
- Oral anticoagulants
- Hypoglycemics.

**Q4. What are the agents whose effects will be decreased by theophylline?**
- Phenytoin
- Lithium

## QUESTIONS

**Q1. What are the conditions in which the dose of theophylline should be reduced?**
- Age more than 60 years (× 0.6)
- Congestive heart failure (CHF) (× 0.6)
- Pneumonia (× 0.4)
- Liver failure (× 0.2–0.4).

**Q2. What are the advantages of theophylline?**
- Theophylline can be used both in acute and chronic asthma
- They can be taken orally
- The drug is cheap.

**Q3. What are the disadvantages of theophylline?**
- Theophylline has a narrow range of safety
- Side effects are common and the blood levels may be needed to monitor for dosing.

**Q4. How dose theophylline affects the blood pressure?**
- ❏ Theophylline will increase the blood pressure by direct action on the vasomotor center and direct cardiac stimulation.
- ❏ Theophylline will decrease the blood pressure by direct vasodilatation and vagal stimulation.

**Q5. What is the danger of rapid infusion of theophylline?**
Rapid intravenous infusion can result in sudden death due to marked fall in blood pressure, ventricular arrhythmias or asystole.

## Terbutaline

Terbutaline is a beta adrenergic receptor agonist used in treatment of asthma.

### Mechanism of Action

It is a short acting beta-2 receptor agonist used as bronchodilator.

### Dosage

- ❖ Children start with 2.5 mg three times a day up to a maximum of 7.5 mg/day.
- ❖ Adults and children more than 15 years of age should not be given more than 15 mg/day.
- ❖ Oral administration three times a day.

### Indications

- ❖ Used as reliever inhaler in asthma and prevention of exercise induced asthma
- ❖ Acute bronchial asthma
- ❖ Bronchitis
- ❖ Chronic obstructive pulmonary disease (COPD)
- ❖ Emphysema.

### Contraindications and Cautions

- ❖ Arrhythmias
- ❖ Blood pressure elevated
- ❖ Cardiac diseases
- ❖ Diabetes
- ❖ Epilepsy
- ❖ Hypokalemia
- ❖ Hyperthyroidism
- ❖ Ischemic heart disease.

### Precautions

The drug may cause dizziness and drowsiness, driving should be avoided.

Over use of short acting beta agonist increases the risk of death or death like episodes.

This drug should be avoided if the child is allergic to this drug or other bronchodilators or sympathomimetic drugs.

### Effects on Pregnancy

- ❖ Category C
- ❖ Use only if clearly indicated. This is a tocolytic preventing uterine contraction. The drug will be passed into breast milk.
- ❖ This can cause fetal tachycardia and hypoglycemia.

### Side Effects

- ❖ Allergic reactions—rash
- ❖ Asthma (paradoxical bronchospasm)
- ❖ Anxiety/nervousness
- ❖ Breathing problems
- ❖ Chest pain
- ❖ Cramps
- ❖ Convulsions
- ❖ Dizziness
- ❖ Drowsiness
- ❖ Dry mouth
- ❖ Emesis
- ❖ Electrolyte imbalance—hypokalemia
- ❖ Elevated/decreased blood pressure
- ❖ Fatigue
- ❖ Flushed feeling
- ❖ Glucose level elevation
- ❖ Headache
- ❖ Itching
- ❖ Insomnia or staying sleep
- ❖ Increased sweating
- ❖ Injection site pain.

*Drug Interactions*

This drug will interact with antidepressants, beta blockers, and diuretics.

## QUESTION

Q. **What are the features of terbutaline overdose?**
- Blood pressure—low or high
- Convulsions
- Dizziness
- Dry mouth
- Gastrointestinal tract symptoms—nausea
- Heart rate—irregular (tachycardia)
- Tremors.

## Corticosteroids

*Steroids*

Steroids are drugs with anti-inflammatory action.

Q1. **What are the mechanisms of action of steroids in asthma?**
- Anti-inflammatory actions
- Suppresses the mediator release
- Prevents formation of leukotrienes by preventing arachidonic acid metabolic derangements
- Increases the action of beta-2 agonists
- Increases the binding sites for cyclic adenosine monophosphate (cAMP)
- Prevent bronchoconstriction by inhibiting phospholipase A2, platelet-activating factor (PAF), leukotrienes, and prostaglandins.

Q2. **What are the commonly used steroids in asthma?**
- Prednisolone
- Hydrocortisone
- Beclomethasone inhalation

**Hydrocortisone:**

Hydrocortisone is a steroid used to treat inflammation in the body.

Q1. **How does hydrocortisone act?**
By its anti-inflammatory and antiallergic actions.

Q2. **What is the dose of hydrocortisone?**
- Parenteral dose: 7–10 mg/kg stratum 4 mg/kg 6th hourly
- Oral dose: 1 mg/kg/dose.

Q2. **What are the complications of steroids in asthma?**
- Oral candidiasis
- Osteoporosis
- Hoarse of voice
- Growth retardation.

*Inhaled Corticosteroids*

- Beclomethasone
- Budesonide
- Fluticasone.

**Mechanism of action:**

- Anti-inflammatory action reduces inflammation and swelling in the air passages
- Decreases mucus production in the airways
- Reduces airway hyper-responsiveness
- Prevents exacerbations of asthma.

**Dosage:**

- *Beclomethasone*: 50–800 µg/day in 2–3 divided doses
- *Budesonide*: 50–800 µg/day in 2–3 divided doses
- *Fluticasone*: 25–400 µg/day in 2–3 divided doses.

**Indications:** Long-term treatment of persistent bronchial asthma.

**Contraindications:** Allergy to steroids like fluticasone.

**Precautions:**

| Infections | • Presence of infections like tuberculosis and herpes, and eye infection<br>• Avoid contact with patients with contagious infections like chickenpox, measles, flu |

*Contd...*

*Contd...*

| | |
|---|---|
| Nose | Nasal problems |
| Hospitalization | Response to physical stress like surgery will be less |
| Acute conditions | Not useful in acute conditions |
| Liver problems | Liver problems |
| Eyes | Avoid spraying into the eyes |

**Effects on pregnancy:** Safe during pregnancy, but should be used only if clearly indicated.

**Side effects:**

- Adrenal suppression [hypothalamic pituitary adrenal (HPA) suppression]
- *Bone metabolism*: Reduced bone mass due to direct effect on bone formation and resorption
- Bleeding of nose irritation and dryness
- Cough
- *Dental problems*: Dry powder formula with pH less than 5.5 will dissolve tooth enamel
- *Eye problems*: Cataracts
- *Fungal infections*: Oropharyngeal candidiasis/oral thrush
- Glaucoma
- Growth retardation (height should be measured periodically)
- Hoarseness of voice/dysphonia due to myopathy of laryngeal muscles
- *Infections*: Pneumonia
- Budesonide and fluticasone are associated with less complications as they are completely metabolized during first pass metabolism
- Long-term use can causes systemic side effects like adrenal suppression, growth retardation, etc.

**Drug interactions:** Some medications can affect removal of steroids from the body.

## QUESTIONS

**Q1. What are the advantages of inhaled corticosteroid treatment?**
- Adverse effects will be less
- Better patient compliance
- Control of asthma will be better
- Decreased rate of hospitalization
- Effective control of asthma
- Flare ups will be less.

**Q2. What are the steps to reduce the incidence of side effects of inhaled corticosteroids?**
- Rinse the mouth after each dose
- Use large volume spacer devices
- Use metered dose inhalers.

### Budesonide

*Inhalation*: 2–4 puffs initially 100 mg/puff followed by 1–2 puffs 2–4 times a day

### Beclomethasone

Beclomethasone is a synthetic halogenated glucocorticoid. Beclomethasone is available as an inhaler, cream, pills, nasal spray.

**Mechanism of action:** Corticosteroid will cross the cell membranes and bind with cytoplasmic receptor protein and forms structural change in steroid receptor complex. Inhibitions of leukocyte infiltration at the site of inflammation, interferes with function of mediators of inflammatory response. Affects biosynthesis of mediators of inflammation like prostaglandins and leukotrienes.

**Pharmacological actions:** Anti-inflammatory, vasoconstrictive effects.

**Indications:**
- Asthma
- Allergic rhinitis
- Inflammatory skin conditions
- Topical form—eczema, psoriasis, dermatitis.

**Contraindications:** Age below 5 years.

**Side effects:**
- Acne
- Body pain/Back pain
- Burning
- Cough
- Dizziness

- Dry skin
- Emesis
- Fast heart rate
- Gastrointestinal upset
- Headache
- Itching
- Irritation of skin

## Anticholinergics

### Ipratropium Bromide
- Semisynthetic derivative
- Nasal inhaler 0.03–0.06%.

**Mechanism of action:** Anticholinergic activity.

**Pharmacological actions:** Acts selectively on smooth muscle.

**Dosage:**
- Used in metered dose inhalers or nebulizer
- 40–80 µg inhalation
- Asthma: Two puffs every 20 minutes.

**Indications:**
- Bronchial asthma
- Chronic bronchitis
- Chronic obstructive pulmonary disease
- Emphysema.

**Contraindications:**
- Benign prostatic hypertrophy
- Narrow angle glaucoma.

**Precautions:**
- Should be kept at room temperature
- Avoid spilling drugs into the eyes as it may cause narrow angle glaucoma.

**Effects on pregnancy:**
Category B

**Side effects:**
- Allergic reactions—rash
- Breathing difficulty
- Bad taste
- Blurred vision
- Cough
- Constipation
- Dryness of mouth
- Dizziness
- Eye pain
- Frequent urination
- Genitourinary problems: Painful urination and dysuria
- Heartburn
- Headache
- Itching.

**Drug interactions:**
- Additive effect with beta-adrenergic drugs
- With atropine side effects will be more.

## Mast Cell Stabilizers

### Sodium Cromoglycate/Cromolyn Sodium

**Mechanism of action:** Mast cell stabilizers that will prevent degranulation of mast cells thus preventing release of histamines and related mediators.

**Dosage:**
- Used in inhalers 5 mg/puff
- Nebulized one to two puffs, three to four times a day 5 mg/puff (remember 1, 2, 3, 4, and 5).

**Indications:**
- Used in prevention of asthmatic attacks
- Continuous prophylaxis for asthma.

**Contraindications:** Age less than 2 years.

**Precautions:**
- Avoid accidental spillage into the eyes
- Should not be swallowed
- The medicine should not be stopped suddenly
- The drug should not be used if the color is changed or had particles in it.

**Effects on pregnancy:**
- Category B
- Not recommended unless clearly indicated.

**Side effects:**
- Hives
- Cough

- ❖ Worsening of asthma
- ❖ Sneezing.

**Drug interactions:** Do not mix with other drugs in the inhalers.

## QUESTION

Q. **How will you use cromolyn to prevent bronchospasm following exercise or environmental factors?**
Cromolyn should be given 10–15 minutes before exercise or exposure to environmental factors that will precipitate bronchospasm.

## Leukotriene Receptor Antagonist

### Monteleukast

### Mechanism of action:
- ❖ Leukotriene receptor antagonist (LTRA)
- ❖ Prevents bronchospasm by preventing the reaction to triggers.

### Pharmacological actions:
- ❖ Decreases inflammation
- ❖ Decreases nasal congestion
- ❖ Prevents exercise induced asthma.

### Dosage:
- ❖ 5 mg tablet once daily in children. Adults dose 10 mg tablet once daily.
- ❖ The drug should be taken at least 2 hours before exercise.

### Indications:
- ❖ Asthma
- ❖ Allergic rhinitis
- ❖ Bronchospasm
- ❖ Exercise induced asthma.

### Contraindications and cautions:
- ❖ Hypersensitivity
- ❖ Allergy to aspirin
- ❖ Be cautious in severe asthma
- ❖ Phenylketonuria (monteleukast tablets contain aspartame, a source of phenylalanine).

### Precautions:
- ❖ Avoid aspirin and NSAIDs
- ❖ Only one dose should be given within 24 hours.

### Effects on pregnancy:
- ❖ Category B
- ❖ Not contraindicated.

### Side effects:
- ❖ Allergy: Rashes
- ❖ Angioedema
- ❖ Behavior and mood changes: Agitation, aggression, and suicidal tendencies
- ❖ Bleeding
- ❖ Cramps
- ❖ Cough
- ❖ Diarrhea
- ❖ Depression
- ❖ Emesis (vomiting)
- ❖ Erythema multiforme
- ❖ Fatigue
- ❖ Flu-like symptoms
- ❖ Fever
- ❖ Gastrointestinal: Nausea
- ❖ Hepatotoxicity
- ❖ Insomnia
- ❖ Irritability
- ❖ Infections
- ❖ Joint pain.

### Drug interactions:
- ❖ Montelukast is an inhibitor of CYP2C8
- ❖ Amodiaquine will increase the plasma concentrate of montelukast.

## SEDATIVES HYPNOTICS

### Benzodiazepines

### Diazepam (Calmpose)
- ❖ Oral availability (F) (%) 100
- ❖ Half-life (h) 43
- ❖ Target concentration 300 ng/mL.

### Mechanism of action of diazepam:
- ❖ Benzodiazepines
- ❖ Acts by enhancing the effect of the gamma-aminobutyric acid (GABA) which is a

neurotransmitter. GABAminergic action in reticular activating system (RAS) by affecting chloride channels.
- Diazepam acts by increasing the effectiveness of the inhibitory neurotransmitter GABA within the CNS.
- Strong action initially for brief period followed by milder effect.
- As active metabolites are produced the biological effects will be longer.

## Pharmacological actions of diazepam:
- Sedation
- Hypnotic
- Muscle relaxant
- Anticonvulsant
- Decreases the blood pressure
- Decreases the respiratory rate.

## Dosage:
- 0.1–0.3 mg/kg/day
- 0.1–0.3 mg/kg/dose intravenously over 15–30 minutes to a maximum dose of 2–5 mg
- 0.1–0.5 mg/kg/dose can be given per rectally.

**Q1. What is the site of absorption of diazepam?**
Diazepam is absorbed rapidly and completely absorbed from proximal small intestine.

**Q2. What are the effects of relatively large doses of diazepam?**
0.2–0.5 mg/kg/dose of diazepam can cause sedation, amnesia, and unconsciousness.

**Indications:** Diazepam will be useful for the following conditions:
- Anxiety states
- Behavior disorders
- Convulsions: Anticonvulsant
- Continuous seizure activity
- Generalized tonic-clonic seizures
- Status epilepticus (drug of choice)
- Control of drug-induced dyskinesia
- Convulsions of nonepileptic origin
- Hypnotic
- Insomnia
- Relieves spasticity in cerebral palsy and multiple sclerosis
- Tetanus spasm control
- Muscle relaxant
- Muscle spasm
- Neurosis
- Night terror
- Psychosomatic disorders
- Preanaesthetic medication
- Tension.

## Contraindications for diazepam:
- Acute narrow-angle glaucoma
- Benzodiazepines hypersensitivity
- Coma
- Depression: Pre-existing CNS depression
- Myasthenia gravis.

**Precautions to be taken while administering diazepam:** Diazepam should be diluted and given very slowly. Observe for respiratory depression or arrest during administration of diazepam.

**Effects on pregnancy:** The adverse effects of digoxin when administered to the mother in the antenatal period. The following may be seen in the newborn:
- Apneic spells
- Reluctance to feed
- Hypotonia.

Problem of using diazepam in pregnant women during labor:
May cause flaccidity and respiratory depression in the newborn.

## Side effects/adverse effects of diazepam:
- Respiratory depression
- Sedation
- Cognitive impairment
- Impairment of motor skills and alertness
- Disinhibition of irritability
- Drug dependence
- Drug abuse
- Vertigo
- Increased appetite and weight gain

- Laryngospasm
- Phlebitis
- Allergy
- Headache
- Impaired sexual function
- Leukopenia
- Menstrual irregularities.

Adverse effects of rapid administration of diazepam:
- Apnea
- Bradycardia
- Cardiac arrest
- Cardiovascular collapse
- Hypotension.

**Q1. What are the adverse effects of diazepam when administered to the mother in the antenatal period?**

The following may be seen in the newborn:
- ❑ Apneic spells
- ❑ Reluctance to feed
- ❑ Hypotonia.

**Q2. What are the adverse effects of rapid administration of diazepam?**

Respiratory depression can be treated by bag and mask ventilation, which may result in death. It can cause respiratory depression. It should be given slowly, 0.3 mg/kg/hour can be given. Give diazepam in a dose of 0.2 mg/kg. More doses may predispose to respiratory depression. Provide bag and mask ventilation. Always dilute the diazepam.

**Drug interactions of diazepam:**
- Quinalones, fluoxetine, fluoxamine, and INH will decrease the metabolism of diazepam
- Phenobarbitone and rifampicin will increase the metabolism of diazepam
- Propranolol will increase the half-life of diazepam
- Diazepam will increase the plasma level of phenytoin
- Diazepam will decrease the metabolism of digoxin
- Valproate will increase the plasma level of diazepam
- Cimetidine will reduce the clearances
- Reduce the efficacy of phenytoin and levodopa.

## QUESTIONS

**Q1. Why diazepam is not used for long-term therapy of epilepsy?**

Diazepam is not used for long-term therapy of epilepsy because of prominent sedative action and rapid development of tolerance.

**Q2. How will you manage respiratory arrest due to calmpose infusion?**

Respiratory depression can be treated by bag and mask ventilation. Provide bag and mask ventilation for few minutes. As the duration of diazepam is of short duration recovery will occur quickly.

**Q3. What is the disadvantage of intramuscular diazepam?**

The absorption will be erratic, slow, and incomplete.

**Q4. What is the problem of using diazepam in a newborn with jaundice?**

The vehicle for intravenous diazepam contains sodium benzoate. This will displace bilirubin from albumin binding sites.

**Q5. What is the danger of using diazepam in a newborn with jaundice?**

Lorazepam and diazepam should be used carefully as sodium benzoate used as a vehicle can uncouple bilirubin-albumin complex, thus enhancing the risk for kernicterus.

**Q6. What is the problem of using diazepam in a newborn with jaundice?**

The vehicle for intravenous diazepam contains sodium benzoate. This will displace bilirubin from albumin binding sites.

**Q7. Why diazepam is not used intramuscularly?**
The absorption will be slow, erratic, and incomplete.

**Q8. What is the disadvantage of using oral diazepam?**
It is not very effective when given orally and rapid development of tolerance.

**Q9. Why diazepam is not used for long-term treatment of seizure disorders?**
It is due to development of tolerance.

**Q10. What is the danger of using diazepam in a newborn with jaundice?**
It can cause respiratory depression. It should be given slowly, 0.3 mg/kg/hour can be given.

**Q11. How will you manage respiratory arrest due to diazepam infusion?**
Provide bag and mask ventilation for few minutes. As the duration action of diazepam is of short duration recovery will occur quickly.

**Q12. What are the precautions you will take while administering diazepam?**
Diazepam should be diluted and given very slowly. Observe for respiratory depression or arrest during administration of diazepam.
Lorazepam and diazepam should be used carefully as sodium benzoate used as a vehicle can uncouple bilirubin-albumin complex, thus enhancing the risk for kernicterus.

**Q13. How will you treat convulsions?**
- Diazepam 0.3 mg/kg given intravenously. It is given slowly after diluting with distilled water. Monitor for respiratory depression.
- Phenobarbitone is given intravenously, in a dose of 20 mg/kg loading dose given over a period of 10–30 minutes. This should be followed by a maintenance dose of 5 mg/kg/day. The rate of infusion should be 1 mg/kg/min.
- Phenytoin is given intravenously, in a dose of 20 mg/kg loading dose followed by a maintenance dose of 5 mg/kg/day.

## Midazolam

It is three times more potent than diazepam and is an nonirritant.

### Mechanism of Action

Increases the activity of GABA on the GABAA receptors.

### Pharmacological Aspects

- Absorption occurs extremely rapidly with peak in 20 minutes.
- Faster acting and shorter duration.

### Dosage

- *Dose*: 0.1–0.4 mg/kg intramuscularly to a maximum dose of 5 mg.
- *Intravenous dose*: 0.02–0.1 mg/kg followed by 0.06–0.4 mg/kg/hour. 200 mg/kg intravenous followed by 30–60 mg/kg/hour. The infusion can be tapered off after 24 hours of seizure control.
- *Dose for sedation*: 0.01–0.1 mg/kg
- *Bolus dose*: 0.05–0.15 mg/kg
- *Dose frequency*: 2–4 hourly
- *Infusion dose*: 0.1–0.6 mg/kg.

### Indications

- Convulsions
- Status epilepticus
- Sedation for procedures
- Insomnia.

### Contraindications

- Pregnancy
- Elderly
- Hypersensitivity
- Acute narrow-angle glaucoma
- Shock
- Hypotension
- Head injury.

## Precautions

- Three times more potent than diazepam
- The drug is used for abuse.

## Effects on Pregnancy

- The drug may cause benzodiazepine withdrawal syndrome in the newborn if administered during the third trimester of pregnancy. The newborn will present with hypotonia, apneic spells, cyanosis, hyperexcitability, tremor, vomiting, and diarrhea.
- Breastfeeding is not recommended during this drug intake.

## Side Effects

- *Central nervous system*: Respiratory depression
- Amnesia
- *Withdrawal syndrome*: Irritability, insomnia, anxiety, seizures, psychosis, nausea, vomiting, diarrhea, tachycardia hypertension, and tachypnea. Reflexes will be abnormal with clonus.
- Paradoxical behavior or effects like increased activity, anxiety, involuntary movements, aggressive behavior, uncontrollable crying, and uncontrollable verbalization.
- Tolerance in chronic users
- Dependence
- Rebound effect.

## Drug Interactions

- The sedative effects of midazolam will be enhanced by anticonvulsants phenytoin, phenobarbitone, and sedative antihistamines.
- Protease inhibitors will prolong the action by inhibit metabolism of midazolam.

# QUESTIONS

**Q1. What is the danger of sudden withdrawal of midazolam?**
The patient may develop withdrawal symptoms. Status epilepticus may occur.

**Q2. How will you prevent withdrawal symptoms?**
The drug should be gradually withdrawn.

## Lorazepam

- Three times more potent than diazepam
- Less irritant
- Shorter action than diazepam.

## Mechanism of Action

- Produces amnesia
- Sedative.

## Pharmacological Aspects

- Absorbed slowly from GIT
- No active metabolite is produced.

## Dosage

- *Bolus dose*: 0.05–0.1 mg/kg
- *Dose frequency*: 4–12 hourly
- Infusion is not recommended
- Intramuscular route.

## Indications

- Anxiety
- Obsessive compulsive neurosis
- Preanesthetic medication.

## Contraindications

- Allergy/hypersensitivity
- Respiratory failure
- Ataxia
- Acute narrow-angle glaucoma
- Myasthenia gravis.

## Precautions

The dose should be reduced in children and elderly.

## Effects on Pregnancy

- Category D and is likely to cause fetal problems
- Benzodiazepine withdrawal syndrome can occur in the newborns if the drug is administered in the late stages of pregnancy or third trimester.

## Side Effects

- Weakness
- Sleepiness
- Hypotension.

Long-term use is associated with the following:
- Tolerance
- Physical dependence
- Psychological dependence
- Benzodiazepine withdrawal syndrome.

## Drug Interactions

Lorazepam with clobazam will increase the risk of CNS and respiratory depression, psychomotor impairment.

Avoid other benzodiazepines and narcotic medications. Alcohol can aggravate the side effects of Lorazepam. Lorazepam and alcohol both have depressive action on the brain. It can cause decreased heart rate and breathing problems.

## QUESTIONS

**Q1. What are the advantages of lorazepam over diazepam?**
- It is three times more potent than diazepam and is less irritant
- Amnesia is more profound than diazepam.

**Q2. What are the differences between diazepam and lorazepam?**

| Features | Diazepam | Lorazepam |
|---|---|---|
| Half-life | More than 24 hours | Short, between 5 hours and 30 hours |
| Absorption | Rapidly and completely from proximal small intestine | Less rapidly absorbed |
| Fate and extent of distribution | Extensively distributed | Less extensive distribution |
| Single dose effect | Reduced | Persist in plasma and brain for many hours after a single dose |

## OPIOIDS

### Morphine (Morphine Sulfate)

It is a natural alkaloid of opium.

### Mechanism of Action

Morphine acts by interacting with specific receptors in the neurons in the central nervous system and peripheral tissues.

### Pharmacological Actions

It has both depressant and stimulant actions.

**Central nervous system:**
- Euphoria
- Sedation
- Hypnosis.

**Analgesia:**
- Raises the pain threshold. Strong analgesia due to raise in the pain threshold
- Alters emotional reaction to pain
- Pupils: Miosis.

**Depressant actions:**
- Depresses respiratory center
- Vasomotor center is depressed at higher doses and causes fall in blood pressure
- Analgesia: Poorly localized dull pain from viscera is better relieved than sharply defined somatic pan.
- Temperature regulating center will be depressed
- Cough center is depressed
- Vasomotor center will be depressed at higher doses and causes fall in blood pressure
- Sedation
- Hypnosis
- Induces sleep
- Calming effect.

**Respiratory system:**
- Depresses respiration by directly depressing the brainstem respiratory center.
- Depresses respiratory center and decreases the sensitivity of medullary respiratory center to increased carbon dioxide.

**Cardiovascular system:** Normal dose does not have any effect, but toxic doses can cause hypotension by dilatation of capillaries by decreasing the tone of blood vessels by direct action, depression of vasomotor center, and histamine release.

**Gastrointestinal tract:**

- Absorption of water is increased resulting in constipation
- Biliary tract: Spasm of sphincter of Oddi
- Constipation by decreasing propulsive movements
- Central action causing inattention to defecation reflex
- Decreases peristaltic propulsive movement
- Decreases hydrochloric acid and intestinal secretion
- Decreases all gastrointestinal secretions
- Spasm of sphincters including pylorus, ileocecal and anal sphincters, and intestinal smooth muscles
- Spasm of smooth muscles of gut reducing the propulsive peristaltic movements.

**Stimulant actions:**

- Stimulates vagal center and causes bradycardia
- Stimulates Edinger-Westphal nucleus of III cranial nerve produces miosis
- Stimulates certain cortical areas and hippocampal cells
- Euphoria
- Stimulate chemoreceptor trigger zone will cause vomiting
- Stimulates autonomic nervous system. Causes mild hyperglycemia by sympathetic stimulation
- Release of ADH will result in decreased urinary output
- Constriction of bronchial smooth muscles.

**Smooth muscles:**

- *Biliary tract*: Morphine causes spasm of sphincter of Oddi in the biliary tract
- *Bladder*: Tone of the detrusor and sphincter are increased producing urinary urgency
- Increase in tone of ureters and detrusor
- Increases the tone of ureters and decreases its peristalsis
- *Uterus*: Will prolong labor.

**Metabolism:** Decreases the metabolic rate.

**Dose in children:**

- 0.2–0.8 mg/kg 12 hourly
- Bolus dose: 0.05–0.2 mg/kg
- Dose frequency: 2–4 hourly
- Infusion dose: 0.1–0.15 mg/kg.

**Route of administration:**

- Subcutaneous
- Absorption from GIT will be slow and incomplete
- Will be completely excreted in urine in 24 hours.

*Indications*

- As analgesic for relief of severe pain
- Sedation
- To relieve cardiac pain
- Cyanotic spells
- Preanesthetic medication
- Acute left ventricular failure and pulmonary edema
- Antitussive.

*Contraindications*

- Respiratory depression
- Paralytic ileus
- Delayed gastric emptying
- Obstructive airway disease
- Morphine sensitivity
- Acute hepatic disease
- Pregnancy.

*Precautions before Administering Morphine*

- Myxoedema with lowered basal metabolic rate (more sensitive and prone to develop coma)

- Old people (more prone to develop respiratory depression and urinary retention)
- *Renal problems*: Impaired kidney function—cumulative toxicity can occur
- Pulmonary problems: Patients with bronchial asthma, respiratory insufficiency like emphysema
- *Hepatic problems*: Impaired liver function—cumulative toxicity can occur
- Infants (more prone to develop respiratory depression)
- Neurological assessment in head injury: Morphine will produce increase in CSF pressure by $CO_2$ retention, miosis, respiratory depression and vomiting. Miosis and altered mentation may interfere with the diagnosis.
- *Endocrine problems*: Morphine should be used with caution in hypothyroidism as the patients are more sensitive to morphine.
- *Acute abdomen with undiagnosed problems*: Morphine will relieve the pain without modifying the underlying problem.

## Effects on Pregnancy

Morphine may evoke excitement in females and care should be exercised when given during pregnancy, lactation or menstruation.

**Q1. What is the effect of morphine on the fetus when given to the mother in the antenatal period? How will you manage?**

Respiratory depression in the fetus can be reversed by injection of 0.1–0.2 mg of nalorphine or 0.05–0.1 mg of levallorphan in the umbilical vein of the newborn.

**Q2. What is the effect of morphine on the fetus when administered to the antenatal mother?**
- Depression of respiration
- Morphine withdrawal syndrome can occur in the newborns. The features will be restlessness, irritability, incessant cry, diarrhea, and convulsions. These babies should be treated by giving small amount of morphine derivatives.

**Q3. What is the effect of morphine on the newborn when given to the mother during labor?**

Apnea in the newborn.

## Side Effects

- Addiction and tolerance when administered repeatedly
- Blurring of vision
- Central nervous system: Dysphoria, mental clouding—paresthesia
- Dysphoria
- Dryness of mouth
- Drug dependence
- Depression of respiration by directly depressing the respiratory center in the brainstem and by reducing the sensitivity of the medullary respiratory center to increased $CO_2$ concentration
- Emesis
- Fatigue
- Gastrointestinal tract: Constipation and nausea
- Headache
- Hypotension due to peripheral vasodilatation
- Idiosyncrasy: Urticaria, itching, and swelling of lips
- Increased intolerance: Delirium and tremors
- Increased pressure in the biliary tract
- Sedation
- Urinary retention
- Vertigo.

## Types of Toxicity

- Acute morphine poisoning
- Cumulative toxicity can occur in patients with impaired renal or hepatic functions.

## Drug Interactions

- Morphine action will be potentiated by phenothiazines, tricyclic antidepressants, MAO inhibitors, amphetamine, and neostigmine
- Morphine will delay the gastric emptying time and will retard absorption of many orally administered drugs.

The drugs that will enhance the sedative effects of morphine are as follows:
- Phenothiazines
- Monoamine oxidase inhibitors
- Tricyclic antidepressants.

## QUESTIONS

**Q1. What are the natural opium alkaloids?**
Morphine and codeine.

**Q2. What are the synthetic morphine substitutes?**
Pethidine and methadone.

**Q3. What is the danger of giving morphine in asthmatics?**
Morphine will cause histamine release and cause bronchoconstriction in asthmatics.

**Q4. What is the effect of morphine on the newborn when given to the mother during labor?**
Apnea in the newborn.

**Q5. What are the features of morphine withdrawal syndrome?**
- After 6–12 hours: After the last dose intense carving for morphine, lethargy, and weakness.
- After 12 hours: Yawning, lacrimation, perspiration, rhinorrhea, tremors, and anorexia.
- After 48 hours: Fever, rise in blood pressure, increase in heart rate, dilatation of previously constricted pupils, and abdominal cramps.
- The features of abstinence syndrome will disappear in 7–10 days.

**Q6. How will you treat morphine withdrawal syndrome?**
Gradual withdrawal of morphine with substitution of another narcotic analgesic is advised. This will decrease the severity of withdrawal syndrome.

**Q7. How will you treat morphine dependence?**
- By substituting methadone
- 1 mg of methadone will substitute 4 mg of morphine.

**Q8. What is the danger of giving morphine in asthmatics?**
Morphine will cause histamine release and cause bronchoconstriction in asthmatics.

**Q9. What are the features of acute morphine poisoning?**
- Altered consciousness and stupor or coma
- Breathing: Shallow, slow, and irregular
- Convulsions
- Cyanosis
- Drowsiness
- Dysuria
- Extreme sleepiness
- Flaccidity
- Gastrointestinal features: Nausea, vomiting, and constipation
- Hypotension
- Incoordination
- Pulmonary edema
- Pinpoint pupil
- Respiratory failure
- Shock
- Death may occur due to respiratory failure.

**Q10. What is the antidote for morphine?**
Naloxone.

**Q11. How will you treat acute morphine poisoning?**
- Gastric lavage using potassium permanganate
- Respiratory support using positive pressure ventilation
- Maintain the blood pressure using intravenous fluids and vasoconstrictors
- Naloxone 0.4–0.8 mg repeated every 2–3 minutes till the respiration picks up.

**Q12. What are the conditions in which morphine should be given carefully or avoided?**
- Infants and elderly people are susceptible for respiratory depression

- Respiratory insufficiency in emphysema, cor pulmonale
- Bronchial asthma
- Head injury
- Hypotensive states
- Diverticulitis, biliary colic, pancreatitis, and inflamed appendix
- Can cause urinary retention in elderly patients
- Hypothyroidism.

**Q13. Why morphine is not used for suppression of cough?**

Cough center is depressed. Cough center is more sensitive than respiratory center.

**Q14. How does morphine causes vasodilatation?**

Morphine causes vasodilatation by the following mechanisms:
- Decreases the tone of blood vessels by direct action
- Histamine release
- Depression of vasomotor center.

**Q15. What is the action of morphine on the pupils?**

It causes constriction of pupil. Morphine will cause pinpoint pupils.

**Q16. How does morphine produces vomiting?**

By stimulation of chemoreceptor trigger zone.

## Naloxone

Naloxone hydrochloride is N-alylnoroxymorphine and is a narcotic competitive antagonist on opioid receptors. This is useful in newborn infants whose mothers had received narcotics within 4 hours of delivery. This will reverse the respiratory depression. Duration of action is 1–2 hours.

### Mechanism of Action

Actions are similar to morphine, but do not produce addiction. It blocks μ receptors. Naloxone has a high affinity to μ opioid binding sites and inhibits μ receptors in the gut.

### Pharmacological Actions

It will antagonize all the effects of morphine.
- Analgesic effect
- Spasmogenic effect on smooth muscles
- Antitussive effect
- Miosis.

### Dosage

- *Dose*: 0.1–0.4 mg/kg of 0.4 mg/mL or 1 mg/mL solution intravenously or subcutaneously
- *Maintenance*: 0.4–0.8 mg/kg intravenously.

### Indications

- Treatment of morphine poisoning
- Diagnosis and treatment of morphine addiction
- Treatment of opioid induced ileus or constipation.
- This is useful in newborn infants whose mothers had received narcotics within 4 hours of delivery. This will reverse the respiratory depression.

### Contraindications

- Hypersensitivity to the drug
- Use cautiously in patients with addiction and cardiovascular diseases.

### Precautions

- The duration of action is short lived. The depressed patient may appear normal after naloxone and may go in to depression after 1–2 hours.
- Naloxone will precipitate morphine withdrawal symptoms in morphine dependent patients.
- Naloxone will impair thinking and reactions.

### Effects on Pregnancy

No evidence of teratogenicity.

### Side Effects

- Abdominal cramps
- Body ache
- Convulsions
- Diarrhea

- ❖ Emesis
- ❖ Excessive crying
- ❖ Fever
- ❖ Goose bumps
- ❖ Hot flushes
- ❖ Hypertension
- ❖ Irregular breathing/breathing difficulties
- ❖ Irritability
- ❖ Insomnia
- ❖ Jerky movements
- ❖ Restlessness.

### Drug Interactions

- ❖ Use of fentanyl and naloxone will result in reversal of effects of fentanyl.
- ❖ Droperidol will increase the risk for conduction abnormalities like irregular cardiac rhythm.

## QUESTIONS

**Q1. Why naloxone is more potent parenterally as compared to oral administration?**
It is because the absorption from gut is poor and this drug is inactivated in liver.

**Q2. Which effect of morphine is not antagonized by morphine?**
Antitussive effect.

**Q3. What are the advantages of naloxone?**
- ☐ Does not produce abstinence symptoms
- ☐ No tolerance to the antagonistic actions.

## ANTICONVULSANTS

Anticonvulsants are the drugs used for the treatment of epileptic seizures.

## Antiepileptics

These are drugs used to treat convulsions.

**Q1. What are the teratogenic effects of antiepileptics?**
The following teratogenic effects will be seen in the fetus if the drugs are given to the mother during antenatal period.

| Antiepileptic drug | Teratogenic effects |
|---|---|
| Carbamazepine | Neural tube defects |
| Phenobarbitone | Withdrawal symptoms, hemorrhagic disease, midfacial hypoplasia |
| Diphenylhydantoin (phenytoin) | Fetal hydantoin syndrome, hypoplastic phalanges, diaphragmatic hernia, cleft lip, coloboma, PDA, pulmonary atresia, hemorrhagic disease, craniofacial anomalies, midfacial hypoplasia, hypoplasia of the distal phalanges |
| Trimethadone | Fetal trimethadione syndrome, growth retardation, abnormal facies, (synophrys with upslanting eyebrows) cleft lip and palate, cardiac anomalies, genital anomalies |
| Benzodiazepines | Drug withdrawal |

### Sodium Valproate
Bleeding due to thrombocytopenia.

### Carbamazepine
- ❖ *Indications*:
    - Temporal lobe epilepsy
    - Trigeminal neuralgia
    - Myoclonus
    - Partial seizures
    - Generalized tonic clonic seizures
- ❖ *Adverse effects*:
    - Cholestatic jaundice
    - Idiosyncrasy
- ❖ *Drug interactions*:
    - Primidone
    - Phenytoin
    - Will decrease the drug level
- ❖ *Dose*:
    - 10 mg/kg/day to 20 mg/kg/day.

| Drug | Therapeutic level (µg/mL) | Toxic level |
|---|---|---|
| Carbamazepine | 8–12 | >15 µg/mL |
| Valproate | 50–100 | >100 µg/mL |
| Phenobarbitone | | |
| Phenytoin | 10–20 | >20 µg/mL |

## Newer Antiepileptics

- Vigabatrin
- Gabapentin
- Felbamate
- Oxcarbazepine
- Lamotrigine
- Lobazam.

**Q. What are the newer antiepileptics?**

Newer antiepileptics are lamotrigine, vigabatrin, and gabapentin.

- *Lamotrigine*:
  - Have carbamazepine like action
  - Side effects: Sleepiness, dizziness, diplopia, ataxia, and vomiting
- *Vigabatrin*:
  - Is an inhibitor of GABA transaminase which degrades GABA
  - Side effects: Behavioral changes, depression, and psychosis
- *Gabapentin*:
  - Is a GABA derivative
  - Lipophilic derivative of GABA and can crosses to the brain and enhance GABA release
  - Side effects: Mild sedation, tiredness, dizziness, and unsteadiness.

## Barbiturates

Barbiturates are sedative–hypnotics that acts as central nervous depressants.

**Q. How will you classify barbiturates?**

Barbiturates are classifies according to the duration of action as follows:
- *Long-acting barbiturates*: Acting for 8 hours or more, e.g. phenobarbitone and mephobarbitone.
- *Intermediate-acting barbiturates*: Acting 4–8 hours, e.g. amylobarbitone and pentobarbitone
- *Short-acting barbiturates*: Acting for less than 4 hours, e.g. secobarbitone and hexobarbitone
- *Ultra-short acting*: Thiopentone, hexobarbitone, and methohexitone.

## Mechanism of Action of Barbiturates

- Barbiturates acts at GABA/benzodiazepine (BZD) receptor Cl– channel complex.
- Barbiturates cause reversible depression of the activity of all excitable tissues. They depress the polysynaptic responses and delay synaptic recovery. Small doses will have GABA like action.
- Reversible depression of activity of all excitable tissues. Reticular activating system is most sensitive which results in inability to maintain wakefulness.
- They facilitate the inhibitory neurotransmission in the CNS.

## Dosage

Dosage of barbiturates will depend upon the type.

## Indications

- Seizure disorder
- Jaundice

## Contraindications and Cautions for Barbiturates

- Acute intermittent porphyria
- Liver disease
- Kidney disease
- Severe pulmonary insufficiency
- Obstructive sleep apnea.

## Precautions

Oral contraceptive failure can occur if given along with barbiturates. Barbiturates will have additive effects with other drugs like alcohol, antihistamines, tranquillizers which slow the functions of central nervous system.

### Effects on Pregnancy

- Administration of barbiturates during pregnancy can cause the following problems in newborn
- Bleeding problems in newborn
- Drug dependence in newborn
- Drug withdrawal symptoms in newborn.

### Side Effects

- Adverse effects of barbiturates:
  - Idiosyncrasy
  - Mental excitement and mental confusion
  - Tolerance
  - Dependence—psychological and physical
  - Hangover
  - Hypersensitivity
- Barbiturates may evoke excitement in females and care should be exercised when given during pregnancy, lactation or menstruation.
- Barbiturate may precipitate an attack of acute intermittent porphyria.

### Drug Interactions of Barbiturates

- Induces metabolism of many drugs like warfarin, steroids, tolbutamide, griseofulvin, chloramphenicol, and theophylline.
- Additive effects with other CNS depressants—alcohol, antihistaminics, opioids, etc.
- Sodium valproate will increase the plasma concentration of phenobarbitone.

## QUESTIONS

**Q1. What are the withdrawal symptoms of barbiturates?**
- Excitement
- Hallucinations
- Delirium
- Convulsions
- Death.

**Q2. What is the lethal dose of barbiturates?**
2–3 g for more lipid soluble short-acting barbiturates and 5–10 g for less lipid soluble barbiturates like phenobarbitone.

**Q3. How does alkalinization help in acute barbiturate poisoning?**
Alkalinization will reduce the plasma concentration of the nonionized and diffusible form of barbiturate. This will lead to withdrawal of barbiturate from the brain and cerebrospinal fluid. Also alkalinization of the urine will prevent reabsorption by ionization of the filtered barbiturate. This will facilitate the elimination.

### Acute Barbiturate Poisoning

Acute barbiturate poisoning will occur due to excessive doses of barbiturates.

**Q1. What are the features of acute barbiturate poisoning?**
- Depression of central nervous system, respiratory depression, and peripheral circulatory collapse.
- Excessive CNS depression—flabby, comatose, shallow, and failing respiration.
- Fall in blood pressure
- Weak, rapid pulse
- Cold clammy skin
- Bullous eruptions
- Rapid pulse
- Pupils will be constricted and reacting to light initially. Later, there will be paralytic dilatation.
- Cardiovascular collapse.

**Q2. What are the fatal complications of acute barbiturate poisoning?**
Fatal complications of acute barbiturate poisoning are respiratory and renal complications.
- *Respiratory complications*:
  - Atelectasis
  - Pulmonary edema
  - Bronchopneumonia
- *Renal complications*: Acute renal shut down

## Q3. How will you treat acute barbiturate poisoning?
Treatment of acute barbiturate poisoning:
- Gastric lavage (if patient is conscious and less than 4 hours after ingestion).
- Endotracheal intubation to maintain adequate ventilation.
- Forced alkaline dieresis using furosemide or mannitol.
- Alkalinization will reduce the plasma concentration of the nonionized and diffusible form of barbiturate.
- Dialysis.

## Q4. What are the contraindications for forced dieresis?
Shock, cardiac failure, and renal impairment.

## Q5. What are the features of chronic barbiturate poisoning?
- Thick slurred speech
- Ataxia
- Impaired superficial and deep reflexes
- Hypotonia
- Nystagmus
- Difficulty in accommodation.

## Q6. What are the features of barbiturate withdrawal syndrome?
- Anxiety
- Restlessness
- Tremors
- Abdominal cramps
- Nausea
- Vomiting
- Orthostatic hypotension
- Prostration
- Convulsions
- Visual hallucinations
- Disorientation
- Delirium
- This may be followed by cardiovascular collapse.

## Q7. How will you treat chronic barbiturate poisoning?
The drug should be gradually withdrawn over 10 days to 3 weeks.

## Phenobarbitone
- This is the first antiepileptic introduced in 1912
- Phenobarbitone sodium
- Trade names—Gardenal
- Injection—200 mg/mL in 1 mL ampoules
- Tablets—15, 30, and 60 mg.

### Mechanism of Action of Phenobarbitone
- Phenobarbital induces microsomal enzymes, which will increase the conjugation and excretion of bilirubin. Phenobarbitone will raise the seizure threshold.
- Phenobarbital lowers the bilirubin levels in the neonate when given to the mother antenatally, but it is not recommended due to its toxicity.
- It will induce hepatic enzymes cytochrome P450.
- It increases the concentration of ligandin, which binds the bilirubin and transports to endoplasmic reticulum.

## Q1. How does phenobarbitone act in controlling seizures?
This drug will raise the seizure threshold.

### Pharmacological Actions
- Respiratory system is depressed in higher doses
- Decreases the blood pressure and heart rate
- Skeletal muscle: Anesthetic doses will cause reduced muscle contraction.
- Smooth muscles: In hypnotic doses, the tone and motility of smooth muscles will be decreased.
- Kidneys: Decreases the urine flow by decreasing blood pressure and increasing ADH release.

### Dosage
*Dose*: 5-8 mg/kg/day.

## Q1. What is the dose for seizures therapy?
- *Loading dose*: 15-20 mg/kg intravenously.

- *Maintenance*: 3–5 mg/kg/day intravenously or intramuscularly.
- Oral one or two divided doses.

**Q2. What is the therapeutic serum concentration of phenobarbitone?**
15–30 mg/mL.

## Convulsions

Phenobarbitone is given intravenously, in a dose of 20 mg/kg loading dose given over a period of 10–30 minutes. This should be followed by a maintenance dose of 5 mg/kg/day. The rate of infusion should be 1 mg/kg/min.

Phenobarbitone 3–10 mg/kg/day induces liver enzymes and promotes excretion of toxic products.

## Indications

- Anticonvulsants
- Cholestasis
- Crigler-Najjar syndrome (type II)
- Gilbert syndrome
- Delirium
- Mania
- Sedative
- Preanesthetic medication
- Neonatal hyperbilirubinemia
- Neonatal seizures
- Seizures—generalized tonic clonic seizures, simple partial seizures, and complex partial seizures
- Focal onset seizures.

**Q1. In which type of seizures phenobarbitone is not useful?**
Absence seizures.

**Q2. Is phenobarbitone useful in status epilepticus?**
In status epilepticus, phenobarbitone can be used parenterally, but the response will be slow to develop.

**Q3. What is the type of seizure which may be aggravated by phenobarbitone?**
Petit mal epilepsy.

## Contraindications

- Acute intermittent porphyria
- Bronchial asthma
- Depression
- Drug dependence
- Diabetes—uncontrolled
- Emphysema
- Hyperkinesia
- Hypersensitivity to barbiturate
- Kidney disease
- Liver disease
- Obstructive sleep apnea
- Severe pulmonary insufficiency.

## Precautions

Should be used with caution in patients with depression, breathing problems, drug dependence, suicidal tendencies, and elderly.

## Effects on Pregnancy

Category D.

## Side Effects

- *Central nervous system*: Agitation, confusion, drowsiness, dizziness, depression, excitement, nightmares, paradoxical excitement or hyperactivity, nystagmus, and ataxia can be seen with larger doses, sedation, and hypnosis
- *Gastrointestinal*: Nausea, vomiting, and constipation
- Respiratory depression (when the serum concentration is >60 mg/mL)
- Hypotension and circulatory collapse
- *Hematological*: Megaloblastic anemia with prolonged phenobarbitone (will respond to folic acid)
- *Hepatitis*: Cholestasis
- Exfoliative dermatitis
- Hypersensitivity
- Sedation (when the serum concentration is >60 mg/mL)
- Hangover
- Tolerance
- Drug dependence

- *Drug automatism*: If hypnotic doses are taken frequently, the patient will fail-to-fall asleep after taking the drug, but will be mentally confused and amnesic.
- Excitement or hyperactivity in children and old people.

## Drug Interactions

- Metabolism of many drugs will be induced by barbiturates
- Phenobarbitone will decrease the absorption of griseofulvin from the gut.
- Sodium valproate will increase the plasma concentration of phenobarbitone.

The following drugs will be associated with CNS depression as addictive effect:
- Alcohol
- Antihistamines
- Opioids.

# QUESTIONS

**Q1. Which drug will enhance the CNS depressant effect of barbiturates?**
The following drugs will cause severe CNS depression when given along with barbiturates:
- Monoamine oxidase inhibitors
- Alcohol
- Benzodiazepines
- Antihistaminics.

**Q2. What is the type of convulsion that is aggravated by the drug phenobarbitone?**
Petit mal epilepsy will be aggravated by phenobarbitone.

**Q2. What are the causes of tolerance?**
Due to hepatic inactivation.

**Q3. What is the effect of phenobarbitone given during the antenatal period?**
- Causes fetal respiratory depression
- Withdrawal symptoms, hemorrhagic disease, and midfacial hypoplasia.

**Q4. What is the fate of barbiturates in the body?**
The barbiturates will be redistributed or metabolically degraded into inactive compounds by the microsomal enzymes in the liver or excreted by the kidneys. As far as phenobarbitone is concerned 25–30% of phenobarbitone will be excreted unchanged.

**Q5. Which is the barbiturate that is completely metabolized in the liver?**
Pentobarbitone is completely metabolized in the liver and is advised in renal failure.

**Q6. What is drug automatism?**
When phenobarbitone is used as hypnotic, may fail-to-fall sleep after taking the drug and get mentally confused and amnesic and will take more phenobarbitone. They will continue to take pills and develop acute poisoning resulting in drug poisoning.

**Q7. What is tolerance? When will it disappear?**
- Tolerance to barbiturates will occur due to repeated doses. Tolerance may be due to increased hepatic inactivation or adaptation of the nervous tissue to the drug.
- Tolerance that is acquired will disappear within 1–2 weeks of abstinence.

**Q8. What is the danger of giving phenobarbitone to asthmatics who are dependent on corticosteroids?**
Exaggerate asthma.

**Q9. What is the disadvantage of stopping phenobarbitone suddenly?**
It will increase the frequency of convulsion and even status epilepticus may be precipitated.

**Q10. What are the conditions in which phenobarbitone and phenytoin should be combined?**
Grand mal epilepsy, resistant cases of focal cortical seizures, and hypsarrhythmia.

**Q11. What are the advantages of combining phenobarbitone and phenytoin?**

The adverse effects of both the drugs can be reduced by keeping the individual doses below the toxicity levels.

**Q12. Why phenytoin should be added before withdrawing phenobarbitone?**

The seizures due to phenobarbitone withdrawal is very difficult to control, hence the dose of phenobarbitone should be gradually reduced and the phenytoin should be increased slowly until the phenytoin takes over fully.

**Q13. What are the disadvantages of sudden cessation of phenobarbitone after prolonged use?**

- There will be increase in frequency of seizures
- Even precipitate status epilepticus.

**Q14. What are the conditions in which phenobarbitone and phenytoin are useful in combination?**

- Grand mal
- Resistant cases of focal cortical seizures
- Hypsarrhythmia.

**Q15. What are the advantages in combining phenobarbitone and phenytoin?**

Both drugs can be used in low doses so that toxicity will not occur.

**Q16. What is the effect of phenobarbitone in petit mal epilepsy and temporal lobe epilepsy?**

- Phenobarbitone is not useful in temporal lobe epilepsy
- Phenobarbitone may aggravate petit mal epilepsy.

## Phenytoin

- Diphenylhydantoin (phenytoin)
- Trade names: Dilantin, eptoin, and epsolin
- Phenytoin sodium:
    - Injection 100 mg/2 mL
    - Suspension—25 mg/mL
- Half-life: 24 hours with wide variation and dose dependent
- Therapeutic range: 10–20 µg/mL.

### Mechanism of Action

Stabilizes the neuronal membrane.

### Pharmacological Actions

- Anticonvulsant abolishes tonic phase of seizures with no effect on clonic phase
- Limits the spread of seizure activity
- Antiarrhythmic: Decreases the permeability of the cardiac muscle to sodium and potassium.

### Dosage

- *Dosage for antiepileptic*:
    - *Loading dose*: 15–20 mg/kg intravenously
    - *Maintenance dose*: 5–7 mg/kg/day given every 6 or 12 hourly by intravenous or oral administration
    - Dilution should be done by adding 1 mL of the drug with 24 mL of normal saline.
    - This results in 2 mg/mL
    - The required dose should be given slowly over 15–20 minutes. The rate of infusion should be less than and equal to 1 mg/kg/min.
- *Convulsions*: Phenytoin is given intravenously in a dose of 20 mg/kg loading dose followed by a maintenance dose of 5 mg/kg/day.
- *Dosage for antiarrhythmic*:
    - Loading dose: 10 mg/kg intravenously
    - Maintenance dose: 5–10 mg/kg/day given every 12 hourly by intravenous administration.
    - Per oral dose loading: 10–15 mg/kg/day in divided doses every 6 hourly
- *Maintenance dose*: 10–15 mg/kg/day given every 12 hourly by intravenous administration.

**Q. What are the precautions you should take before injection phenytoin?**

The line should be in the vein. Intra-arterial injection may result in gangrene.

## Indications
- Antiepileptic
- Antiarrhythmic
- Partial seizures
- Generalized tonic clonic seizures
- Grand mal epilepsy
- Psychomotor seizures
- Focal cortical epilepsy
- Focal onset seizures
- Cardiac arrhythmias
- Trigeminal neuralgia (first choice carbamazepine)
- Status epilepticus
- Digitalis induced arrhythmias
- Migraine.

## Contraindications for Phenytoin
- Heart block
- AV block
- Sinus bradycardia
- Pregnancy and lactation.

## Precautions
- Electrocardiogram should be monitored during this drug administration
- Dose should be adjusted in hepatic dysfunction
- History of allergy to any other drugs should be enquired. As this drug causes dizziness or drowsiness, do not drive or any other activity needing alertness
- In diabetics, this drug may increase glucose levels
- Products containing calcium will decrease the absorption of phenytoin.

## Effects on Pregnancy
- Will cause fetal hydantoin syndrome
- Folate supplements should be given
- The dose should be reduced in the elderly patients.

## Side Effects/Adverse Reactions of Phenytoin at Therapeutic Levels
- Acne
- Allergic rashes
- Blood dyscrasias (aplastic anemia, pancytopenia, leucopenia, neutropenia, agranulocytosis)
- Anemia due to folic acid deficiency
- Methemoglobinemia
- Coarsening of facial features
- Constipation
- Discoid lupus erythematosus (DLE)
- Dizziness
- Dermatitis
- Emesis
- Fetal hydantoin syndrome
- Fever
- Gum hyperplasia and hypertrophy with edema and bleeding. Gingival hyperplasia is more common in children. This is not related to dose. It will return to normal within 1 year after discontinuation of the drug.
- Gastrointestinal disturbances
- Hirsutism
- Hypersensitivity reaction
- Insomnia
- Intolerance (urticaria, scarlatiniform, and measles like rash)
- Idiosyncrasy
- Lymphadenopathy: Lymphoid hyperplasia (generalized lymphadenopathy—pseudolymphoma)
- Megaloblastic anemia responding to folic acid
- Nystagmus
- Osteomalacia
- Hyperglycemia by inhibiting insulin release
- Anemia due to folic acid deficiency. Megaloblastic anemia responding to folic acid.

Adverse reactions of phenytoin at high plasma levels:
- Cardiac arrhythmias
- Blood pressure: Fall in blood pressure (hypotension)
- Cerebellar and vestibular manifestations (ataxia, vertigo, diplopia, and nystagmus)
- Drowsiness, behavioral alterations, mental confusion, and hallucinations

- ❖ Epigastric pain
- ❖ Nausea and vomiting
- ❖ Vascular injury.

*Other complications*:
- ❖ Agranulocytosis
- ❖ Liver damage
- ❖ Peripheral neuropathy
- ❖ Behavioral changes
- ❖ Secondary rickets
- ❖ Morbilliform rash
- ❖ Hepatosplenomegaly
- ❖ Nausea
- ❖ Lupus like reaction
- ❖ Methemoglobinemia.

**Q. What are the dreaded complications during phenytoin administration?**
- ❑ Cardiovascular collapse
- ❑ Central nervous system depression
- ❑ Stevens-Johnson syndrome
- ❑ Systemic lupus erythematosus like syndrome
- ❑ Vestibulocerebellar syndrome
- ❑ Extravasations will cause dermal necrosis and tissue sloughing
- ❑ Seizures will be associated with high serum concentration
- ❑ Rarely toxic hepatitis.

## Drug Interactions

- ❖ Phenytoin is highly protein bound. Other protein bound drugs like sulfonamides and phenylbutazone can replace phenytoin from its binding site
- ❖ Phenytoin will induce microsomal enzymes responsible for metabolism of many drugs like steroids, oral contraceptives, digitoxin, doxycycline, and theophylline.
- ❖ Phenytoin will alter the effect of warfarin
- ❖ Phenytoin will reduce the effectiveness of oral contraceptives
- ❖ Ethosuximide will increase the plasma level of phenytoin
- ❖ Chloramphenicol will increase the serum levels of phenytoin and may increase the risk of toxicity.
- ❖ Rifampicin will decrease the serum levels of phenytoin
- ❖ Phenytoin will decrease the serum level of cyclosporine
- ❖ Other drugs like phenylbutazone and sulfonamides will displace phenytoin from binding sites and increase the plasma concentration. In hypoalbuminic states the total phenytoin level will be decreased but the free phenytoin level may not be affected.
- ❖ Drugs that will increase the metabolism of phenytoin and each other: Phenobarbitone and carbamazepine will induce hepatic microsomal enzymes.
- ❖ Drugs that will decrease the metabolism of phenytoin and thereby precipitate its toxicity:
  - Isonicotinylhydrazide (INH)
  - Chloramphenicol
  - Cimetidine
  - Dicumarol
  - Warfarin.

**Q1. What are the effects of giving phenytoin and valproate together?**
Valproate will replace protein bound phenytoin and decreases the metabolism and thereby increases plasma level of unbound phenytoin.

**Q2. What are the effects of giving phenytoin and tolbutamide together?**
Phenytoin will inhibit tolbutamide metabolism which may cause hypoglycemia.

**Q3. What are the effects of giving phenytoin and sucralfate together?**
Sucralfate will bind phenytoin and decrease its absorption.

**Q4. What are the drugs that will prolong the half-life of phenytoin by inhibiting phenytoin metabolism?**
Isoniazid, chloramphenicol, coumarin anticoagulants, and sulfonamides.

**Q5. What are the drugs that are metabolized rapidly due to enzyme inducing activity of phenytoin?**

- Contraceptive steroids, coumarin anticoagulants, glucocorticoids, and vitamin D.
- Phenytoin will induce microsomal enzymes and increase degradation of steroids, digitoxin, doxycycline, and theophylline.

**Q6. What are the drugs that will inhibit phenytoin metabolism and precipitate its toxicity?**
Chloramphenicol, isoniazid, cimetidine, dicumarol, and warfarin.

## QUESTIONS

**Q1. What are the factors that will affect serum levels of phenytoin?**
- Uremia
- Hypoalbuminemia.

**Q2. What is the diluent that should be used to dilute phenytoin?**
Only normal saline is compatible with this drug. All other solutions are not compatible.

**Q3. What are the precautions to be taken while administering phenytoin by intravenous route?**
- One should confirm that the needle is in the vein. After the administration of the drug, the cannula should be flushed with normal saline to prevent phlebitis.
- If the solution looks cloudy do not administer it.

**Q4. What are the steps you will take to prevent precipitate formation?**
- 0.9% NaCl should be used for infusion solution
- Dilute to less than 6.7 mg/mL
- Start infusion immediately after preparation
- Infuse slowly over 30 minutes
- Use a 0.22 µm in line filter
- Observe for precipitate.

**Q5. What is the therapeutic serum concentration of phenytoin?**
Free plus bound phenytoin 10–20 mg/L or free phenytoin 1–2 mg/L.

**Q6. What are the earliest features of phenytoin toxicity?**
- Nystagmus
- Loss of smooth extraocular pursuit movements.

**Q7. What are the dose related features of phenytoin toxicity that requires adjustment of dose?**
Ataxia and diplopia.

**Q8. What are the features of toxicity associated with long-term use of phenytoin?**
- Coarse facies
- Mild peripheral neuropathy associated with diminished deep tendon reflexes in lower extremities
- Affects vitamin D metabolism resulting in osteomalacia
- Decreases folate levels predisposing to megaloblastic anemia.

**Q9. What are the factors predisposing to phenytoin toxicity?**
- Increased oral intake
- Renal disease.

**Q10. What are the steps to prevent gum hypertrophy?**
Massage the gums twice daily after brushing the tooth will prevent gum hypertrophy.

**Q11. What are the steps to prevent megaloblastic anemia?**
Supplementation of folic acid 5 mg daily.

**Q12. What are the steps to prevent osteomalacia?**
Supplementation of vitamin D, 6 lacs units intramuscularly once in 6 months.

**Q13. What are the dreaded complications during phenytoin administration?**
- Cardiovascular collapse
- Central nervous system depression.

**Q14. What is the step to be taken to prevent vascular injury?**
The rate of infusion should not exceed 25 mg/minute.

**Q15. What are the teratogenic effects of phenytoin?**
Fetal hydantoin syndrome.

**Q16. What are the features of fetal hydantoin syndrome?**
Fetal hydantoin syndrome—diaphragmatic hernia, cleft lip and palate, coloboma, CVS malformations like PDA, pulmonary atresia, hemorrhagic disease, craniofacial anomalies, microcephaly, midfacial hypoplasia, hypoplasia of the distal phalanges, nail hypoplasia, ocular hypertelorism, and flat nasal bridge.

**Q17. What is the danger of giving phenytoin in diabetics?**
Dangerous hyperglycemia probably due to inhibition of insulin secretion by phenytoin.

**Q18. What is the effect of folic acid on phenytoin?**
Chronic administration of folic acid will reduce the effectiveness of phenytoin.

**Q19. What are the effects of giving phenytoin and phenobarbitone together?**
- Phenobarbitone will competitively inhibit phenytoin metabolism
- Both will induce enzymes and facilitate degradation of other drugs.

## Valproic Acid/Sodium Valproate

### Mechanism of Action of Valproate
Blocks sustained high frequency repetitive firing of neurons. In high doses, it will block degradation of GABA.

### Pharmacological Actions
Broad spectrum anticonvulsant with little central acts and little sedation.

### Dosage
- 15 mg/kg in divided doses can be increased by 5 mg per week up to 30 mg/kg/day
- 20-25 mg/kg orally
- Therapeutic levels 50 mg/mL to 100 mg/mL.

### Indications
- Focal onset seizures
- Absence seizures with concomitant GTCS
- Generalized tonic clonic seizures
- Atonic seizures
- Partial seizures: Simple partial seizures (SPS)/complex partial seizures (CPS)
- Mania and bipolar illness
- Migraine prophylaxis
- Petit mal
- Temporal lobe epilepsy
- Psychomotor epilepsy
- Myoclonic epilepsy.

### Contraindications
- Pregnancy
- Hepatic decompensation.

### Precautions
Sodium valproate should be stared gradually.

**Q1. What is the precaution to be taken to prevent the toxicity of valproate?**
- Food will delay the absorption of valproate, hence the drug should be given after food to decrease the incidence of its toxicity.
- Liver function tests should be performed before staring sodium valproate.

### Effects on Pregnancy
Increases the incidence of spina bifida, cardiovascular, orofacial, and digital abnormalities.

**Q1. What are the teratogenic effects of valproic acid?**
- Spina bifida and neural tube defects
- Neural tube defects—myelomeningocele, facial dysmorphism, learning disability, and motor incoordination
- Cardiovascular defects

- Orofacial defects
- Digital defects.

**Q2. What is the risk of pregnant women giving birth to a baby with spina bifida?**
1-2%.

## Side Effects
- Anorexia
- Sedation
- Ataxia
- Incoordination
- Hyperammonemia
- Inhibition of platelet aggregation
- Fulminant liver failure
- Pancreatitis
- Thrombocytopenia.

**Q1. What are the dose-related adverse effects of valproic acid?**
- Nausea
- Vomiting
- Abdominal pain
- Heart burn
- Fine tremors
- Idiosyncrasy—hepatotoxicity.

**Q2. What are the reversible side effects of sodium valproate?**
- Weight gain
- Increased appetite
- Alopecia—hair loss.

**Q3. What are the nondose-related adverse effects of valproic acid?**
- Idiosyncratic hepatic damage is more in children aged less than 2 years and those who are on multiple drugs. Most of the patients develop this complication within 4 months after initiation of the drug therapy.
- Idiosyncratic thrombocytopenia.

## Drug Interactions
Will cause rise of barbiturates resulting in stupor or coma.
- Valproate will increase the plasma level of phenobarbitone by inhibiting its metabolism.
- Valproate and carbamazepine will induce each other's metabolism.
- Will displace phenytoin from the plasma proteins and binding sites.
- Will inhibit the metabolism of drugs like phenobarbitol, phenytoin, and carbamazepine.
- When added to phenobarbitol sedation may occur.

The following drugs will decrease the serum levels of valproate:
- Carbamazepine
- Phenobarbitone
- Phenytoin
- Primidone.

**Q1. How does valproate precipitate phenytoin toxicity?**
Valproate will displace phenytoin from protein binding site and decrease the metabolism.

**Q2. What are the effects of giving clonazepam and valproate together?**
Absence status may be precipitated.

**Q3. What are the effects of giving carbamazepine and valproate together?**
Fetal abnormalities are more, blood level of valproate will be reduced.

**Q4. What are the effects of giving aspirin and valproate together?**
Blood level of valproate will be increased.

**Q5. What is the drug to be given to patients developing idiosyncratic hepatotoxicity?**
Intravenous L-carnitine should be given.

## Carbamazepine (Tegretol)

### Mechanism of Action
- It is a sodium channel blocker
- Carbamazepine acts by blocking sodium channels
- Raises threshold to pentylenetetrazole (PTZ)
- Inhibits kindling.

### Pharmacological Actions
- Anticonvulsive antipsychotic activity
- Inhibits kindling

- Antidiuretic action by enhancing antidiuretic hormone (ADH) action on renal tubules.

## Dosage
- 15–25 mg/kg/day
- 10–20 mg/kg/day in two to three divided doses
- Adult dose: 100–200 mg twice a day.

**The therapeutic level of carbamazepine:** 4–8 mg/mL.

## Indications
- This drug is used in combination of other anticonvulsants:
  - Complex partial seizures
  - Generalized tonic clonic seizures
  - Focal onset seizures
  - Trigeminal neuralgia
  - Bipolar mania
  - Diabetes insipidus of primary origin.
- Used as an adjuvant when phenobarbitone and diphenylhydantoin fail to control the following:
  - Temporal lobe epilepsy
  - Grand mal epilepsy
  - Complex partial seizures
  - Generalized tonic-clonic (GTC)
  - Simple partial seizures (SPS)
  - Myoclonus
- Prophylactic therapy in manic depressive psychosis (alternative to lithium).

## Contraindications
- Allergy—hypersensitivity
- AV block
- Acute intermittent porphyria
- Bone marrow depression.

## Precautions
- Monitor blood pressure and liver function tests
- Use with caution in patients with liver and renal impairment
- Use with caution on severe cardiac problems
- Pregnancy and lactation.

## Effects on Pregnancy
- Teratogenic effects of carbamazepine include increased incidence of minor malformations in the fetus
- Neural tube defects.

## Side Effects
- Dose-related adverse effects of carbamazepine:
  - Ataxia
  - Ankle swelling
  - Ataxia
  - Blood dyscrasia—agranulocytosis and aplastic anemia
  - Blurred vision (visual accommodation problems)
  - Constipation
  - Cholestatic jaundice
  - Diarrhea
  - Diplopia
  - Drowsiness
  - Edema due to water retention
  - Exfoliative dermatitis
  - Gastrointestinal upset (mild)
  - Headache
  - Hepatotoxicity
  - Hyponatremia
  - Itching
  - Idiosyncrasy
  - Loss of appetite
  - Leukopenia
  - Lupus like syndrome
  - Neurotoxicity
  - Photosensitivity
  - Rash
  - Stevens-Johnson syndrome
  - Somnolence
  - Unsteadiness
  - Water intoxication.
- Hypersensitivity reactions—rashes, photosensitivity, lupus-like syndrome, rarely agranulocytosis, and aplastic anemia.

## Drug Interactions

- Carbamazepine will induce hepatic enzymes which will increase its own metabolism. Hence a steady state carbamazepine concentration is not possible. It will also reduce the efficacy of haloperidol and oral contraceptives.
- Carbamazepine increase the metabolism of drugs like phenytoin, primidone, ethosuximide, valproic acid, and clonazepam.
- Will shorten the half-life of doxycycline.
- Carbamazepine will reduce the effect of anticoagulants and oral contraceptives.
- Cimetidine and verapamil will increase the effect of carbamazepine.
- Erythromycin will inhibit the metabolism of carbamazepine.
- Should not be administered if MAOI is administered within 2 weeks.
- With lithium it will be neurotoxic.
- In combination with valproate the rate of teratogenicity will be more
- Enzyme inducer
- Reduces the efficacy of haloperidol and oral contraceptives.

The drugs that inhibit carbamazepine clearance:
- Valproic acid, propoxyphene, and troleandomycin
- Phenytoin, phenobarbitone will induce enzymes and decrease the steady state concentration of carbamazepine.

# QUESTIONS

Q1. **What is the earliest sign of toxicity?**
Diplopia may be observed from 7 mg/mL in some patients and above 10 mg/mL in most patients.

Q2. **What is the earliest sign of carbamazepine toxicity?**
Diplopia which may last for less than 1 hour during a particular time of the day.

Q3. **What is the idiosyncratic reaction of carbamazepine?**
Erythematous skin rash.

## Ethosuximide

- Half-life: 60 hours
- Therapeutic range: 40–100 µg/mL

### Mechanism of Action

Neuron excitability is affected by blocking T-type calcium channels.

### Dosage

- 20–40 mg/kg
- 750–1,250 mg/day.

### Indications

Absence (petit mal) seizures.

### Contraindications

- Liver disorders
- Myasthenia gravis
- Depression
- Systemic lupus erythematosus (SLE)
- Pregnancy
- Kidney diseases
- Allergy.

### Precautions

- When used alone may increase the frequency of grand mal seizures
- Abrupt withdrawal may precipitate petit mal seizures (absence seizures)
- Avoid driving or tasks that require skills.

### Effects on Pregnancy

Will cross placenta and cause birth defects.

### Side Effects

- Ataxia
- Bone marrow suppression
- Blood dyscrasia—pancytopenia
- Constipation
- Drowsiness
- Eyes—myopia
- Gastrointestinal irritation
- Hepatotoxicity—abnormal liver functions
- Insomnia
- Mental confusion
- Nephrotoxicity

- ❖ Systemic lupus erythematosus
- ❖ Suicidal behavior
- ❖ Stevenson-Johnson syndrome
- ❖ Skin—urticaria.

## Drug Interactions

- ❖ Ethosuximide will elevate the serum levels of phenytoin
- ❖ Valproic acid may increase or decrease etosuximide levels.

## Newer Antiepileptics

### Gabapentin

**Mechanism of action:** Gabapentin structurally resembles the neurotransmitter gamma amino butyric acid.

**Pharmacological actions:**

- ❖ Pain relief in herpes zoster
- ❖ Entire drug is excreted unchanged through urine.

### Dosage:

Oral dose:
- ❖ 40 g/kg/day
- ❖ More than 12 years: 300–800 orally three times a day
- ❖ Up to 900–2,400 mg/day.

**Indications:**

- ❖ Focal onset seizures
- ❖ Depression
- ❖ Mania
- ❖ Anxiety
- ❖ Tardive dyskinesia
- ❖ Postherpetic neuralgia.

**Contraindications:**

- ❖ Allergy to gabapentin
- ❖ Depression
- ❖ Myasthenia gravis
- ❖ Pregnancy
- ❖ Renal impairment.

**Precautions:**

- ❖ Antacids with aluminum or magnesium will interfere with absorption of gabapentin
- ❖ Take gabapentin 2 hours after taking antacid
- ❖ There are different forms of gabapentin like immediate release, sustained release, and switch over from one form to other should be avoided.
- ❖ Doses should be decreased in renal insufficiency.

**Effects on pregnancy:** Contraindicated as teratogenic effects are present.

**Side effects:**

- ❖ Allergy
- ❖ Blurred vision
- ❖ Clumsiness
- ❖ Coordination problems
- ❖ Constipation
- ❖ Diarrhea
- ❖ Dizziness
- ❖ Drowsiness
- ❖ Depression
- ❖ Edema
- ❖ Fatigue
- ❖ Gain in weight
- ❖ Headache
- ❖ Itching.

**Drug interactions:** Alcohol will increase the side effects.

## QUESTION

Q. What are the features of gabapentin overdose?
- ☐ Double vision
- ☐ Drowsiness
- ☐ Dysarthria (slurred speech)
- ☐ Decreased activity (lethargy)
- ☐ Diarrhea.

### Lamotrigine

**Mechanism of action:**

- ❖ Sodium channel blocker stabilizing neuronal membranes.
- ❖ Decreases presynaptic glutamate and aspartate release.

**Pharmacological actions:** Anticonvulsant.

**Dosage:** 150–500 mg/bd.

**Indications:**
- Partial/focal onset seizures
- Generalized tonic clonic seizures
- Absence seizures
- Bipolar disorder
- Myoclonic
- Lennox-Gastaut syndrome.

**Contraindications:**
- Hypersensitivity/allergy to previous dose
- Anemia
- Bone marrow failure
- Depression
- Liver problems
- Kidney impairment.

**Precautions:** Should not be stopped abruptly.

**Effects on pregnancy:**
- Not associated with birth defects
- Folic acid in high doses of 5 mg/day should be taken along with antiepileptic.

**Side effects:** Rash.

**Serious side effects:**
- Allergic reactions
- Steven-Johnson syndrome
- Drug reaction with eosinophilia and systemic symptoms (DRESS)
- Toxic epidermal necrolysis.

**Drug interactions:** The following drugs will induce glucuronidation and decrease the lamotrigine concentration:
- Oral contraceptives with estrogen
- Phenobarbitone
- Phenytoin
- Rifampin.

The following drug will inhibits glucuronidation and increases the lamotrigine concentration: Valproate

Lamotrigine should not be used along with valproic acid as it will cause serious rash.

## Levetiracetam

**Mechanism of action:** This drug binds to a synaptic vesicle glycoprotein and inhibit presynaptic calcium channels.

**Dosage:**
- 1–6 months old: 4–7 mg/kg in two divided doses
- 6 months to 4 years: 20–50 mg/kg in two divided doses
- 4–16 years: 20–60 mg/kg in two divided doses.

**Indications:**
- Convulsions
- Partial seizures
- Generalized tonic clonic seizures
- Myoclonic seizures.

**Contraindications:**
- Allergy
- Kidney problems.

**Precautions:**
- This drug may cause suicidal tendencies
- Sudden withdrawal of this drug may precipitate status epilepticus.

**Effects on pregnancy:**
- Category C
- The drug is teratogenic. This should be used only if clearly indicated.

**Side effects:**
- Anxiety
- Agitation
- Allergy—skin rash
- Breathing difficulty
- Cough
- Drowsiness
- Dizziness
- Depersonalization
- Emotional lability
- Euphoria
- Fatigue
- Gastrointestinal problems—diarrhea

- Headache
- Hives
- Hostility
- Irritability
- Suicidal behavior
- Stevens-Johnson syndrome
- Toxic epidermal necrolysis (TEN).

**Drug interactions:** No significant interactions noted.

## CORTICOSTEROIDS (GLUCOCORTICOIDS)

- Prednisone
- Prednisolone
- Dexamethasone
- Hydrocortisone
- Betamethasone.

### Steroids

- Prednisolone
- Dexamethasone 0.25 mg/kg/dose intravenously every 8 hourly.
- Hydrocortisone 1–2 mg/kg/dose intravenously every 8 hourly.
- Placenta will metabolize hydrocortisone and prednisolone to less active cortisone and prednisone.
- Dexamethasone and betamethasone will cross placenta and can achieve higher concentration to suppress fetal hypothalamic-pituitary-adrenal (HPA) axis.

### Mechanism of Action

- *Carbohydrate metabolism*: Promote gluconeogenesis and deposition of glycogen in the liver.
- *Protein metabolism*: Will increase the breakdown of proteins
- *Fat metabolism*: Increases the mobilization of fat from peripheral fat deposits
- *Electrolyte and water*: Water retention
- *Calcium*: Increases calcium excretion
- *Muscle*: Weakness in Addison disease will be corrected
- *Hematological*: Decreases eosinophils and lymphocytes
- *Gastrointestinal tract*: Stimulation of pepsin and hydrochloric acid secretion
- Anti-inflammatory
- Antiallergic
- *Central nervous system*: Elevation of mood in large doses, euphoria, and restlessness
- *Miscellaneous*: Uricosuric and antipyretic.

### Pharmacological Actions

The pharmacological actions of glucocorticoids are widespread and includes alterations in the carbohydrate, protein, fat metabolism, modulation of electrolyte and fluid balance.

Q. **What are the pharmacological actions of glucocorticoids?**
- Antianabolic action: Inhibits incorporation of amino acids into protein in the peripheral tissues (results in wasting, lympholysis, loss of osteoid from bones, and thinning of skin).
- Amino acids will be mobilized into the liver and will be used for gluconeogenesis
- Antiallergic
- Anti-inflammatory
- Bone
- Calcium metabolism: Steroids will inhibit calcium absorption from intestines and enhance renal excretion of calcium
- Antagonizes the activity of vitamin D on the gut, there by reduces absorption of calcium from gut.
- Electrolyte balance
- Fluid balance
- Fat mobilization of fat from peripheral fat depots, promotes lipolysis, deposited over face (moon face), neck (fish mouth), and shoulder (buffalo hump).
- Glucocorticoids will promote glycogen deposition in liver.

- Stimulates gluconeogenesis in the liver (by inducing hepatic glycogen synthetase).
- Gastric acid secretion increased: Increases secretion of gastrin and pepsin, thereby aggravates peptic ulcer.
- Hypothalamo-hypophyseal: Adrenal axis is inhibited
- Inflammatory response will be suppressed
- Hydrocortisone will have a feeble salt retaining activity
- Impair immunological competence
- Inhibit glucose utilization by tissues.

## Dosage
Depends upon the type of glucocorticoids and conditions for which they are used.

## Indications
- Arthritis
- Allergy
- Autoimmune hemolytic anemia
- Bronchial asthma
- Bronchitis
- Colitis
- Substitution therapy in adrenal insufficiency
- Rheumatoid arthritis
- Rheumatic fever
- Anti-inflammatory
- Allergic diseases: Asthma
- Acute viral hepatitis
- Inflammatory bowel disease: Ulcerative colitis
- Neoplastic diseases: Myeloma, hemolytic anemia, thrombocytopenic purpura
- Immune disorders
- Eye
- Skin.

## Contraindications
- Allergic to glucocorticoids
- Cushing's syndrome
- Diabetes mellitus
- Epilepsy
- Failure: Congestive heart failure (CHF)
- Gastritis/peptic ulcer
- Hypertension
- Infections like tuberculosis, herpes simplex, fungal infections, measles, and chickenpox
- Immunodeficiency
- Increased risk of infections
- Osteoporosis
- Psychosis
- Renal failure.

## Precautions to be followed during Treatment with Corticosteroids
- Watch for anemia as blood loss can occur due to erosive gastritis.
- Rule out peptic ulceration
- Urine should be examined for sugar periodically
- Monitor weight
- Monitor blood pressure
- Do not stop therapy abruptly
- Rule out infections, steroids will aggravate infections.

## Effects on Pregnancy
Cleft palate/lip and cardiac defects.

## Side Effects
- It depends upon the individual susceptibility, dose, and duration of treatment
- Single large doses are harmless
- Prolonged therapy with dose higher than 20–30 mg/day of hydrocortisone or equivalent doses of other steroids will cause adverse effects.
- Acne/acneiform eruptions
- Aggression
- Anxiety
- Blurred vision
- Bruising—easy bruising
- Blood sugar increased
- Cataract—subcapsular cataract
- Cushing's syndrome—moon face
- Diabetes—worsening of diabetes

- Dermatitis—perioral
- Dizziness
- Depression
- Euphoria
- Edema due to sodium retention
- Electrolyte imbalance—hypokalemia
- Fluid imbalance/fluid retention—sodium and water retention
- Fat deposit in the body
- Folliculitis
- Gastritis
- Glaucoma
- Glycosuria
- Growth retardation
- Gain in weight
- Gastrointestinal upset—dyspepsia
- Hypertension
- Hyperglycemia
- Headache
- Healing of wound delayed
- Hypopigmentation
- Hypertrichosis
- Hirsutism
- Irritability
- Insomnia
- Immunity decreased
- Increased sweating
- Increased susceptibility to infection—secondary infections
- Increased intracranial pressure
- Immunosuppression
- Infections—candidiasis
- Joint problems—arthralgia and joint pain
- K+ loss
- Long bone fractures
- Muscular weakness due to potassium loss/steroid myopathy
- Mood changes—anxious, irritable, and depression
- Neuropsychiatric problems—euphoria
- Ophthalmic problems—increased intraocular pressure, glaucoma, papilledema, and cataracts
- Osteoporosis
- Osteonecrosis of femoral head
- Peptic ulceration
- Psychological disorders
- Skin atrophy
- Striae
- Suppression of adrenals
- Suppression of hypothalamo-hypophyseal—adrenal axis.
- Suppression of immune response
- Suppression of inflammation
- Tendon rupture
- Thinning of skin
- Weight gain due to fluid retention and fat deposition.

| System | Side effects |
|---|---|
| General | Prolonged treatment will cause central obesity, moon face, buffalo hump<br>Growth retardation: Retardation of liner growth |
| Eyes | Glaucoma, posterior subcapsular cataract |
| Gastrointestinal tract | Acute erosive gastritis<br>Peptic ulcer, perforation, hemorrhage |
| Cardiovascular system | Hypertension |
| Central nervous system | Acute psychotic reactions, benign intracranial hypertension, aggravation of epilepsy in children |
| Renal system | Salt and water retention, hypokalemic alkalosis |
| Metabolic effects | Ketoacidosis, nonketotic hyperglycemic, hyperosmolar coma, hypokalemic alkalosis, hyperglycemia |
| Endocrine changes | Diabetes mellitus |
| Androgenic effects | Hirsutism, amenorrhea |
| Skeletal system | Interfere with development of cartilage, inhibits linear growth<br>Severe osteoporosis, spontaneous fractures |
| Psychiatric disturbances | Euphoria, excitation |

*Contd...*

*Contd...*

| System | Side effects |
|---|---|
| Skin | Striae formation, bruising |
| Miscellaneous | Hirsutism, thromboembolism, hypercoagulability of blood, loss of scalp hair, subcutaneous atrophy, delayed wound healing |

## Drug Interactions

Anticonvulsants, phenytoin, barbiturates, and rifampicin will accelerate the metabolism of glucocorticoids.

## QUESTIONS

**Q1.** What are the steps to prevent suppression of hypothalamo-hypophyseal—adrenal axis?
- ❏ Use short-acting steroids
- ❏ Use steroids for short duration
- ❏ Give the entire dose as one dose in the early morning
- ❏ Switchover to alternate dose as early as possible and then taper the dose before stopping.

**Q2.** What are the natural glucocorticoids?
- ❏ Hydrocortisone
- ❏ Cortisone
- ❏ Corticosterone.

**Q3.** What are the synthetic glucocorticoids?
- ❏ Prednisone
- ❏ Prednisolone.

**Q4.** What are the advantages of synthetic glucocorticoids?
- ❏ Less salt and water retention
- ❏ More anti-inflammatory action
- ❏ More effective in small doses
- ❏ Easy diffusion into tissues.

## Hydrocortisone

- ❖ Has glucocorticoid and significant mineralocorticoid activity also
- ❖ 25 mL/5 mL vials
- ❖ 10–20 mg/kg/dose IV 6th hourly
- ❖ Rapid action but short duration of action.

### Dosage

- ❖ *Intractable hypoglycemia*: 10–25 mg/kg
- ❖ *Adrenal crisis*: 3–10 mg/kg/day in divided doses every 6 hourly
- ❖ *Congenital adrenal hyperplasia*: Initial dose 0.5–0.7 mg/kg/24 hours. One-fourth dose in the morning and one-fourth dose in the evening
- ❖ *Dilution*: Can be given undiluted
- ❖ *Hypercalcemia*: 1 mg/kg every 6 hourly will be helpful in lowering serum calcium level
- ❖ *Dilution*: Can be given undiluted.
- ❖ Depends upon the route and condition treated
- ❖ *Asthma*: 1–2 mg/kg intravenously
- ❖ *Adrenal crisis*: 100 mg bolus intravenously followed by 20 mg over 24 hours by infusion
- ❖ *Chronic adrenal insufficiency*: 15–25 mg/day in divided doses.

### Systemic therapy in children:

- ❖ *Dose*: 20–50 mg/kg/dose iv 6 hourly
- ❖ *Up to 1 year*: 25 mg
- ❖ *1–5 years*: 50 mg
- ❖ *6–12 years*: 100 mg.

### Indications for Hydrocortisone
### (Mnemonic A–I)

- ❖ Acute adrenocortical insufficiency
- ❖ Asthma: Status asthmaticus
- ❖ Addison's disease: Can be used for replacement therapy in adrenal insufficiency
- ❖ Arthritis: Rheumatoid arthritis
- ❖ Blood disorders
- ❖ Congenital adrenal hyperplasia
- ❖ Cancer
- ❖ Calcium: Hypercalcemia
- ❖ COPD
- ❖ Dermatitis
- ❖ Endotoxic shock
- ❖ Fatal asthma
- ❖ Gram-negative shock
- ❖ Hypoglycemia
- ❖ Hypercalcemia
- ❖ Infections: Tuberculous meningitis

- ❖ Inflammatory bowel disease: Can be used as enema in ulcerative colitis.

Can be used topically:
- ❖ Lupus
- ❖ Psoriasis.

### Contraindications for the Use of Hydrocortisone
- ❖ Hypersensitivity
- ❖ Systemic infections
- ❖ Live viral infections
- ❖ Peptic ulcer.

### Precautions
- ❖ Should not get immunized with live vaccines like chickenpox, measles, mumps, and rubella when the patient is on long-term steroids.
- ❖ The steroids should not be stopped suddenly if the drugs were used for more than 3 weeks as it will precipitate adrenal insufficiency. The dose should be tapered slowly.
- ❖ Should not be used to treat cerebral edema associated with head injury.

### Effects on Pregnancy
- ❖ Hydrocortisones will cross placenta readily. Prolonged use may cause intrauterine growth retardation.
- ❖ Hydrocortisone will be secreted in breast milk. It may cause adrenal suppression.

### Drug Interactions of Hydrocortisone
- ❖ Will reduce the efficacy of carbamazepine, phenytoin, barbiturates, and primidone
- ❖ Nonsteroidal anti-inflammatory drug will increase the risk of peptic ulcer
- ❖ Will increase the requirement of insulin and oral hypoglycemic agents.

## Dexamethasone
Very potent, long active, highly selective glucocorticoid.

**Q1. What is the dose of dexamethasone?**
- ❑ Bacterial meningitis 0.15 mg/kg/dose every 6 hours (0.6 mg/kg/day in four divided doses) intravenously for first 4 days of the antibiotic treatment. The first dose should be administered 20 minutes before the administration of the antibiotics. Alternatively, 0.4 mg/kg can be given every 12 hourly for 2 days.
- ❑ Asthma: 0.2–0.4 mg/kg/dose IM/IV 8th hourly.

**Q2. What are the indications for dexamethasone?**
- ❑ Inflammation
- ❑ Allergic conditions
- ❑ Shock
- ❑ Cerebral edema
- ❑ Bronchopulmonary dysplasia
- ❑ Adrenocortical insufficiency
- ❑ Refractory neonatal hypoglycemia
- ❑ While extubation.

**Q3. What are the contraindications for the use of dexamethasone?**
Active untreated infections.

**Q4. What are the adverse effects of dexamethasone?**
- ❑ Short-term adverse effects: Seizures, hypokalemia, hypocalcemia, alkalosis, sodium and water retention, gastric and duodenal ulceration/perforation, and gastrointestinal hemorrhage.
- ❑ Long-term side effects: Nephrolithiasis, osteopenia, osteoporosis, fractures, Cushing's syndrome, marked pituitary adrenal axis suppression, growth suppression, cataracts, transient hypertrophic cardiomyopathy, pseudotumor cerebri, fragile skin, telangiectasis, and hirsutism.
- ❑ Pituitary—adrenal axis suppression: Will reduce the pituitary–adrenal axis response to stress.

**Q5. What are the adverse effects of cutaneous dexamethasone?**
- ❑ Cutaneous atrophy hyperglycemia and glycosuria
- ❑ Muscular weakness
- ❑ Delayed healing of wounds.

**Q6. What are the conditions in which dexamethasone should be given carefully?**
- Elderly
- Function of liver decreased
- Glaucoma
- Hypertension.

**Q7. What are the advantages of dexamethasone?**
Does not cause fluid retention or hypertension.

**Q8. What are the drug interactions of dexamethasone?**
- Phenytoin, phenobarbitone, and ephedrine will reduce the efficacy.
- Magnesium trisilicate will reduce the gastrointestinal absorption.

## Prednisolone
Synthetic adrenal corticosteroid.

### Dosage
- 1–2 mg/kg/24 hours orally in divided doses
- Prednisolone is four times more potent than hydrocortisone
- More selective glucocorticoid
- Fluid retention does not occur with high doses.

### Indications
Arthritis, allergy, ulcerative colitis, lupus, inflammatory conditions, autoimmune diseases.

### Contraindications for the Use of Prednisolone
- Hypersensitivity
- Systemic infections
- Live viral infections
- Peptic ulcer.

### Precautions
The conditions in which the drug should be given with precautions are as follows:
- Osteoporosis
- Pregnancy
- Diabetes mellitus
- Glaucoma
- Diverticulitis
- Myasthenia gravis
- Congestive cardiac failure
- Renal failure.

### Effects on Pregnancy
Prematurity.

### Drug Interactions of Prednisolone
- Rifampicin will accelerate the metabolism
- Antiepileptics will blunt the action
- Estrogens and oral contraceptives will increase the bioavailability
- Antacids in larger doses will impair the absorption
- Will increase the requirement of insulin and oral hypoglycemic agents
- Methylprednisolone is slightly more potent and more selective than prednisolone
- Methylprednisolone is high doses can be given as pulse therapy 1 g intravenously every 6–8 weeks will be useful in treating active rheumatoid arthritis.

## Betamethasone
- Available as tablet, injection, and cream
- Betamethasone is about 8–10 times more potent than prednisolone on weight-to-weight basis.

### Dosage
Depends upon the condition treated.

### Indications
- Acute allergic conditions
- Anaphylactic reaction
- Addison's disease
- Arthritis: Rheumatoid arthritis
- Bronchial asthma: Status asthmatics
- Bursitis
- Circumscribed scleroderma
- Dermatitis
- Eczema
- Erythema multiforme
- Tennis elbow and tenosynovitis
- Severe shock

- Hypopituitarism following adrenalectomy
- Inflammation of skin
- Intralesional injections
- Keloids
- Prophylaxis for hyaline membrane disease in newborn. This drug is administered to the mother during antenatal period.

## Contraindications for the Use of Betamethasone
- Systemic infections
- Live viral infection or immunizations
- Hypersensitivity to betamethasone.

## Precautions
The conditions in which the drug betamethasone should be given with caution:
- Osteoporosis
- Pregnancy
- Diabetes mellitus
- Hypertension
- Glaucoma
- Diverticulitis
- Myasthenia gravis
- Congestive cardiac failure (due to fluid retention)
- Renal failure
- History myopathy and peptic ulcer.

## Effects on Pregnancy
- Category C
- Secreted in the breast milk.

## Drug Interactions of Betamethasone
- Carbamazepine, phenytoin, primidone, and barbiturates will reduce the efficacy
- Rifampicin will reduce efficacy
- Dose of antidiabetics and antihypertensives should be increased.

# QUESTION

**Q1. What are the drugs to accelerate the fetal lung maturity?**
Steroids: Two doses of betamethasone, 12 mg intramuscularly in an interval of 24 hours. Four doses of dexamethasone, 6 mg intramuscularly between 24 weeks and 34 weeks of gestation given at least 24 hours to 7 days before delivery will enhance the lung maturity. This will reduce the incidence of hyaline membrane disease, intraventricular hemorrhage, and NNEC. Betamethasone is preferred as it has less side effects.

# HORMONES

## Insulin
- Insulin is a hormone secreted by the islets of Langerhans in pancreas. It is stored in the beta cells and released in response to blood glucose.
- Polypeptide.
- Contains 51 amino acids arranged in two chains linked by disulfide bridges.

## Mechanism of Action
- Underutilization and overproduction of glucose
- Acts on specific receptors on the cell membrane of all cells. Liver and fat cells are rich in these receptors.
- Lowers blood glucose by facilitating transport of glucose across the cell membranes.
- Insulin stimulates the enzyme glycogen synthetase and promotes glycogen synthesis from glucose in the liver, muscles, and fat.
- Prevents gluconeogenesis in liver by inhibiting phosphorylase.
- Promotes uptake and utilization of glucose in the skeletal muscles.
- Promotes conversion of glucose to fat in adipose tissue.

## Pharmacological Actions
- Glycogen synthetase
- Decreases the activity of the following two enzymes:
  1. Phosphorylase and cyclic AMP
  2. Enzymes associated with gluconeogenesis

- The effects of insulin on the muscles:
  - Increases protein synthesis
  - Increases glycogen synthesis and glycogen synthase
  - Inhibits phosphorylase.
- Skeletal muscle: Anabolic effect—stimulation of uptake of glucose. Stimulates entry of amino acids and incorporation into protein.
- The effects of insulin on the liver:
  - Inhibits glycogenolysis
  - Inhibits conversion of amino acids to glucose
  - Anabolic action—increases glycogen and triglyceride synthesis
  - Liver—increases the activity of glucokinase which increases glucose intake.
- The effects of insulin on the adipose tissue:
  - Increases triglyceride storage
  - Increases the glucose utilization by fat tissue
  - Induces lipogenesis
  - Antilipolytic effect—prevents breakdown of fat
  - Induces lipoprotein lipase which hydrolyzes triglycerides from lipoproteins.

## Dosage

60-75% of the dose should be given in the morning before breakfast and 25-40% in the evening dose before dinner.

The sites in which insulin can be given:
- Posterior aspect of the upper arm
- Lateral and anterior aspect of thigh
- Buttocks
- Anterior abdominal wall.

The route of administration of insulin:
- Subcutaneous
- Regular insulin can be given by intravenous or intramuscular route.

## Indications

- Diabetes mellitus—insulin dependent
- Diabetic ketoacidosis
- Treatment of hyperkalemia—insulin with glucose infusion
- Diagnosis of growth hormone deficiency.

## Contraindications

- Hypoglycemia
- Insulinoma.

## Precautions

- Insulin should not be freezed
- Can be kept in room temperature up to 1 month
- Should be protected from excess sunlight and heat.

The conditions in which insulin should be given precautiously:
- Pregnancy
- Renal failure
- Hepatic failures.

## Effects on Pregnancy

Can be given during pregnancy.

## Side Effects

- Hypoglycemia
- Edema in dependent areas due to sodium retention
- Loss of visual accommodation due to alteration of in the physical properties of lens
- Presbyopia
- Insulin allergy—urticaria, angioedema, anaphylaxis (may be due to contaminating proteins)
- Neuropathy
- Obesity can occur if insulin is used without dietary restriction.

Local reactions:
- Lipodystrophy—at the injection sites after prolonged use
- Erythema
- Swelling
- Stinging.

## Drug Interactions

Beta blockers like propranolol, atenolol with mask the symptoms of hypoglycemia. They will inhibit the compensatory mechanisms acting through β2-receptors.

During general anesthesia, the insulin needs will be increased, so it is better to switch over to plain insulin even if the patent is on oral hypoglycemic drugs.

The following agents will increase the blood sugar levels and reduce the effectiveness of insulin:
- Frusemide
- Thiazides
- Corticosteroids
- Oral contraceptives
- Salbutamol
- Calcium channel blockers.

The following agents will enhance insulin secretion and peripheral utilization of glucose and predispose to hypoglycemia:
- Salicylates
- Lithium
- Theophylline.

## QUESTIONS

**Q1. What is the half-life of insulin?**
5–6 minutes.

**Q2. How will you classify insulin?**
- Short-acting insulin: Plain insulin and semilente insulin (insulin zinc suspension).
- Intermediate-acting insulin: Lente insulin and isophane insulin
- Long-acting insulin: Protamine zinc insulin and ultralente insulin.

**Q3. What are the types of insulin?**
- Plain insulin
- Semilente insulin
- Lente insulin
- Ultralente insulin.

**Q4. What is the time of onset of action of various insulins?**
- Plain insulin: 5–7 hours
- Semilente insulin: 12–16 hours
- Lente insulin: 2–4 hours
- Ultralente insulin: 10–30 hours.

**Q5. What is the duration of action of various insulins?**
- Plain insulin: 5–7 hours
- Semilente insulin: 12–16 hours
- Lente insulin: 24–28 hours
- Ultralente insulin more than 36 hours
- Protamine zinc insulin more than 36 hours.

**Q6. How can the duration of action of insulin be prolonged with preservation of its biological activity?**
By combining with protamine and zinc.

**Q7. How will you divide the doses of insulin?**
60–75% of the dose should be given in the morning before breakfast and 25–40% in the evening dose before dinner.

**Q8. What are the sites in which insulin can be given?**
- Posterior aspect of the upper arm
- Lateral and anterior aspect of thigh
- Buttocks
- Anterior abdominal wall.

**Q9. What is lente insulin?**
Intermediate acting insulin in zinc suspension.

**Q10. What is semilente insulin?**
Short-acting insulin.

**Q11. What is ultralente insulin?**
It is a long-acting insulin with onset of action by 4–6 hours and duration of 28–36 hours.

**Q12. What are the advantages of newer insulins?**
- Pure
- Neutral
- Less antigenic
- Less likely to cause subcutaneous fat atrophy.

**Q13. What are the organs involved in insulin degradation?**
Liver and kidneys.

**Q14. Which are stimulus for insulin synthesis and release?**
- Glucose
- Mannose

- Amino acids—leucine and arginine
- Hormones—glucagon-like polypeptide
- Gastrin
- Secretin
- Pancreozymin
- Enteroglucagon
- Catecholamines
- Vagal stimulation
- Selective beta adrenergic stimulation
- Drugs—xanthines, sulfonylureas, meglitinides, and D-phenylalanine.

**Q15. Which is the most potent stimulus for insulin synthesis and release?**
Glucose is the most potent stimulus for insulin synthesis and release.

**Q16. What are the drugs that inhibit insulin secretion?**
Thiazides, diazoxide and diphenylhydantoin.

**Q17. What are the newer insulins?**
- Actrapid
- Rapitard
- Monotard
- Humulin insulin.

**Q18. What are the advantages of newer insulins?**
- Pure
- Neutral
- Less antigenic
- Less likely to cause subcutaneous fat atrophy.

**Q19. What are the insulin delivery systems?**
- Insulin syringes
- Insulin Pen
- Jet injections
- Insulin pumps
- Implantable pumps
- External artificial pancreas.

## Thyroxin

L-thyroxine is available as 100 mg tablets.

## Mechanism of Action

It is used as replacement therapy.

## Pharmacological Actions

- Increase in metabolism
- Increase in oxygen consumption
- Increase in heat production
- Increase in basal metabolic rate
- Anabolic effects—protein synthesis
- Increase in glucose absorption and utilization
- Myelination of CNS.

## Dosage

For treatment of hypothyroidism, neonates are given L-thyroxine (levothyroxine) in a dose of 10–15 mg/kg/day. Older children require 4–8 mg/kg/day.

## Treatment of Hypothyroidism

- L-thyroxine (levothyroxine) is given orally in a dose of 10–15 µg/kg/day for neonates. L-thyroxine is available as 100 µg tablets.
- Sodium L-thyroxine is given lifelong as once a day, dose in early morning empty stomach.
- Thyroxine replacement therapy should be started as early as possible.
- The levels of T4 and thyroid-stimulating hormone (TSH) should be monitored every 2 weeks.

## Recommended Daily Dosage

| Age | Dose (µg/kg/day) |
|---|---|
| 0–3 months | 10–15 |
| 3–6 months | 8–12 |
| 6–12 months | 6–8 |

The dose should be adjusted so that the level of T4 is maintained at a level of 10–16 µg/dL and TSH below 5 mU/L.

## Effects of Treatment

- The first sign of improvement is onset of diuresis. Coarse facies will improve in 2–3 weeks time
- Increase in the activity
- Decrease in the weight
- Hemoglobin level will improve.

## Indications

- Hypothyroidism
- Cretinism
- Myxedema coma
- Nontoxic goiter—endemic goiter
- In papillary carcinoma of thyroid not resectable cases full dose of thyroxine will suppress TSH and cause regression of the tumor.
- Thyroxine is used empirically in the following conditions:
  - Refractory anemia
  - Obstinate constipation
  - Chronic nonhealing ulcers.

## Contraindications

Thyroxine should not be used to lower blood cholesterol as it will increase the cardiovascular problems.

## Precautions

- Sodium L-thyroxine should be given lifelong as once a day dose early morning empty stomach.
- The tablet should be swallowed and should not be bitten, crushed or chewed.
- L-thyroxine should be taken at least 2 hours before or 4 hours after the intake of binding agent.

## Effects on Pregnancy

Thyroxine should be given and the dose should be increased in the first trimester.

## Side Effects

Side effects from levothyroxine are rare and occur usually due to over dosage, which causes thyroid over activity:

- Diarrhea
- Bone pain
- Craniosynostosis
- Hair loss
- Temperamental problems.

**Q. What are the effects of overdose of L-thyroxine?**

Side effects from levothyroxine are rare and usually due to overdosage, which causes thyroid over activity.

Symptoms of overdose include:
- Anxiety
- Agitation
- Diarrhea
- Weight loss or gain
- Excessive sweating
- Flushed skin
- Tiredness
- Tachycardia, wide pulse pressure, risk of CCF and arrhythmia
- Excitability and craniosynostosis.

In older children, side effects include:
- Pseudotumor cerebri (benign intracranial hypertension)
- Temperamental problems
- Nervousness
- Chest pain
- Tremors and palpitations
- Insomnia
- Hyperkinetic child
- Irritable child.

## Drug Interactions

The following drugs can decrease the absorption of thyroxine:
- Iron
- Cholestyramine
- Calcium supplements
- Antacids
- Proton pump inhibitors by increasing gastric pH.

# QUESTIONS

**Q1. What are the types of hypothyroidism?**
- Primary hypothyroidism: The defect is in the thyroid gland. As the defect is in the thyroid gland the secretion of TSH is increased.
- Secondary hypothyroidism: This is due to decreased secretion of TSH, which may be due to the defect in the pituitary gland (hypopituitarism).
- Tertiary hypothyroidism: This is due to decreased secretion of thyrotropin-releasing hormone (TRH), which may be due to the defect in the hypothalamus.

## Drugs

**Q2. Why thyroxine should be taken in empty stomach?**
The absorption is complete when taken in empty stomach, but variable when taken with food.

**Q3. What are the differences between T3 and T4?**
- Overall effects will be similar qualitatively
- T3 has a quicker onset of action
- 25 µg of T3 will have the same effect of 100 µg of T4.

| Properties | T3 | T4 |
| --- | --- | --- |
| Onset of action | Within 6–8 hours | Within 7–10 days |
| Effect after cessation of treatment | Wears off quickly | Lasts for several days |
| Suppression of elevated TSH to normal | 0.1 µg of T3 for 3–10 days | 0.3 µg of T4 for 7–21 days |

**Q4. What is the first sign of improvement?**
Onset of diuresis is the first sign of improvement.

**Q5. What are the other signs of improvement?**
- Increase in the activity
- Decrease in the weight
- Hemoglobin level will improve.

**Q6. What is the duration for improvement of coarse facies after starting treatment?**
Coarse facies will improve in 2–3 weeks time.

**Q7. What are the conditions associated with bad prognosis?**
- Prenatal onset
- Diagnosis and treatment are delayed.

**Q8. What are the complications associated with delayed diagnosis and treatment?**
- Growth retardation
- Neurological problems ataxia, incoordination, spastic diplegia, sensorineural hearing loss, and strabismus
- Intellectual disability.

### Mnemonics Features of Hypothyroidism

| | |
| --- | --- |
| A | Anemia and anorexia |
| | Ascites |
| B | Bowel habits altered—constipation |
| | Bradycardia |
| C | Cold and clammy skin |
| | Carpal tunnel syndrome |
| D | Deafness |
| | Delayed dentition |
| | Depression |
| E | Extremities cold |
| | Expressionless face |
| F | Fontanel closure delayed |
| | Fatigue |
| G | Gynecological problems—menorrhagia |
| | Growth retardation—short stature |
| H | Hoarseness of voice |
| | Hair loss |
| I | Intolerance to cold |
| | Intellectual impairment |
| J | Jaundice |
| | Jerks |
| K | Kinesthesia |
| L | Lethargy |
| | Libido decreased |
| | L-thyroxine is the drug of choice |
| M | Myxedema |
| | Mononeuritis multiplex |
| | Memory loss |
| | Muscle cramps |
| N | Neuralgia |
| O | Oedema (nonpitting) |
| P | Pulse rate decreased |
| | Pleural effusion and pericardial effusion |
| | Puffiness around the eye |
| | Pallor |
| | Puberty delayed |
| Q | Quebec scoring |
| | Quickness of actions absent |
| R | Rheumatologic pain |
| | Reaction time slow |
| | Reflexes—delayed relaxation |
| S | Skin thick, coarse, and dry |
| T | Tongue—macroglossia |
| | Temperature—decreased |
| U | Umbilical hernia |
| V | Vitiligo |

*Contd...*

*Contd...*

| W | Weight gain<br>Weakness<br>Common in women |
|---|---|
| X | Xanthelasma<br>X-ray delayed bone age |
| Y | Younger the age of replacement therapy, better will be the prognosis |
| Z | Basal metabolic rate (BMR) moves towards zero |

## DIURETICS

### Classification of Diuretics

- Weak diuretics—osmotic diuretics (mannitol, glycerol), carbonic anhydrase inhibitors (acetazolamide)
- Moderately potent diuretics—benzothiadiazine
- Very potent diuretics—furosemide
- Potassium-sparing diuretics—spironolactone, amiloride, triamterene.
- Loop diuretics are:
  - Furosemide
  - Bumetanide
  - Ethacrynic acid

Loop diuretics act on the ascending loop of Henle where about 30% of the salt secreted is reabsorbed.

### Furosemide

- Furosemide—Lasix
- Injection 20 mg/2 mL ampoule
- Tablets 40 mg
- Furosemide is high ceiling diuretic
- Furosemide is a weaker antihypertensive than thiazide.

### Mechanism of Action of Furosemide

- Furosemide will inhibit the reabsorption of sodium and water in the distal tubules and the loop of Henle.
- Onset of action is rapid within 0.5–1 hour
- Duration of action is short from 4–6 hours.

### Pharmacological Actions

Strong diuretic lacks antihypertensive effect.

### Dosage

- Dosage: 1–2 mg/kg/day, oral or intravenous route
- Compatible with normal saline, 5% dextrose
- Rapidly absorbed by oral administration
- On intravenous administration, the effect will start in 2 minutes and will last for 2–3 hours.
- Furosemide (Lasix) 1 mg/kg (can be increased up to 6 mg/kg).
- Furosemide 1 mg/kg/dose is given if there is pulmonary edema. Spironolactone, an aldosterone antagonist, given in a dose of 2–3 mg/kg/day orally in two divided doses. Hydrochlorothiazide (2 mg/kg/day orally in two divided doses, metolazone (0.2 mg/kg/dose orally).

### Indications

- Acute pulmonary edema
- Blood transfusion (to prevent adverse hemodynamic effects)
- Congestive cardiac failure (CCF)
- Cerebral edema
- Calcium excess (hypercalcemia)—increases calcium excretion and urinary flow.
- Diuresis in patients with oliguria due to renal failure
- Edema/acute pulmonary edema associated with CCF, hepatic and renal disease—nephrotic syndrome.
- Forced diuresis in poisoning
- Fluid overload
- Glomerulonephritis—acute glomerulonephritis
- Hypertension in presence of renal insufficiency
- Hyperkalemia.

### Contraindications

- Anuria
- Allergic to furosemide
- Azotemia
- Blockage of urinary tract

- Coma—hepatic coma
- Dehydration
- Electrolyte imbalance—hyponatremia, hypokalemia
- Renal failure with anuria
- Gout/Hyperuricemia
- Hearing problems—hearing loss
- Hypovolemia with or without hypotension
- Hypersensitivity to furosemide
- Hypersensitivity to sulfonamides—furosemide may exhibit allergic cross-reactivity in patients who are sensitive to other sulfonamides.

## Precautions
Prevention of hypokalemia in patients with Lasix:
- Potassium chloride (KCl) supplementation
- Potassium-sparing diuretic or angiotensin-converting enzyme (ACE) inhibitor can be used along with Lasix.

## Effects on Pregnancy
Contraindicated in pregnancy, may affect the fetus.

## Side Effects/Adverse Effects of Furosemide
- Agranulocytosis
- Anemia
- Allergic manifestations
- Bone marrow depression
- Cholelithiasis
- Dehydration
- Ear problems—potential ototoxicity (hearing loss), tinnitus, deafness
- Fluid and electrolyte imbalance (hypokalemia, hyponatremia, hypochloremic alkalosis)
- Gastrointestinal (GI) tract disturbances—nausea, vomiting, diarrhea
- Hypotension
- Hypocalcemia
- Hypercalciuria
- Hyperglycemia
- Hypomagnesemia
- Hyperuricemia and gout
- Interstitial nephritis
- Liver and bone marrow changes
- Muscle weakness and cramps due to loss of electrolytes
- Nephrocalcinosis
- Pancreatitis
- Prerenal azotemia
- Resistance to diuretics
- Thrombocytopenia
- Skin rashes
- Vertigo.

| System | Adverse effects |
| --- | --- |
| General | Allergic manifestations |
| Ear problems | Potential ototoxicity (hearing loss), tinnitus, deafness, vertigo |
| Cardiovascular | Hypotension |
| Gastrointestinal tract | Nausea<br>Cholelithiasis<br>Diarrhea<br>Vomiting |
| Renal | Nephrocalcinosis |
| Hematological | Agranulocytosis<br>Anemia<br>Thrombocytopenia<br>Bone marrow depression |
| Metabolic | Hypocalcemia<br>Hypercalciuria<br>Hyperglycemia<br>Hypomagnesemia<br>Hyperuricemia and gout |
| Fluid and electrolyte imbalance | Dehydration<br>Hypokalemia<br>Hyponatremia<br>Hypochloremic alkalosis |
| Skin | Rashes |

**Q1. What is the complication associated with intravenous administration of furosemide?**
Intravenous administration can result in cardiac arrest.

**Q2. What is the most common complication of furosemide?**
Hypokalemia.

**Q3. What precaution should be taken to prevent ototoxicity?**
Injection furosemide 1 mg/kg can be given. The rate should not be more than 4 mg/minute to prevent ototoxicity.

### Drug Interactions
- Compatible with normal saline, 5% dextrose
- Potentiates antihypertensives
- Causes lithium toxicity
- Cotrimoxazole—thrombocytopenia
- Aminoglycosides will increase the risk of ototoxicity resulting in deafness
- Nonsteroidal anti-inflammatory drugs (NSAIDs) will decrease the diuretic effect of furosemide.

## QUESTIONS

**Q1. How can you prevent hypokalemia in patients with Lasix?**
- KCl supplementation
- Potassium-sparing diuretic or ACE inhibitor can be used along with Lasix.

**Q2. What is the problem of administration of furosemide to the mother antenatally?**
It increases fetal urinary sodium and potassium levels.

## Mannitol
- Osmotic diuretic
- 25% in 50 mL vial
- It is a sugar polyhydroxy aliphatic alcohol.

Contents and characteristics of mannitol:

| Concentration (%) | Grams/ 100 mL | mOsmol/L | pH |
|---|---|---|---|
| 5 | 5 | 274 | 6.3 (4.5–7) |
| 10 | 10 | 549 | 6.3 (4.5–7) |
| 15 | 15 | 823 | 6.3 (4.5–7) |
| 20 | 20 | 1098 | 6.3 (4.5–7) |
| 25 | 25 | 1372 | 5.9 (4.5–7) |

**Q1. What are the properties of mannitol?**
- Nonelectrolyte
- Low-molecular-weight of 182
- Pharmacologically inert
- Poorly absorbed from gut and should be given by parenteral route
- Freely filtered at glomerulus by filtration within 30–60 minutes
- Undergoes limited reabsorption
- Limits tubular water and electrolyte reabsorption
- Increases glomerular filtration rate (GFR) by expanding extracellular fluid (ECF) volume.
- Inhibits renin release
- Increases renal medullary blood flow.

**Q2. What is the principle for osmotic diuresis?**
The proximal tubule and descending limb of loop of Henle in the kidney are freely permeable to water. Any agent like mannitol filtered by glomerulus and not absorbed will promote water diuresis.

### Mechanism of Action
- Expansion of ECF: When given intravenously mannitol will remain in the extracellular space. Mannitol will not be metabolized and is rapidly filtered by the glomeruli. This will prevent back diffusion of water and reabsorption of sodium result in osmotic diuresis.
- Increases GFR
- Inhibits renin release
- Mannitol will also act on the loop of Henle and reduces medullary hypertonicity probably by increasing the medullary blood flow. This will reduce the reabsorption of water from that site.

*The sites of action of mannitol:*
- Glomeruli
- Loop of Henle.

### Pharmacological Actions
- Pharmacologically inert
- Will expand the extracellular volume and thereby increases the GFR

- Increases the renal medullary blood flow thereby reducing the medullary hypertonicity.

## Dosage

*For increased intracranial tension*: 20% mannitol in a dose of 0.5-1 g/dose, intravenously over a period of 20 minutes. This can be in a dose of 0.25-0.5 g/dose repeated every 4-6 hours. Mannitol should be given for 2-3 days.

*The route of administration of mannitol*: Intravenous route.

## Indications

- Acute renal failure during oliguric phase
- Barbiturate poisoning—forced alkaline diuresis along with sodium bicarbonate.
- Cerebral edema—increased intracranial tension
- Diagnostic—measurement of GFR
- Excretion of toxic substances through urine
- Forced diuresis in certain poisonings like hypnotics
- Glaucoma—increased intraocular tension
- Glomerular filtration rate and urine flow maintenance in impending renal failure due to shock, severe trauma.
- Hemolysis—to maintain urine volume in hemolysis and rhabdomyolysis.
- Hemodialysis or to counteract low osmolality of plasma due to hemodialysis or peritoneal dialysis.
- Increased water excretion in preference to sodium.

## Contraindications

- Acute tubular necrosis
- Anuria
- Bleeding—intracranial bleeding
- Cerebral hemorrhage
- Dehydration
- Edema—pulmonary edema
- Failure—acute left ventricular failure (LVF)
- Hypersensitivity to mannitol.

## Precautions

- Mannitol does not contain any antibacterial agents and should be used for one use only. The unused portion should be discarded.
- Mannitol should be given parenterally only and is not effective orally.
- Few cases with oliguria may not respond to Mannitol.

**Q. Why a test dose of mannitol should be given before continuous infusion of mannitol?**

Mannitol is given as a test dose of 12.5 g intravenously and observed for 3 hours

If there is no increase in urinary flow rate to more than 50 mL/hour, mannitol infusion is contraindicated.

## Effects on Pregnancy

Category C.

## Side Effects/Adverse Effects of Mannitol

- Arrhythmias
- Angina like chest pains
- Blurring of vision
- Chills
- Convulsions
- Dehydration
- Dry mouth
- Dizziness
- Extracellular volume depletion
- Fluid and electrolyte imbalance—acidosis
- Gastrointestinal tract—nausea, vomiting, diarrhea
- Headache
- Hypotension
- Excessive use without water replacement will cause severe dehydration, free water loss, hypernatremia, hyperkalemia.

## Drug Interactions

Combination of mannitol and amikacin or gentamicin or kanamycin can damage the kidneys and increases the effects of nephrotoxic drugs.

## QUESTIONS

**Q1. What will happen if mannitol is administered orally?**
It will cause osmotic diarrhea.

**Q2. What is the condition in which mannitol is not useful?**
Cardiac edema with sodium retention because mannitol increases ECF volume. This will increase the load on the heart.

**Q3. How is mannitol helpful in hypnotics and other poisonings?**
By decreasing water resorption, the poison is also not reabsorbed.

By diluting the urine, the toxic substances are also diluted.

## Potassium-Sparing Diuretics—Spironolactone

**Q1. What are potassium-sparing diuretics?**
- Spironolactone (aldosterone antagonist)
- Amiloride
- Triamterene.

Spironolactone can be used with furosemide so that potassium supplementation can be avoided.

**Q2. What is spironolactone?**
- It is a potassium-sparing diuretic
- Its active component is canrenone
- Lag period of 2–3 days before diuresis occurs.

### Mechanism of Action
- Aldosterone antagonist competitively antagonizes the effect of aldosterone on the distal tubules. It combines with an intracellular mineralocorticoid receptor.
- Acts by competitive antagonism of aldosterone
- Slow onset of action
- Acts only on the distal tubule and collecting duct where 10% of salt resorption occurs.

### Pharmacological Actions
It has antihypertensive effects like thiazides.

### Dosage
Dose: 2–3 mg/kg can be increased up to 6 mg/kg/day or up to 600 mg/day as single morning dose.

### Indications for Spironolactone
- Edema in CCF, hepatic cirrhosis, nephritic syndrome.
- Along with thiazides to counteract potassium loss.
- Hypertension along with other drugs.

### Contraindications for Spironolactone
Use of beta-blockers or ACE inhibitors will blunt the renin-angiotensin system and increases the likelihood of hyperkalemia.

### Precautions
- It is a weak diuretic and should be used with other diuretics. Spironolactone will not be effective in treatment of edema which is not associated with rise in aldosterone.
- Dose should be reduced in elderly.
- Renal, hepatic impairment.
- Not active in normal individual or edema not associated with elevate aldosterone levels resulting in hyperkalemia.
- In renal insufficiency can cause retention of potassium.

**Q1. What are the conditions in which spironolactone should be used carefully?**
- Chronic renal insufficiency
- Hepatic failure.

**Q2. What are the precautions for spironolactone?**
Oral potassium should be avoided.

### Effects on Pregnancy
Contraindicated may affect the fetus.

## Side Effects/Adverse Reactions for Spironolactone

- Ataxia
- Breast gynecomastia
- Confusion—mental confusion
- Drowsiness
- Electrolyte imbalances—hyperkalemia
- Failure—acute renal failure
- Gastrointestinal upset—nausea, vomiting
- Headache
- Hyperchloremic metabolic acidosis
- Hirsutism (when used for a prolonged period)
- Impotence
- Joint problems (gout) due to increased uric acid levels
- Kidney stones
- Menstrual irregularities.

## Drug Interactions

- Increases blood levels of digoxin
- Will reduce the effect of warfarin
- ACE inhibitors, potassium-sparing drugs amiloride, triamterene, potassium supplements will predispose to hyperkalemia.
- Aspirin will block the spironolactone action
- Side effects of nephrotoxic or ototoxic drugs will be aggravated
- Will potentiate the action of lithium, tubocurarine
- Salicylates, NSAIDs will reduce the efficacy of spironolactone.

# QUESTIONS

**Q1. What are the predisposing factors for hyperkalemia?**
- ☐ Potassium supplements
- ☐ ACE inhibitors.

**Q2. What is the use of combining spironolactone with thiazides?**
Spironolactone will act slowly, hence it can be combined with thiazides.

**Q3. What are the differences between furosemide and spironolactone?**

| Features | Furosemide | Spironolactone |
|---|---|---|
| Type | Loop diuretic | Potassium-sparing diuretic |
| Site of action | Ascending loop of Henle | Distal loop and collecting duct |
| Dose | 1 mg/kg | 2 mg/kg |
| Maximum dose | 240 mg/day | 600 mg/day |
| Onset of action | 0.5–1 hour | 2–4 days |
| Duration of action | 4–6 hours | Long half-life of 48–72 hours |

# CARDIAC GLYCOSIDES

## Digoxin

Digoxin is a purified digitalis glycoside.

### Mechanism of Action

- Atrioventricular (AV) node—increases the refractory period and decreases the conduction.
- It decreases the heart rate and increases the myocardial contractility.
- Digoxin acts by inhibiting sodium-potassium adenosine triphosphatase ($Na^+/K^+$-ATPase) pump. This will result in increase in cytosolic (sarcoplasmic) calcium which leads to enhance myocardial contractility. It increases the force of contraction of heart which is dose-dependent. Systole will be prolonged and diastole will be shortened.
- Reduces sympathetic flow from the central nervous system (CNS)
- Reduces absorption of sodium by the kidneys which results in suppression of renal renin secretion.
- Digoxin will increase the vagal tone which results in increase in refractory period and slow in conduction through sinus node and the AV node.
- Digoxin increases the myocardial contractility.

## Pharmacological Actions

- Heart: Digoxin will reduce the heart rate, increase the diastolic time.
- Conduction system—will be depressed.
- The size of the normal and failing heart will be decreased.
- Cardiac output—will be decreased.
- Blood pressure—if it is low, it will be raised to normal.
- Coronary circulation will be improved due to improvement in cardiac output.
- Diuresis.

## Dosage

### Oral dose of digoxin:

- Oral loading dose—0.5 mg 6 hourly
- Maintenance dose—0.125 mg once a day.

### Intravenous dose of digoxin:

- Intravenous loading dose—0.02 mg/kg
- Maintenance dose—0.125-0.5 mg once a day.

**Digitalization:** Digitalization means to build up the blood levels of digoxin rapidly by giving large initial dose. Digoxin is given in a dose depending on the age of the child. Half of this dose is given initially and one-fourth after 6 hours. The remaining one-fourth is given after the next 6 hours. Maintenance dose is 25% of the total digitalization dose which should be given for 5 days in a week and should be given once in 24 hours. In children with mild CCF, directly maintenance dose can be started orally without giving the loading dose.

| Age | Dose |
|---|---|
| Premature | 0.02-0.025 |
| Newborn | 0.03-0.04 |
| Infant or child | 0.04-0.06 |
| Adolescents | 1.0-1.5 |

The total dose should not exceed 0.2-0.5 mg/24 hours. When digitalization is done intravenously, 75% of the total oral dose should be given.

Digoxin is given in a dose of 0.04-0.05 mg/kg orally. Of this half of this dose is given stratum and one-fourth after 6 hours. The remaining one-fourth is given after the next 6 hours.

The digitalizing dose should be administered over 24 hours—50% of dose initially, 25% at 12 hours and 25% at 24 hours. If used intravenously, 80% of the above said dosage should be employed. Maintenance dose is generally one-fourth of total, digitalizing dose.

Intravenous digitalization can be done by using 75% of the oral dose.

The loading dose should be given over 12-18 hours. This should be followed by maintenance dose. A pharmacokinetic steady state will be attained in 3-4 days.

**Q1. How will you administer the total digitalizing dose (TDD)?**

Total digitalizing dose should be administered over 24 hours in three divided doses.

Half of the total digitalizing dose (½ TDD) should be given as first dose. The second dose should be given after 8 hours which is one-fourth the third dose should be half of TDD, the second dose which should be given 8 hours after the third dose after maintenance dose is one-fourth of TDD should be given 24 hours.

- 1 dose = ½ of TDD
- 2 dose = ¼ of TDD
- 3 dose = ¼ of TDD.

*Intravenous dose of digoxin:*
Intravenous dose should be 75% of the oral dose.

*Maintenance dose of digoxin:*
Maintenance dose 0.01 mg/kg is given for 5 days in a week (1/4th to 1/5th of digitalizing dose). Potassium supplements are given to prevent hypokalemia.

*Slow digitalization*:
0.125–0.25 mg/day.

*Rapid digitalization*:
0.5–0.75 mg every 8 hours for 3 days followed by 0.125–0.25 mg/day.

**Q. What is the serum concentration of digoxin?**

The maternal serum digoxin concentration will be lower in pregnancy. The fetal serum concentration will be 40–90% of the maternal serum level.

*Therapeutic level of digoxin*:
- 0.8–2 µg/mL
- The mortality rate is low in patients with a digoxin concentration around 0.8 µg/mL as compared to around 1.5 µg/mL.

*Drugs given along with digoxin in cardiac failure*: Digoxin is given along with Lasix and an ACE inhibitor.

*Conditions in which half the dose of digoxin is administered*:
- The digoxin dose should be reduced in renal failure and preterm babies.
- In dilated cardiomyopathy when combined with carvedilol.

## Indications

Conditions in which digoxin can be used are:
- Congestive cardiac failure associated with reduced systolic function of heart
- Left ventricular failure
- Cardiac arrhythmias:
    - Atrial fibrillation
    - Atrial flutter
    - Atrial and supraventricular (SV) nodal paroxysmal atrial tachycardia (PAT)

Slows the ventricular rate in SV tachycardia (SVT), atrial flutter and atrial fibrillation:
- Paroxysmal AV nodal tachycardia
- Supraventricular tachycardia.

## Contraindications for Digoxin Use

The contraindications for digoxin are:

| | |
|---|---|
| A | Adverse effects to digoxin—hypersensitivity<br>AV block<br>Acute myocarditis—the response will be poor and may precipitate arrhythmia<br>Atrial fibrillation/flutter with slow ventricular rates<br>Arrhythmias—ventricular dysrhythmias<br>Ventricular tachycardia may precipitate ventricular arrhythmia |
| B | Blocks—AV blocks, partial or complete heart block |
| C | Carditis—acute myocarditis<br>Constrictive pericarditis |
| D | Decreased oxygen—hypoxia<br>Diphtheritic myocarditis<br>Digoxin toxicity |
| E | Electrolyte disorders—hypokalemia |
| F | Fibrillation (ventricular) |
| G | Green vision (for drivers, pilots)<br>Gross myocardial damage |
| H | Hypertrophic obstructive cardiomyopathy (HOCM)<br>Hypothyroidism |
| I | Infarction (acute myocardial infarction)—recent myocardial infarction<br>Idiopathic hypertrophic subaortic stenosis |

Absolute contraindication is digitalis toxicity. The other contraindications for digoxin are:
- Sick sinus syndrome
- Wolff-Parkinson-White (WPW) syndrome
- Stokes-Adams syndrome
- Tight mitral stenosis.

| | |
|---|---|
| A | Acute decompensated cardiac failure |
| B | Bronchial asthma; Bradycardia |
| C | Cardiogenic shock |
| D | Decreased blood pressure—hypotension |
| E | Endocrine—hypothyroidism |

Conditions in which digoxin are not useful:
- No use in tachycardia due to fever
- Active rheumatic fever
- High output circulatory states like thyrotoxicosis, anemia, beri-beri, arteriovenous aneurysm.
- Chronic cor pulmonale.

## Precautions

- Old age
- Patients with renal failure
- Severe hepatic disease
- Myocardial infarction
- Thyrotoxicosis
- Calcium will precipitate toxicity.

## Effects on Pregnancy

- There is no risk.
- The drug will be present in the breast milk. Hence should be given to lactating mothers only if needed.

## Side Effects/Adverse Effects of Digoxin

The adverse effects can be cardiac and extra-cardiac.

Cardiac toxicity:
- Cardiac arrhythmias due to disturbed impulse formation or conduction or both. Multifocal extrasystoles and bigeminy are common followed by partial or complete AV block
- Less common cardiac side effects are AV dissociation, sinoatrial block, PAT with block, sinoatrial arrest, ventricular tachycardia, ventricular fibrillation.

Extracardiac adverse effects are:
- Gastrointestinal—anorexia, nausea, vomiting, diarrhea, abdominal pain due to gastritis, mesenteric vasoconstriction.
- Central nervous system—headache, mental confusion, restlessness, disorientation, visual disturbances, chemoreceptor trigger zone (CTZ) stimulation.
- Psychosis
- Respiratory system—hyperpnea
- Skin rashes
- Hematological—increased coagulability of the blood resulting in thromboembolic manifestations.
- Electrolyte disturbances—hyperkalemia
- Miscellaneous—gynecomastia, fatigue.

Digoxin has a narrow therapeutic range in children the adverse effects of digoxin are:

| | |
|---|---|
| A | Arrhythmias<br>Anxiety |
| B | Blocks—heart blocks<br>Blurred vision |
| C | Confusion |
| D | Delirium<br>Disorientation<br>Depression |
| E | Ectopic beats<br>Eye—blurred vision, photophobia, color defects, yellow/green vision, haloes |
| F | Flashing lights<br>Fatigue |
| G | Gastrointestinal tract—nausea, vomiting |
| H | Hyperkalemia<br>Headache<br>Hallucinations |

Nontoxic cardiac effects of digoxin:
- Shortening of QTc interval, sagging ST segment
- Diminished T wave.

Toxic cardiac effects of digoxin:
- Prolongation of PR interval, sinus bradycardia, SA block
- Atrial or nodal ectopic beats
- Ventricular arrhythmias—ventricular trigeminy, ventricular tachycardia/fibrillation, ventricular ectopics
- Paroxysmal atrial tachycardia
- Pulsus bigeminus.
- Ventricular extrasystoles
- Partial to complete blocks.

## QUESTIONS

**Q1. What is cumulative toxicity? How will you prevent?**
Digoxin will be excreted slowly and is prone to develop increased concentration resulting in toxicity.

**Q2. Precautions that can prevent cumulative toxicity.**
Give digoxin only for 5 days of the week
Monitor the digoxin levels frequently.

**Q3. What are the features of digitalis toxicity?**

- Digoxin has a narrow therapeutic range
- Heart block
- Ectopics are common in adults.

### Q4. How will you treat a case of digitalis toxicity?
- Stop the digitalis and electrocardiography (ECG) monitoring should be done.
- Mild toxicity may present with stable, ventricular premature beats or bigeminy can be treated by using potassium supplementation to the intravenous fluids.
- The predisposing factors should be identified and eliminated.

### Q5. What are the factors that will modify cardiac toxicity of digitalis?
- Age—children will tolerate more dose than the older people. In older people, decreased muscle mass and kidney function will predispose to c toxicity at a lower dose.
- Blocks—partial AV block will be converted into total AV block.
- Cardiac status recent myocardial infarction will predispose to cardiac arrhythmias.
- Calcium—excess calcium ion will predispose to cardiac arrest in systole. Digoxin will act synergistically with calcium. Hence calcium will enhance digitalis toxicity.
- Drugs—hormones—adrenergic drugs, adrenaline will enhance the toxicity.
- Hypoxia will enhance the cardiac toxicity

The following factors will enhance digitalis toxicity:
- Hypokalemia—will enhance the toxicity
- Hypomagnesemia
- Hypocalcemia
- Cardiac inflammation due to myocarditis
- Thyrotoxicosis
- Myxoedema.

Conditions predisposing to digitalis toxicity:

| | |
|---|---|
| A | Acidosis |
| B | Babies (premature) are more prone for toxicity Bicarbonate |
| C | Calcium—digitalis acts synergistically with calcium by increasing the force of contraction of heart. Excess calcium will result in cardiac arrest in systole |
| D | Drug interactions—quinidine, verapamil, amiodarone |
| E | Electrolyte imbalances—hypokalemia, hypercalcemia, hypomagnesemia. Hypokalemia enhances myocardial uptake of digitalis. Hypokalemia can be precipitated by intravenous infusion of large doses of glucose, insulin or sodium |
| F | Fasting (food in the stomach will slow the absorption of digoxin) |
| G | Geriatric age—elderly |
| H | Hypothyroidism Hypoxia |
| I | Inflammatory changes/ischemia in myocardium |
| K | Kidney disease (decreases the excretion of digitalis) |
| L | Liver disorders resulting in decreased detoxification |

### Q6. What are the factors that predispose to digoxin toxicity?
- Overdose
- Renal insufficiency
- Intake of drugs that interfere with elimination of digoxin.

### Q7. What are the features of digoxin toxicity?
- Vomiting
- Cardiac rhythm disturbances—sinus bradycardia, AV block, premature ventricular beats, bidirectional ventricular tachycardia, atrial tachycardia with block.

### Q8. What is the toxic effect of digoxin on eye?
Xanthopsia.

**Q9. How will you monitor for digitalis toxicity?**
- Clinical manifestations—anorexia, nausea, vomiting, decrease in pulse less than 60/min.
- ECG—disturbances the formation and conduction of impulse resulting in arrhythmia or conduction disturbances, extrasystoles or ventricular bigeminy.
- Serum electrolytes especially potassium
- Serum digoxin levels.

**Q10. What is the treatment of digoxin toxicity?**
- Stop the drug digoxin
- Digoxin immune Fab
- Treat hypokalemia if present. Infuse KCl 20 mmol/hour (maximum of 100 mmol/hour) intravenously. In milder cases, KCl can be given orally.
- Beta-blockers (propranolol) for SV arrhythmia
- Atropine in AV block and bradycardia
- Lignocaine.

## Drug Interactions

- Diuretics can cause hypokalemia and precipitate arrhythmias.
- Calcium will synergize with digitalis and precipitate toxicity.
- Quinidine will reduce binding of digoxin
- Potassium-sparing diuretics will reduce renal excretion of digoxin.
- Succinylcholine will cause arrhythmias in digitalized patients.
- Phenobarbitone will increase digoxin metabolism by inducing enzymes and thereby decrease the half-life of digoxin.

The following drugs will increase the plasma concentration of digoxin:
- Calcium channel blockers—verapamil
- Diltiazem
- Captopril
- Amiodarone
- Spironolactone
- Quinidine
- Calcium salts.

The following drugs will decrease the absorption of digoxin:
- Antacids
- Neomycin
- Sulfasalazine
- Metoclopramide (GI hurrying)
- Sucralfate (adsorbs digoxin).

The following drugs will depress AV conduction and oppose positive inotropic action:
- Propranolol
- Verapamil
- Diltiazem
- Disopyramide.

## QUESTIONS

**Q1. What is digoxin?**
Digoxin is a purified digitalis glycoside.

**Q2. What is the half-life of digoxin?**
Half-life of digoxin is 24–36 hours.

**Q3. What is the serum concentration of digoxin?**
The maternal serum digoxin concentration will be lower in pregnancy. The fetal serum concentration will be 40–90% of the maternal serum level.

**Q4. What is the action of digoxin in a normal heart?**
In normal heart, the cardiac glycosides like digoxin will augment the strength and speed of myocardial contractility.

**Q5. What is the action of digoxin in a failing heart?**
It improves the myocardial contractility by direct action on the myocardium.

**Q6. What are the conditions in which digoxin is not useful?**
- No use in tachycardia due to fever
- Active rheumatic fever
- High output circulatory states like thyrotoxicosis, anemia, beri-beri, arteriovenous aneurysm.
- Chronic cor pulmonale.

**Q7. What are the drugs given along with digoxin in cardiac failure?**
Digoxin is given along with Lasix and an ACE inhibitor.

**Q8. What are the conditions in which half the dose of digoxin is administered?**
The digoxin dose should be reduced in renal failure and preterm babies.

## CHELATING AGENTS

### Deferiprone (L1)—Kelfer

- Orally active iron chelator
- High affinity for iron
- Hydrophilic
- One molecule of L1 will bind to 1 molecule of iron neutral complex
- One molecule of desferrioxamine (DFO) will bind to 1 molecule of iron positive charged complex
- Efficacy: 70–100% effective as DFO.

### Mechanism of Action
Chelates iron.

### Dosage
- 50–100 mg/kg daily in divided doses
- 25–33 mg/kg orally three times a day.

### Indications
- Acute iron poisoning
- Hemochromatosis
- Transfusion siderosis
- Repeated blood transfusions causing iron overload in thalassemia patients.

### Contraindications
- Hypersensitivity to deferiprone
- Absolute neutrophil count (ANC) less than 1,500

### Precautions
- Monitor serum ferritin every 2–3 months
- At 4-hour gap should be present before taking iron, aluminum, zinc-containing preparations like antacids.

### Effects on Pregnancy
Category D fetal defects were noted.

### Side Effects/Adverse Effects
- Anorexia
- Arthropathy
- Arthralgia
- Altered taste
- Blood dyscrasia—neutropenia (reversible), thrombocytopenia, rarely agranulocytosis
- Chromaturia
- Drug-induced lupus
- Emesis
- Fever
- Gastrointestinal symptoms—abdominal pain, nausea, diarrhea
- Hepatotoxicity—elevation of alanine aminotransferase
- Increased heart rate (tachycardia)
- Joint problems—joint pain, synovial thickening and effusion
- Zinc deficiency.

### Drug Interactions
It will bind to polyvalent cations.

## QUESTIONS

**Q1. What are the advantages of combination of chelating agents DFO and deferiprone (L1)?**
Advantages:
- Chelates iron from different sites and do not compete for same site
- L1 will shuttle iron from DFO
- Decreases the side effects of both.

### Desferrioxamine

- Potent and specific iron chelator
- 1 g is capable of chelating 85 mg of elemental iron.
- Ferrioxamine is a long chain containing complex chemical removal of iron will yield desferrioxamine which has a very high affinity for iron. The desferrioxamine molecule which is straight will turn round

and form stable nontoxic complex which will be excreted in urine.

## Mechanism of Action
- Readily binds to ferric iron to form ferrioxamine which is a stable and water-soluble chelate.
- Removes iron from hemosiderin except that in the bone marrow.
- 100 mg of desferrioxamine will bind to 8.5 mg of iron.

## Dosage of Desferrioxamine
Dose: 0.5–1 g/day.

## Indications for Desferrioxamine
- Acute iron poisoning
- Hemochromatosis
- Transfusion siderosis
- Repeated blood transfusions causing iron overload in thalassemia patients.

## Contraindications for Desferrioxamine
- Severe renal disease
- Anuria
- Pregnancy.

## Precautions
Iron will oxidize vitamin C resulting in deficiency of vitamin C in those receiving iron-chelating therapy. Supplementation of vitamin C should be given. Vitamin C in a dose of 50 mg in children and 100 mg for older children and adults should be given along with desferrioxamine.

## Effects on Pregnancy
Avoided due to its potential teratogenic toxicity.

## Side Effects/Adverse Effects of Desferrioxamine
- Allergic reactions (erythema, urticaria, itching, rashes)
- Abdominal pain
- Bleeding
- Bruising
- Blurred vision
- Breathing problems—shortness of breath, wheezing
- Convulsions
- Cramps—muscle cramps
- Dizziness
- Diarrhea
- Dysuria
- Emesis (vomiting)
- Fever
- Flushing
- Gastrointestinal discomfort
- Hypotension
- Hives
- Itching
- Irritability.

Q. **What are the adverse effects of chronic administration of desferrioxamine?**
 ❑ Allergic reactions, cataract formation
 ❑ Changes in retina and lens.

## Drug Interactions
Vitamin C will increase the availability of iron for chelation.

# QUESTIONS

Q1. **How is ferrioxamine excreted?**
 About two-third of ferrioxamine will be excreted by urine and one-third by the bile.

Q2. **Which is an orally effective iron chelator?**
 Deferiprone.

# H2-RECEPTOR BLOCKERS

Cimetidine, ranitidine and all other H2 antagonists will block the histamine induced gastric secretions.

## Proton-pump Inhibitors

Proton pump inhibitors are potent inhibitors of gastric acid secretion.

**Q. What are the proton-pump inhibitors (PPIs)?**
- ❑ Omeprazole
- ❑ Lansoprazole
- ❑ Rabeprazole
- ❑ Pantoprazole
- ❑ Esomeprazole.

## Mechanism of Action
- ❖ Proton pump is the terminal stage in gastric secretion by parietal cells.
- ❖ Reduces stomach acid production by blocking the gastric hydrogen/potassium adenosine triphosphate ($H^+/K^+$-ATPase) enzyme system in the stomach.
- ❖ Potent inhibitors of acid secretion.

## Dosage
**Oral dose:**

Omeprazole:
- ❖ Infants 0.7 mg/kg/day
- ❖ 5–10 kg—5 mg daily
- ❖ 10–20 kg—10 mg daily
- ❖ Greater than 20 kg—20 mg orally daily.

Lansoprazole:
- ❖ Less than 10 kg—7.5 mg twice daily or 15 mg daily
- ❖ Greater than 30 kg—30 mg daily.

Pantoprazole: 40 mg daily

Esomeprazole: 20–40 mg daily.

## Indications
- ❖ Aspiration pneumonia
- ❖ Barrett's esophagus
- ❖ Chronic acid peptic disease
- ❖ Duodenal ulcer
- ❖ Drug-induced ulcer like NSAID
- ❖ Esophageal ulcer
- ❖ Erosive reflux esophagitis/gastritis
- ❖ Functional dyspepsia
- ❖ Gastroesophageal reflux disease/gastric ulcer
- ❖ Hiatus hernia
- ❖ Hypersecretory conditions
- ❖ Hypersecretion of acid—gastrinomas, Zollinger-Ellison syndrome
- ❖ Infections—used along with antibiotics for eradicating *Helicobacter pylori*.

## Contraindications
- ❖ Hypersensitivity
- ❖ Hepatic problems.

## Precautions
- ❖ The effects will be delayed for 5–7 days until the proton pumps are fully blocked.
- ❖ Rebound GI symptoms and rebound acid hypersecretion can occur after discontinuation.
- ❖ Avoid long-term use for more than 8 weeks.
- ❖ The drugs should be tapered before stopping the drugs.

## Effects on Pregnancy
- ❖ Category C for omeprazole
- ❖ Category B for other PPIs.

## Side Effects
- ❖ Abdominal pain
- ❖ Allergic reactions
- ❖ Anxiety
- ❖ Bone problems—osteoporosis, fractures of hip, wrist, spine (long-term use >1 year)
- ❖ Constipation
- ❖ Cardiac problems (in long-term use)
- ❖ Diarrhea
- ❖ Emesis
- ❖ Flatulence
- ❖ Gastrointestinal tract upset—nausea
- ❖ Gastric carcinoma (in long-term use)
- ❖ Headache
- ❖ Hypomagnesemia
- ❖ Hypocalcemia
- ❖ Infections with *Clostridium difficile*, community-acquired pneumonia
- ❖ Itching
- ❖ Iron and vitamin B12 deficiency.

## Drug Interactions
- ❖ Drugs that need acid in the stomach for better absorption will be affected

as these drugs decrease the acid in the stomach.
- ❖ Reduces the absorption of ketoconazole, iron salts, griseofulvin, vitamin B12
- ❖ Increases the absorption and thereby concentration of digoxin, nifedipine
- ❖ Reduces the metabolism of drugs like omeprazole by liver
- ❖ Increases the drug levels of diazepam, warfarin, and methotrexate.

## QUESTIONS

**Q1. What are the adverse effects of PPIs due to decreased acidity?**
Adverse effects due to decreased acidity are:
- ❑ Infections due to ingested flora
- ❑ Decreases vitamin B12 absorption
- ❑ Iron, calcium, zinc absorption.

**Q2. What are the adverse effects of long-term use of PPIs?**
- ❑ Absorption of minerals affected
- ❑ Bone problems
- ❑ Cardiac problems
- ❑ Community-acquired pneumonia
- ❑ *Clostridium difficile* infection
- ❑ Cancers—gastric carcinoma
- ❑ Chronic kidney disease
- ❑ Dementia.

**Q3. How PPIs differ from H2 blockers?**
Proton-pump inhibitors will shut down the acid pumps whereas H2 blockers will block the signals that trigger acid production. The duration of H2 blockers will last for about 12 hours whereas the PPIs will last for 24–72 hours.

## Ranitidine

### Mechanism of Action

- ❖ It is a long-acting antagonist for histamine H2 receptor.
- ❖ Competitive and reversible inhibitor of interaction of histamine on H2 receptors. Ranitidine does not have any action on other H2 receptors.

### Pharmacological Actions

Ranitidine reduces basal and nocturnal acid secretion. Ranitidine also will inhibit acid secretion induced by histamine and gastrin. Ranitidine will decrease the volume of gastric acid secretion also.

### Dosage

- ❖ Oral dose: 5–10 mg/kg/day in two divided doses
- ❖ Parenteral dose: 2–4 mg/kg every 12–24 hours.

### Indications

- ❖ Duodenal ulcer
- ❖ Dyspepsia
- ❖ Esophagitis
- ❖ Gastroesophageal reflux disease/gastric ulcer
- ❖ Hypersecretory conditions
- ❖ Zollinger-Ellison syndrome.

### Contraindications

- ❖ Age less than 1 month
- ❖ Hypersensitivity
- ❖ Acute porphyria.

### Precautions

- ❖ Dose should be reduced in conditions associated with decreased GFR, liver problems
- ❖ Rule out gastric malignancy.

### Effects on Pregnancy

Although no side effects are noted, it should be given only clearly indicated.

### Side Effects

- ❖ Allergic reactions—skin rash
- ❖ Arthralgia
- ❖ Agitation
- ❖ Blurred vision
- ❖ Constipation
- ❖ Mental confusion
- ❖ Diarrhea
- ❖ Dizziness

- Depression
- Emesis
- Fast heart rate
- Gastrointestinal discomfort
- Headache
- Hallucination
- Icterus (due to inflammation of liver).

## Drug Interactions
- Nonsteroidal anti-inflammatory drugs should be used carefully especially in patients with renal failure
- Antacid will delay absorption
- Warfarin with ranitidine will increase the risk of bleeding.

# QUESTIONS

**Q1. What is the amount of acid produced in the stomach?**
Human stomach can produce 20–40 mEq of hydrochloric acid per hour.

**Q2. Which is more potent cimetidine or ranitidine?**
Ranitidine is five times more potent than cimetidine in inhibiting acid secretion.

# MISCELLANEOUS

## Acetazolamide

### Mechanism of Action
- They are carbonic anhydrase inhibitors which inhibits bicarbonate ($HCO_3$) reabsorption in proximal tubular cells.
- It will affect secretion of $H^+$ in the distal tubule and collecting duct.
- Hydrogen ions will not be available for exchange with sodium. This results in loss of sodium and water is also eliminated along with it.

### Pharmacological Actions
- It will decrease synthesis of aqueous humor
- Decrease intraocular tension
- Inhibits bicarbonate reabsorption which results in mild alkaline diuresis.

### Dosage
0.25–0.5 g.

### Indications
- Altitude sickness
- Benign/idiopathic intracranial hypertension
- Congestive cardiac failure
- Drug-induced edema
- Drug poisoning (alkalinization of urine)
- Epilepsy
- Familial periodic paralysis
- Glaucoma—Open angle, secondary, acute angle closure
- Hyper-/hypokalemia
- Idiopathic endolymphatic hydrops (Meniere's syndrome).

### Contraindications
- Hepatic disorders—Liver disease may precipitate hepatic coma
- Hypoadrenalism—Adrenal insufficiency
- Hyperchloremic acidosis (renal)
- Hyponatremia
- Hypokalemia
- Hypersensitivity to acetazolamide.

### Precautions
- Gout, diabetes
- Potassium supplements may be needed
- Side effects are more in elderly.

### Effects on Pregnancy
It is contraindicated in pregnancy since it may affect the fetus.

### Side Effects
- Allergy—Rashes
- Blood dyscrasias
- Bone marrow suppression
- Cramp—Abdominal cramps
- Drowsiness

- Electrolyte imbalances—hypokalemia, hyponatremia, and metabolic acidosis
- Fever
- Fatigue
- Gustatory problems—bitter or metallic taste
- Gastrointestinal—nausea, vomiting, and diarrhea
- Headache
- Hypersensitivity
- Increased urination (polyuria)
- Stevens-Johnson syndrome
- Kidney stones
- Libido decreased
- Myopia (transient)
- Neurological—Paresthesia, flaccid paralysis.

### Drug Interactions

- It potentiates the effects of folic acid, oral hypoglycemic agents, and oral anticoagulants
- It can cause osteomalacia with phenytoin
- Hypokalemia with corticosteroids.

## QUESTION

Q1. How acetazolamide is useful in treating epilepsy?

Increasing the level of carbon dioxide results in acidosis in the brain and raises the threshold for seizures.

## Caffeine Citrate (Methylxanthine)

*Plasma concentration*: 5–20 µg/mL.

### Mechanism of Action

It stimulates central nervous system (CNS).

### Pharmacological Actions

- Stimulant for CNS, heart, and muscles
- It will raise the blood pressure
- Diuretic
- Increase the frequency of urination.

### Dosage

- Loading dose—20 mg/kg (10 mg caffeine base)
- Maintenance dose—2.5–5 mg/kg
- Route—Oral/intravenous (IV).

### Indication

Apnea of prematurity.

### Contraindications

- Anxiety
- Bipolar disorder
- Bleeding disorders
- Cardiac disorders
- Diabetes
- Epilepsy
- Failure—Hepatic/renal failure
- Glaucoma
- Hypertension
- Irritable bowel syndrome
- Osteoporosis.

### Precautions

Very high doses can cause irregular heartbeats and death. Caffeine may increase the blood sugar.

### Effects on Pregnancy

- It is safer to use less than 200 mg/day. High doses are contraindicated.
- Caffeine will cross the placenta and affect the sleep and movement pattern in the fetus during later stages of pregnancy.
- Also caffeine can cause birth defects, premature labor.
- Caffeine can cause miscarriages.

### Side Effects

- Agitation
- Breathing problems
- Crying
- Dry skin
- Emesis (vomiting)
- Fast breathing
- Gastric irritation
- Headache
- Increased heart rate and respiratory rate

- Insomnia
- Jitteriness
- Nausea
- Nervousness
- Restlessness
- Large doses—Anxiety, agitation, headache, chest pain, and ringing in the ears.

## Drug Interactions

Caffeine and ephedrine are stimulants and may cause too much stimulation.

The following drugs will decrease the caffeine metabolism:
- Alcohol
- Birth control contraceptive
- Cimetidine
- Disulfiram
- Estrogen
- Fluconazole
- Fluvoxamine.

## Calcium Gluconate

- Oral calcium
- Parenteral calcium—Available as 10% solution, 1 g/10 mL
- 1 g of calcium gluconate will contain 90 mg of calcium which is equal to 4.6 mEq.

## Mechanism of Action

It regulates the release and storage of neurotransmitters.

## Pharmacological Aspects

Calcium will be absorbed in the small intestines. The following factors will affect the absorption of calcium:
- Achlorhydria
- Blood pH
- Calcium deficiency
- Vitamin D
- Diet low in calcium
- Calcium binding fibers
- Phytates.

## Dosage

- 2 mL/kg of 10% calcium gluconate is diluted with equal volume of 5% gram dry weight (GDW) or distilled water and given intravenously by slow infusion followed by a continuous infusion of 5–8 mL/kg/24 hours
- Infuse in 5% dextrose
- Cardiac monitoring should be done.

**Dose of calcium gluconate:**
- 100–200 mg/kg/dose
- 1–2 mL/kg/dose
- 10% calcium gluconate and 1–2 mL/kg should be given intravenously over 3–5 minutes.
- Up to a total of 10 mL, calcium gluconate can be diluted in 5% dextrose and given very slowly with cardiac monitoring.
- Calcium gluconate contains 0.98 mg/mL or 0.45 mEq/mL of elemental calcium.

Q1. **What is the maximum dose of calcium gluconate?**
10 mL/dose.

Q2. **How will you dilute calcium gluconate?**
Dilute with equal amount of water or 5% dextrose in the ratio of 1:1.

Q3. **What is the route of administration?**
- Intravenous only
- Subcutaneous or intramuscular administration will cause severe sloughing.

## Indications for Calcium

- Antidote for calcium channel blocker, verapamil overdosage
- Bone problems—Osteoporosis (long-term corticosteroid therapy), osteomalacia
- Cardiac arrest
- Vitamin D deficiency rickets
- Exchange transfusion
- Generalized osteoporosis
- Hyperkalemia
- Hypoparathyroidism
- Hypermagnesemia

- Hypocalcemia—Symptomatic like tetany
- Intestinal colic (nonspecific)
- Urticaria.

## Contraindications for the Use of Calcium Gluconate

- Hypercalcemia
- Renal calculi
- Ventricular fibrillation.

## Precautions

- Rapid infusion of IV calcium may cause bradycardia, cardiac arrhythmias, or cardiac arrest.
- Bolus doses should be given only in cases of hypocalcemia.
- Continuous infusion should be preferred to bolus doses.
- Duration of infusion should be over 72 hours.
- It should not be given intramuscularly. Extravasation of calcium into the subcutaneous tissues can cause necrosis and subcutaneous calcifications.

## Factors to be remembered while administering calcium gluconate:

- Heart rate and rhythm should be monitored—monitor for bradycardia during administration.
- Use with caution in digitalized patients
- This should not be mixed with sodium bicarbonate as it can result in the formation of calcium carbonate precipitate.
- Should not be given intramuscularly as it can lead to sterile abscess.
- If given by umbilical vein catheter ensure that the tip of the catheter is in the inferior vena cava.
- Calcium should not be give through umbilical artery as it can cause arterial spasm, intestinal necrosis.

**Effects of sudden rise in calcium:** Sudden elevation of calcium will lead to arrhythmias, bradycardia, and dysrhythmias.

## Effects on Pregnancy

Category C.

## Side Effects/Adverse Effects of Calcium

- Arrhythmia
- Bradycardia
- Constipation
- Dysrhythmias
- Extravasation of calcium salts during IV administration can result in necrosis and local sloughing of the skin and subcutaneous tissue
- Frequent urination
- Gustatory—chalky taste
- Hypercalcemia
- Hepatic necrosis can occur [if the tip of the umbilical venous catheter (UVC) lies in the portal vein].
- Intestinal obstruction due to formation of calcium concretions.

## Drug Interactions

- Calcium and bicarbonate should not be mixed in the same solutions. When given along with sodium bicarbonate, it will be precipitated to calcium carbonate.
- Calcium carbonate is used as an antacid
- Thiazide diuretics will facilitate tubular reabsorption of calcium.
- Ceftriaxone will cause particulate precipitate in the lungs and kidneys.

The following will form an insoluble complex in the intestines and interfere with absorption of calcium:

- Phytates
- Phosphates
- Oxalates
- Tetracyclines.

The following drugs will reduce absorption of calcium:

- Glucocorticoids
- Phenytoin
- Doxycycline.

# QUESTIONS

**Q1. Can we use sodium bicarbonate with calcium gluconate?**
No, it will form precipitates.

**Q2. How will you treat hypocalcemia?**
It is treated by slow infusion of calcium gluconate 1-2 mL/kg IV with equal amount of dextrose.

**Q3. What is the rate of infusion of calcium gluconate?**
Give at a rate of 0.5 mL/min.

**Q4. How will you treat hypocalcemia in newborn?**
*Hypocalcemia*—10% calcium gluconate 1-2 mL/kg diluted with normal saline (1:1 dilution) and given slowly (it forms calcium carbonate when given along with sodium bicarbonate. Hence, it should be avoided along with it). Monitor the heart rate during the loading dose.

**Q5. What will you suspect if convulsion persists in spite of calcium transfusion?**
Suspect hypomagnesemia and treat with magnesium sulfate infusion. Symptomatic hypocalcemia, which is not responding to calcium, may be due to hypomagnesemia. 50% magnesium sulfate in a dose of 0.1-0.2 mL/kg can be given deep intramuscularly.

**Q6. How will you treat convulsions not responding to calcium?**
If magnesium is low, 50% magnesium sulfate can be given as 0.1-0.2 mL/kg intramuscularly every 12-24 hours as needed.

**Q7. What are the conditions in which oral calcium can cause hypercalcemia?**
Milk alkali syndrome and hypothyroidism.

**Q8. What are the complications associated with calcium transfusion?**
- Arrhythmia
- Bradycardia
- Cardiac arrest, if given rapidly
- Calcium level increase (hypercalcemia)
- Damage to tissues—Tissue necrosis due to extravasations
- Hepatic necrosis can occur (if the tip of the UVC lies in the portal vein)
- Intestinal necrosis (if infused through umbilical artery).

## Cyclopam

It is a combination of dicyclomine and paracetamol.

### Mechanism of Action

- Antispasmodic drug
- Dicyclomine is a anticholinergic which will relax the smooth muscles of the stomach and intestines.
- This drug will increase the pain threshold

### Dosage

- *Children*:
  - 6 months to 2 years—5-10 mg orally in three to four divided doses up to maximum of 20 mg/day.
  - 2-12 years—10 mg/kg/day.
- *Adults*: 80 mg/day in 4 divided doses.

### Indications

Treatment of pain due to smooth muscle spasms in the following conditions:
- Abdominal pain
- Bowel spasm
- Bloating
- Cramps (intestinal cramps)
- Dysmenorrhea (painful menstruation)
- Ear pain
- Fever
- Gastrointestinal tract (GIT) disorders with pain
- Headache
- Irritable bowel syndrome
- Joint pain.

### Contraindications and Cautions

- Age less than 6 months
- Allergy to cyclopam

- Bowel obstruction
- Breastfeeding mothers
- Cardiovascular instability
- Deep or puncture wounds
- Glaucoma
- Hypersensitivity
- Hepatic impairment
- Inflammatory bowel diseases, ulcerative colitis
- Myasthenia gravis.

## Precautions
- Should be taken 1 hour before food
- Should be used cautiously in patients with kidney diseases
- If used with antifungals like ketoconazole, it should be taken 2 hours before
- Avoid driving or working in machinery after taking this medicine
- Intake of alcohol should be avoided.

## Effects on Pregnancy
- Should be used cautiously during pregnancy
- Not safe during lactation.

## Side Effects
- Allergic reactions
- Bloating
- Blurred vision
- Constipation
- Dizziness
- Drowsiness
- Dryness of mouth
- Dysuria
- Eye problem—blurred vision
- Nausea
- Sleepiness
- Weakness
- Nervousness.

## Drug Interactions
This will interact with the following drugs:
- Antacids
- Antihistamines
- Benzodiazepines
- Corticosteroids
- Digoxin
- Ketoconazole
- Monoamine oxidase inhibitor (MAOI).

## QUESTION

**Q. What are the problems of overdosage of cyclopam?**
Overdoses of cyclopam will cause muscle weakness or paralysis.

## Diclofenac Sodium

### Mechanism of Action
- Analgesic, antipyretic, and anti-inflammatory
- Nonsteroidal anti-inflammatory drug inhibits prostaglandin synthesis
- Antiplatelet action of short duration.

### Dosage
- 25 mg four times a day
- 35 mg thrice daily
- 50 mg orally twice a day
- 100 mg once daily.

### Indications
- Arthritis
- Pain relief.

### Contraindications and Cautions
- Allergy reactions
- Bleeding—active bleeding
- Clotting disorders
- Coronary artery bypass graft
- Dengue fever
- Duodenal ulcer
- Elderly and debilitated patients
- Fluid retention
- Gastrointestinal bleeding
- Gestational period—3rd trimester after 30 weeks of gestation
- Gastric bypass surgery
- Gastrointestinal ulcers
- Hypersensitivity
- Hepatotoxicity

- Inflammatory bowel diseases (Crohn's disease, ulcerative colitis)
- Jaundice due to hepatic dysfunction
- Kidney failure
- Porphyria.

### Precautions
- The tablet should be swallowed as a whole and should not be chewed or bitten.
- Patient should not lie down for at least 10 minutes after taking the tablet.
- This drug can cause fatal gastrointestinal bleeding.

### Effects on Pregnancy
Contraindicated in the 3rd trimester of pregnancy.

### Side Effects
- Abdominal pain
- Bloating of abdomen
- Constipation
- Dyspepsia
- Emesis
- Exfoliative dermatitis
- Fluid retention
- Gastrointestinal problems
- Headache
- Indigestion
- Itching
- Stevens-Johnson syndrome
- Toxic epidermal necrolysis.

### Drug Interactions
- Aminoglycosides—Nephrotoxicity
- Amphotericin B, cisplatin, capreomycin, and vancomycin will cause nephrotoxicity.

## QUESTION

Q. What are the features of overdose of diclofenac sodium?
- ❑ Agitation
- ❑ Blurred vision
- ❑ Breathing problems
- ❑ Consciousness altered
- ❑ Confusion
- ❑ Convulsions
- ❑ Depression
- ❑ Irritability.

## Dicyclomine
Anticholinergics, antispasmodics.

### Mechanism of Action
- Muscarinic antagonist
- Relaxes the smooth muscles.

### Dosage
20 mg four times a day.

### Indications
- To relieve spasms due to irritable bowel syndrome
- Urinary incontinence.

### Contraindications and Cautions
- Age less than 6 months
- Bowel obstruction
- Breastfeeding.

### Precautions
- The drug will cause decreased sweating and can predispose to heatstroke.
- Dicyclomine can impair the thinking
- Avoid driving or using machinery as this will cause blurring of vision, dizziness.

### Effects on Pregnancy
- Use only if clearly indicated during pregnancy
- Contraindicated during breastfeeding.

### Side Effects
- Abdominal bloating
- Blurred vision
- Constipation
- Dizziness
- Drowsiness
- Dry eyes
- Dry mouth
- Delusion
- Disorientation

- Eye problems—photosensitivity
- Fever
- Forgetfulness
- Gas or bloating
- Heatstroke
- Itching
- Insomnia or excessive sleep
- Withdrawal symptoms.

## Drug Interactions

Antacids will delay the absorption of dicyclomine. Dicyclomine will affect the absorption of levodopa, ketoconazole.

## QUESTION

Q. What are the withdrawal symptoms?
- ☐ Dizziness
- ☐ Sweating
- ☐ Vomiting.

## Ferrous Sulfate

- Iron is absorbed in ferrous form from the gut. It is transported in the blood as ferric form attached to transferrin. Monoamine oxidase is an iron-dependent enzyme which plays an important role in neurochemical reaction in the CNS.
- Ferrous sulfate elemental iron content—15 mg/0.6 mL drops, 18 mg/5 mL in the syrup, and 44 mg/5 mL in the elixir.
- Ferrous sulfate tablets.

### Dosage

- 4-6 mg/kg/day in two divided doses for 3 months are recommended for treatment of iron deficiency in children. Smaller dose of 3 mg/kg/day is equally effective and better tolerated. So, it is better to use iron in a lower dose. Prophylaxis is 1 mg/kg/day
- Iron can be given for 6 months.

### Indications

- Iron-deficiency anemia
- Supplementation during pregnancy.

## Contraindications for the Treatment with Oral Iron

- Allergy
- Acid—peptic ulcer disease
- Blood transfusions (repeated).
- Colitis—ulcerative colitis
- Diverticular disease
- Enteritis
- Failure of treatment with oral iron (may be due to malabsorption of iron)
- Gastric ulcer
- Hemochromatosis, hemolytic anemia
- Iron overload syndrome.

### Precautions

The tablet should not be chewed, it should be swallowed.
- Peptic ulcer
- Severe renal failure
- Patients will pass black colored stools
- Administered after meals.

At bedtime as decreased motility of gut during sleep will increase the absorption, iron has to be converted into ferrous salts before it is absorbed. Gastric acid will reduce ferric to ferrous ions. Hence, ferrous salts are preferred for ferric salts.

### Effects on Pregnancy

Not contraindicated.

### Side Effects of Oral Iron

- Allergy
- Anorexia
- Black colored stools
- Constipation
- Diarrhea
- Discoloration of teeth (temporary)
- Epigastric pain
- Emesis
- Fever
- Gastrointestinal intolerance
- Gastrointestinal irritation
- Gustatory problem—metallic taste.

## Drug Interactions

- Iron and tetracycline will bind together
- Iron will decrease L-thyroxine absorption
- Vitamin C will facilitate iron absorption from gut
- Cholestyramine will bind with iron and prevent absorption.

**Q1. What is the role of vitamin C in treating iron-deficiency anemia?**
Vitamin C 200 mg per 30 mg of elemental iron will enhance iron absorption.

**Q2. What are the drugs that will decrease iron absorption?**
Tetracycline, antacids, and chloramphenicol.

# QUESTIONS

**Q1. What are the clinical features of iron deficiency?**
- Iron-deficiency anemia
- Hypochromic, microcytic anemia
- Growth retardation.

**Q2. What are the preventive steps for gastrointestinal intolerance after ferrous sulfate?**
- Administered after meals
- At bedtime as decreased motility of gut during sleep will increase the absorption.

**Q3. Why ferrous salts are preferred for ferric salts?**
Iron has to be converted into ferrous salts before it is absorbed. Hence, ferrous salts are preferred for ferric salts.

**Q4. What are the signs of recovery from iron deficiency?**
*Response to iron therapy after initiation of therapy*:

| Hours/days | Response to iron therapy |
|---|---|
| 12–24 hours | Mentation improved, decreased irritability, and improvement in appetite |
| 36–48 hours | Bone marrow changes—Erythroid hyperplasia |

*Contd...*

*Contd...*

| Hours/days | Response to iron therapy |
|---|---|
| 48–72 hours | Reticulocyte count increases |
| 4–30 days | Hemoglobin (Hb) level increases |
| 1–3 months | Repletion of iron stores |

**Q5. What is the earliest sign of recovery in iron-deficiency anemia?**
Decreased irritability, improvement in appetite.

**Q6. What are the foods rich in iron?**
- Animal sources—Liver, red meat
- Plant sources—Jaggery, dates, Ragi and green leafy vegetables, drumstick leaves are rich sources of iron, amaranth, mint, whole grain, legumes, and nuts.

Positive response to treatment raises of hemoglobin (Hb) 0.1 g/dL daily.
Hemoglobin level raises to normal in 2 months and in another 2 months, the stores will be replenished.

**Q7. What are the causes for failure to respond to oral iron?**
Failure to respond to iron therapy is seen in the following conditions:
- Inadequate iron dose
- Poor patient compliance
- Persistent blood loss
- Impaired intestinal absorption
- Associated infections/infestations.

**Q8. What are the features of iron overdose?**
Gastrointestinal irritation, erosion of gastrointestinal mucosa, hematemesis, lethargy, acidosis, hepatic and renal function, circulatory collapse, coma, and death.

**Q9. How will you treat iron overdose?**
- Iron chelation therapy using deferoxamine
- Gastric lavage using sodium bicarbonate (as iron absorption will be poor in alkaline medium) or sodium phosphate solution.

**Q10. What is the serum level of iron that requires iron chelation therapy?**
Serum iron level more than 300 µg/mL.

**Q11. What are the forms of iron available for treatment of iron deficiency?**
Oral and parenteral forms.
- ❑ Oral forms are ferrous sulfate, ferrous gluconate, and ferrous fumarate
- ❑ Parenteral forms are iron dextran, iron sorbitol.

**Q12. What are the oral preparations of iron?**
- ❑ Ferrous gluconate
- ❑ Ferrous fumarate.

## Haloperidol

### Mechanism of Action
It inhibits the effects of dopamine (DA) by competitively blocking postsynaptic D2 receptors in the brain.

### Dosage
- ❖ Children—0.05–0.15 mg/kg/day up to a maximum of 6 mg/day in two to three divided doses
- ❖ Adult—0.5–2 mg two to three times a day.

### Indications
- ❖ Acute psychosis
- ❖ Bipolar disorders
- ❖ Behavioral disorders in children
- ❖ Chorea
- ❖ Confusion associated with cerebral sclerosis
- ❖ Delirium (agitation component)
- ❖ Drug-induced psychosis [lysergic acid diethylamide (LSD), amphetamines, ketamine, and phencyclidine]
- ❖ Emesis
- ❖ Fever-induced psychosis
- ❖ Gilles de la Tourette syndrome
- ❖ Hyperactivity
- ❖ Intractable hiccups
- ❖ Mania
- ❖ Mood disorders
- ❖ Nausea
- ❖ Psychosis
- ❖ Schizophrenia.

### Contraindications and Cautions
- ❖ Age less than 3 years
- ❖ Allergy to haloperidol
- ❖ Acute stroke
- ❖ Butyrophenone allergy
- ❖ Coma
- ❖ Drugs—Central depressant drugs, drugs that prolong QT interval
- ❖ Depression of CNS system
- ❖ Elderly patients with dementia
- ❖ Familial long QT syndrome
- ❖ Gestational period
- ❖ Hypokalemia
- ❖ Hypomagnesemia
- ❖ Impaired liver function
- ❖ Parkinsonism.

### Precautions
- ❖ Intravenous administration will be associated with hypotension or orthostatic collapse
- ❖ Use cautiously in hepatic dysfunction as the drug is metabolized and eliminated by liver.
- ❖ Avoid abrupt cessation of the drug
- ❖ With anticholinergics, it will increase the intraocular pressure.

### Effects on Pregnancy
Not teratogenic but embryotoxic in high doses. The drug is secreted in the breast milk and may cause extrapyramidal symptoms in breastfed babies.

### Side Effects
- ❖ Anxiety
- ❖ Anorexia
- ❖ Blurred vision
- ❖ Bronchospasm
- ❖ Constipation
- ❖ Chorea
- ❖ Diaphoresis
- ❖ Dizziness
- ❖ Drowsiness
- ❖ Emesis

- Extrapyramidal side effects—akathisia, dystonia, rigidity, and parkinsonism
- Facial edema
- Gynecomastia
- Hyperactivity
- Hypotension
- Hepatitis
- Insomnia
- Jaundice
- Kidney failure
- Leukopenia
- Motor restlessness
- Neuroleptic malignant syndrome
- Edema
- Priapism
- QT prolongation
- Rash
- Retinopathy
- Sleep disturbances
- Tardive dyskinesia
- Tics
- Urinary retention
- Ventricular fibrillation, tachycardia.

| Systems | Adverse effects |
|---|---|
| General | Anxiety<br>Anorexia<br>Hyperactivity |
| Cardiovascular | QT prolongation<br>Ventricular fibrillation, tachycardia |
| Respiratory | Bronchospasm |
| Nervous system | • Motor restlessness<br>• Neuroleptic malignant syndrome<br>• Extrapyramidal side effects—Akathisia, dystonia, rigidity, and parkinsonism<br>• Chorea<br>• Tardive dyskinesia |
| Gastrointestinal tract | Emesis, constipation |
| Renal/genitourinary | Urinary retention |
| Eye | Blurred vision, retinopathy |
| Skin | Rash |
| Miscellaneous | Priapism<br>Insomnia |

## Drug Interactions
- Amiodarone will cause Q-Tc prolongation
- Epinephrine will antagonize the action of haloperidol
- There will be paradoxical decrease in blood pressure
- Haloperidol will decrease the effects of levodopa.

## QUESTION

Q. What are the autonomic effects of haloperidol?
- ❏ Blurred vision
- ❏ Diaphoresis
- ❏ Urinary retention
- ❏ Priapism.

## Anticoagulants

### Heparin

Heparin is a naturally occurring anticoagulant. It is secreted by the mast cells and is degraded by tissue macrophages.

**Heparin sodium:**
- It is a powerful and instantaneously acting anticoagulant
- Also, heparin will bind to the endothelial cell surfaces and a variety of plasma proteins
- Antithrombin will inhibit the clotting factor proteases especially thrombin.

**Mechanism of action:** It indirectly acts by activating plasma antithrombin III and other cofactors. The complex will bind to the clotting factors Xa, IIa, IXa, and XIIa and inactivates them.

In low doses, conversion of prothrombin to thrombin, which is mediated by Xa, is affected.

**Pharmacological actions:**
- Blood coagulation—it prevents blood clotting

- Heparin will prevent formation of fibrin monomer and inhibit the polymerization.
- It will prolong the clotting time but the bleeding time will not be affected.

**Dosage**
- 5,000-10,000 units every 4-6 hours.
- 10 units/mL made in normal saline
- 50-100 U/kg every 4-6 hours
- Dose and frequency can be controlled by activated partial thromboplastin time (aPTT) measurement which should be kept at 50-80 seconds or 1.5-2.5 times of the pretreatment value.

**Q1. What is the ideal dose of heparin?**
- A plasma concentration of 0.2-0.4 units of heparin per mL
- This concentration of heparin will prolong the activated partial thromboplastin time (aPTT) by 2-2.5 times.

**Q2. Why heparin should not be given intramuscularly?**
Hematoma formation can occur after intramuscular injection.

**Q3. What is the ideal dose of heparin for stroke?**
Loading dosage 75-100 µg/kg intravenously over 10 minutes followed by initial maintenance dose—maintenance dose of 28 µg/kg/h for infants and 18 µg/kg/h for older children.

This concentration of heparin will prolong the activated partial thromboplastin time (aPTT) by 2-2.5 times.

**Q4. What is the indication for adjustment of dosage of heparin?**
The dose of heparin should be adjusted so that the activated partial thromboplastin time (aPTT) should be maintained at 60-85 seconds.

**Indications:**
- Prophylaxis in deep vein thrombosis
- Thromboembolic complications
- Stroke.

**Uses:**
- Continuous infusion for patency of arterial line
- 1 unit/mL in total parenteral nutrition
- 5 units/mL for washing syringes during exchange transfusion
- 70 units/10 mL of blood to prevent coagulation of blood.

**Contraindications for heparin:**
- Allergy to heparin
- Bleeding disorders
- Cirrhosis/advanced hepatic disease
- Severe hypertension
- Gastrointestinal bleeding
- Thrombocytopenia [heparin-induced thrombocytopenia (HIT)]
- Subacute bacterial endocarditis
- Ulcerative lesions in the gut
- Renal failure
- Chronic alcoholics
- Threatened abortion
- Visceral carcinoma
- Avoid heparin in patients who had undergone brain, spinal cord, or eye surgery recently.
- Lumbar puncture
- Regional anesthesia.

**Precautions:**
- Observe for bleeding during or following heparin administration
- Should be used carefully in renal or hepatic impairment
- Decrease the dose in children.

**Effects on pregnancy:**
- Contraindicated. Category C
- Preservative may be secreted in the breast milk. Preservative-free heparin should be administered in lactating women.

**Side effects:**
- Allergic and anaphylactoid reactions
- Asthma
- Bleeding
- Urticaria
- Rhinitis
- Fever

- Thrombocytopenic purpura
- Osteoporosis
- Hypersensitivity reactions
- Transient alopecia
- Prolong hemorrhage from peptic ulcer
- Adrenal hemorrhage and necrosis.

**Drug interactions:**
- The activity will be enhanced by salicylates and dipyridamoles.
- Oral anticoagulants will enhance the effect
- Avoid aspirin and aspirin containing drug during administration of heparin.
- Aspirin and antiplatelet drugs should not be given during heparin therapy.

## QUESTIONS

**Q1. What are the richest sources of heparin?**
Lung, liver, and intestinal mucosa.
Heparin is present in all tissues containing mast cells. The heparin released from mast cells will be degraded by macrophages.

**Q2. What is the mechanism of action of heparin?**
Low dose of heparin will prolong activated partial thromboplastin time (aPTT) without significantly prolonging prothrombin time (PT) by affecting the intrinsic pathway but high dose will prolong both by affecting common pathway also.

**Q3. What is the heparin antagonist?**
Protamine sulfate which is strongly basic protein.

**Q4. What is the heparin antagonist?**
Protamine sulfate.

**Q5. How will you treat excessive anticoagulant action of heparin?**
For every 100 units of heparin, 1 mg of protamine sulfate should be given intravenously.

**Q6. What is the ideal dose of heparin?**
A plasma concentration of 0.2–0.4 units of heparin per mL. This concentration of heparin will prolong the activated partial thromboplastin time (aPTT) by 2–2.5 times.

**Q7. How will you monitor the effects of heparin?**
The patients on heparin therapy should be closely monitored by monitoring activated partial thromboplastin time (aPTT).

**Q8. What are the adverse effects of heparin?**
- Bleeding
- Thrombocytopenia
- Osteoporosis
- Hypersensitivity reactions like urticaria, rigor, and anaphylaxis.

**Q9. What are the adverse effects associated with long-term use of heparin?**
- Osteoporosis
- Spontaneous fractures
- Mineralocorticoid deficiency.

**Q10. What are the low-molecular-weight heparins?**
Low-molecular-weight heparins are heparins with molecular weight less than 8,000 kDa which are obtained by fragmentation or depolymerization of polymeric heparin. They are safe during pregnancy. They have long half-life, fewer side effects.

**Q11. What is tyndall effect?**
Administration of heparin will abolish the cloudiness of hyperlipemic plasma.

## Indomethacin

It is an indole acetic acid derivative.

### Mechanism of Action

Indomethacin acts by reducing prostaglandin E (PGE) levels by inhibiting prostaglandin synthesis. It also inhibits phosphodiesterase which results in increased concentration of cyclic adenosine monophosphate (AMP) which will interfere with migration of leukocytes into the site of inflammation.

## Pharmacological Actions
- Anti-inflammatory
- Analgesic
- Antipyretic.

## Dosage
Dose 0.1–0.2 mg/kg at 12 hourly intervals for three doses.

## Indications
- **In children less than 14 years:** Closure of patent ductus arteriosus (PDA).
- **In adolescents:**
    - Rheumatoid arthritis not responding to aspirin
    - Ankylosing spondylitis
    - Acute gout
    - Osteoarthritis.

## Contraindications for Indomethacin

| | |
|---|---|
| A | • Anuria/oliguria<br>• Allergy to indomethacin<br>• Allergy to salicylates, nonsteroidal anti-inflammatory drugs (NSAIDs) |
| B | • Bilirubin increased (hyperbilirubinemia)<br>• Bleeding tendency<br>• Blood urea nitrogen >25 mg/dL. |
| C | • Creatinine levels >1–8 mg/dL<br>• Coagulation disorders |
| D | Decreased platelet count <50,000/mm³ |
| E | Enterocolitis—Neonatal necrotizing enterocolitis (NNEC) |
| F | Fallot's tetralogy |
| G | Gastrointestinal bleeding |
| H | • Hypertension<br>• Hypersensitivity |
| I | Infections |
| J | Jobs—Drivers |
| K | Kidney diseases/dysfunction |
| L | Liver dysfunction |
| M | Machine operators |
| N | NNEC |
| O | Edema due to fluid retention |
| P | • Pregnancy<br>• Psychotic disorders |

## Precautions
*Precautions before giving indomethacin:*
- Before giving indomethacin, investigate for neutropenia, renal function, and NNEC
- Active peptic ulcer
- Renal or hepatic dysfunction.

## Effects on Pregnancy
Indomethacin given to mother can lead to tricuspid regurgitation, closure of PDA in utero, renal dysfunction, ileal perforation, and necrotizing enterocolitis.

## Side Effects
- Allergy—Skin rashes
- Anorexia
- Blood dyscrasia
- Blurring of vision
- Central nervous system—Mental confusion
- Depression
- Diarrhea
- Dyspepsia
- Disseminated intravascular coagulation (DIVC) (in neonates)
- Electrolyte imbalance—Sodium retention (hyponatremia, hyperkalemia in neonates)
- Emesis
- Frontal headache
- Giddiness
- Gastric irritation, bleeding, and nausea
- Gastric ulcer/perforation
- Hallucination
- Masks signs and symptoms of infection
- Joint pain
- Kidney failure
- Liver damage
- Myocardial infarction
- Nephrotoxicity—Transient rise in blood urea and creatinine
- Psychosis
- Peptic ulceration.

| Systems | Adverse effects |
|---|---|
| General | Anorexia |
| Cardiovascular | Myocardial infarction |

*Contd...*

Contd...

| | |
|---|---|
| Nervous system | • Frontal headache<br>• Giddiness |
| Gastrointestinal tract | • Diarrhea<br>• Dyspepsia<br>• Emesis<br>• Gastric ulcer/perforation<br>• Peptic ulceration |
| Renal | Kidney failure |
| Hematological | Blood dyscrasia |
| Eye | Blurring of vision |
| Fluid and electrolyte imbalance | Sodium retention (hyponatremia, hyperkalemia in neonates) |
| Skin | Rashes |
| Miscellaneous | • DIVC (in neonates)<br>• Hallucination |

## Drug Interactions

- Anticoagulants will cause gastrointestinal hemorrhage
- Beta-blockers
- Corticosteroids
- Diuretics—Indomethacin will cause renal failure if given with triamterene.
- Probenecid—It will not interfere with the uricosuric effect of probenecid.
- Indomethacin will decrease the antihypertensive effect of thiazides, beta blockers.
- Indomethacin will replace warfarin from protein binding sites.
- Lithium—It reduces renal clearance of lithium.
- Salicylates.

## QUESTION

**Q1. Why indomethacin is not useful for closure of ductus arteriosus in term babies?**

The ductus arteriosus in a term baby is not sensitive to prostaglandin.

## Lactulose

- Synthetic, nondigestible sugar 2.5–10 mL/24 h
- 40–90 mg/24 h may be administered as an enema.

## Mechanism of Action of Lactulose

- Lactulose is not absorbed in the intestines and is degraded by the colonic bacteria to lactic and acetic acids resulting in an acid pH. It is converted to lactic acid which will bind to ammonia (ammonium ion trapping). This improves ammonia (NH3) generation by bacteria and conversion of the ammonia to inabsorbable ammonium (NH4). This also increases transit of bowel content through the gut. This is effective in decreasing systemic ammonia concentrations in patients with liver failure.
- Lactulose is broken down into monosaccharide sugars in the colon. This will increase the acidity and osmolality. The acidity will have a bacteriostatic effect on ammoniagenic bacteria.
- Cathartic effect of lactulose results in bacterial elimination—diarrhea.
- Altering the bowel flora—decreased fecal pH will promote lactose fermenting organisms. Also, the growth of NH3 forming organisms will be inhibited. In the acidic media, NH3 will be converted to NH4. Thus, absorption of ammonia is less.
- Lactulose will bind with ammonium
- Lactulose promotes lactic acid production which promotes growth of lactobacillus and suppresses the proteolytic and urealytic bacteria.
- Lactulose inhibits bacterial metabolism of amino acids
- Nonbacterially mediated breakdown of glutamine will be inhibited.
- Lactulose detoxifies short chain fatty acids
- Lactulose promotes incorporation of N2 into the bacteria.
- Decreases the time of stasis of proteins in the gut. Thus, the degradation and production of ammonia is decreased.

- Synthetic nonabsorbable disaccharide by its osmotic effect draws water into the colon. Increases the osmotic volume which has a laxative effect and bowel cleaning.

## Dosage

- Oral lactulose—40-90 mg/24 h may be administered as an enema
- 2 mL/kg with the goal of two to three soft stools per day.
- Rectal enema—Mix the lactulose in 700 mL of saline and keep it for 30-60 minutes.

## Indications

- Portosystemic encephalopathy
- Chronic constipation
- Habitual constipation.

## Contraindications

- Galactosemia
- Disaccharidase deficiency
- Patients on galactose free or low galactose diet
- Patients allergic to any ingredients.

## Precautions

- Do not refrigerate or freeze
- The drug effect should be known in 24-48 hours
- Drink plenty of water or oral fluid while taking lactulose
- The patient on lactulose should take a low protein diet
- Lactulose should be avoided in the following conditions:
    - Acute inflammatory bowel disease
    - Bowel obstruction
    - Children
    - Diabetics—Lactulose will raise the blood sugar
    - Disaccharidase deficiency
    - Elderly
    - Fructose intolerance
    - Galactosemia
    - History of allergy
    - Intolerance to lactose and galactose.

## Effects on Pregnancy

Although no side effects are seen, it is better to avoid during pregnancy and lactation.

## Side Effects

- Allergic reaction (rash, itching, difficulty in breathing, tightness in the chest, swelling of face, tongue, throat, etc.)
- Abdominal pain
- Bloating
- Belching
- Cramps (muscles, intestinal, etc.)
- Diarrhea
- Dehydration
- Emesis (vomiting)
- Flatulence
- Fluid loss
- Gastrointestinal problem—nausea
- Hypernatremia
- Hypokalemia.

## Drug Interactions

- Antacids will decrease the effectiveness of lactulose
- Do not take laxatives along with lactulose as this will predispose to dehydration especially in children and old-aged patients
- Neomycin will interact with lactulose and make it less effective.

## QUESTIONS

**Q1. What is the bowel cleaning?**
Lactulose is given orally in a dose of 1-2 mL/kg/dose four times a day. Dose—2.5-10 mL/24 h (it should produce two to four loose acidic stools per day). 40-90 mg/24 h may be administered as an enema.

**Q2. What are the actions which makes lactulose useful in liver failure?**
- Ammonia binding property
- Cathartic effect.

**Q3. What are the doses of lactulose for bowel cleaning?**
The dose can be adjusted to get two to three soft stools per day.

## Liquid Paraffin

- It is a highly refined mineral oil
- Mixture of petroleum hydrocarbons.

### Mechanism of Action
It is an inert, nonirritable substance which coats the surface and protects the surface.

### Pharmacological Actions
Pharmacologically inert.

### Dosage
15–30 mL/day.

### Indications
- Topical application for diaper rash, eczema irritation
- Emollient for dry skin
- Constipation
- Laxative
- Used in cosmetics like detergent creams, cold creams, eye lubricants, etc.
- Used to warm up a body part by submerging the part like hand into a tub of paraffin.

### Contraindications
- Should not be used as a laxative for regular use as it will seep from the anus causing perianal irritation
- Sensitivity to liquid paraffin.

### Precaution
Do not inhale the liquid paraffin as it can cause pneumonitis.

### Effects on Pregnancy
- No effect
- Should not take when pregnant or planning to become pregnant or during breastfeeding.

### Side Effects
- Perianal irritation
- Interfere with healing of wounds in perianal region
- Can be absorbed in the intestines.

### Complications
- Rarely lipoid pneumonia if aspirated
- Small amount may be absorbed and get deposited in the intestinal mucosa.
- Given orally, it will cause decreased absorption of vitamin A and many nutrients
- It will interfere with absorption of essential fat-soluble substances
- Predisposes to deficiency of vitamins A, D, and K.

### Drug Interactions
In combination with magnesium salts, it acts as an osmotic laxative.

## QUESTIONS

**Q1. What are the features of liquid paraffin?**
- Colorless, transparent, and oily liquid
- No organisms can grow in liquid paraffin
- Not digested
- Mineral oil contains a mixture of hydrocarbons obtained from petroleum
- Emollient laxative.

**Q2. What are the advantages of liquid paraffin?**
*Advantages*:
- Straining during defecation can be avoided
- Liquid paraffin is used to make apples shiny and glossy by applying over them.

## Magnesium Sulfate

- 2 mL vial (4 mEq/mL)
- 500 mg/mL.

### Mechanism of Action
Suppression of neuromuscular transmission in the CNS and neuromuscular junction.

### Dosage
**Hypomagnesemia:** Magnesium sulfate ($MgSO_4$) (50%) should be given intramuscular (IM) or IV in a single dose of 0.3 mL/kg (up to a maximum of 2 mL) or 0.1–0.2 mL/kg/dose can

be given in two divided doses for 1–3 days. This should be followed by daily oral administration of 0.4–0.6 mmol/kg. Magnesium supplements can be added to the food.

25–50 mg/kg/dose four to six times a day. The dose can be repeated if hypomagnesemia persists.

**Anticonvulsant:** 20–40 mg/kg/dose parenterally.

**Cathartic:** Oral 250 mg/kg/dose four to six times per day.

**Q. How will you treat hypomagnesemia in newborn?**
*Hypomagnesemia*—Magnesium 50% (500 mg/mL), 0.2 mg/kg intramuscularly (100 mg/kg at 12-hour interval for 3 days).

## Indications

- Magnesium deficiency
- Gastritis—Antacid
- Ingredient of universal antidote
- To control seizures in acute nephritis, toxemia of pregnancy
- Digitalis-induced cardiotoxicity resistant to potassium
- Antiarrhythmic—Ventricular arrhythmias
- Seizure prevention
- Bronchodilator.

## Contraindications

- Severe abdominal pain
- Nausea
- Vomiting
- Bowel obstruction
- Perforation of bowel
- Severe constipation
- Colitis
- Toxic megacolon
- Sudden changes in bowel habits lasted for more than 2 weeks.

## Precautions

- Take plenty of water with oral $MgSO_4$.
- Too much use of $MgSO_4$ can predispose to serious complications
- If there is rectal bleeding or absent bowel movements after taking $MgSO_4$, the drug should be stopped.
- Injections should be diluted more for IV use.

## Effects on Pregnancy and Lactation

- Can cause fetal abnormalities, hypocalcemia, osteopenia, and skeletal abnormalities
- Magnesium will be secreted in the breast milk.

## Side Effects

- Allergy
- Bleeding time—Increased
- Confusion
- Diarrhea
- Diplopia
- Dizziness
- Excessive sleepiness
- Ventricular fibrillation
- Gastrointestinal—nausea
- Hypotension—low blood pressure
- Hypersensitivity.

| Serum magnesium level (mEq/L) | Side effects |
| --- | --- |
| More than 4–7 mEq/L | Decreased tendon reflexes, muscle weakness, mental confusion, and sedation |
| 7–10 mEq/L | Slow respiratory rate, decreased blood pressure |
| 10–15 mEq/L | Profound mental depression, are flexia, and coma |
| 15 mEq/L | Death |

**Q1. What are the features of overdose of magnesium?**
Overdose can result in the following:
- Nausea
- Vomiting
- Flushing
- Depression
- Respiratory arrest.

**Q2. What are the clinical features of hypermagnesemia in newborn?**
Hyporeflexia, respiratory depression, drowsiness, and coma.

**Q3. What are the conditions associated with hypermagnesemia in newborns?**
Hypermagnesemia is seen in newborn babies in renal failure or when the mother receives magnesium antenatally.

## Drug Interactions

- In patients with digoxin, it may cause abnormal heart beats.
- Barbiturates, narcotics, and hypnotics will slow the brain function.
- Neuromuscular blocking drugs—Magnesium will add to the effect.
- Magnesium sulfate will interfere absorption of antibiotics.
- Avoid taking other drugs 2 hours before and after intake of $MgSO_4$.

# QUESTIONS

**Q1. What are the functions of magnesium?**
- Magnesium is a depressant of central nervous system
- Local anesthetic activity
- Depresses myoneural transmission by reducing quantal release of acetylcholine and by antagonizing its depolarizing effect at the motor end-plates.

**Q2. How can the depressant effect of magnesium on central nervous system and myocardium can be antagonized?**
By calcium administration.

**Q3. What are the conditions associated with magnesium deficiency?**
- Continued diarrhea
- Chronic alcoholism
- Intestinal malabsorption
- Hyperparathyroidism
- Diuretic therapy
- Renal tubular acidosis
- Malnutrition
- Pancreatitis
- Chronic renal failure
- Diabetes.

**Q4. What are the clinical features of magnesium deficiency?**
- Magnesium will have an inhibitory effect on the nervous system. Hypomagnesemia will present as irritability, confusion, and convulsions
- Involuntary movements
- Tetany may develop
- Tetany (calcium resistant), hyperexcitability, and convulsions.

A child with convulsions not responding to calcium infusion should be suspected to have hypomagnesemia.

# Metoclopramide

## Mechanism of Action

- Dopamine antagonist
- Enhances gastric emptying and to be of lower esophageal sphincter
- Relaxes the pylorus and first part of duodenum
- Blocks apomorphine-induced vomiting by acting on chemoreceptor trigger zone (CTZ) in the CNS.

## Dosage

10–20 mg intramuscularly will reduce postoperative vomiting.

## Indications

- Antiemetic
- Diabetic gastroparesis
- Early satiety
- Fullness after feeding
- Gastrointestinal symptoms—nausea and vomiting in uremia, radiation sickness
- Gastroesophageal reflux
- Heartburn
- Hyperemesis gravidarum
- Headache due to migraine.

## Contraindications and Cautions

- Bowel obstruction
- Newborn babies
- Pheochromocytoma.

### Precautions
- As it causes movement disorders, the drug should not be taken for more than 12 weeks
- Should be used cautiously in parkinsonism
- Long-term use will be avoided in depression.

### Effects on Pregnancy
- Not contraindicated
- Secreted in breast milk and can cause diarrhea, dystonia, and myoclonus in newborn babies.

### Side Effects
- Agitation
- Akathisia
- Blood pressure will be elevated
- Breast tenderness
- Congestive cardiac failure
- Diarrhea
- Extrapyramidal symptom—dystonia
- Feeling tired
- Focal dystonia
- Galactorrhea, gynecomastia due to hyperprolactinemia
- Headache
- Insomnia
- Movement disorder—Tardive dyskinesia
- Motor restlessness
- Neuroleptic malignant syndrome
- Oculogyric crisis.

### Drug Interactions
- This will enhance absorption of aspirin, diazepam
- The effects of levodopa will be abolished by blocking the DA receptors in the basal ganglia.

## Metoprolol
Oral tablets.

### Mechanism of Action
Beta-blocker prevents action of noradrenaline on the β-receptors in the blood vessels and heart.

### Dosage
- Children—12.5-25 mg once a day
- Adults—18-64 years 50-100 mg once a day.

### Indications
- Angina pectoris
- Blood pressure elevation
- Congestive cardiac failure.

### Contraindications and Cautions
- Allergy/hypersensitivity to drug
- Bronchial asthma
- Chronic obstructive pulmonary disease (COPD)
- Cardiac failure
- Diabetes
- Hypotension
- Heart blocks
- Sick sinus syndrome.

### Precautions
This drug should not be stopped abruptly as it can cause severe chest pain, elevation of blood pressure, or even heart attack. The drug should be tapering the dose.

### Effects on Pregnancy
- Category C
- This drug is secreted in breast milk.

### Side Effects
- Allergic rash
- Breathing problem—bronchospasm
- Bradycardia
- Congestive cardiac failure
- Constipation
- Diarrhea
- Depression
- Decreased libido
- Dizziness
- Erection problems
- Fatigue
- Generalized itching
- Hypotension
- Infarction (myocardial).

## Drug Interactions

- Alpha-blockers, which also will decrease the blood pressure, will further decrease the blood pressure
- Calcium channel blockers will reduce the contraction of heart
- Dipyridamole
- Ergot alkaloids will cause severe narrowing of blood vessels.

## Nitroglycerin

Administered sublingually, transdermally, rectal, or intravenously. Extended release oral tablets are also available.

## Mechanism of Action

- It acts by vasodilatation.
- The drugs decrease both preload and afterload and blood pressure.
- At low doses, this will dilate the veins and decrease the preload and at higher doses, it will dilate the arteries also and decrease the afterload.

## Dosage

It depends upon the route of administration.

## Indication

Angina pectoris.

## Contraindications and Cautions

- Age under 12 years
- Allergy/hypersensitivity to drug
- Blood pressure low (hypotension)
- Cardiac tamponade
- Drugs for hypertension
- Erectile dysfunction on treatment
- Hypertrophic obstructive cardiomyopathy (HOCM)
- Hypovolemia
- Inferior myocardial infarction
- Increased intracranial tension.

## Precautions

- The tablet should be swallowed as whole and should not be bitten or chewed
- To avoid dizziness, the patients should get up from the bed slowly
- The drug should not be discontinued abruptly as it will precipitate more frequent angina.

## Effects on Pregnancy

It should be used only if clearly indicated during pregnancy.

## Side Effects

- Dizziness
- Flushing
- Headache
- Hypotension
- Reflex tachycardia.

## Drug Interaction

Interacts with aspirin.

# QUESTIONS

**Q1. What is the advantage of sublingual administration?**
Sublingual drug is absorbed quickly and acts quickly.

**Q2. What is the advantage of transdermal administration?**
Transdermal drugs acts slowly but the duration of action is more.

**Q3. What is the indication for intravenous administration?**
Intravenous routes are used for those who do not respond to sublingual or other routes.

**Q4. What is the complication of overdose of nitroglycerin?**
Overdose can cause:
- Bradycardia
- Cold, clammy skin
- Cyanosis due to methemoglobinemia
- Emesis
- Visual problems
- Sweating.

## Ondansetron

- Oral tablets 4 mg, 8 mg, and 24 mg
- Oral solution 4 mg/mL
- Injection 2 mg/mL.

### Mechanism of Action
Selective serotonin 5-HT3 receptor antagonist.

### Dosage
- Oral:
  - 4–11 years—4 mg orally three times a day
  - More than 12 years—8 mg orally twice a day.
- Intravenous dose diluted in 50 mL of:
  - Less than 40 kg 0.15 mg/kg
  - More than 40 kg—4 mg intravenously over 2–5 minutes.

### Indications
Nausea and vomiting during chemotherapy or radiotherapy.

### Contraindication and Caution
Allergy to the drug.

### Precautions
- The tablets should be allowed to dissolve in saliva and then swallowed. Do not swallow it with water as it may cause headache.
- Parenteral forms should not be given for children below 6 months and oral forms below 4 years.

### Effects on Pregnancy
- Category B
- Breastfeeding should not be continued during administration of this drug.

### Side Effects
- Anxiety
- Anaphylaxis
- Bradycardia
- Blurred vision
- Constipation
- Diarrhea
- Dizziness
- Drowsiness
- Emesis
- Fainting
- Fatigue
- Gynecological problems
- Headache
- Itching
- Joint pain
- QT prolongation
- Stevens-Johnson syndrome
- Toxic epidermal necrolysis.

### Drug Interactions
Other drugs which may cause QT prolongation like amiodarone, quinidine, and sotalol should not be used along with ondansetron.

## Oral Rehydration Solutions

### Mechanism of Action
Glucose-dependent sodium cotransporter.

### Dosage
One packet should be dissolved in 1 L or potable water.
- Less than 2 years—50–100 mL per loose stool
- 2–10 years—100–200 mL per loose stool
- More than 10 years—Much as the child wants as.

Q. **What are the indications of oral rehydration solution (ORS)?**
- ❏ To treat some dehydration due to diarrhea (plan B). Treatment of children with diarrhea with no dehydration.
- ❏ As maintenance fluid in severe dehydration.

### Contraindications
Oral rehydration solution (ORS) is contraindicated in the following conditions:
- Abdominal distension
- Altered sensorium
- Acidosis
- Bowel movements more (high purge rate)

- Coma
- Convulsion
- Dehydration—Severe
- Electrolyte disturbances (severe)
- Emesis—Persistent vomiting
- Feeding refusal
- Gastrointestinal tract obstruction
- Hypovolemic or septic shock
- Infections/sepsis
- Inability to drink
- Ileus—Paralytic ileus.

## Precautions to be taken while Giving Oral Rehydration Solution

Oral rehydration solution should be given in sips by spoon at short intervals as large volumes will induce vomiting.

The ORS prepared should be used within 24 hours or else discarded.

- Avoid giving high fiber diet along with ORS
- If there is vomiting, give ORS after 10 minutes.
- If vomiting is severe, intravenous fluids should be given.
- Staple food should be given. Rice with milk or curd and sugar can be given.

## QUESTIONS

**Q1. What is the principle of oral rehydration?**

Glucose-dependent sodium cotransporter is unaffected in acute diarrheal diseases.

**Q2. What are the other channels of sodium absorption?**

Short chain peptides, amino acids, short chain fatty acids, and vitamin B complex molecules operate through separate channels are used in food-based oral rehydration solution (ORS).

**Q3. What are the qualities of an ideal oral rehydration solution (ORS)?**
- It should contain adequate quantities of glucose to achieve maximum sodium absorption. The amount should not be more than 20 g/dL (110 mOsmol/L).
- The ratio of glucose to sodium should be 1:1.
- The total osmolarity should be equal or less than that of plasma osmolarity.
- It should contain adequate amount of electrolytes like sodium, potassium, etc. to replenish the loss.
- It should contain adequate amount of bicarbonate or citrate to combat acidosis.

**Q4. What are the steps in preparation of oral rehydration solution (ORS)?**
- Wash the hand thoroughly
- Clean the container
- Take 1 L of clean potable drinking water in the container
- Put whole of one packet of ORS into the container
- Stir well until all the salt is dissolved
- Cover the container
- Should be consumed on the same day.

**Q5. How long the prepared oral rehydration solution (ORS) can be used?**

The ORS should be used within 24 hours of preparation or within the same day of preparation.

**Q6. How the oral rehydration solution (ORS) should be given to the child?**

Oral rehydration solution should be given in small sips or by spoon.

**Q7. Why oral rehydration solution (ORS) should not be given in large quantities?**

Large quantities of ORS will induce vomiting.

**Q8. What are home available fluids (HAFs)?**

Home available fluids, which contain water, electrolytes, and foods, can be given at the beginning stages of diarrhea.
- Salt sugar solution
- Rice water with added salt
- Dal with water and added salt

- Smashed puffed rice in water with added salt.

**Q9. What are the fluids that cannot be used as home available fluid (HAF)?**
- Lemon water
- Weak tea.

**Q10. What is homemade oral rehydration solution (ORS)?**
- 4 g salt + 40 g sugar in 1 L of water
- Food-based ORS contains rice water (50 g) + salt (40 g)
- Lemon water
- Coconut water
- Rice kanji
- Dhal water.

**Q11. What is sugar salt solution (SSS)?**
- Sugar salt solution: 40 g of cane sugar will liberate 20 g of glucose in 1 L of oral rehydration solution (ORS).
- 200 mL of water (one glass)
- 8 g sugar (one heaped teaspoonful)
- Two finger pinch of common salt.

**Q12. What is rice-based oral rehydration solution (ORS)?**
Glucose in standard ORS is replaced by starch.

**Q13. What are the good qualities of oral rehydration solution (ORS)?**
- Oral rehydration solution should contain adequate amount of glucose.
- Ratio of glucose to sodium (Na) should be 1:1 molar ratio.
- The total osmolarity of the ORS should be same or less than that of plasma.
- It should contain adequate amount of electrolytes like Na, K, Cl to replenish loss.
- It should contain adequate amount of bicarbonate or citrate to combat acidosis.

**Q14. What are the types of World Health Organization (WHO) approved oral rehydration solution (ORS)?**
- World Health Organization standard ORS
- Rice-based ORS
- Hypo-osmolar ORS.

**Q15. What is glucose-based oral rehydration solution (ORS)?**

**What are the advantages of rice based ORS?**
- Add more substrate to the gut lumen
- Better taste
- Culturally acceptable
- Caloreis provided will be more
- Duration of diarrhea will be reduced

**What are the advantages of citrate based ORS?**
- Stability—more stable, discoloration is not seen
- Shelf life 2–3 years
- Stool output—less especially in high output diarrhea as in cholera
- Sodium and water—increased intestinal absorption

**What are the disadvantages of citrate based ORS?**
Hypertonicity in the net fluid absorption

**What is polymer-based ORS?**
Polymer based ORS are prepared using rice or wheat will release glucose slowly.

**Q16. What are the ranges of concentration of the constituents in the World Health Organization (WHO) recommended oral rehydration solution (ORS)?**
World Health Organization recommended:

| Constituents | World Health Organization (WHO) recommended range of concentration (mEq/L) |
|---|---|
| Sodium | 60–90 |
| Chloride | 50–80 |
| Potassium | 15–25 |
| Citrate | 8–12 |
| Glucose | 75 (should be equal to sodium but should not exceed 111 mmol/L) |
| Osmolarity | 200–311 mOsm/L |

The total substance concentration should be within the range of 200–311 mmol/L.

**Q17. What is World Health Organization-oral rehydration solution (WHO-ORS) (conventional)?**

| Ingredients | Ingredients (g) per liter | Concentration of ingredients (mmol/L) per liter | |
|---|---|---|---|
| Sodium chloride | 3.5 | Sodium | 90 mmol/L |
| | | chloride | 80 mmol/L |
| Trisodium citrate dehydrate | 2.9 | Citrate | 10 mmol/L |
| Potassium chloride | 1.5 | Potassium | 20 mmol/L |
| Glucose | 20 | Glucose | 111 mmol/L |
| Water | 1 L | | |
| Total osmolality | 330 mOsm/L | | |

**Q18. What is the difference between bicarbonate oral rehydration solution (ORS) and citrate-based ORS?**

In bicarbonate ORS, 2.5 g of sodium bicarbonate is used and in citrate-based ORS, 2.9 g of trisodium citrate dehydrate is used.

**Q19. What are the disadvantages with the World Health Organization-oral rehydration solution (WHO-ORS)?**
- There is a potential risk of hypernatremia with the WHO-ORS.
- Normal WHO-ORS with sodium concentration of 90 mEq will provide too much sodium which is dangerous in edematous children. Congestive cardiac failure can occur in these patients when associated with anemia
- The potassium in the standard WHO-ORS may be too low to replace the losses in stool during diarrhea.

**Q20. What is the oral rehydration solution (ORS) (currently recommended)?**

Hypo-osmolar ORS or reduced osmolarity ORS.

**Q21. What is hypo-osmolar oral rehydration solution (ORS) or reduced osmolarity ORS?**

| Ingredients | | Ingredients | |
|---|---|---|---|
| NaCl | 2.6 g | Sodium | 75 mEq/L |
| Trisodium citrate | 2.9 g | Chloride | 65 mEq/L |
| Glucose (anhydrous) | 13.5 g | Glucose (anhydrous) | 75 mEq/L |
| KCl | 1.5 g | Potassium | 20 mEq/L |
| | | Citrate | 10 mEq/L |
| Total weight | 20.5 g | Osmolality | 245 mOsm/L |

**Q21. What are the advantages of hypo-osmolar oral rehydration solution (ORS)?**
- Absorption of water and sodium will be good. Reduced osmolarity ORS promotes more effective water and sodium absorption than the World Health Organization-oral rehydration solution (WHO-ORS).
- Bulk of stools decreased by favoring movement of water from to the body
- Cost of manufacture will be low
- Duration of diarrhea decreased
- Efficacy increased
- Frequency of loose stools or vomiting will be low
- Good acceptance by the parents or caretakers
- No additional risk for developing hyponatremia/hypernatremia
- Infections like cholera—The reduced osmolarity as effective as standard ORS in adults with cholera
- Acute diarrheal disease in newborn and young infants can be treated effectively
- Decreases stool output
- More stability of reconstituted solution

- Advantage of the reduced osmolarity ORS formulation for general use including malnutrition is that, a single formulation would be promoted for all ages, irrespective of etiology or nutrition status. Severely malnourished children have low total body potassium content, which is associated with high mortality
- Number of hospitalizations decreased.

**Q22. What are the disadvantages of hypo-osmolar oral rehydration solution (ORS)?**

This will not be useful in cholera patients where the sodium requirement is more.

**Q23. What is low sodium oral rehydration solution (ORS)?**
- Sodium—60 mEq/L
- Glucose—250 mEq/L
- Osmolality like conventional ORS
- Advantages—Decreases vomiting and decrease the purge rates.

**Q24. What is citrate-based oral rehydration solution (ORS) [World Health Organization (WHO)]?**
- Trisodium citrate is used instead of bicarbonate
- This is more effective in controlling diarrhea. Also, it increases the shelf-life of ORS.

**Q25. What is cereal-based/rice-based oral rehydration solution (ORS)? How is it prepared?**

The rice-based ORS is clearly superior to World Health Organization-oral rehydration solution (WHO-ORS) in efficacy in adults with cholera, the two solutions had similar efficacy in noncholera diarrhea.

Rice-based ORS can be prepared as follows:
50 g of puffed rice + 1 L of water.

**Q26. What is super ORS?**

ORS contains more complex sugars instead of monosugars.

**What are the advantages of super ORS?**
- Allows early introduction of feeding
- Bulk of stools decreased (stool output/volume)
- Complex sugars are present
- Calories provided will be more (180 Kcal/liter)
- Duration of diarrhea shortened
- Endogenous secretions in the intestines are reabsorbed
- Frequency of stools decreased
- Gradual release of glucose
- Gain in weight as it provided extra nutrition
- Hydrolyses glucose, aminoacids and oligopeptides are formed.

**What are the disadvantages of super ORS ?**
- Cooking using fuel in required
- Decreased shelf life of less than 10 hours
- Fermentation of ORS occurs within 8-24 hours
- Grounding of the rice is required.

**Q27. What are the advantages of glycine-based oral rehydration solution (ORS)?**

*Advantages*:
- Decreased purged rate
- Slow release of glucose from starch.

**Q28. What are the advantages of oral rehydration solution (ORS) with micronutrients?**

Micronutrients will help in absorption of water and sodium.

**Q29. What is the dose of zinc in patients with diarrhea? What are the advantages?**

10 mg for 0–14 days
20 mg for 0–14 days

Advantages in diarrhea:
- Reduces diarrhea
- Modifies the course of diarrheal illness
- Decreases severity of diarrhea
- Prevents diarrhea.

**What is super ORS?**
Zinc added to ORS.

**What are the advantages of super ORS?**
- Absorption of water and electrolytes from the intestines will be improved
- Brush border enzymes increased
- Clearance of pathogens
- Diarrhea will be reduced
- Enhanced immune response
- Faster regeneration of gut epithelium

**What are the advantages of low osmolarity ORS?**
- Cost effective
- Decrease stool output by 25%
- Emesis incidence decreased by 30%
- Effective in noncholera diraahea
- Safe

**Q30. What is oral rehydration solution (ORS) fortified with amino acids?**
Oral rehydration solutions fortified with amino acids such as L-alanine, glycine, and glutamine with high osmolarity. This has been more efficacious in adult cholera but is not as effective in noncholeric diarrhea in children.

**Q31. What is amylase-resistant starch oral rehydration solution (ORS)?**
Glucose in the ORS is replaced with starch [cereal powder (50 g/L)].

**Q32. What is ReSoMaL?**
*Re*hydration *S*olution for *Mal*nutrition.
This is a rehydration solution for the severely malnourished children. They have potassium deficiency but have high levels of sodium.

**Q33. What is the composition of ReSoMaL?**
- Glucose—125 mmol/L
- Sodium—45 mmol/L
- Potassium—40 mmol/L
- Chloride—70 mmol/L
- Citrate—7 mmol/L
- Magnesium—3 mmol/L
- Zinc—0.3 mmol/L
- Copper—0.045 mmol/L
- Osmolarity—300 mOsm/L.

**Q34. What is the type of oral rehydration solution (ORS) in severely malnourished children with dehydration?**
As severely dehydrated children have low body potassium content, potassium supplements are needed.
Potassium concentration of standard World Health Organization-oral rehydration solution (WHO-ORS) cannot replace the potassium. Hence, a ORS solution with potassium 40 mEq/L and sodium 45 mEq/L with magnesium, zinc, and copper is recommended.

**Q35. What is hypo-osmolar oral rehydration solution (ORS)?**
Hypo-osmolar ORS is the ORS with osmolarity less than that of plasma osmolarity.

**Q36. What are the two types of hypo-osmolar oral rehydration solution (ORS)?**
1. Hypo-osmolar ORS with osmolarity of 245 mOsmol/L which is approved by World Health Organization (WHO)
2. Hypo-osmolar ORS with osmolarity of 224 mOsmol/L.

**Q37. What are the advantages of hypo-osmolar oral rehydration solution (ORS)?**
Hypo-osmolar ORS will decrease the total stool output, frequency of the stools, and volume per purging especially in noncholera diarrhea in children.

**Q38. What are the differences between conventional and low osmolarity oral rehydration solution (ORS)?**
The differences between conventional and low osmolarity ORS:

| Conventional | | Low osmolarity ORS | | |
| --- | --- | --- | --- | --- |
| Ingredients | mEq/L (mmol/L) | mEq/L (mmol/L) | mEq/L (mmol/L) | mEq/L (mmol/L) |
| Sodium | 90 | 50 | 60–70 | 75 |
| Chloride | 80 | 40 | 60–70 | 65 |
| Potassium | 20 | 20 | 20 | 20 |
| Citrate | 10 | 30 | 10 | 10 |
| Glucose (anhydrous) | 111 | 111 | 75–90 | 75 |
| Osmolarity | 311 | 251 | 210–260 | 245 |

**Q39. What is the amount of oral rehydration solution (ORS) to be used?**
- Less than 2 years—50-100 mL per loose stool
- 2-10 years—100-200 mL per loose stool
- More than 10 years—Much as the child wants as.

| Age | Amount of ORS to be given after loose stool |
| --- | --- |
| <24 months | 50–100 mL/loose stool |
| 2–10 years | 100–200 mL/loose stool |
| 10 years or more | As much as the child wanted |

If ORS is not available, home available fluids can be used.

**Q40. What is the plan B treatment in diarrhea?**
Plan B is followed in children with some dehydration. Oral rehydration solution (ORS) is used for the same.

**Q41. What is the amount of oral rehydration solution (ORS) to be used in plan B?**

| Age | <4 months | 4–11 months | 12–23 months | 2–4 years | 5–12 years |
| --- | --- | --- | --- | --- | --- |
| Approximately (weight in kg) | <5 | 5–8 | 8–11 | 11–16 | 16–30 |
| ORS (in mL) | 200–400 | 400–600 | 600–800 | 800–1,200 | 1,200–2,200 |
| Local measure (glass) | 1–2 | 2–3 | 3–4 | 4–6 | 6–11 |

World Health Organization-oral rehydration solution (WHO-ORS) is given over 4-6 hours. In infants below 6 months, clear watery fluids are given along with ORS to prevent hypernatremia. The child should be reassessed at the end of 6 hours.

**Q42. What are the conditions in which oral rehydration solution (ORS) will be ineffective?**
Oral rehydration solution will be ineffective in the following cases:
- Emesis—Persistent vomiting
- Faulty/incorrect preparation
- Glucose malabsorption
- High purge rate.
- Improper administration of ORS
- Paralytic ileus
- Shock.

**Q43. Why boiling of water is not necessary to prepare oral rehydration solution (ORS)?**
There is no need of boiling the water because boiling and cooling will take some precious time by which the treatment will be delayed and the condition of the dehydrated patient will become worse.

## Pralidoxime
- Pyridine-2-aldoxime
- Intravenous administration slowly
- Cholinesterase (ChE) reactivators.

### Mechanism of Action
This drug has a quaternary nitrogen that will attach to the anionic site of the enzyme. The oxime-phosphonate will diffuse leaving the reactivated ChE.

Organophosphorus compounds will bind to the hydroxy component of the active site of acetylcholinesterase enzyme and block its activity.

Pralidoxime will bind to the other unblocked site and reverse the paralysis. Irreversible inhibition of ChE produced by organophosphorus compounds. This is due to phosphorylation of esteratic site of the enzymes.

Pharmacological actions restores neuromuscular transmission in organophosphate anti-ChE poisoning. It reverses the neuroparalysis by organophosphorus compounds.

## Dosage
- Children—20-50 mg/kg followed by maintenance of 5-10 mg/kg/h.
- Adults—30 mg/kg by IV route over 15-30 minutes.
  - 500 mg/20 mL is given slow intravenously 20-40 mg/kg. It can be repeated after 60 minutes.

## Indications
Organophosphorus poisoning overdose of anticholinesterase drugs.

## Contraindications
- Hypersensitivity to the drug.
- Carbamate poisoning.

## Precautions
This will be effective when administered immediately after poisoning. Hence, it should be administered as early as possible. Rapid infusion can result in respiratory or cardiac arrest. The drug should be given within 24 hours because the phosphorylated enzyme will undergo and become resistant to hydrolysis. Maximum dose of 12 g in first 24 hours.

## Effects on Pregnancy
### Category C
The drug will cross the placenta. The drug will be excreted in the breast milk and breastfeeding should be avoided for 6-7 hours after administration of the drug.

### Side Effects
- Allergic reaction
- Blurred vision
- Choking feeling
- Drowsiness
- Eye problems—diplopia
- Fast heart rate
- Giddiness
- Headache
- Hypotension
- Local irritation

### Drug Interactions
When given along with atropine, signs of atropinization like flushing, tachycardia, mydriasis, and dry mouth and nose will occur. Actions of barbiturates will be potentiate by ChEs.

The following drugs should be avoided in patients with organophosphorus poisoning:
- Morphine
- Theophylline
- Aminophylline
- Phenothiazine
- Succinylcholine.

## QUESTIONS

Q1. Why pralidoxime is not useful as an antidote to carbamate antiches like physostigmine, neostigmine, etc.?
The anionic site is not free for attachment to pralidoxime.

Q2. Why pralidoxime is not useful as an antidote to carbamate poisoning?
- ❏ It does not reactivate carbamylated enzyme
- ❏ It has a weak anti-ChE activity.

## Paracetamol
Analgesic, antipyretic.

## Mechanism of Action

- Analgesic and antipyretic activity
- Paracetamol is mainly excreted in the urine as conjugation products
- The ability of liver of an infant for glucuronidation is poor
- Analgesic
- Antipyretic.

## Pharmacological Actions

- Analgesic
- Antipyretic
- Paracetamol is mainly excreted in the urine as conjugation products
- The ability of liver of an infant for glucuronidation is poor.

## Dosage

Dose is 15 mg/kg/dose.

## Indication

Treatment of fever.

## Contraindications

- Liver failure
- Preterm babies less than 2 kg.

## Precautions

- Acute paracetamol poisoning can occur in small children with low hepatic glucuronide conjugating ability.
- Glucuronidation of paracetamol in the liver is poor and may lead to enhanced toxicity in the neonates.

## Effects on Pregnancy

It can be used in pregnancy.

## Side Effects/Adverse Effects of Paracetamol

- Methemoglobinemia
- Hemolytic anemia especially in glucose-6-phosphate dehydrogenase (G6PD) deficiency.
- Neutropenia
- Thrombocytopenia
- Anemia as a result of hemolysis.

## Drug Interactions

No major drug interactions.

## QUESTIONS

**Q1. What are the features of acute paracetamol poisoning?**
Early manifestations:
- [ ] Abdominal pain
- [ ] Nausea
- [ ] Vomiting.

After 12–18 hours—centrilobular hepatic necrosis and renal tubular necrosis and hypoglycemia, jaundice after 2 days.

Fulminant hepatic failure will be seen if the 200 µg/mL at 4 hours and 30 µg/mL at 15 hours.

**Q2. What is the mechanism of paracetamol toxicity?**
The metabolite of paracetamol will be detoxified by conjugation with glutathione. When more paracetamol is taken, the capacity for glucuronidation will be saturated. The metabolite will bid to hepatic and renal cells causing necrosis.

**Q3. What is the fatal dose of paracetamol?**
More than 250 mg/kg is fatal.

**Q4. What is the treatment of paracetamol poisoning?**
- [ ] Gastric lavage
- [ ] Activated charcoal can be given orally that will prevent further absorption
- [ ] Administration of antidote N-acetylcysteine.

**Q5. What is the antidote of paracetamol?**
N-acetylcysteine 150 mg/kg should be infused over 15 minutes. This is followed by infusion of same dose over 20 hours or 75 mg/kg can be given orally every 4–6 hours for next 2–3 days.

**Q6. What is the significance of paracetamol ingestion—treatment interval?**
Prognosis depends upon the ingestion—treatment interval, the shorter the interval, better will be the prognosis. If the treatment is started after 16 hours, the prognosis will be bad.

**Q7. What is the mechanism of action of N-acetylcysteine?**
N-acetylcysteine acts by replenishing the glutathione stores in the liver. This will prevent the binding of toxic metabolite to the cell constituents.

**Q8. What are the differences between salicylates and paracetamol?**
- Do not have anti-inflammatory and uricosuric effects
- Paracetamol will not produce acid-base imbalance, gastrointestinal irritation, and electrolyte imbalance
- Paracetamol will not affect blood clotting
- Cytochrome P450
- Liver cell injury which may require orthotopic liver transplantation.

## Potassium Chloride

### Mechanism of Action
Supplement to treat to levels of potassium.

### Dosage
- 1 mL should be added in 100 mL of the drip
- Do not give directly in the IV route
- Oral potassium 2 mEq/kg/day.

**Q1. What is the dose of potassium for acute symptomatic hypokalemia?**
0.5–1 mEq/kg can be given with suitable dilution over 1 hour with continuous monitoring.

**Q2. What is the maximal concentration that can be given by various routes?**
- 80 mEq/L in central vein
- 40 mEq/L in peripheral vein.

### Indications for Potassium Chloride
- Hypokalemia
- Hypochloremia
- Maintenance of potassium.

**Q. What are the indications for rapid correction?**
Rapid correction of hypokalemia is indicated in the following conditions:
- Cardiac arrhythmias
- Bradycardia
- Shallow respiration
- Severe muscular weakness
- Patients on digoxin
- Critically-ill children at risk for arrhythmia.

### Contraindications

**Q. What are the contraindications of potassium administration?**
- Severe renal impairment
- Hyperkalemia
- Severe tissue necrosis
- Potassium-sparing diuretics
- Severe burns
- Systemic acidosis
- Adrenal insufficiency.

### Precautions
- This drug should not be given directly through IV route, undiluted or as a bolus. This can result in fatal cardiotoxicity.
- Potassium should not be infused in presence of decreased urine output or renal failure.
- Hypokalemia should be corrected slowly. Oral correction is safer.
- Daily administration should not exceed 4 mEq/kg/day
- Maximum concentration of potassium without electrocardiogram (ECG) monitoring can be up to 40 mEq/L.
- Under ECG monitoring up to 80 mEq/L can be given
- Persistent low serum potassium may be due to accompanying hypomagnesemia.

- Correction of magnesium levels will restore potassium levels.
- Administration of calcium in hypokalemia will precipitate cardiotoxicity.
- Correction of hypocalcemia or metabolic acidosis should be done after correction of hypokalemia.
- Hypokalemia should be corrected slowly, rapid correction can lead to hyperkalemia predisposing to fatal cardiac arrhythmias.
- Monitor the child with an ECG while giving potassium infusion
- This should be given in the IV infusion 1 mL added to 100 mL of IV fluid.

*Oral administration* of potassium chloride solution—supplementation of potassium at 3–4 mmol/kg/day for at least 2 weeks. Administration of modified ORS with less sodium and extra potassium. Add 1 mL of potassium chloride to each 100 mL of IV fluid. The fluid infused should not contain potassium more than 40 mEq/L. IV potassium is given only if the child is passing urine normally.

In severe hypokalemia (serum potassium less than 2 mmol/L or <3.5 mmol/L) with ECG changes—correct by starting potassium chloride in IV fluids at 0.3–0.5 mmol/kg/h. If arrhythmias are present, provide 1 mmol/kg/h of potassium chloride until the serum potassium normalizes.

*Dose*: 1 mEq/kg/day 8 hourly with a maximum dose 20 mEq/h.

### Effects on Pregnancy
Not contraindicated.

### Side Effect/Adverse Effect of Potassium Administration
Cardiotoxicity.

Q. **What are the adverse effects of potassium chloride?**
- Arrhythmias
- Respiratory paralysis
- Hypotension
- Diarrhea, vomiting, and bleeding due to gastric irritation.

*Serious side effects*:
- Mental confusion
- Lethargy.

### Drug Interactions
- Angiotensin-converting enzyme inhibitors like captopril, enalapril, and lisinopril
- Angiotensin receptor blocking drug like losartan
- Diuretics
- Potassium-sparing diuretics—Spironolactone, amiloride, and triamterene.

## QUESTIONS

Q1. **What are the cardioprotective measures in hyperkalemia?**
- Calcium gluconate 0.5–1 mL/kg over 5 minutes can be repeated once more. This acts by membrane stabilization. This can cause asystole. Stop the drug of the heart rate that is less than 100 beats/min.
- Sodium bicarbonate 1 mEq/kg diluted over 10–15 minutes.
- Glucose with insulin 0.5–1 g/kg of glucose with 0.1 µg/kg as infusion over 30 minutes.
- β2 agonist salbutamol 5–10 mg nebulization
- Kayexalate 1 g/kg per mouth (PO) or PR in sorbitol
- Calcium-potassium exchange resin 1 g/kg PO or PR.

Q2. **What are the causes of hypokalemia?**
- Adrenal gland disorders
- Barter syndrome
- Corticosteroids
- Diarrheas
- Diuretics
- Diabetic ketoacidosis
- Diabetes insipidus
- Dialysis
- Emesis (vomiting)
- Furosemide
- Gastrointestinal problems

- Gitelman syndrome
- Hyperaldosteronism—Renal artery stenosis, Conn syndrome, and Cushing's syndrome
- Hypomagnesemia
- Inadequate intake.

**Q3. What are the features of potassium overdose?**
- Bradycardia
- Breathing shallow
- Convulsions
- Confusion
- Heaviness of arms and legs
- Lightheadedness
- Heart block, periodic paralysis.

**Q4. What are the predisposing factors for hyperkalemia?**
Intravenous infusion of potassium, cell injury, and renal failure.

## Pregnancy Category

| Category | |
|---|---|
| A | Generally acceptable. No evidence of risk to the fetus |
| B | May be acceptable. Animal studies showed minor risk or no risk. Human studies are not available |
| C | Should be used with caution if benefits outweigh risks |
| D | There is positive evidence of human fetal risk |
| X | Should not be used in pregnant females |
| NA | No information available |

## Promethazine

This is a phenothiazine derivative with the following effects:
- Antihistamine
- Sedative
- Hypnotic effects.

### Mechanism of Action
- Antagonizes the central histamine, serotonin, and acetylcholine receptors and causes sedation
- Central anticholinergic action for antiemetic, antimotion sickness, and antivertigo effects.

### Dosage
1 mg/kg/24 hours in four divided doses.
- Less than 1 year—2.5-5 mg
- 1-6 years—5-10 mg
- 6-12 years—10-15 mg
- 12-18 years—10-20 mg.

### Indications
- Nausea induced by drugs
- Motion sickness
- Pruritis
- Urticaria
- Angioedema
- Sedative effects in preoperative and postoperative period.

### Contraindications and Cautions
- Age less than 2 years
- Asthma
- Abnormal ECG with QT changes
- Bone marrow depression
- Bladder problems
- Closed angle glaucoma
- Coma
- Cardiovascular disorders—Arrhythmias, myocardial infarction
- Drugs—Along with MAOIs
- Enlarged prostate
- Electrolyte abnormalities
- Fits
- Gastrointestinal obstruction
- Genitourinary obstruction
- Hepatic problems
- Idiopathic hypertrophic pyloric stenosis
- Jaundice.

### Precautions
- As the drug causes blurring of vision, avoid driving or working in machinery
- Decreases sweating and predisposes to heat stroke
- Elderly people are more prone to develop side effects.

## Effects on Pregnancy
It should be used only if indicated.

## Side Effects
- Abdominal pain
- Blurred vision
- Constipation
- Dry mouth
- Dermatitis
- Drowsiness
- Emesis
- Fainting
- Fatigue
- Gastrointestinal problems
- Hallucinations
- Hyperexcitability
- Insomnia
- Incoordination
- Jaundice.

## Drug Interactions
- It should not be used along with sedatives/hypnotics, narcotics, and general anesthetics as this drug will intensify the sedative actions
- Dose of barbiturates should be reduced when given along with promethazine hydrochloric acid (HCl)
- Promethazine HCl will reverse the effects of epinephrine
- Promethazine HCl with MAOI will cause extrapyramidal side effects.

## Sodium Bicarbonate
- Available strengths—7.5%
- Injection of 7.5% solution in 10 mL and 100 mL quantities
- Also available in 8.4%, 1 cc = 0.9 mEq
- Preparation—2 mL (0.5 mEq/mL)
- Dilution—Dilute each ml of solution in 3 mL of water (1:3 dilution)
- Give by IV route slowly over 15 minutes.

### Mechanism of Action
Alkalinization of blood.

### Dosage
**Dose:** 1–2 mEq/kg of a 0.5 mEq/mL solution given by IV route slowly.

*Dose of sodium bicarbonate depending upon the weight:*

| Weight | Total dose |
|---|---|
| 1 kg | 2 mEq (4 mL) |
| 2 kg | 4 mEq (8 mL) |
| 3 kg | 6 mEq (12 mL) |
| 4 kg | 8 mEq (16 mL) |

Sodium bicarbonate 4.2% solution in a dose of 2 mEq/kg can be given to correct acidosis.

**Route:** Intravenously, ideally through umbilical vein.

- Recommended route—It should be given through a large vein with good venous return, usually through umbilical vein.
- Recommended preparation—0.5 mEq/mL in 4.2% solution.
- Recommended rate of administration—To avoid complications, sodium bicarbonate should be given very slowly at a rate not more than 1 mEq/kg/min.

**Rate of administration of sodium bicarbonate:** Sodium bicarbonate should be administered slowly over 5 minutes and not more than 1 mEq/kg/min.

### Indications
- Acidosis—metabolic acidosis in renal failure, diabetic ketoacidosis, after resuscitation, cyanotic spell, inborn errors of metabolism, and renal tubular acidosis.
- Barbiturate overdose
- Cyanotic spell
- Drug intoxication—salicylate poisoning
- Diarrhea when more bicarbonate is lost
- Electrolyte imbalance—Hyperkalemia
- Gastric wash in iron poisoning.

### Contraindications
- Allergy
- Alkalosis

- Cardiac problems
- Hypocalcemia
- Kidney problems
- Peripheral edema
- Inadequate ventilation during cardiopulmonary resuscitation
- Patients on salt restricted diet.

## Precautions

- Diluted with 5% dextrose
- Check the patency of the IV line as extravasation can cause tissue necrosis.

**Q1. What is the precondition to administer sodium bicarbonate during neonatal resuscitation?**
The baby should be adequately ventilated.
This should not be given before the respiration is established and confirmed by arterial blood gas (ABG) and significant metabolic acidosis and normal level of carbon dioxide ($CO_2$) confirmed on ABG analysis.
Sodium bicarbonate will correct acidosis by producing $CO_2$ and water. To remove this, $CO_2$ adequate ventilation should be given. Without adequate ventilation, this will not improve the pH.

**Q2. When should you give sodium bicarbonate in newborn resuscitation?**
Only after the respiration is established. It may cause cerebral hemorrhage.
Sodium bicarbonate should be given only when severe metabolic acidosis is confirmed by blood gas analysis.

**Q3. In centers where there is no facility for arterial blood gas analysis, when will you administer sodium bicarbonate?**
When the Apgar is less than 3 after 5 minutes.

## Effects on Pregnancy

- Category C
- It can increase the blood pressure in pregnant women.

## Side Effects/Adverse Reactions of Sodium Bicarbonate

- Metabolic alkalosis
- Hypernatremia
- Hypokalemia
- Hypocalcemia, decreased plasma ionized calcium concentration
- Edema
- Intracranial hemorrhage—Cerebral hemorrhage/intraventricular hemorrhage
- Decreased fibrillation threshold
- Intracranial acidosis
- Tissue necrosis following extravasation
- Impaired cardiac function
- Tetany.

## Drug Interactions

- Rapid infusion may predispose to pulmonary or intraventricular hemorrhage.
- Do not infuse this drug until respiration is established.
- Compatible with water and 5% dextrose
- Along with calcium, it can cause milk alkali syndrome.

## QUESTIONS

**Q1. What are the drugs with which sodium bicarbonate should not be mixed with?**
Do not mix with calcium salts, catecholamines, and atropine.

**Q2. What are the things to be monitored during the administration of sodium bicarbonate?**
- Acid-base status
- Ventilation.

**Q3. How will you calculate the amount of sodium bicarbonate?**
The amount of sodium bicarbonate (mEq) to be given can be calculated by:

$$\frac{\text{Body weight} \times \text{Base deficit} \times 0.35}{18 - \text{Observed bicarbonate} \times \text{body weight in kg} \times 0.5}$$

## Pulmonary Surfactant

Surfactant is active lipoprotein complex formed by type 2 alveolar cells. Surfactant synthesis starts in the terminal saccular stage of lung development and it forms a meshwork of tubular myelin.

### Mechanism of Action

It lowers the surface tension between two liquids, or liquid and gas or a liquid and solid. The surfactant contains proteins and lipids. They have both hydrophilic and hydrophobic regions. They adsorb to the air-water interface of alveoli with hydrophilic toward the water and hydrophobic part toward the air.

### Functions

- Decreases the surface tension
- To promote lung expansion during inspiration
- To prevent alveolar collapse and loss of lung volume in end expiration
- Facilitates recruitment of collapsed alveoli. Respiratory distress syndrome (RDS) is more common in preterm babies as they have surfactant storage pool of 4–5 mg/kg compared to 100 mg/kg in term babies.

### Types of Surfactant

- Natural surfactant (Beractant/Porcine/Calfactant)
- Synthetic surfactant (Colfosceril/Lucinactant).

### Dose

- 100 mg/kg of phospholipid
- Timing of surfactant therapy can be prophylactic (surfactant given at birth before distress sets in), early rescue (within 2 hours of life after distress), and late rescue (after 2 hours of life with distress)

**Number of doses:** Evidence for three doses at 6 hours interval and the indication being same as first dose of surfactant.

### Technique of Administration

- Insure technique:
  - Intubation
  - Intratracheal surfactant administration
  - Extubation.
- Minimally invasive surfactant therapy: Surfactant administration via vascular catheter when the baby is breathing spontaneously
- Surfactant administration during mechanical ventilation.

### Indications

- Premature babies with evidence of surfactant deficiency
- Hyaline membrane disease in newborn (RDS)
- Congenital surfactant deficiency
- Continuous positive airway pressure (CPAP) failure.

### Contraindication

Severe hemodynamic instability.

### Side Effects

- Apnea
- Air embolism
- Air leak syndromes
- Bradycardia
- Desaturation
- Endotracheal tube reflux/obstruction
- Air embolism
- Hypotension
- Hypocarbia
- Hypercarbia
- Pulmonary hemorrhage
- Retinopathy of prematurity
- Patent ductus arteriosus
- Volutrauma.

### Drug Interactions

No drug interactions.

## QUESTIONS

**Q1. What are the advantages of pulmonary surfactant?**
- Increases the pulmonary compliance
- Prevents atelectasis
- Facilitates recruitment of collapsed airways.

**Q2. What is pulmonary surfactant?**
Pulmonary surfactant is phospholipoprotein formed by type II alveolar cells.

**Q3. What is preventive strategy?**
Give first dose as soon as possible after birth within 15 minutes of delivery.

## Tramadol

It is a synthetic pain reliever.

### Mechanism of Action

This will be changed into an opioid drug in the body. Like morphine, tramadol will bind to narcotic or opioid receptors in the brain.

### Dosage

100 mg up to a maximum of 400 mg.

### Indication

Relief of moderate to severe pain.

### Contraindications and Cautions

- Age under 12 years
- Breathing problem—obstructive sleep apnea
- Bronchial asthma
- Coma
- Chronic obstructive pulmonary disease
- CYP2D6 deficient patients, CYP3A4 deficient patients
- Drug—MAOIs
- Excessive or overweight
- Ear-nose-throat (ENT) surgery—removal of adenoids, tonsils
- Fits
- Gastrointestinal obstruction
- Hypersensitivity to drug
- Impairment of pulmonary, kidney, or liver functions.

### Precautions

- It should not be used to relieve pain in children under the age of 12 years.
- This drug is associated with addiction, abuse
- Overdosage can result in death
- It should be used cautiously in elderly, patients with liver failure, and kidney failure.

### Effects on Pregnancy

When used in pregnancy, it can cause life-threatening withdrawal symptoms in the newborn.

### Side Effects

- Abdominal pain
- Breathing problems
- Blood pressure elevated
- Constipation
- Drowsiness
- Dry mouth
- Diarrhea
- Emesis
- Euphoria
- Fever
- Gastrointestinal symptom—Nausea
- Headache
- Indigestion
- Withdrawal symptoms.

### Drug Interactions

- Carbamazepine will reduce the effect of tramadol.
- Quinidine will increase the concentration of tramadol by reducing the inactivation of tramadol.
- Tramadol will cause CNS and respiratory depression when combined with alcohol, sedative hypnotics.

## QUESTIONS

**Q1. What are the withdrawal symptoms of tramadol?**

Withdrawal symptoms are:
- Anxiety
- Abdominal cramps
- Backache
- Chills
- Diarrhea
- Excessive tear production
- Insomnia
- Joint pain
- Sweating
- Yawning.

**Q2. What are the features of overdosage of tramadol?**
- Addiction
- Convulsions
- Depression.

**Q3. What is the action of tramadol on the immune system?**

Tramadol may enhance the function of immune system.

# 5
## CHAPTER

# Vitamins

## CHAPTER OUTLINE

- Vitamin A
- Vitamin $B_{12}$ (Cyanocobalamin)
- Vitamin D
- Vitamin E
- Vitamin K

## INTRODUCTION

Vitamins are a group of essential organic micronutrients needed in small quantities for proper functioning of its metabolism. Deficiency of these vitamins will result in specific disorders. They may contain weakened or inactivated forms or killed forms of the diseases causing agent or one of its toxins or surface proteins. The vaccines will provide acquired immunity to particular diseases. The process of introducing a vaccine into the body is known as vaccination.

## VITAMIN A

Vitamin A is absorbed well for the gut and stored in hepatic stellate (ITO) cells of the liver as retinyl palmitate. These stores will last for 6 months. Retinol is transported in the blood and bound to retinol binding protein (RBP). β-carotene is also known as provitamin A and gets converted into retinol in the intestinal wall. Out of the many different carotene pigments, the β-carotene yields the highest amount of retinol. β-carotene is also known as provitamin A and gets converted into retinol in the intestinal wall. Both retinol and carotenes are fat-soluble. Cooking or frying in oil improves the absorption of carotenes.

### Actions

- *Antioxidant activity:* Beta carotene has antioxidant properties. This reduces the incidence of lung, breast, oral, esophageal and bladder cancers.
- Bone turnover increased—suppresses osteoblast activity and stimulates osteoclastic activity.

### Daily Requirement

Daily requirement depends upon the age.

#### Daily Requirements of Vitamin A

- 1,000–1,500 IU/day
- Under 1 year—1,500 IU
- 1–3 years—2,000 IU
- 4–6 years—2,500 IU
- 7–9 years—3,500 IU
- 10–12 years—4,500 IU/day.

### Recommended Daily Allowance of Vitamin A, Retinol and β-carotene

Recommended daily allowance (RDA) of vitamin A is given in Table 5.1.

**Table 5.1:** Recommended daily allowance of vitamin A.

| Recommended daily allowance (RDA) | | |
|---|---|---|
| Age | µg/day of retinol | β-carotene |
| 0–1 year | 350 | 1,400 |
| 1–5 years | 400 | 1,600 |
| 7–12 years | 600–750 µg/day | 1,400 |
| >12 years | 750 µg/day | 2,400 |
| Adults | 750 µg/day | 2,400 |
| Pregnant women | 750 µg/day | 2,400 |
| Lactating mothers | Add 400 µg more (1,150 µg) | 3,800 |

## Dosage for Treatment of Vitamin A Deficiency

- Less than 6 months—50,000 IU
- 6 months to 1 year—100,000 IU
- More than 1 year—200,000 IU

The above dose is given on day one and day two. The same dose is repeated again on day 14.

## Vitamin A Prophylaxis Program

- Dose at 9 months (6-11 months) one lakh units
- 2 lakhs units once in 6 months from 12-36 months up to 3 years of age
- From 2006 the program was revised to 6-59 months of age

## Indications

- Vitamin A deficiency.
- During treatment of measles.
- Vitamin A prophylaxis program.

## Contraindications and Cautions

- Hypersensitivity
- Hepatic diseases
- *Malabsorption*: Oral vitamin a will not be useful in patients with fat malabsorption.

## Effects on Pregnancy

Teratogenic.

## Side Effects

### Features of Hypervitaminosis A

Excessive intake of vitamin A containing solutions or therapeutic overdose. Intake of more than 8,000 IU/day.

Acute toxicity (acute hypervitaminosis A):

- Abdominal pain
- Benign intracranial hypertension or pseudotumor cerebri (bulging anterior fontanelle)
- Blurring of vision.
- *Changes in consciousness*:
  - Coma
  - Dizziness
- *Double vision*:
  - Emesis
  - Emotional lability
  - Fatigue
  - Gastrointestinal—nausea, headache, irritability.

Chronic toxicity (Chronic hypervitaminosis A):

- Anorexia
- Alopecia or sparse hair
- Arthralgia
- Benign intracranial hypertension
- Bone pains
- Confusion
- Calcium levels increased
- Dry skin
- Desquamation of skin
- Emesis
- Fractures
- Gastrointestinal—nausea
- Gastric mucosal calcinosis
- Headache
- Hepatotoxicity
- Hepatosplenomegaly
- Hypoplastic anemia
- Hyperostosis of bone
- Irritability

- Itching
- Jaundice
- Knee joint pain
- Lips—dry or cracked
- Loss of weight
- Muscular weakness
- Neurological features—delirium, coma
- Ophthalmological features—visual disturbances
- Psychiatric changes
- Pruritus

Hypercalcinosis with calicification of ear valves, gastric mucosa, etc.

Excess intake of carotenoids does not result in toxicity.

## Drug Interactions
- Long-term use of liquid paraffin will predispose to vitamin deficiency.
- Vitamin E will promote storage and utilization of vitamin A.
- Long-term use of neomycin will cause steatorrhea and will predispose to vitamin deficiency.
- Vitamin A and vitamin D will have synergistic and antagonistic interactions.

## QUESTIONS

**Q1. What are the forms of vitamin A available in foods?**
- Carotene from plant sources.
- Retinal from animal sources.

**Q2. What is the richest source of retinol?**
β-carotene (provitamin A) yields the highest amount of retinol. β-carotene gets converted into retinol in the intestinal wall. Both retinol and carotenes are fat-soluble.

**Q3. How does cooking or frying affect the absorption of carotenes?**
Cooking or frying in oil improves the absorption of carotenes.

**Q4. How is retinol transported?**
Retinol is transported in the blood, bound to RBP.

**Q5. Where is vitamin A stored?**
Absorbed vitamin A is stored in the ITO cells of the liver as retinyl palmitate. These stores last for 6 months.

**Q6. What are the precursors of vitamin A?**
Vitamin A or retinol is obtained from the diet as carotene from plant sources and as retinal from animal sources. Out of the many different carotene pigments, the β-carotene yields the highest amount of retinol.

**Q7. What is provitamin A?**
Carotene is also known as provitamin A and gets converted into retinol in the intestinal wall. Both retinol and carotenes are fat-soluble.

**Q8. How does cooking affect the absorption of carotene?**
Cooking or frying in oil improves the absorption of carotenes.

**Q9. What are the functions of vitamin A?**
- Normal maintenance and functioning of body tissues.
- Maintains cellular integrity.
- Enhances the immune competence and thus prevents infections.

*Antioxidant activity:* β-carotene has antioxidant properties. This reduces the incidence of lung, breast, oral, esophageal and bladder cancers.

**Q10. What are the sources of vitamin A?**
Sources of carotene including β-carotene are *plant sources:*
- Carrot
- Drumstick leaves
- Papaya
- Pumpkin
- Tomatoes
- Green leafy vegetables
- Yellow fruits.

**Q11. What are the sources of retinol?**
*Sources of retinol are*—Animal sources:
- Liver
- Egg
- Fish liver oils.

**Q12. What are the conditions predisposing to vitamin A deficiency?**

Conditions predisposing to Vitamin A deficiency are:
- Biliary duct obstruction which affects fat absorption:
  - Celiac disease—fat malabsorption is a feature.
  - Drugs—excess use of liquid paraffin will coat the intestines there by interfering with absorption of vitamins.
- *Exanthematous fever*: Infections—measles.
- *Fat malabsorption*: Tropical sprue—fat malabsorption is a feature.
- *Gastrointestinal disorders*: Hepatic disorders will result in decreased bile secretion which will predispose to fat malabsorption. As vitamin A is a fat soluble vitamin, the absorption will be affected intake less than required.

**Q13. What are the symptoms of vitamin A deficiency?**
- Poor dark adaptation
- Night blindness
- Photophobia (due to xerosis or corneal ulcer).

**Q14. What are Bitot's spots?**

*Bitot's spot* is a small plaque of silver gray color with a foamy surface. It is seen in the lateral half of the bulbar conjunctiva just close to the limbus. The shape is triangular and usually. The spots vary in size from 2 mm to 10 mm. These are usually seen bilaterally.

**Q15. What are the signs and symptoms of Vitamin A deficiency?**
- *Signs*:
  - Guttural pigmentation
  - Bitot's spots
  - Xerosis (corneal and conjunctival)
  - Ulcer (Corneal and conjunctival)
  - Keratomalacia
  - Phrynoderma (toad skin)
- *Symptoms*: Night blindness, decreased dark adaptation.
- *Clinical Investigation*: Defective dark adaptation can be detected by dark adaptometry or electroretinography in the early stages before night blindness appears.

**Q16. What are the ocular manifestations of vitamin A deficiency?**
- Defective dark adaptation
- Night blindness
- Xerophthalmia (dry eyes)
- Bitot's spots
- Corneal xerosis
- Corneal ulceration
- Keratomalacia
- Pigmentation—guttural pigmentation is one of the early signs of vitamin A deficiency.

**Q17. What are the conjunctival findings in vitamin A deficiency?**

The lesions occur characteristically in the bulbar conjunctiva:
- Conjunctival xerosis—seen at the bulbar conjunctiva, lateral to limbus
- Hazy conjunctiva
- Thickening of the conjunctiva
- *Pigmentation*: Guttural pigmentation
- Bitot's spots.

**Q18. What are the corneal findings in vitamin A deficiency?**
- Corneal xerosis occurs after conjunctival xerosis and Bitot's spots.
- Corneal ulceration.
- Perforation of the eyes—iris prolapses in the lower and central part of the cornea.
- Keratomalacia
- Fundal changes (xerophthalmia fundus)—small white spots on the retina do not interfere with the vision.

**Q19. What are the skin changes in vitamin A deficiency?**

Phrynoderma is a skin disorder which results in follicular keratosis.

**Q20. What are respiratory tract changes in vitamin A deficiency?**
Squamous metaplasia of the respiratory mucosa and ciliary damage occurs. The children are prone for respiratory infections.

**Q21. What is World Health Organization (WHO) classification of vitamin A deficiency?**
- *Primary signs:*
  - X1A: Conjunctival xerosis.
  - X1B: Bitot's spots.
  - X2: Corneal xerosis.
  - X3A: Corneal ulceration or keratomalacia (less than 1/3 of cornea involved).
  - X3B: Corneal ulceration or keratomalacia (more than 1/3 of cornea involved).
- *Secondary signs:*
  - XN: Night blindness.
  - XF: Fundal changes—xerophthalmic fundus.
  - XS: Corneal scars.

**Q22. What is vitamin A prophylaxis program?**
Vitamin A is given orally to all children aged 6 months to 5 years (60 months) at an interval of 6 months. The dose is 50,000 units for less than one year, 1 lakh units for one year and 2 lakhs units for more than one year.

# VITAMIN $B_{12}$ (CYANOCOBALAMIN)

Cyanocobalamin and hydroxycobalamin are referred as vitamin $B_{12}$.

Ionic calcium is necessary for initial binding of intrinsic factor—B complex to the ileal binding site. Cyanocobalamin can get absorbed without the intrinsic factor when given in milligrams.

This is due to simple diffusion due to mass action. Vitamin $B_{12}$ will be absorbed and transported in the serum is a bound form bound to transcobalamin.

## Functions of Vitamin $B_{12}$

- Vitamin $B_{12}$ helps in synthesis of nucleic acid along with folic acid.
- Vitamin $B_{12}$ is essential for formation and maturation of red blood cells.
- Vitamin $B_{12}$ maintains normal activity of nervous system.
- It is essential for formation and maturation of red blood cells.
- Maintains normal activity of nervous system.

## Daily Requirement of Vitamin $B_{12}$

- 1–3 µg per day.
- Pregnancy and lactation: 3–5 µg per day.

## Dosage

- For treatment of vitamin $B_{12}$ deficiency—parenteral dose 1,000 µg.
- 30–50 µg once daily for 2 weeks.

## Indications

- Megaloblastic anemia.
- Pernicious anemia.

## Contraindications

- Allergy to cobalt.
- Hypokalemia.
- Leber's hereditary optic atrophy
- Atrophic gastritis
- Gastrectomy
- Polycythemia.

## Conditions Caused by Deficiency of Vitamin $B_{12}$

- Megaloblastic anemia.
- Pernicious anemia.

## Precautions

When both vitamin $B_{12}$ and folate deficiency coexist, first provide vitamin $B_{12}$ and then give folate. If folate is given first; it will increase the turnover of cells and precipitate acute deficiency of vitamin $B_{12}$ presenting a subacute combined degeneration.

### Effects on Pregnancy
- Can be given in recommended doses during pregnancy or lactation.
- High doses can harm the baby during pregnancy and lactation.
- Vitamin $B_{12}$ will be secreted in the milk and is not recommended to lactating mothers.

### Side Effects
- Anaphylaxis
- Anxiety
- Burning skin
- Blood clots in the limbs
- Congestive cardiac failure
- Cramps
- Diarrhea
- Eye pain
- Fatigue
- Facial flushing
- Gout flare up
- Hypokalemia
- Hypertension
- Itching
- Involuntary movements.

### Drug Interactions
The following drugs can decrease the absorption or serum levels of vitamin $B_{12}$:
- Aspirin
- Chloramphenicol
- $H_2$-blockers

## QUESTIONS

**Q1. What is the site of absorption of vitamin $B_{12}$?**
Vitamin $B_{12}$ is absorbed in the lower part of the ileum.

**Q2. What are the forms of vitamin $B_{12}$?**
- Cyanocobalamin and hydroxocobalamin.
- Vitamin $B_{12}$ is not synthesized by animals or plants.
- Ultimate source of vitamin $B_{12}$ is from microbial synthesis.

**Q3. What are the sources of vitamin $B_{12}$?**
- Liver, kidneys, meat.
- It is a vitamin that is synthesized by microorganisms it is not found in plants. The children are dependent on the animal sources. Strict vegetarians, who do not consume milk or milk products, are prone to develop this vitamin deficiency.

**Q4. How vitamin $B_{12}$ is produced in humans?**
Vitamin $B_{12}$ is produced by microorganisms in soils, water and intestine of humans.

**Q5. What is the plant source of vitamin $B_{12}$?**
- Vitamin $B_{12}$ is absent in plant products. The only vegetable source of vitamin $B_{12}$ is legumes (pulses). The microorganism harbored in the root nodules will provide this vitamin.
- Vitamin $B_{12}$ will be absorbed only in the presence of intrinsic factor.

**Q6. What are the dietary sources of vitamin $B_{12}$?**
Liver, kidney, sea fish, egg yolk, meat, cheese.

**Q7. What are the causes of vitamin $B_{12}$ deficiency?**
- Addisonian pernicious anemia.
- Decreased intake.
- Malabsorption—bowel resection, gastric mucosal damage, gastrectomy.
- Increased demand—pregnancy, infancy.
- Increased consumption by abnormal flora in the gut—blind loop syndrome, fish tape worm.

**Q8. What is primary and secondary vitamin $B_{12}$ deficiency?**
- Primary deficiency is due to decreased intake
- Secondary deficiency:
  - Inadequate absorption (addisonian pernicious anemia due to failure of secretion of intrinsic factor in the stomach, after resection of stomach results in intrinsic factor deficiency,

- diseases of terminal ileum, bacterial colonization of small intestine)
- Inadequate utilization of the vitamin $B_{12}$
- Increased requirement
- Increased excretion—due to inadequate binding of this vitamin in the serum. This occurs in the liver and kidney diseases.

**Q9. What are the types of pernicious anemia?**
- *Congenital pernicious anemia*: Pernicious anemia is due to defect in absorption of vitamin $B_{12}$.
- Pernicious anemia is due to defect in absorption of vitamin $B_{12}$.
- Acquired pernicious anemia [small bowel diseases, drugs: Para-aminosalicylic acid (PAS), neomycin]. Methylmalonic acid excretion is increased in deficiency of $B_{12}$.
- *Worm infestation causing $B_{12}$ deficiency*: Diphyllobothrium latum.

**Q10. What are the features associated with vitamin $B_{12}$ deficiency?**

*Neurological manifestations:*
- Peripheral neuropathy paresthesia—pins and needles sensation in the fingers and toes or numbness.
- Subacute combined degeneration due to involvement of the posterior column (distal sensory loss, absent ankle reflex, exaggerated knee jerk, extensor plantar).
- Weakness in peripheral nerves, progressing to spasticity, ataxia, central nervous system (CNS) dysfunction, convulsions.
- *Mental changes*: Mental retardation, poor memory, mood changes, hallucinations, irritability.
- Retrobulbar neuropathy.
- Personality changes.

*Skin:*
- Hyperpigmentation over the back of the hands, fingers, nose, the knuckles and nail beds.

*Hematological system:*
- Megaloblastic anemia, pernicious anemia, macrocytic anemia.
- Glossitis.
- Bald tongue.

**Q11. What are the causes of megaloblastic anemia?**
- Vitamin $B_{12}$ deficiency.
- Folic acid deficiency.

**Q12. What are the typical features of megaloblastic anemia?**
- Moderate leukopenia.
- Thrombocytopenia.
- Hypercellular bone marrow with megaloblastic erythroid and other precussor cells.

**Q13. How will you treat vitamin $B_{12}$ deficiency?**
- 100 µg of cyano- or hydroxycobalamin is given three times a week till the hemoglobin is normal. Following this the child can be given 100 µg intramuscularly (IM) weekly and then monthly.
- In patients with neurological complications the dose can be increased to 500 µg.

# VITAMIN D

Calcitriol—1α,25-dihydroxyvitamin D3.

## Mechanism of Action

Alfacalcidol is activated by the enzyme 25-hydroxylase in the liver. The active form is calcitriol which binds to intracellular receptors regulation of calcium and bone metabolism.

## Pharmacological Actions

Increases calcium and phosphorus absorption' from the gastrointestinal tract.

## Functions of Vitamin D

- Enhances absorption of calcium from the gut and maintains normal serum calcium.
- Stimulation of normal bone mineralization. Promotes mineralization of bone

collagen, maturation and remodeling, increases tubular absorption of calcium and phosphorus in kidneys.
- Bone resorption and release of calcium from bone.
- Helps in maintenance of growing skeleton and adult bones throughout the life.
- Differentiation of keratinocytes.
- Antiproliferative action against the cells in the skin.

## Dosage

- Physiological replacement: 5–15 ng/kg
- Oral 0.25 µg/day
- Once a day
- *Renal rickets*: 10–30 ng/kg.

## Indications

- Used for physiological replacement
- Rickets
- Hypocalcemia in hypoparathyroidism
- Osteomalacia in adults
- Renal osteodystrophy
- Osteoporosis
- Corticosteroid induced osteoporosis
- Secondary hyperparathyroidism.

## Contraindications

- Monitor serum calcium levels every 2–4 weeks.
- Once the alkaline phosphatase levels become normal reduce the dose.

## Conditions Caused by Deficiency of Vitamin D

Rickets, osteomalacia.

## Precautions

Drink plenty of water.

## Effects on Pregnancy

- It is not contraindicated. The fetus derives vitamin D exclusively from the mother. So, vitamin D should be given to the mother if needed.
- Calcitriol is secreted in breast milk and should be avoided in nursing mothers.

## Side Effects

Vitamin D toxicity is due to excess intake of vitamin D:
- Anorexia
- Abdominal pain
- Arrhythmias
- Bone pain
- Constipation
- Clouding of cornea
- Drowsiness
- Dry mouth
- Diarrhea
- Ectopic calcification: Nephrocalcinosis, aortic or myocardial calcification, kidneys, lungs, arteries, soft tissues.
- Emesis (vomiting)
- Fatigue
- Gustatory changes: Metallic taste
- Headache
- Hypertension
- Hypercalcemia or hypercalciuria.
- Hypotonia
- Irritability
- Itching or pruritus
- Joint pain
- Kidney damage
- Libido decreased
- Muscle pain
- Nausea
- Ocular calcification
- Polyuria or frequent urination
- Sweating
- Somnolence
- Hyperparathyroidism.

*Late manifestations:*
- Anorexia
- Albuminuria
- Apathy
- Blood urea nitrogen (BUN) elevated
- Cardiac arrhythmias
- Calcific conjunctivitis
- Dehydration
- Ectopic calcification—nephrocalcinosis
- Growth arrest or retardation
- Hypertension
- Hyperthermia

- Hepatic—elevated aspartate aminotransferase (AST), alanine aminotransferase (ALT)
- *Infections*: Urinary tract infection (UTI)
- Libido decreased
- Muscle weakness
- Nocturia
- Pancreatitis
- Photophobia
- Polyuria
- Polydipsia
- Photophobia
- Psychosis
- Pruritis
- Weight loss.

**Drug Interactions**
- Antacids should be avoided.
- *Anticonvulsants*: Phenytoin and phenobarbitone will accelerate the metabolism of calcitriol and reduce the endogenous levels.
- *Barbiturates*: Phenobarbitone will accelerate the metabolism of calcitriol.
- Corticosteroids—will have functional antagonism by inhibiting calcium absorption.
- Cholestyramine will reduce the absorption of fat-soluble vitamins.
- *Diuretics*: Use along with thiazides will predispose to hypercalcemia.
- Digoxin—hypercalcemia caused by calcitriol will predispose to arrhythmias in patients with digoxin.
- Ketoconazole will inhibit synthetic and catabolic enzymes of calcitriol and decrease the serum levels of calcitriol.

## QUESTIONS

**Q1. What are the sources of vitamin D?**
- Egg, liver, milk, fish liver oils, butter and cheese.
- Foods fortified with vitamin D.
- *Exposure to sunlight*: Whole body exposure 30 min/week or head exposure 2 h/week to UV rays (296–310 nm) lead to synthesis of 10 µg of vitamin D.

**Q2. What is the daily requirement of vitamin D?**
Daily requirements depend upon the age:
- *Preschool children*: 400 IU/day (10 µg)
- *Children*: 200 IU/day (5 µg)
- *Pregnancy and lactation*: 400 IU/day (10 µg).

**Q3. What are the sources of vitamin D?**
- *Plant sources*: Cereals
- *Animal sources*: Milk, egg yolk, fish, liver.

**Q4. What are the types of rickets?**
- Vitamin D deficiency—responds to normal doses of vitamin D.
- Vitamin D dependent—responds to high doses of vitamin D.
- Vitamin D resistant—will not respond to high doses of vitamin D.

**Q5. What are the clinical features of nutritional rickets?**
*During 1st year:*
- Cranium—craniotabes, widening of sutures, frontal bossing.
- Wrist—widening.
- Ribs—rachitic rosary, Harrison's sulcus.
- Teeth-delayed eruption, pit grooves enamel hypoplasia.
- Muscle weakness—unable to stand till 3 years (motor mile stone delay).

**Q6. What are the clinical features of rickets when the age of onset is after 1 year?**
- Long bones deformities (legs have most deformities).
- Genu varum or valgum
- coxa vara
- Rachitic saber shin.
- Up to 4 years of age they resolve with treatment.

**Q7. What are the complications associated with nutritional rickets?**
- ☐ Recurrent respiratory infection—pneumonia.
- ☐ Tetany (or) stridor—in hypocalcemia.

## VITAMIN E

- ❖ Fat soluble vitamin
- ❖ *Sources*:
  - Vegetable oils are the richest sources of vitamin E.
  - Wheat germ oil, sunflower oil, cotton seed oil, safflower, palm, rape seeds oil.
  - Whole meal cereals.
  - Eggs, butter.
  - Meat, poultry.
- ❖ *Recommended intake*: 4 IU for infants and 15 IU for adolescents.

## Predisposing Factors for Vitamin E Deficiency

- ❖ Premature babies
- ❖ Low birth weight babies
- ❖ Abnormal α-tocopherol transfer protein
- ❖ Metabolic syndrome.

## Mechanism of Action

- ❖ *Reduces free radical damage*: Vitamin E is an antioxidant, which prevents the injury to cells by oxygen radicals induced peroxidase damage of the body cells like muscles, nerves, red blood cells, sperms, etc.
  - Essential for structural functional maintenance of skeletal, cardiac and smooth muscle.
  - Antioxidant
  - Antiaging
  - Positive effect on immune health.

## Clinical Features of Vitamin E Deficiency

- ❖ Neuropathy
- ❖ Male sterility
- ❖ In the deficient conditions of this vitamin the body cells are prone to be damaged and causes the following symptoms:
  - *RBCs*: Hemolytic anemia
  - *Muscle*: Muscle weakness, myopathy.
  - *Nerve cells*: Reflexes diminished (neuropathy) posterior column degeneration (causes ataxia).
- ❖ Prevents cataract
- ❖ Prevents Alzheimer's disease.

## Dosage

### Recommended Daily Allowance

- ❖ *Infants 0–6 months*: 4 mg/day (6 IU/day)
- ❖ *7–12 months*: 5 mg/day (7.5 IU/day)
- ❖ *Children*: 1–3 years—6 mg/day (9 IU/day)
- ❖ *4–8 years*: 7 mg/day (10 IU/day)
- ❖ *9–13 years*: 11mg/day (16 IU/day)

## Indications

- ❖ Vitamin E deficiency
- ❖ Ataxia.

## Contraindications and Cautions

- ❖ Allergic reactions
- ❖ Anemia
- ❖ *Angioplasty*: Avoid immediately before and after angioplasty.
- ❖ Bleeding in the brain.
- ❖ Bleeding disorders—increases the risk of bleeding in associated vitamin K deficiency.
- ❖ *Cardiac failure*: In high doses increase the risk of heart failure in diabetics.
- ❖ Diabetics
- ❖ *Eye problems*: Retinitis pigmentosa.
- ❖ (Do not take more than 400 IU in diabetics or cardiac diseases)
- ❖ Hypersensitivity to drug
- ❖ Liver disorders
- ❖ Kidney disorders.

## Precautions

- ❖ Parenteral intravenous administration in preterm babies in high dose.
- ❖ Increases the risk of hemorrhagic stroke.
- ❖ Use cautiously in iron deficiency anemia.
- ❖ Use cautiously in hypoprothrombinemia.

## Effects on Pregnancy

*Category C:*
- Safe during pregnancy in recommended in daily amount.
- In early pregnancy it may be harmful and can cause fetal resorption, encephalomalacia.
- Safe during breastfeeding in recommended levels.

## Side Effects
- Allergy—rash
- Bleeding
- Blurred vision
- Cramps (abdominal or stomach cramps)
- Dizziness
- Diarrhea
- Emesis
- Enterocolitis (necrotizing enterocolitis)
- Fatigue
- Gastrointestinal (GIT) symptoms—nausea
- Gonadal dysfunction
- Headache
- Healing of wounds impaired
- Intestinal cramps
- Weakness.

## Vitamin E Excess
Anticoagulant effect.

## Metabolic Side Effects

*Urine*
- Creatinuria
- Urinary androgens and estrogens increased.

*Serum*
- Cholesterol increased.
- Serum cholesterol increased.
- Serum triglycerides increased.

## Drug Interactions
- If on statins do not exceed the dose of 400 NIU Reduce the effect of cholesterol drugs.
- Cholestyramine will alter absorption of vitamin E.
- High dose of vitamin E will increase the requirement of vitamin K.
- Increased omega-6-fatty acids will increase the requirement of vitamin E.

## VITAMIN K
- Phylloquinone (vitamin k1)
- Menaquinone (vitamin K2)
- Menadione (vitamin K3)
- Vitamin K is required for the synthesis of clotting factors II, VII, IX, and X. This is synthesized by a process of carboxylation of glutamic acid in vitamin K-dependent proteins.
- The half-life of plasma is 72 hours. Vitamin K is stored in the liver up to one month.

## Functions of Vitamin K
- This is a fat-soluble vitamin required for synthesis of vitamin K-dependent clotting factors.
- Vitamin K acts as a cofactor of at a later stage of synthesis of prothrombin, factors VII, IX, and X.
- Coagulation factors 2, 7, 9, 10 are vitamin K dependent.
- Vitamin K is synthesized in the gut by the microorganisms in the gut. It is a fat-soluble vitamin and bile is required for absorption in the gut.
- Breast milk is a poor source of vitamin K.
- Acts as a cofactor in the synthesis of coagulation factors by the liver.

## Daily Requirement of Vitamin K

*Infants:*
- 0-6 months—15 µg/kg
- 7-12 months—15-25 µg/kg.

*Children:*
- 1-3 years—30 µg/kg
- 4-8 years—55 µg/kg
- 9-13 years—60 µg/kg.

*Adolescents:*
- 14–18 years—75 µg/kg
- More than 19 years—90 µg/kg.

## Dosage

### Prophylaxis
- 0.5–1 mg/kg IM, at birth.
- 1 mg at birth IM, at birth.

**Q. What is the dose for prevention of hemolytic disease of the newborn (HDN) in newborn in term and preterm babies?**
- Prophylaxis in newborn—0.5–1mg
- 0.5 mg for preterm or babies weighing less than 2 kg
- 1 mg for term babies
- 1 mg for babies weighing more than 2 kg.

### Treatment of HDN
- Dose of vitamin K for HDN is 1 mg intramuscularly or 5 mg intravenously.
- If bleeding is not controlled the dose can be continued for 3 days.

**Q. What is the dose of vitamin K for treatment of HDN?**
Vitamin K in babies with vitamin K deficiency:
- 1–2 mg orally daily for infants.
- 5 mg IM for bleeding until bleeding is controlled.
- Adults—2.5–25 mg/day.

## Indications
- Prophylaxis and treatment of vitamin k deficiency.
- Hemorrhagic disease of the newborn (HDN).
- Treatment of liver failure.

## Contraindications for Vitamin K
- Vitamin E deficiency
- Hepatic disorders
- Glucose-6-phosphate dehydrogenase (G6PD) deficiency.

## Precautions
- Menadione can cause hemolysis in patients with G6PD deficiency.
- Gallbladder disease—high dose should be given, as absorption will be affected.
- Liver disease.

## Effects on Pregnancy
Although birth defects are not reported, jaundice in newborn can occur. So vitamin K is not recommended during pregnancy.

## Side Effects
*Local:*
- Pain, swelling
- Flushing
- Taste changes
- Dizziness
- Hypotension.

**Q. What are the complications of vitamin K excess?**
Effects of vitamin K excess are:
- *Hemolytic anemia*: Hyperbilirubinemia and kernicterus, (competitively inhibits glucuronidation of bilirubin).
- *Hepatomegaly*: This usually occurs in newborn babies.

## Drug Interactions
Menadiones will interacting oral anticoagulants, warfarin and reverse the anticoagulant activity.

# QUESTIONS

**Q1. What are the coagulation factors that are vitamin K dependent?**
Coagulation factors 2, 7, 9, 10 are vitamin K dependent.

**Q2. What is the daily requirement of vitamin K?**
5–10 µg.

**Q3. What are the sources of vitamin K?**
- *Plant sources:* Green leafy vegetables, cabbages, spinach, tomato, soyabeans.

- *Animal sources*: Liver (pork liver) is a good source, it is also synthesized in the colon.

**Q4. What are the features of vitamin K deficiency?**
Deficiency symptoms are:
- Hemorrhage
- Bleeding tendencies (clotting factors 2, 7, 9 and 10 are dependent on the normal functioning liver. The deficiency of these factors will lead to bleeding tendencies).
- Hemorrhagic disease of newborn.
- Hematuria.

**Q5. What are the clinical features of vitamin K deficiency?**
Bleeding tendencies.

**Q6. What are the common sites of bleeding?**
- Nose
- Under the skin (ecchymosis).

**Q7. What is the importance of breastfeeding to prevent vitamin K deficiency?**
Breast milk is a poor source of vitamin K.

**Q8. Why newborn babies are prone for vitamin K deficiency?**
Vitamin K is synthesized in the gut by the microorganisms in the gut. The number of microorganisms will be less in newborn babies.

**Q9. What are the types of hemorrhagic disease of the newborn (HDN)?**
Hemorrhagic disease of the newborn has three distinct patterns of presentation. They are:
1. *Early HDN:* Early HDN is seen within 24 hours of birth.
2. *Classic HDN:* Classic HDN occurs between the 2-5 days of life.
3. *Late hemorrhagic disease:* Late HDN is characterized by bleeding in infants aged 2-16 weeks.

**Q10. What are the predisposing factors for early HDN?**
In infants whose mothers have been on anticonvulsant or antituberculosis drugs or oral anticoagulant during pregnancy.

**Q11. What are the predisposing factors for Classic HDN?**
- Most of the cases being idiopathic.
- Malabsorption
- Total parenteral nutrition without vitamin K.

**Q12. What are the predisposing factors for late hemorrhagic disease of newborn?**
- Due to severe vitamin K deficiency, occurring primarily in exclusively breastfed infant.
- Human newborn are prone for vitamin K deficiency due to the following reasons:
  - Inefficient placental transfer of vitamin K.
  - Poor hepatic storage of vitamin K (1/5th of adult storage).
  - Low vitamin K in breast milk (15 µg/L compared to 60 µg/L in cow's milk).
  - Presence of *Lactobacilli* and bifidus factor in gut flora of breastfed babies, both are poor synthesizers of vitamin K.

## Summary Table

| Vitamin | Source | Mechanism of action | RDA | Deficiency |
|---|---|---|---|---|
| A (Retinol, retinal, beta carotene) | Dark green leafy vegetables, carrots Liver, meat, fish liver oil | Normal vision, integrity of epithelial cells, reproduction, growth, immune response | <1 year-1000: 1500 IU<br>1-3 years: 2000 IU<br>4-8 years: 2500 IU<br>7-9 years: 3500 IU | Bitot's spots, corneal/conjunctival xerosis/ulcer, nyctalopia, xerophthalmia |
| B<br>B1–Thiamine | Whole brain, cereals, legumes, meat, milk, liver | Component of coenzyme in carbohydrate metabolism | Infants: 0.2-0.4 mg<br>Children: 0.5-1 mg | Beriberi, Wernicke's encephalopathy, Korsakoff's psychosis |
| B2–Riboflavin | Whole grains, green leafy vegetables, meat, milk, egg | Component of coenzyme in carbohydrate metabolism | Infants: 0.5 mg/1000 kcal<br>Children: 0.6-1.2 mg/1000 kcal | Angular stomatitis, glossitis, dyssebacia, vascularization of cornea, dermatitis |
| Niacin | Whole grains, green leafy vegetables, beans, meat, fish, liver | Component of coenzyme in carbohydrate metabolism | Infants: 5-6 mg<br>Children: 6-12 mg<br>Adolescents: 14-16 mg | Dermatitis, diarrhea, dementia |
| Pantothenic acid | Cereals, legumes, meat, liver, egg | Component of coenzyme A essential for metabolism of carbohydrate, protein, fat. Cofactor for elongation of fatty acids | Infants: 1.7 mg<br>Children: 2-4 mg<br>Adolescents: 5 mg | Burning feet syndrome, cornification of skin, depigmentation of hair |
| Biotin | Peanuts, cereals, legumes, yeast | Cofactor for carbohydrate, fatty acid and amino acid metabolism | Infants: 20 µg/kg<br>Children: 20-100 µg/kg<br>Adolescents: 150-200 µg/kg | Seborrhoeic dermatitis, anorexia, paresthesia |
| B6–Pyridoxine | Whole grain, nuts, green leafy vegetables liver, meat, kidney | Component of coenzyme in amino acid metabolism, synthesis of hemoglobin | Infants: 0.2-0.5mg<br>Children: 0.5-1.5 mg<br>Adolescents: 1.5-2 mg | Anemia, glossitis, cheilosis, peripheral neuropathy, irritability |
| Folic acid (folate, pteroylglutamic acid) | Green leafy vegetables, legumes, peas, beans liver, meat, egg, kidney | Component of coenzyme in DNA synthesis, maturation of RBCs | Infants: 25-35 µg/kg<br>Children: 50-1502 µg/kg<br>Adolescents: 100-200 µg/kg | Anemia, anorexia, glossitis, neural tube defects in the fetus |
| B12 (Coblamin, cyanocobalamin) | Yeast extract, milk, meat, egg, liver | Component of coenzyme in aminoacid metabolism | Infants: 0.3-0.5µg<br>Children: 1-2 µg | Anemia, sub-acute combined degeneration |

*Contd...*

*Contd...*

| Vitamin | Source | Mechanism of action | RDA | Deficiency |
|---|---|---|---|---|
| C (Ascorbic acid) | Citrus fruits | Antioxidant, synthesis of collagen, amino acids, hormones, enhances absorption of nonheme iron | Infants: 35 mg<br>Children: 40-45 mg | Scurvy–irritability, spongy gums, scorbutic rosary, hemorrhages, poor wound healing |
| D (Calciferol, cholecalciferol, calcitriol) | Milk, egg, yolk, fish, liver oil | Maintenance of blood calcium, and phosphorus, mineralization of bones | Infants: 400 IU<br>Older children: 200 IU | Rickets, osteomalacia |
| E (alpha tocopherol) | Cereals, legumes, vegetable oils, dairy products, egg, fish | Antioxidant, interruption of free radical chain reactions, protection of poly unsaturated fatty acids | Infants: 304 mg<br>Children: 6-7 mg<br>Adolescents: 5-5 mg | Myopathy, neuropathy, hemolytic anemia, infertility |
| K (Phylloquinone, menaquinone, menadione) | Whole grain, cereals, legumes, nuts, oil seeds, meat, yolk, liver | Synthesis of proteins involved in blood coagulation and bone metabolism | 15 -25 µg/kg | Bleeding |

# CHAPTER 6

# Intravenous Fluids

## CHAPTER OUTLINE

- Intravenous Fluid Requirements
- Crystalloids
- Colloids
- Blood Products

## INTRODUCTION

Intravenous fluids are the liquids that are infused directly in to the vein. The type of fluid to be infused should depend upon the condition treated. The knowledge of composition of various fluids will be helpful to select the correct fluid to be used.

Intravenous fluids can be classified as:
1. *Maintenance fluids*: Which is used to replace insensible fluid loss
   5% dextrose, 0.45% normal saline
2. *Replacement fluids* is used to correct the fluid deficit caused by vomiting, diarrhea, burns, trauma, gastric drainage, etc.
3. *Special fluids*:
   - 25% dextrose to treat hypoglycemia
   - Potassium chloride to treat hypokalemia
   - Sodium bicarbonate to treat metabolic acidosis.

## Types of Intravenous Fluids

- Crystalloids
- Colloids
- Blood products.

## Crystalloids

Crystalloids are clear fluids made up of water and electrolytes solutions. These fluids will cross the semipermeable membrane.

They are classified as isotonic, hypotonic, and hypertonic.

### Intravenous Crystalloids Fluids

- *Dextrose solutions*:
  - 5% dextrose
  - 10% glucose
  - 25% dextrose
- Isolyte P
- Ringer lactate (RL)
- *Saline*:
  - Normal saline 0.9%
  - Hypertonic saline
  - Dextrose normal saline (DNS)
  - ½ DNS.

Uses:
- Intravascular resuscitation and replacement of salt loss
- Treatment of dehydration due to fluid loss as in diarrhea and vomiting

- To dilute packed red blood cells (RBCs) before dilution
- Used to dilute drugs.

**Advantages:**
- Cheap
- Easily available
- More effective
- Preferred fluids in shock.

**Disadvantage:** Multiple boluses will be needed as only 30% of the fluid will be retained.

**Complications:**

Excess volume transfusion can result in the following:
- Extravascular accumulation of fluid in the skin, connective tissue, lungs, etc.
- Inhibits gastrointestinal motility
- Hypercoagulability.

## Colloids

The fluid consists of large molecular weight substances which will remain in the intravascular compartment. This will result in generation of oncotic pressure. They will not cross the semipermeable membranes and will stay in the intravascular compartment for a longer time.

### Intravenous Colloids Fluids
- Albumin
- Hetastarch
- Dextran
- Haemaccel
- Gelatin 4%.

**Advantages:**
- Colloids contain larger molecules
- Expansion of intravascular compartment for longer time.

**Disadvantage:** Risk of anaphylaxis.

## Blood Products
- Red blood cells
- Platelets
- Fresh frozen plasma.

## Uses of Intravenous Fluids
- Acute fluid resuscitation in hypovolemia like sepsis, hemorrhage, diarrhea, vomiting, burns, etc.
- Maintenance fluids in bowel obstruction and perioperative period.

## INTRAVENOUS FLUID REQUIREMENTS

Holliday Segar formula for maintenance fluid requirements.

| Weight (kg) | Fluid requirement (mL/day) |
|---|---|
| <10 kg | 100 mL/kg |
| 11–20 | 1,000 mL +50 mL/kg for each kg >10 |
| >20 | 1,500 + 20 mL/kg for each kg >20 |

- The patients receiving intravenous fluids should be weighed daily. An increase of body weight by more than 5% will indicate fluid overload
- A decrease of body weight by more than 5% will indicate dehydration
- Check for edema:
  - If the patient receives more than 50% of the maintenance fluid through intravenous route, the serum electrolytes should be checked daily. If the serum sodium is less than 130 mmol/L, the fluid should be changed.
  - If the serum sodium is more than 150 mmol/L, dehydration or sodium excess should be suspected.

**Calculation of rate of transfusion of the fluid**
- 1 mL = 60 microdrops
- 1 mL = 15 macrodrops

Calculate the amount of fluid to be infused in one hour. Suppose you have to transfuse 600 mL in 6 hours. Then it will be 100 mL per hour

The rate of drip can be calculated as follows:

*Microdrops:*

$$100\ mL = 100 \times 60 = 600\ microdrops$$

Drops for 1 minute—

$$6000/60 = 100\ drops$$

(Calculate the mL to be transfused in 1 hour. If 60 mL is to be transfused in 1 hour, it will be 60 microdrops per minute. Divide this by 4 to calculate the macrodrops)

*Macrodrops:*

$$100 \text{ mL} = 100 \times 15 = 1{,}500 \text{ macrodrops}$$

Drops for 1 minute—

$$1{,}500/60 = 25 \text{ drops}$$

*Calculate the fluid needed for one hour:*

*Microdrops:* The rate of transfusion for one minute will be equal to the fluid needed for 1 hour. If the fluid needed is 50 mL per hour, then the rate of microdrops will be 50 drops per minute.

*Macrodrops:* The rate of transfusion for 1 minute will be equal to the fluid needed for 1 hour divided by 4. If the fluid needed is 60 mL per hour, then the rate of microdrops will be 60 divided by 4, i.e. 15 drops per minute.

**Composition of commonly used parenteral solutions**

| Fluids | Osmolarity (mOsm /L) | Glucose (g/L) | Na (mEq/L) | Cl (mEq/L) | K (mEq/L) | Others |
|---|---|---|---|---|---|---|
| 5% D/W | 252 | 50 | – | – | – | – |
| 10% D/W | 505 | 100 | – | – | – | – |
| 50% D/W | 2520 | 500 | – | – | – | – |
| Isolyte P | 368 | 50 | 25–26 | 22 | 20 | Acetate: 23 |
| DNS | 432 | 50 | 154 | 154 | – | – |
| ½ DNS | | 50 | 77 | 77 | | |
| 0.45% NaCl ½ Isotonic saline | 154 | 25 | 77 | 77 | – | – |
| 0.9% NaCl isotonic saline | 308 | 50 | 154 | 154 | – | – |
| 3% NaCl | 1026 | – | 513 | 513 | – | – |
| 5% saline | 1616 | – | 855 | 855 | – | – |
| Ringer's lactate | 273 | | 130 | 109 | 4 | Bicarbonate/lactate: 28 mEq/L Calcium: 2.7 |

## QUESTIONS

**Q1. What are the hydrating fluids?**
Hydrating fluids are the following:
- ☐ 5% DNS
- ☐ Normal saline
- ☐ Acetated ringer

**Q2. What are the fluids used as volume expanders?**
- ☐ Normal saline
- ☐ Ringer lactate
- ☐ "O" group Rh negative blood

**Q3. What is the rate of administration of volume expanders?**
Volume expanders should be administered over 5 to 10 minutes.

**Q4. What are precautions to be taken while administering volume expanders in a preterm baby ?**
Too rapid administration of volume expanders will result in increased cerebral blood flow which will result in bleeding in immature germinal matrix.

# Intravenous Fluids

**Q5. How will you treat hyponatremia?**
Sodium deficit can be calculated by the following formula:

*Sodium deficit = (135 - observed sodium) × weight in kg × 0.6*

Part of this deficit should be corrected by using 3% NaCl until the sodium level raises to 125 mEq/L. Then the deficit should be corrected slowly over 24 hours.

**Q6. How will you treat hypokalemia?**
Serum potassium less than 3.5 mEq/L should be treated. The concentration of potassium in the fluid can be increased to 20 mEq/L by adding potassium into the intravenous fluid. It should not be pushed directly intravenously. 1 mL can be added only when the urine output is good.

**Q7. What are the intravenous fluids used as volume expanders?**
Volume expanders are:
- Whole blood (O negative Rh-negative blood crossmatched with mother's blood)
- Normal saline
- Ringer's lactate
- 5% albumin

**Q8. What is the amount for volume expanders used in newborn babies? What are the indications and precautions?**
Dosage—10 mL/kg
The amount of the volume expanders required will depend upon the weight of the child:

| Weight | Total |
| --- | --- |
| 1 kg | 10 mL |
| 2 kg | 20 mL |
| 3 kg | 30 mL |
| 4 kg | 40 mL |

*Indications*:
- Baby not responding to resuscitation
- Evidence of blood loss like pale color, weak pulses, persistently high or low heart rate.

*Precautions*: Give over 5–10 minutes.

**Q9. Which is the most physiological intravenous fluid?**
Ringer lactate.

**Q10. Which intravenous fluid is rich in sodium?**
Normal saline, DNS.

**Q11. Which intravenous fluid is rich in potassium?**
Isolyte P.

**Q12. Which intravenous fluid does not contain glucose?**
Normal saline.

**Q13. Which intravenous fluid does not contain sodium?**
Dextrose.

**Q14. Which intravenous fluid does not contain potassium?**
Normal saline, DNS, dextrose.

**Q15. What are the intravenous fluids useful in correcting acidosis?**
Ringer lactate, Isolyte P.

**Q16. How much amount of colloids or crystalloids is needed to replace 1 mL of blood loss?**
1 mL of blood loss can be replaced by 1 mL of colloid or 3 mL of crystalloids.

## CRYSTALLOIDS

### ½ DNS

- Half normal saline with 5% dextrose
- Used in conditions where $Na^+$ and $K^+$ are normal.

### Contents

- 4.5 g of NaCl is dissolved in 1,000 mL of water.
  - Contains 75 mEq/L of sodium ion
  - Contains 75 mEq/L of chloride ion

- pH: 5.5 (4.5 to 7.0)
- Osmolarity 154 mOsm /L
❖ ½ DNS will contain 5 g/100 mL
❖ Contains no potassium.

## Indications

Used in conditions with elevated potassium.

## Half Normal Saline (½ NS)

❖ 0.45 NaCl
❖ Hypotonic saline
❖ With 5% dextrose contains 77 mEq/L of sodium and chloride.

## Contents

Half normal saline contains:
❖ 0.45 normal saline
❖ $Na^+$ 77 mmol/L
❖ Cl 77 mmol/L
❖ Osmolarity 154 mOsm/L
❖ 50 g/L dextrose.

## Uses

Maintenance fluid therapy.

## Complications

❖ Hyponatremia
❖ Cerebral edema
❖ Central pontine demyelinosis
❖ Precautions
❖ Should be used cautiously in patients with normal or decreased sodium levels

## 5% Dextrose

*Contents*:
❖ Contains 50 mg/mL of glucose (5 g/L of glucose)
❖ Electrolyte-free fluid containing no sodium, potassium, chloride, and calcium
❖ *Osmolarity*: 252 mOsm/L
❖ pH: 4-4.5.

## Mechanism of Action

This fluid will supply glucose and calories for metabolism.

## Pharmacological Actions

❖ Will replace fluids and provide carbohydrates
❖ Replace fluids and provide glucose
❖ Diluents for certain medicines.

## Indications

❖ Used in conjunction with salt retaining fluids
  - Renal failure
  - Hypoglycemia
  - Shock
  - *Nutritional support*: Prevents ketosis in starvation, vomiting, etc.
❖ It can be used as diluents and vehicle for administration of various drugs.

## Contraindications

❖ Allergy to dextrose
❖ Breathing problems
❖ Cerebral edema
❖ Diabetes
❖ Electrolyte imbalance—hypokalemia
❖ Food allergy
❖ Glucose levels high (severe, uncontrolled hyperglycemia)
❖ Hypovolemic shock
❖ Hyponatremia
❖ Intoxication with water
❖ Ischemic stroke (acute)
❖ Kidney disease
❖ Liver disease

Should not be given for patients on regular blood transfusion.

## Precautions

Solution should be colorless and clear. Do not use if the color is changed or any particles are seen. 5% dextrose without electrolytes should not be used for treatment of dehydration.

## Effects on Pregnancy

FDA pregnancy category C.

## Side Effects
- Allergic reactions—hives
- Burning pain—severe
- Cough
- Fever
- Glucose level increased—hyperglycemia
- Headache
- Hypokalemia
- Hyponatremia.

## Drug Interactions
- Rapid dehydration of hydralazine will occur if infused with 5% dextrose.
- If amoxicillin is diluted with 5% dextrose, use it within 1 hour.
- Compatibility—not compatible with blood and will cause hemolysis.

## Disadvantage
This fluid cannot be used for fluid resuscitation because only 10% of the fluid will stay in the intravascular compartment.

## QUESTIONS

**Q1. What is the nutritive value of 5% dextrose?**
200 kcal/L

**Q2. Why 5% dextrose is not useful in fluid resuscitation?**
It is because only less than 10 of this fluid will stay in the intravascular space.

## 10% Dextrose
- It is a hypertonic solution of dextrose
- Contains 100 g of glucose per liter
- Electrolyte-free fluid containing no sodium, potassium, chloride, and calcium
- *Osmolarity*: 505 mOsm/L.

### Mechanism of Action
- Provides calories
- Oxidized into carbon dioxide and provide 3.4 cal G of glucose.
- Peak plasma glucose level will occur in 40 minutes.

### Indications
- Parenteral nutrition
- Hypoglycemia in newborn babies especially preterm.

### Contraindications
- Intracranial or intraspinal hemorrhage
- This should not be sued as maintenance fluid.

### Precautions
- As it is a hypertonic fluid, it should be infused slowly through a small bore needle into a large vein.
- Should not be infused along with blood transfusion as pseudoagglutination of red cells may occur.
- Rapid administration may predispose to hyperosmolar syndrome.
- Should be used cautiously in patients with diabetes.

### Effects on Pregnancy
Category C.

### Side Effects
- Diarrhea
- Electrolyte imbalance
- Extravasation, tissue necrosis
- Fever
- Glucose level increased—hyperglycemia
- Hypervolemia
- Hyperosmolar syndrome
- Hypomagnesemia
- Hypophosphatemia
- Infection—phlebitis
- Increased thirst—polydipsia
- Pulmonary edema
- Venous thrombosis.

## 25% Dextrose
- Hypertonic solution of dextrose in water
- Contains 250 g of glucose per liter.

### Mechanism of Action
Provides glucose, a source of calories.

### Pharmacological Actions
- Provides calories
- Supplies water for hydration
- Helps in sparing body proteins
- May produce diuresis.

### Dosage
Newborn—1-2 mL/kg/dose only for correction of hypoglycemia. Should not be sued as a maintenance fluid.

### Indications
- Treatment of acute episodes of symptomatic hypoglycemia
- Used as a source of energy in total parenteral nutrition.

### Contraindications
- Intracranial or intraspinal hemorrhage
- Increased intracranial tension
- Hypovolemic states
- Hyperglycemia
- Patients at risk for shift of fluid into third space
- Do not use in patients with head injury as its tonicity is slow.

### Precautions
- Should not be administered subcutaneously or intramuscularly
- Monitor blood glucose frequently
- Rapid infusion may cause hyperglycemia or hyperosmolar syndrome with loss of consciousness
- Monitor electrocardiograph (ECG) continuously
- Monitor the blood pressure, pulse, and respiratory rates.

### Side Effects
- Phlebitis
- Thrombosis
- Hyperosmolar syndrome
- Hyperglycemia
- Fluid overload
- Hyponatremia
- Hypokalemia
- Water intoxication.

## DNS
- Contains dextrose and normal saline 0.9%.
- Infusion of fluids with low osmolality can cause problems hence dextrose is added to normal saline. This will maintain same osmolarity levels and at the same time provide sodium chloride.

### Composition
- Contains 154 mEq/L of sodium ion
- Contains 154 mEq/L of chloride ion
- pH: 5.5 (4.5 to 7.0)
- 5% DNS will contain 5 g of glucose/100 mL (50 g/L)

### Osmolarity
- 154 mOsml/L
- *pH: 4.0 (3.2 to 6.5)*
- Calorie content: 170 kcal/L

### Pharmacological Actions
- Source of water
- Fluid and electrolyte replenishment
- Supplies glucose and restores blood glucose levels
- Can induce diuresis
- Source of carbohydrate
- Supplies extracellular electrolytes
- Increases blood volume.

### Dosage
Depends upon the age, weight, and clinical condition.

### Indications
- Hypovolemia: Blood and fluid loss—correction of fluid deficit

- Maintenance fluid in suspected meningitis cases
- Acute neurological conditions
- Hypoglycemia
- Vomiting induced alkalosis or hypochloremia.

## Contraindications

- Anasarca (cardiac, hepatic, renal)
- Congestive cardiac failure
- Hypertension
- Intracranial hemorrhage
- Intraspinal hemorrhage
- Liver cirrhosis
- Renal dysfunction
- Edema due to sodium retention
- Severe hypovolemic shock.

## Precautions

- This should be used carefully in the conditions such as congestive cardiac failure
- Severe renal insufficiency will predispose to edema with sodium retention
- DNS should be used cautiously in overt or subclinical diabetes
- Should not be injected intramuscularly or subcutaneously.

## Side Effects

- Fever
- Hypokalemia
- Hypervolemia
- Hyperosmolar syndrome
- Infections: Phlebitis
- Overhydration
- Pulmonary edema
- Sodium retention in patients with renal failure
- Venous thrombosis.

## Drug Interactions

- Compatible with blood
- Dextrose with low electrolyte should not be infused with blood which may cause hemolysis
- Should not be used along with indomethacin, oxytocin, and terbutaline.

## Compatibility

Compatible with blood.

# QUESTIONS

**Q1. What is the problem with excess administration of DNS?**
Excess use of DNS will predispose to hypokalemia.

**Q2. Can DNS be used to correct renal failure?**
Dextrose containing fluids may cause hyperglycemia and should not be used for bolus administration to correct shock.

## Isolyte P

Isotonic pediatric maintenance solution.

*One liter of Isolyte P will contain the following:*

- Sodium ion: 26 mEq/L
- Chloride: 21 mEq/L
- Potassium ion: 20 mEq/L
- Magnesium: 03
- Phosphate: 03
- Acetate: 23
- Glucose: 5 g/100 mL
- pH—5.0 (4.0 to 6.0)
- Osmolarity 340 mOsm/L

## Mechanism of Action

It will provide electrolytes, calories and water for hydration.

## Dosage

Depends upon the age, weight, and health status.

## Indications

- Dehydration in children who require less electrolytes and more water.

- Electrolyte imbalance
- Isolyte P is used as maintenance fluid in treatment of diarrhea.

### Contraindications
- Hyponatremia
- Renal failure.

### Precaution
Should be used cautiously in renal impairment.

### Side Effects
- Allergic reactions
- Weakness
- Muscle twitching
- Seizures
- *Volume overload*: Edema of hands and feet.

## Ringer Lactate
- Isotonic with blood
- Crystalloids
- *One liter of RL will contain the following:*
  - Sodium ion: 130 mEq/L
  - Chloride: 109 mEq/L
  - Lactate: 28 mEq/L
  - Potassium ion: 4 mEq/L
  - Calcium ion: 1.5 mEq/L
  - Osmolarity: 273–275 mOsm/L
  - pH: 5.1–6.5

The electrolyte composition is similar to extracellular fluid.

### Mechanism of Action
*Corrects metabolic acidosis*: The lactate will be converted into bicarbonate in the liver. The by-product bicarbonate of lactate metabolism in the liver will counteract acidosis and provide buffering capacity.

### Pharmacological Actions
Can induce diuresis. It is the most physiological fluid and can be used to expand intravascular volume. This will maintain normal extracellular fluid and electrolyte balance.

### Dosage
- 20–30 mL/kg body weight/hour
- Can be given intravenously or subcutaneously.

### Indications
- Hypovolemia
- Blood loss after trauma, surgery, burns injury
- Diabetic ketoacidosis
- Severe dehydration
- Acidosis due to renal failure

*Ringer lactate* used in treating severe dehydration to correct intracellular dehydration.

### Contraindications
- Addison's disease
- Should not be given along with blood or blood products
- In severe congestive cardiac failure
- Drugs—along with amphotericin, thiopental, ampicillin, doxycycline
- Emesis or NGT aspiration induced alkalosis
- Liver diseases (impair conversion of lactate)
- Hypoxia (severe)
- Hypersensitivity to sodium lactate
- Severe metabolic acidosis which will impair conversion of lactate
- Shock—impair conversion of lactate
- Should not be used for maintenance therapy.

### Precautions
- The sodium content is too low about 130 mEq/L and the potassium content is low about 4 mEq/L.
- Should be given carefully in patients with hyperkalemia or conditions predisposing to hyperkalemia like severe renal failure, adrenocortical insufficiency, acute dehydration, extensive tissue injury, burns, and cardiac diseases.

- As potassium level is similar to plasma, this should not be used to treat hypokalemia.
- Should be given carefully in patients with alkalosis or conditions predisposing to alkalosis.
- Should be given carefully in patients with sodium or potassium retention or conditions predisposing to edema.
- Lactate is a substrate for gluconeogenesis and should be given cautiously in patients with type 2 diabetes.
- Should be given carefully in patients with hypercalcemia or conditions predisposing to hypercalcemia.

## Effects on Pregnancy
Not known.

## Side Effects
- Anaphylactic reactions
- Anaphylactoid reactions
- Lactate will be converted to bicarbonate and will predispose to alkalosis
- Fluid overload
- Pulmonary edema
- Acid–base imbalance
- Dilution of serum electrolytes
- Hyperlactatemia can occur in patients with liver failure due to failure of metabolism of lactate
- Thiazides and vitamin D can cause hypercalcemia and RL should be administered cautiously.

## Drug Interactions
- Ceftriaxone and RL should not be given together in same line.
- Corticosteroids will cause sodium and potassium retention.
- Renal clearance of lithium, salicylates, and barbiturates will be increased.

## Compatibility
Should not be used with blood as the calcium binds with citrate. Also the anticoagulant activity will be decreased.

## QUESTIONS

**Q1. What is the advantage of RL over isotonic saline?**
Ringer lactate will maintain a stable pH as compared to isotonic saline.

**Q2. Can acetate be used instead of lactate?**
Yes, it will be useful in severe shock.

## Normal Saline
- Physiological saline or isotonic saline
- It is a solution of 0.9% strength of sodium chloride in water.
- *Contents of physiological or isotonic saline:*
  - 0.90% w/v of NaCl
  - 9 g of NaCl is dissolved in 1,000 mL of water.
- *Electrolyte concentration:*
  - Contains 154 mEq/L of sodium ion
  - Contains 154 mEq/L of chloride ion
  - pH: 5.5–6.0 (4.5 to 7.0)
  - Osmolarity 308 mOsm/L which is slightly higher than that of plasma.
- Iso-osmolar compared to plasma
- Normal saline will not contain any glucose
- 5% DNS will contain 5 g/100 mL.

## Mechanism of Action
- This will correct water and electrolyte deficit.
- Provide major extracellular electrolytes and increase the intravascular volume.

## Dosage
Depends on the age, weight, and the clinical condition of the patient.

## Indications
- Used as a source of water and electrolytes
- Alkalosis with dehydration
- Bolus administration in hypovolemic shock
- Cleaning of wounds
- Diabetic ketoacidosis
- Eye drops

- Fluid challenge in prerenal failure
- Gastrointestinal water and salt loss in vomiting and diarrhea
- Hypovolemia (Most appropriate fluid for bolus)
- Hypercalcemia
- Hyponatremia
- Initial volume resuscitation on septic shock, trauma
- Used in correcting hyponatremia, diabetic ketoacidosis
- Used in administration of vasopressor agents like noradrenaline
- Vehicle for drugs.

### Contraindications
- Allergic to normal saline
- Blood urea nitrogen (BUN) elevated in renal disease
- Congestive cardiac failure
- Cirrhosis
- Dehydration with severe hypokalemia
- Eclampsia or preeclampsia.

### Precautions
In patients with decreased renal functions, sodium retention can occur. It should be used carefully in patients with congestive cardiac failure, edema, and others stated with sodium retention.

### Side Effects
- Fever
- Phlebitis
- Thrombosis
- Larger volume infusion can result in the following:
  - Hypervolemia
  - Metabolic acidosis (Hyperchloremic)
  - Hypernatremia
  - Osmotic demyelination syndrome.

### Complications
- Rapid administration will predispose to pulmonary edema.
- Due to excess chloride ions and lack of buffering capacity, metabolic acidosis can occur. Excess chloride loading will lead to disproportionate urinary bicarbonate loss. Excess chloride will suppress renin release, reduced aldosterone, and decreased bicarbonate retention.
- When large quantities are administered, hyperchloremic metabolic acidosis can occur due to high sodium and chloride content.

### Drug Interactions
- Will interact with corticosteroids and corticotropin.
- Compatible with most drugs and blood products.

## QUESTIONS

**Q1. What is normal saline?**
0.9% sodium chloride.

**Q2. What is half normal saline?**
0.45% sodium chloride is known as half normal saline. It contains 4.5 g/L sodium chloride. It contains 77 mEq/L of sodium and 77mEq/L of chloride.

**Q3. What is hypertonic saline?**
7.5% sodium chloride is known as hypertonic saline.
This will replace sodium and water lost during dehydration.

**Q4. What are the conditions in which normal saline is used?**
☐ Diabetic ketoacidosis
☐ Shock therapy—20 mL/kg.

## Hypertonic Saline
3% NaCl.

### Contents
- Contains 513 mEq/L of sodium and chloride
- $Na^+$ 513 mmol/L

- Cl⁻ 513 mmol/L
- Osmolality—1026 mOsm/L
- pH—5.0
- 1 mL of 3% saline will provide 0.5 mEq of sodium.

## Indications
- Treatment of symptomatic hyponatremia when sodium less than 120 mEq/L
- 3-4 mL/kg over 1-2 hours
- Severe hyponatremia
- Resuscitation of severe hypovolemic shock
- Mucoactive agents which will hydrate thick secretions.

## Side Effects
- Phlebitis
- Necrosis
- Hemolysis.

## Precautions
- Should be administered slowly
- Hypertonic solutions should be infused through a central line
- Rapid correction of hyponatremia using hypertonic saline will increase the risk for central pontine myelinosis
- Should be used cautiously in patients with congestive cardiac failure, severe renal insufficiency, and edema with sodium retention.

# COLLOIDS

Colloids are mixtures where a solid phase is dispersed in a liquid phase. The size of dispersed solid particle may range from 1 nanometer to 1,000 nanometers. Liquid that exerts osmotic pressure due to large particles with molecular weight more than 30,000 in the solution. The colloids can be natural or artificial.

The following are some of the colloids used:
- *Natural colloids:*
  - 5% albumin
- *Artificial colloids:*
  - Dextran (6% dextran 70, 10% dextran 40)
  - Haemaccel
  - Starch derivatives
  - Hydroxyethyl starch
  - Pentastarch
  - Hetastarch
  - Plasma
  - Gelatin.

## Advantages
- Colloids contain certain particles which do not cross the permeable membranes like capillary membrane. Thus the whole volume infused will stay in the intravascular compartment for a prolonged time than crystalloids.
- Colloids preserve high colloid osmotic pressure in the blood.
- These particles stay longer in the intravascular compartment.
- More effective in restoring blood volume as compared to crystalloids.
- Dextrans have osmotic pressure similar to plasma.
- Interfere with normal coagulation by hemodilution of clotting factors and coating platelets and vascular endothelium.

## Disadvantages
- Since colloids have gelatinous properties, they will cause platelet dysfunction.
- Colloids can interfere with fibrinolysis and coagulation factors like factor VIII resulting in coagulopathy.
- Can cause coagulopathy in large volumes.
- Increased adverse reactions.
- Not readily available.
- Costly.

## Precautions
- Colloids should not be used as sole fluid replacement.
- In cases of severe injury to the capillary membranes like trauma and burns, colloids will leak out.

## Uses
Colloids are used as volume expanders in patients with fluid loss.

| Colloid | Effective plasma volume expansion/100 mL | Duration (Hours) |
|---|---|---|
| 5% albumin | 70–130 mL | 16 |
| 25% albumin | 400–500 mL | 16 |
| Hetastarch | 100–130 mL | 24 |
| Pentastarch | 150 mL | 8 |
| Dextran 40 | 100–130 mL | 6 |
| Dextran 70 | 80 mL | 12 |

## 5% Albumin

- It contains plasma protein fractions from human plasma comprising of 50-60% of all plasma proteins.
- 100 mL of 25% albumin is equal to 25 g of albumin
- 500 mL of 5% albumin is equal to 25 g of albumin
- Available as 5%, 20%, and 25% albumin
- They are natural colloids
- Albumin is synthesized only in the liver
- Half-life is approximately 20 days.

### Mechanism of Action

- Both 5% and 25% albumin are volume expanders
- 5% solution will increase 80% of volume
- 25% solution will increase 200-400% increase in volume
- It will draw about 3-4 times its volume of additional fluid into the circulation in about 15 minutes.
- Mobilize fluid from the interstitial compartment to intravascular space
- It causes volume expansion and protein replacement
- It increases intravascular oncotic pressure.

### Dosage

- 25 g can be repeated after 15–30 minutes
- The total dose should not exceed 250 g/48 h
- *Rate of infusion*:
  - 5% albumin: 1-2 mL/min
  - 25% albumin: 1 mL/min
- Hypovolemic shock—initial bolus can be given rapidly. Once a normal volume is achieved.
- 5% albumin—5–10 mL/min
- 20% solution—2 mL/min
- 25% albumin—2-3 mL/min.

### Indications

- 5% infusion can be given for volume replacement.
  - Acute liver disease
  - Albumin less than 1.5 g/kg body weight
  - Burns
  - Cardiothoracic surgery
  - Cardiopulmonary bypass
  - Decreased blood volume in hypovolemic shock
  - Exchange—plasma exchange transfusion
- 25% albumin can be used for increasing the oncotic pressure.
  - Acute nephrosis
  - Acute respiratory distress syndrome
  - Burns with fluid loss
  - Cardiopulmonary bypass
  - Dialysis
  - Extremely low albumin in critically ill patients (Albumin <1.5 g/kg body weight)
  - Fluid resuscitation in emergencies
  - Gross ascites tap more than 6 L
  - Hepatic failure
  - Hypoproteinemia or hypoalbuminemia
  - Hypovolemic shock
  - Hemodialysis.

### Contraindications

- Hypersensitivity to albumin and albumin products
- Cardiac failure
- Severe anemia
- 25% albumin may cause intraventricular hemorrhage in preterm babies.

### Precautions

- These should be used within 4 hours of dilution or else should be discarded.
- 5% albumin should not be diluted.
- Should be stored at less than 30°C (86°F) and should not freeze.

- Should not be used, if the solution is turbid or contains any deposits.
- Facilities for cardiopulmonary resuscitation should be available during infusion of albumin.
- Infusion of 25% albumin instead of 5% albumin will predispose to volume overload. Hypervolemia and pulmonary edema can occur here.
- Sterile water should be used along with albumin.
- Should be used cautiously in chronic renal insufficiency, chronic anemia, and patients with low cardiac reserve.
- In patients with sodium restriction, it should be used cautiously because it contains 130–160 mEq/L of sodium.
- Rapid infusion of albumin can lead to increase in protein bound calcium and decrease in ionized calcium.

### Effects on Pregnancy

Risk category C, use with caution as it benefits outweigh risks.

### Side Effects

- Anaphylaxis
- Bronchospasm
- Congestive cardiac failure
- Coagulation problems
- Decreased myocardial contractility
- Edema
- Fluid retention
- Fever
- Gastrointestinal problems—nausea, vomiting
- Headache
- Hypotension
- Hypertension
- Hypervolemia
- Itching/pruritus/urticaria.

### Drug Interactions

- 25% albumin should be diluted with normal saline or D5W.
- Do not use sterile water as diluents.
- With protein hydrolysates or ethanol will precipitate.

## QUESTIONS

**Q1. What is the normal distribution of plasma albumin?**
30–40% in the plasma and 67% in extravascular compartment.

**Q2. What is the elimination half-life of albumin?**
15–20 days.

**Q3. What is the route of excretion of albumin?**
Intestinal mucosa.

## Dextran

Dextrans are highly branched polysaccharide molecules made from natural resources of sugar.

Available in various strengths as 6% dextran, 10% dextran; dextran 40; and dextran 70.

### Composition

- *Dextran 40 (10%)*:
  - Sodium—154 mEq
  - pH—6.7
  - Osmolarity—320
- *Dextran 70 (6%)*
  - Sodium—154 mEq
  - pH—6.3
  - Osmolarity—310

### Mechanism of Action

- Plasma volume expander
- Reduces red cell aggregation by coating the RBCs and increasing the electronegativity
- Restores blood volume which has lost through bleeding
- Reduces blood viscosity and improves microcirculation
- Excretes by kidneys
- Improves microcirculatory flow.

## Advantages

- More volume expansion than 5% albumin and hydroxyethyl strach (HES)
- Improves microcirculation
- Inhibits platelet aggregation.

## Disadvantage

Precipitate acute renal failure.

## Indications

- Hypovolemia
- During microsurgery
- Used in extracorporeal circulation (ECC) during cardiopulmonary bypass
- Prophylaxis for deep vein thrombosis
- Myocardial ischemia
- Cerebral ischemia
- Priming in extracorporeal circulation.

## Contraindications

- Kidney disease or acute renal failure
- Congestive cardiac failure
- Uncontrolled bleeding
- Hypersensitivity reaction to dextran.

## Precautions

- Asthma
- Allergy
- Breathing problems
- Bleeding or blood clotting disorders
- Cardiovascular disorders
- Circulatory overload
- Congestive cardiac failure
- Diabetes
- Dehydration (severe)
- Epilepsy
- Food allergy
- Fluid retention
- Gastrointestinal tract (GIT) disorders.
- Hematological problems—hemophilia and thrombocytopenic purpura
- Intestinal disorders
- Joint pain
- Kidney disorders
- Liver disorders
- Migraine
- Patients on low salt diet.

## Side Effects

- Anaphylactic reactions
- Bruising
- Breathing problems—weak breathing and wheezing
- Coagulation abnormalities
- Chest tightness
- Cerebral edema
- Dysfunction of platelets
- Emesis
- Electrolyte disturbances
- Fluid overload—pulmonary edema
- Gastrointestinal problems—nausea
- Hyponatremia
- Infection at the site of injection causes phlebitis which extends from the site of injection
- Joint pain
- Kidney failure
- Pain
- Swelling.

## Drug Interactions

- Dextran will interfere with blood grouping and cross matching.
- Will enhance the effect of heparin.

# QUESTIONS

**Q1.** What are the disadvantages of dextran infusion?
- ❑ Cheap
- ❑ Shelf life about 10 years
- ❑ Reduces blood viscosity
- ❑ Circulation and microcirculation are improved.

**Q2.** What are the advantages of dextran infusion?
- ❑ Dextrans will interfere with blood grouping and cross matching.
- ❑ Higher volume expansion as compared to HES and 5% albumin.

### Q3. How will you administer dextran?
- Rapid infusion in patients with shock
- Should not exceed 20 mL/kg in the first 24 hours and 10 mL/kg/day in the next 5 days.

## Haemaccel

### Composition
- Contains degraded gelatin polymers
- NaCl—145 mEq
- Ca—2.5 mEq

### Mechanism of Action
- Plasma expander that will replace the lost blood volume and it increases calcium levels.
- Plasma substitutes for volume replacement will improve the microcirculation.
- Contains calcium chloride, potassium chloride, and sodium chloride.
- 50% will be excreted in 4-8 hours of administration. Complete excretion will occur in 48 hours.

### Dosage
- Dose should be adjusted depending upon the response to treatment.
- The rate and duration of infusion will depend upon the existing volume deficit.
- In shock due to hypovolemia up to 2,000 mL can be given.
- In emergencies, the fluid can be used rapidly about 500 mL in 5-15 minutes.

### Indications
- Used for prevention of shock due to reduction in effective circulating volume due to hemorrhage.
- Blood loss and loss of blood volume
- Hypovolemic shock
- Used in heart lung machine
- Hypocalcemia
- Hypokalemia.

### Contraindications
- *Allergic disorders*: Hypersensitivity
- Atrioventricular (AV) block
- Anuria-renal or postrenal
- Bleeding disorders
- Congestive cardiac failure (on rapid infusion)
- Dehydration
- Esophageal varices
- Fluid overload, sodium retention, edema, and pulmonary edema
- Geriatric age
- Hypersensitivity to the constituents
- Hypertension
- Hyperkalemia.

### Precautions
- Do not infuse in cold state
- Do not mix with citrated blood
- Only clear fluids should be infused reactions caused by histamine release can be prevented by use of histamine $H_1$ and $H_2$ receptor antagonists
- The haemaccel should be used carefully in patients with congestive cardiac failure, esophageal varices, bleeding diathesis, pulmonary edema, postrenal anuria, and renal insufficiency.

### Effects on Pregnancy
Not contraindicated.

### Side Effects
Reactions can be caused by histamine release:
- Anorexia
- Abdominal pain
- Bloating of abdomen
- Cardiac toxicity
- Constipation
- Diarrhea
- Emesis
- Flush—hot flush
- Gustatory problems—chalky taste
- Hypotension.

## Drug Interactions
With cardiac glycosides, calcium in haemaccel will have a synergistic effect.

## Compatibility
Haemaccel can be used with saline, glucose solutions, and Ringer's lactate, etc.

## Advantages
- Antibody is not produced since it is not immunogenic
- Blood grouping is not affected
- Coagulation is not impaired
- Degraded by endogenous proteases
- Eliminated completely and unchanged through kidneys and intestines and no retention occurs
- Freezing and thawing will not affect haemaccel
- Does not get stored in the tissues
- Lowers viscosity of blood.

# Hetastarch
Hydroxyethyl starch is made from the natural sources of highly branched starch like amylopectin. This is a highly branched compound of starch.

## Mechanism of Action
- Increases the blood plasma volume
- Increases blood volume by increasing the blood plasma volume
- The improvement in volume will last for 24 hours or more.
- 6% hetastarch will be iso-oncotic.

## Dosage
- 500–1,000 mL/kg up to a maximum of 1,500 mL/day.
- Maximum dose 20 mL/kg.

## Indications
Hypovolemia due to blood loss from injury, surgery, burns, trauma, etc.

## Contraindications
- Allergy to hetastarch and corn
- Acidosis—lactic acidosis
- Bleeding disorders
- Clotting disorder
- Congestive cardiac failure
- Critically, ill patients
- Dialysis patients
- Intracranial bleeding
- Kidney dysfunction
- Liver dysfunction.

## Precautions
- Monitor complete blood count, differential count, hemoglobin, hematocrit, prothrombin time, and partial thromboplastin time.
- Hetastarch can damage kidneys. If creatinine clearance is less than 10 mL/minute, further dose should be reduced by 20–50%. Monitor the renal function for at least 90 days after infusion.
- Hetastarch and citrate should be mixed thoroughly for effective anticoagulation.
- Hetastarch is not eliminated by hemodialysis or peritoneal dialysis.
- Do not freeze and avoid excessive heat.
- Change in color or formation of crystalline precipitate is a contraindication for its use.

## Effects on Pregnancy and Lactation
Category C.

## Side Effects
- Anxiety
- Allergy
- Anaphylaxis
- Anaphylactoid reactions
- Breathing problems
- Coagulation abnormalities
- Chest pain
- Chills
- Cardiovascular—bradycardia, tachycardia, circulatory overload, and peripheral edema
- Drooping of eyelids
- Easy bruising

- Edema (pulmonary/peripheral)
- Emesis
- Fever
- Flu-like symptoms
- Fluid overload
- Glandular enlargement (submaxillary, parotid)
- Headache
- Hemodilution
- Hypersensitivity reactions
- Hematologic—bleeding, bruising, coagulopathy, and hemodilution
- Itching
- Kidney impairment or injury
- Light-headed feeling
- Musculoskeletal—muscle pain
- Metabolic acidosis
- Noncardiogenic pulmonary edema
- Pruritus due to deposition of hydroxyl ethyl starch in the peripheral nerves
- Skin—severe skin reactions and skin rash
- Features of kidney dysfunction include:
    - Amount of urine altered—anuria or oliguria
    - Blood in the urine
    - Breathing problems
    - Color of urine changed
    - Dysuria
    - Edema of legs, ankles, feet, hands
    - Fatigue
    - Flapping tremors in renal failure
    - Facial puffiness
    - GIT symptoms—nausea and vomiting.

## Drug Interactions
- Use with normal saline is contraindicated as it will increase sodium and chloride levels.
- The following drugs will interact with hetastarch:
    - Warfarin
    - Digoxin
    - Diuretics.

## Advantages
- Cheap
- Cost effective
- Good volume expansion.

## Disadvantages
- Coagulation problems
- Expensive
- Rapidly expands the intravascular volume.

# Gelatin
- Gelatins are formed by hydrolysis of collagen.
- Low molecular weight proteins.

## Mechanism of Action
Volume expander used as plasma replacement increases blood volume, flow, cardiac output, and oxygen transportation.

## Indications
- Blood loss
- Rapid volume expansion
- Hypotension
- Dehydration.

## Contraindications
- Hypersensitivity
- Liver disease.

## Advantages
- 70–80% volume expansion
- Can be used in renal impairment
- Does not affect coagulation.

## Disadvantages
- Unpleasant taste
- Heartburn

## Side Effects
- Anaphylactoid reactions
- Hypersensitivity
- Hypotension or hypertension
- Dyspnea.

## Complications
- Arrhythmias
- Belching
- Bloating

## BLOOD PRODUCTS

Whole blood is not used often for transfusion. Blood products are therapeutic substance prepared from human blood. These include blood components including packed cells, plasma, cryoprecipitate, fresh frozen plasma, etc.

## Red Blood Cells
- Dose of packed red cells 10 mL/kg
- Fresh blood 20 mL/kg.

## Platelets Concentrate

Platelets are produced by apheresis.

### Indications

Thrombocytopenia—platelet count $10 \times 10^9$/L.

### Precautions

Blood cross matching should be done before transfusion of platelet concentrates.

### Side Effects
- Allergic reactions
- Infection
- Lung injury.

## Fresh Frozen Plasma

Plasma is frozen within 24 hours after collection by phlebotomy.

### Indications
- Replacement of clotting factor in deficiency
- Antithrombin III deficiency
- Plasma exchange
- Thrombotic thrombocytopenic purpura.

### Precautions

This should not be used as a volume expander.

### Side Effects
- Allergy
- Blood clotting
- Infections
- Transfusion related lung injury.

# CHAPTER 7

# Vaccines

## CHAPTER OUTLINE

- Vaccines for General Use
- Vaccines Used on Special Occasions
- Combination of Vaccines
- Duration of Protection Offered by Vaccines
- Contradictions Precautions for Immunization
- Vaccination Failure
- Vaccine Storage
- Adverse Events following Vaccination
- National Vaccine Injury Compensation Program

## INTRODUCTION

### Immunization and Vaccines–A View

Every year number of new vaccines are added to already overloaded schedule. There are lot of confusions among the public and the medical practitioners regarding the immunization schedule and vaccines. Number of vaccines are pouring into the market. Many manufacturers are advertising them in a manner which threatens the public and even the medical people. First of all one should have the basic knowledge of vaccines. Also a number of disorders like autism, dyslexia, asthma, and diabetes mellitus are on the rise. It is well known that environmental factors will predispose to these conditions. It is important to verify if vaccines or adjuvants used for vaccines play a role.

Immunization is introduction of any substance or organism (live attenuated, killed or a part of the organism), thereby inducing a primary immune response

There are two types of immunization, active and passive.

1. *Active immunization* involves stimulating the host to produce prolonged humoral (antibodies) and/or cellular immune response to the pathogenic agent causing disease by administering a vaccine or toxoid.
2. *Passive immunization* is immunity induced passively by administration of antibody containing preparations to induce protection against an infectious agent.

### Vaccines

The vaccines will contain an agent that will resemble the disease causing microorganism and are made from weakened or killed form of the microorganism or toxins or one of its surface proteins.

### Live Vaccines (Live Attenuated Vaccines)

The virulent organism is weakened by multiple subcultures in unfavorable conditions so that it will induce antigenic response without disease which produces immunity by causing mild infection.

Live vaccines containing inactivated microorganisms are—BCG, polio, measles, mumps, and rubella, varicella, rotavirus, hepatitis A, and live attenuated influenza which produce immunity by causing mild infection.

| Type | Example |
|---|---|
| Bacterial | BCG, oral typhoid |
| Viral | Polio, measles, mumps, rubella. Varicella, rotavirus, hepatitis A, live attenuated influenza |

*The advantages of live vaccines:*
- Extremely potent
- Usually produce life-long immunity
- Single dose provides adequate immunity.

*The disadvantages of live vaccines:*
- Cannot be given to immunocompromised individuals
- Potential danger of transmitting disease
- Possible reactivation in the host.

*The contraindications of live vaccines:*
- Hypogammaglobulinemia
- Leukemia
- Lymphoma
- Drugs (corticosteroids, immunosuppressant drugs)
- Immunosuppressive states: HIV with low CD4 count, 8 weeks post IVIg therapy.

### killed/Inactivated Vaccines

*Killed vaccines (killed or inactivated vaccines)* are prepared from virulent organisms inactivated by heat, phenol, formaldehyde, or some other means.

*Killed vaccines are:*

| Type | Example |
|---|---|
| Bacterial | DTwP, Pertussis vaccine, Whole cell killed Typhoid vaccine |
| Viral | Polio (inactivated) vaccine—IPV, Influenza (killed) vaccine, Rabies vaccine, Hepatitis B vaccine, Hepatitis A vaccine, Japanese B encephalitis vaccine |

*The advantages of killed vaccines:*
- Can be given to immunocompromised individuals
- No potential danger of transmitting disease.

*The disadvantages of killed vaccines:*
- Poorly immunogenic
- Require multiple dose for protection
- Short duration of immunity.

*Vaccines containing part of microorganisms:* Acellular Pertussis vaccine, HPV, and hepatitis B vaccine.

*Vaccines containing polysaccharide capsule vaccine:*
- Meningococcal C vaccine
- Pneumococcal vaccine.

*Vaccines containing polysaccharide capsule conjugated to protein carriers:*
- *Haemophilus influenzae* type b vaccine (Hib)
- Pneumococcal vaccine
- Meningococcal vaccine
- S typhi Vi—polysaccharide.

*Vaccines containing protein component known as subunit vaccine:*

| Types | Vaccines |
|---|---|
| Bacterial | Acellular pertussis vaccine |
| Viral | Influenza vaccine Hepatitis B vaccine |

**Toxoids** are modified bacterial toxins that are made nontoxic but are still able to induce active immune response against the toxin.
- Tetanus toxoid and diphtheria toxoid.

*Differences between live and killed vaccines:*

| Features | Live vaccines | Killed vaccines |
|---|---|---|
| Infection | Can cause infection | Cannot cause infection |
| Heat sensitivity | Heat labile | Heat stable |
| Number of dose | Single (3 for MMR, more for polio) | Multiple |
| Duration of immunity | Longer duration. May be lifelong | Short duration |
| Dose interval | Minimum of 4 weeks between two doses | Can be administered simultaneously |
| Booster dose | Not needed | Needed |

*Contd...*

Contd...

| Features | Live vaccines | Killed vaccines |
|---|---|---|
| Breakthrough infections | Can occur | Cannot occur |
| Immunodeficiency | Contraindicated | Can be given |
| Contraindications | Immunodeficiency | |
| Adverse reactions | Less severe May revert to virulent | More severe |

*Excipients used in a vaccine:*
- Aluminum salts and gels are used as adjuvants
- Antibiotics
- Egg protein is present in influenza and yellow fever vaccines
- Formaldehyde
- Monosodium glutamate and 2-phenoxyethanol are used as stabilizers
- Thimerosal is a mercury containing preservative used in vials that will prevent contamination and growth of potentially harmful bacteria.

*Preservatives used in a vaccine are*: Thiomersal, phenoxyethanol, and formaldehyde.

## Expanded Program on Immunization

The Government of India started the Expanded Program on Immunization (EPI) in January 1978 to reduce the incidence of common infectious diseases such as diphtheria, tetanus, pertussis, polio, tuberculosis, and Measles. The target populations were children under 1 year of age and pregnant women.

## Universal Immunization Program

In 1985, Universal Immunization Program (UIP) was introduced in India. The target populations were the children under 16 years of age and pregnant women. The vaccines recommended were BCG, DPT, OPV, and Measles.

*Catch-up vaccination:* When a vaccine is missed for a child, the vaccine can be administered at a later age. The upper age up to which the vaccine can be administered should be known.

*Lapsed immunization:* A lapse in providing the doses as per schedule is not an indication for reinitiation of the entire schedule. But if the immunization status is not known or uncertain it is better to start the schedule.

*Availability of a vaccine is not an indication for immunization:*

Availability of vaccine should not be considered as an indication for immunization of the child. One has to take into consideration of various factors like prevalence, infectivity, outcome, etc. To immunize a person against an organism, the following four criteria should be satisfied:
1. The infection should be prevalent in the area
2. The disease should be easily spread to the contacts
3. No treatment should be available
4. The disease should cause death or deformities.

Vaccines do not guarantee complete 100% protection from any diseases. No vaccine is 100% effective. No drug or vaccine is perfectly safe and adverse effects can occur following any drug or vaccination. Both doctors and parents should be aware of the indications, contraindications, and side effects of various drugs and vaccines before deciding to administer the drug or vaccine.

Report any abnormal event following a drug or vaccine so that further administration of that drug or vaccine can be prevented.

## VACCINES FOR GENERAL USE

### Bacillus Calmette–Guérin Vaccine
- A live attenuated vaccine, Bacillus Calmette-Guérin (BCG), induces cell-mediated immunity.
- BCG is given to protect against tuberculosis.

### Technical Aspects

Bacillus Calmette-Guérin vaccine contains a live attenuated strain of bovine mycobacteria prepared by 231 repeated cultures once every 3 weeks. Vaccine is derived from bovine tuberculosis strain. It was first developed in the year 1921 by French microbiologist Albert Calmette by performing 231 repeated subcultures. Two common strains in use are Copenhagen (Danish 1331) and Pasteur.

**Contents:** Freeze dried live attenuated bovine mycobacterium tuberculosis.

Vaccine contains 0.1–0.4 million live viable bacilli per dose.

**Strain:** Copenhagen and Pasteur

**Nature:** This vaccine is supplied as a lyophilized (freeze dried) in vacuum sealed multi-dose, dark colored vials with normal saline as diluent.

**Diluents used for BCG:** 20 dose vial to be diluted with 2 mL normal saline. Distilled water is not used as it will act as an irritant to the skin. Do not shake vigorously.

**Ideal age at immunization:** At birth

**Dose and schedule:**

Dose:
- 0.05–0.1 mL as suggested by the manufacturer.
- 0.05 mL for children below 4 weeks of life
- 0.1 mL after 28 days of life.
- Dose will not depend upon the age and weight of the baby. For preterm and low birth weight more than 2 Kg or after 1 month in clinically stable babies.

**Syringe:** Tuberculin syringe with 26G/27G gauge needle is used.

**Schedule:** *See* Annexure.

**Catch-up vaccination:** *See* Annexure.

**Route of administration:** Intradermal route.

**Site of administration:** In the left arm at the level of insertion of deltoid.

**Preparation of the site of administration:** Is not required. Do not use antiseptics. It was told BCG should not be given along with measles, mumps, and rubella (MMR) where a gap of 4 weeks between the two vaccines should be present but now it is said that they can be given.

**Precautions:** Do not give subcutaneously, which may result in abscess. Do not rub after injection.

**Protective efficacy:** Tuberculin conversion is almost 100%. The clinical efficacy as per various studies is 0–80%. Efficacy is 50–80% for prevention of miliary and meningeal form of tuberculosis. 50% efficacy for pulmonary tuberculosis.

**Storage:** +2 to +8°C. Reconstituted vaccine should be stored at 2–8°C.

Keep away from light.

**Precautions:** Syringe and needle used. Use tuberculin syringe with 26G/27G needle.

Should be protected from light. BCG is stored in Amber coloured vials. Vaccine is light-sensitive and deteriorates on exposure to ultraviolet rays in lyophilized form. The reconstituted vaccine should be discarded within 4–6 hours of reconstitution.

**Compatibility:** Can be concurrently given with other live vaccine, but if not given should be given only after 3 to 4 weeks of BCG vaccination.

BCG can be given with all vaccines on the same day with exception of MMR where an interval of 4 weeks is recommended.

Should not be given along with measles or MMR vaccine because MMR may cause immunosuppression facilitating dissemination of tuberculous bacilli in the vaccine.

## Clinical Aspects

BCG induces cell-mediated immunity.

## Natural History of BCG

- Evolution stages:
  - Wheal
  - Papule
  - Pustule
  - Ulceration

- Evolution of BCG scar after BCG injections is as follows:
  - Wheal: 20-30 minutes
  - Papule by 2-3 weeks increases to size of 4-8 mm by the end of 5-6 weeks
  - Induration: 3$^{rd}$ to 4$^{th}$ week
  - Lump: 6$^{th}$ week
  - Ulcer: 8$^{th}$ week
  - Scar: 10-12 weeks
  - Ulcer may persist for few weeks.
- Healing with scarring in 3 months.

## Indications: To all babies

## Contraindications and Cautions for BCG Vaccination

- AIDS
- Anaphylaxis or hypersensitivity or angio-edema to vaccine components
- Bone marrow suppression
- Cell-mediated immunodeficiency
- Congenital immunodeficiency
- Drugs—immunosuppressives, steroids, alkylating agents
- Eczema (Give at another site)
- Family history of immunodeficiency
- Generalized malignancy
- Gestational period (Pregnancy)
- Hypogammaglobulinemia
- Immunosuppressive disorders –Subacute combined immunodeficiency
- Infections like HIV infections causing immunodeficiency
- Keloid or lupoid reactions at the site of injection
- Leukemia
- Malignant lymphoma
- Sarcoidosis.

The risk of disseminated BCG infection is more in the following conditions:
- Severely immunosuppressed especially cellular immunity
- Symptomatic HIV infection
- Up to 12 weeks after measles infection (contraindicated in conditions with immunodeficiency as the risk for clinical disease is high and poor immune response will be seen).

## Side Effects of BCG

**Local:**
- Abscess formation at the site of inoculation
- Granuloma formation
- Hypertrophic scar
- Keloid formation
- Lupoid reactions
- Lupus vulgaris
- Local nonhealing ulcer
- Necrosis.

**Regional:**
- Axillary lymphadenitis—ipsilateral BCG adenitis (solitary, multiple, soft, fluctuant with sinus formation)
- Abscess due to Suppurative adenitis
- BCG complex
- Cervical adenitis (ipsilateral)
- Disseminated BCG infection in children with cellular immunodeficiency.

**Systemic:**
- Generalized dissemination (Disseminated TB)
- Scrofuloderma
- Tuberculous osteomyelitis or BCG osteitis
- BCG disease.

Severe adverse effects:
- Erythema nodosum
- Lupus like symptoms.

## Complications of BCG Vaccination

- Disseminated BCG infection in an immunocompromised child especially with cellular immunodeficiency.
- Secondary infections: Infection at the injection site. As the BCG contains no preservative, bacterial contamination can occur if it is kept for a long time after reconstitution. Toxic shock syndrome can occur.

The asymptomatic HIV-infected patients who were routinely immunized with BCG developed AIDS and showed an increased risk of developing systemic or disseminated BCG disease.

## QUESTIONS

**Q1. What is BCG test?**
BCG can be used to diagnose tuberculous infection. In already infected patients, natural response to BCG after injection of BCG vaccine will be accelerated. In conditions like severe malnutrition where Mantoux will be false negative, BCG can be used to diagnose tuberculosis.

**Q2. Doses BCG contain any preservative?**
No, BCG has no preservative, hence bacterial contamination can occur if kept for a long time after reconstitution.

**Q3. What is BCG complex?**
Local lymphadenitis, paratracheal node with positive Mantoux test.

**Q4. Why deltoid is used for BCG administration?**
- The convex surface facilitated easy observation of scar.
- Optimal lymphatic drainage of the area.

**Q5. Can BCG be given with vaccines?**
BCG can be given along with other vaccines on the same day or at any interval.

**Q6. What is the sign of successful administration of intradermal injection?**
A wheal of 5 mm at the injection site.

**Q7. What is the complication of subcutaneous administration of BCG?**
Subcutaneous administration is associated with increased incidence of BCG adenitis.

**Q8. Can BCG be given in the thigh? Why?**
No it should not be given in the thigh. Regional complications like lymphadenitis may predispose to rupture and spread of tubercular infection into the abdomen.

**Q9. Can BCG be given to babies born to HIV mothers?**
Yes it can be given at birth.

## Poliomyelitis Vaccine

Polio infection will result in paralysis of limbs which will result in lifelong handicap.

*Types of vaccines:* Two types of vaccines are available—oral live attenuated polio vaccine (OPV) and injectable killed polio vaccine.

### Oral Live Attenuated Polio Vaccine

**Technical aspects:**

Contents:
- Type 1: $10^5$ TCID 5.9
- Type 3: $10^5$ TCID 5.7

Type 2 is not used now as this strain is not prevalent also type 2 is associated with VAPP.

Nature: Liquid vaccine.

Stabilizing agent: $MgCl_2$.

Indications: Recommended to all infants and children under the age of 5 years.

Dose: Two drops.

Route of administration: Oral.

Schedule: *See* Annexure.
- On all national immunization days (NIDs) for children less than 5 years of age.
- On all sub-national immunization days (SNIDs).
- Pulse polio immunization (irrespective of the immunization status).

Ideal age of initiating primary vaccination: At birth.

Boosters: One and half years and 4–5 years.

Instructions to the mother after administration of vaccine:
- If the child regurgitates or vomits immediately within 1 hour after the dose, repeat the polio dose.

Seroconversion rate of oral polio vaccine: 90–95% after multiple doses.

For polio there is variation in seroconversion amongst different regions of the world. The immunogenicity is good in developed countries as compared to developing countries.

Protective efficacy 70–80%: 15% per dose in India and 30% dose in the world. The efficacy is more in temperate regions than in tropical regions.

Storage:
- Freezer
- OPV should be stored below 8°C
- Unopened vials can be stored up to 6 months at temperature between 0°C to 8°C
- Primary health centers: + 2°C to + 8°C for 1 month
- Regional level: –20°C for a maximum of 3–6 months.

Catch-up vaccination: Can be given up to the age of 5 years.

### Clinical aspects:

The live attenuated polio virus will multiply in the intestines and produce active immunity simulating natural infection without producing symptoms of disease.

Indications: To all infants and children below the age of 5 years.
- Poliomyelitis prophylaxis
- Poliomyelitis eradication.

Contraindications and cautions to oral polio vaccination:

Oral polio should be avoided or postponed in the following conditions—
- Allergy/anaphylactic reactions to previous dose
- AIDS/HIV
- Biological immunosuppressive therapy (e.g anti-TNF therapy like alemtuzumab, ofatumumab, rituximab)
- Corticosteroids or immunosuppressant or radiotherapy
- Diarrhea, dysentry, dysgammaglobinemia (moderate to severe)
- Drugs: Immunosuppressive drugs
- Hep E
- Enteritis
- (Fever Above 38.5°C): Acute febrile illness
- Gestational period (Pregnancy)
- Hypersensitivity to neomycin
- Household contacts with immunodeficiency disorders
- Immunodeficiency disorders both congenital and acquired/immunocompromised (especially humoral immunodeficiencies) and their household contacts/abnormal immunoglobulin synthesis agammaglobulinemia/hypogammaglobulinemia/combined humoral and cell-mediated immunity
- Lymphoma and leukemia
- Neoplasm.

### Side effects
- Appetite lost
- Anaphylactic shock (Rare)
- Black out
- Conjunctivitis
- Drowsiness
- Emesis
- Fatigue
- Guillain-Barré syndrome (rare)
- High fever
- Itching
- Irritability.

### Complications of oral poliomyelitis immunization:

- *Vaccine associated paralytic poliomyelitis (VAPP):* Vaccine associated paralytic poliomyelitis is defined as cases of AFP which have residual weakness 60 days after the onset of paralysis and from whose stool samples, vaccine-related poliovirus but no wild polio virus is isolated. Vaccine associated paralytic poliomyelitis is seen in vaccine recipient occurring within 4–40 days of receiving OPV or contact with vaccine recipient which is known as contact VAPP. VAPP occurs due to loss of attenuating mutations and reversion to neurovirulence during replication of the vaccine virus in the gut. The risk is more with the first dose.

❖ *Emergence of vaccine derived polio virus:* Due to mutation and recombination in the human gut. They are 1-15% divergent from the parent vaccine virus. These viruses are neurovirulent and are transmissible and are capable of causing outbreaks.

Vaccine-induced poliomyelitis or vaccine associated paralytic poliomyelitis can occur even 6 months after the immunization.

Inefficient transmissibility of the vaccine virus is reversible. With both neurovirulence and transmissibility reacquired, the vaccine virus is virtually wild virus like (vaccine derived wild like virus).

## QUESTIONS

**Q1. What are the conditions in which Oral polio vaccine is postponed?**
Oral polio vaccine is postponed in the following conditions:
- 8 weeks following injection of immunoglobulin
- 1 month after an attack of chicken pox
- 1 month after an attack of measles.

**Q2. What is switch over polio?**
Administration of trivalent polio vaccine (tOPV) was stopped and bivalent polio vaccine (bOPV) was started from 25th April 2016. This is known as Switch over polio.

This is because of the following reasons:
- Type 2 polio virus was not found since 1999.
- Type 2 polio causes VAPP.
- Type 2 polio virus interferes with formation of antibodies to other two polio viruses types 1 and 3.

**Q3. What is pulse polio immunization?**
Intermittent polio immunization vaccinates all children below the age of 5 years irrespective of previous immunization status.

**Q4. What is global polio eradication initiative?**
Global polio eradication initiative was launched in the year 1988.
- Four-pronged strategy
- High routine immunization coverage.

**Q5. What is Mop-up immunization?**
Mop-up immunization is door to door immunization carried out in specific priority areas where the virus is suspected to be circulating. The strain should be identified and the vaccine for mop-up monovalent vaccine should be used.

Priority areas are areas where the polio cases were found in the last three years and the access to healthcare is difficult.
- High population density
- High population mobility
- Poor sanitation
- Low routine immunization coverage.

**Q6. What is four-pronged strategy?**
Four-pronged strategy includes:
- Routine immunization
- National immunization days
- Acute flaccid paralysis surveillance
- "Mop-up" immunization.

## Hepatitis B Vaccine

There are two types of vaccines:
1. Plasma derived and recombinant DNA vaccine
2. Killed vaccine.

### Recombinant DNA Vaccine

Recombinant vaccine is produced by cloning the HBV S gene in yeast cells.

Seroconversion—Protective anti-HBs antibody levels of at least 10m IU/mL in 90% of healthy adults and 95% of infants and children. Recombinant vaccine has excellent immunogenicity and safety.

**Duration of protection:** The anti-HBs levels will decrease over time. About 50-80% of vaccines may have levels below 10 mIU/mL 12 years after vaccination. This may be due to priming of memory cells which are capable of eliciting an anamnestic response when challenged.

## Technical aspects:

Contents: 1 mL dose contains 10 μg/mL (Recombivax) 20 μg/mL of (Engerix B) and 40 μg/mL (Recombivax HB) of hepatitis B surface antigen (HBsAg) and 0.5 mg of aluminum per mL of vaccine

Nature: Liquid vaccine.

Preservative: Thimerosal.

Dose and schedule:

Dose:
- 0.5 mL (10 μg) in children less than 18 years
- 1 mL (20 μg) (10 μg) in adults more than 18 years.

Schedule and catch-up vaccination: See Annexure.

Route of administration: Intramuscular.

Site of administration: Deltoid or anterolateral aspect of thigh.

Hepatitis B vaccine should be injected intramuscularly, avoiding the gluteal region since it has been shown to be sometimes less immunogenic at this site. It is believed that the microgram dose of HbsAg might be deposited within the fat tissue, thereby reducing its bioavailability to antigen-presenting cells.

Protective efficacy: More than 90%.

Storage: + 2°C to + 8°C
- When vaccine is not in use: + 2°C to + 8°C in the upper most compartment of the refrigerator
- During immunization: At room temperature.
- Storage of vaccine in case of power failure: Keep in an ice box

## Clinical aspects:

The vaccine is not useful for carriers of HbSAg.

## Hepatitis B Vaccine Indications

Recommended to all infants but there is a controversy in administering this vaccine to already infected individuals, HbsAg carriers.

## Contraindications and Cautions to the Hepatitis B Vaccine

- Allergic reaction (severe): Severe allergic reaction to Baker's yeast
- Breathing difficulties
- Edema over mouth and throat
- Hypotension
- Hypersensitivity to yeast.
- Shock.

## Side Effects of Hepatitis B Vaccine

Mild side effects are:
- Local: Pain, soreness, induration and erythema at local site
- Systemic:
  - Anaphylaxis
  - Fever
  - Headache
  - Irritability
  - Joint pain
  - Loss of appetite
  - Lymphadenopathy
  - Myalgia
  - Nausea.

Serious side effects of hepatitis B vaccine:
- Anaphylaxis (Rare)
- Autoimmune disorders (SLE, Lupus like syndrome, vasculitis, polyarteritis nodosa)
- Alopecia
- Arthritis, arthralgia of knee joint (mono-articular)
- Anorexia
- Bell's palsy
- Chronic fatigue syndrome
- Convulsions
- Diabetes Type I
- Diarrhea
- Demyelinating neurological disorders
- Eye problems
- Ear ache
- Eczema
- Erythema multiforme
- Fever
- Guillain-Barré syndrome
- Headache
- Hypersensitivity
- Hypotension
- Hypotensive-hyporesponsive episode
- Inflammatory polyneuropathy
- Irritability
- Insomnia

- Juvenile idiopathic arthritis/Rheumatoid arthritis
- Keratitis
- Leukoencephalitis
- Lupus
- Multiple sclerosis
- Myalgia
- Myasthenia gravis
- Numbness
- Neck stiffness
- Optic neuritis
- Pharyngitis
- Rhinitis-Running nose
- Stevens-Johnson syndrome
- Somnolence
- Syncope
- Tinnitus
- Thrombocytopenia
- Transverse myelitis
- Uveitis
- Urticaria
- Visual disturbances
- Vertigo

Since the recombinant vaccines contain tiny quantities of yeast proteins, there is a risk of anaphylactic reaction.

*Vaccine scares:* Multiple sclerosis, lupus, diabetes.

## QUESTIONS

**Q1. What is active and passive immunization?**
- Active: Hepatitis B vaccine (0.5 mL, three doses)
- Passive: Immunoglobulin HBIG in a dose of 0.5 mL should be given intramuscularly, immediately after birth. If not given it should be given within 48 hours of age.

**Q2. What is postexposure prophylaxis?**
Postexposure prophylaxis can be given for the following persons:
- If mothers HBsAg status unknown
- Administer Hep B vaccine regardless of birthweight.
  - Birth weight <2 kg administer HBIg within 12 hours of birth.
  - Birth weight >2 kg determine mothers HBsAg, if positive administer HBIg.
- Newborns born to HbsAg positive mothers. For babies born of Hepatitis B positive mothers, the vaccine should be given from birth onward followed by three doses at 6,10 and 14 weeks of age. Also hepatitis B immunoglobulin should be given within 12 hours of birth. If hepatitis B immunoglobulin is not available, HB vaccine alone should be given as four doses schedule at birth, 6 weeks, 10 weeks, and 12 months.
- Healthcare workers.

**Q3. What is passive immunization?**
Routine screening of pregnant women for HBV carrier status should be done wherever feasible. If the mother is found to be a carrier and especially so for hepatitis e antigen carrier, the baby must be protected with passive immunization soon after birth with Hepatitis B immunoglobulins given within 12 hours of birth along with active hepatitis B vaccination.

**Q4. What are the causes of hepatitis b vaccination failure?**
- Anticancer therapy
- Blood transfusion or antibody containing blood products transfusion
- Cold chain problems—non-maintenance of cold chain
- Drugs: Patients on certain drugs like steroids, immunosuppressants Anticancer chemotherapy, prolonged steroid therapy, etc.
- Elderly people: Old age more than 50 years
- Faulty or poor storage
- Faulty technique of administration
- Gluteal injections
- Genetic predisposition
- Hemodialysis patients
- HLA B8, DR3, SCO1
- HB mutants
- Immunosuppressed state of the host. Some persons with T cell suppression without obvious immunodeficiency

- Leukemia patients
- Mutant strains: Infection with surface mutant strain which will escape neutralization by surface antibodies
- Normal individuals: 10% of normal individuals.

**Q5. What is the indication of good protection?**
Anti-HBs titre should be measured after 9–18 months of age of the dose. Level more than 10 mIU/mL indicates a good protection against infection.

**Q6. What is the management of nonresponders to hepatitis B vaccination?**
0.06 mL/kg as soon as possible second dose at an interval of 1 month.
If there is no response after two completed schedule. It is considered as vaccine failure.

**Q7. When should the level of protective antibodies tested after the immunization?**
Serological testing should be done 4–8 weeks after completion of primary course of vaccination. Anti-HbsAg antibody levels should be measured.

**Q8. What are the tests to be done to the nonresponders?**
For nonresponders, presence of current infection should be tested by Anti-HBsAg and Anti-HBs antibody levels.

**Q9. What are the conditions that are not contraindications to the hepatitis B vaccination?**
- Asthma
- Allergy
- Breastfeeding
- Convulsions
- Cerebral palsy
- Down syndrome
- Drugs—treatment with antibiotics
- Enteritis with diarrhea
- Family history of convulsions
- Fever (Temperature below 38.5°C)
- Gestational age—preterm or low-birth weight
- HIV infection
- Infection of respiratory system
- Immaturity
- Jaundice at birth
- Kidney diseases
- Liver diseases.

## DPT Vaccine

### Types of DPT (Diphtheria, Pertussis and Tetanus) Vaccines

- DTwP vaccine (whole cell vaccine)
- DTaP vaccine (acellular vaccine).

### Diphtheria Tetanus Whole Cell Pertussis Vaccine

It is a combined vaccine.

**Technical aspects:**
- Killed vaccine
- Contents: Each 0.5 mL contains—
  - 20–30 Lf of diphtheria toxoid and 5–25 Lf tetanus toxoid, and > 4 IU of whole cell killed pertussis
- Nature: Liquid vaccine
- Dose and schedule:
  - Dose: 0.5 mL
  - Schedule: *See* Annexure
- Catch-up vaccination: Up to 5 years
  - Catch-up ≤ 7 years—0, 1 and 6 months
  - Catch-up ≥ 7 years—Tdap at 0 months and Td at 1 and 6 months
- Site of injection: Anterolateral aspect of thigh or deltoid
- Route of administration: Intramuscular
- Preparation of the site: Clean with spirit. Do not rub vigorously after injection.
- Efficacy of vaccine: Diphtheria and tetanus—95% after three doses. Pertussis—70–90%.

Efficacy of three doses: 82–96%
Antibody levels will decline over time. This will result in increased susceptibility of adolescents and adults to diphtheria. Tdap is advised at the age of 10–12 years. Catch-up vaccination is advised till the age of 18 years.

- ❖ Duration of immunity: Up to 6–8 years
- ❖ Storage: + 2°C to +8°C. Do not freeze.

**Clinical aspects:**

- ❖ Indications: Recommended to all infants below the age of 5 years
- ❖ Contraindications and cautions for the use of DTwP vaccine:
  - Anaphylaxis: History of anaphylaxis within 7 days following previous DTwP vaccination
  - Age below 6 weeks: Should not be given after 6 years of age because of the dangers of reactions to diphtheria
  - Brain disorders
  - Bronchospasm
  - Convulsions (Uncontrolled) or seizures within 3 days
  - Crying: History of persistent or high pitched crying following previous DTwP vaccination
  - CNS problems: Evolving neurological disease or severe neurological reactions (convulsions or acute encephalopathy) within 3 days to the first dose or subsequent doses
  - Degenerative or demyelinating disorders: Progressive neurological disease in the child
  - Encephalopathy occurring within 7 days following previous DTwP vaccination
  - Fever >40.5°C/105°F
  - Generalized collapse
  - Hypotonic–hyporesponsive episode (collapse/shock-like state)
  - Inconsolable crying or screaming for more than 3 hours within 2 days of DTwP injection
  - Infantile spasms or any progressive neurological disorder
  - Prolonged unresponsiveness.

**Two absolute contraindications for the use of DTwP vaccine:**

- ❖ Severe reactions to previous dose of DTwP
- ❖ Progressive neurological disease or uncontrolled convulsions.

*The conditions in which DTwP is not contraindicated:*
- ❖ Febrile fits
- ❖ Family history of seizures
- ❖ Cerebral palsy

**Vaccine scares of Pertussis whole cell vaccine:**

Encephalopathy, epilepsy, learning disorders, and sudden death (cot death or sudden infant death syndrome).

*Contraindications for first dose of DTwP vaccine:*
- ❖ Progressive neurological disease
- ❖ Uncontrolled seizures.

**DTwP vaccine—side effects or complications of DTwP vaccine:**

Local reactions: Redness and swelling
General reactions:
- ❖ Acute encephalopathy
- ❖ Anaphylactic shock
- ❖ Autism
- ❖ Brain damage: Vaccine associated seizures may produce brain damage
- ❖ Crying: Persistent inconsolable crying for more than 3 hours duration
- ❖ Deafness
- ❖ Encephalitis/Encephalopathy: Post-pertussis vaccine encephalopathy
- ❖ Excessive somnolence
- ❖ Fever (hyperpyrexia ≥40.5°C)
- ❖ Generalized seizures (Febrile convulsions)
- ❖ Generalized collapse
- ❖ Hyporesponsive hypotensive episodes (HHE) shock like state within 48 hours of DTwP
- ❖ Induration
- ❖ Infantile spasms
- ❖ Local pain
- ❖ Learning disorders
- ❖ Prolonged unresponsiveness
- ❖ Reye's syndrome
- ❖ Screaming episodes
- ❖ Shock
- ❖ Sudden infant death syndrome (SIDS)
- ❖ Seizures with or without fever within 72 hours of administration of DTwP.

**Catastrophic complications of DTwP vaccine:**
- Sudden infant death syndrome
- Autism
- Chronic neurologic damage
- Infantile spasms
- Learning disorders
- Reye's syndrome.

## QUESTIONS

**Q1. What is the contraindication for first dose of DTwP?**
Progressive or evolving neurological illness

**Q2. What are the conditions considered as precautions and not contraindications to future doses of DTwP vaccination?**
- Persistent inconsolable crying for more than 3 hours duration following vaccination
- Seizures with or without fever within 72 hours of administration of DTwP
- Should not be used in children aged 7 years or more due to reactogenicity.

## Polio—Inactivated Polio Vaccine

### Technical Aspects

Inactivated polio vaccine is an inactivated or killed vaccine. Containing poliovirus grown in monkey kidney, human diploid or Vero cell culture.

### Contents:
- Type 1: 40 D
- Type 3: 32 D (Dalton antigen units)

Inactivated polio vaccine contains streptomycin, neomycin, and polymyxin B; allergic reactions may be seen. Use of this vaccine should be avoided in children with hypersensitivity to these antimicrobials.

*Ideal age of initiating primary vaccination:* 8 weeks.

*Boosters:* One and half and 4–5 years.

*Nature:* Liquid vaccine.

*Dose:* 0.5 mL.

*Route of administration:* Intramuscular or subcutaneous.

Fractional IPV is given in a dose of 0.1 mL, intradermal.

*Site of administration:* Anterolateral aspect of thigh or right upper deltoid.

*Preparation of the site of administration:* Clean with spirit.

*Schedule for IPV for children:* See Annexure

*Seroconversion rate of IPV:* Seroconversion rates of IPV is 95–100%.

*Protective efficacy of IPV:* 95–100%.

*Storage:* + 2°C to + 8°C
- *When vaccine is not in use:* Should be kept in the lowermost compartment of the refrigerator
- *During immunization:* Can be kept at room temperature.

### Clinical Aspects

**Indications for IPV:**
- Immunodeficient children and their close contacts
- Primary immunization in adults.

**Contraindications:**
- Anaphylaxis
- Hypersensitive reactions to any of the components of the vaccine like neomycin.

### Side Effects of IPV Vaccination
- Local reactions—erythema, induration, pain
- Systemic reactions
- Allergic reactions
- Arthralgia
- Agitation
- Body ache
- Convulsions
- Crying
- Drowsiness
- Emesis
- Fever
- Hypersensitive reactions
- Somnolence.

## QUESTIONS

**Q1. Why injectable polio is used in developed countries like USA, Germany?**

Recent recommendations from American Academy of Pediatrics and Center for Disease Control and Prevention were to utilize inactivated polio vaccine instead of live vaccine. This was due to the fact that most of the recent paralytic polio cases were associated with vaccine virus. Many countries like USA, Germany have switched over from oral polio to injectable polio. This is due to the fact that the incidence of vaccine-induced poliomyelitis was on the rise. In India, a proposal to add injectable polio is put forward.

### Haemophilus Influenzae Type B Vaccine

*It is a killed vaccine.*
During first 3 months of life, the infants are protected by antibodies that are passively transferred from the mother.

### Technical Aspects

Conjugated *Haemophilus influenzae* type B (Hib) vaccine contains group B meningococcal outer membrane protein (OMP) or tetanus toxoid (PRO-T), PRP conjugated to tetanus toxoid (PRP-D), CRM mutant diphtheria toxoid (HbOC). This will improve.

There are three types of conjugate Hib vaccine depending upon the protein carrier used:
i. PRP-OMP: Outer membrane of meningococcus
ii. PRP-D using diphtheria toxoid
iii. PRP-T
iv. HbOC

**Contents:** 10 μg of PRP-T, HbOC.

**Nature:** Liquid or lyophilized powder.

**Diluent:** Sterile water 0.5 mL volume.

**Dose:** 0.5 mL in children, 1 mL in adults.

**Schedule:** *See* Annexure.

**Route of administration:** Intramuscular.

**Site of administration:** Deltoid/thigh.

### Precautions

- *Protective efficacy:* >90%
- *Storage:* + 2°C to +8°C
- Route of administration: Subcutaneous
- Stored in the middle rack
- Should not be frozen.

### Clinical Aspects

**Indications:**

- To all infants more than 6 weeks old
- Before splenectomy
- HIV
- Sickle cell anemia
- Leukemia.

**Contraindications and cautions to Hib vaccine:**

- Anyone who had life-threatening adverse reactions to previous dose of Hib like serious hypersensitivity
- Children below 6 weeks of age
- Children more than 5 years of age should not receive this vaccination
- People who are moderately or severely ill at the time of vaccination.

**Mild to moderate side effects:**

- Local: Local pain, swelling, redness will be mild nature and will last for 1–2 days
- Systemic: Fever over 101°F, loss of appetite, restlessness, excessive crying, vomiting, and diarrhea
  - Appetite loss
  - Behavior—restlessness
  - Crying—excessive
  - Diarrhea
  - Emesis—vomiting
  - Fever over 101°F.

**Severe side effects:**

- Severe allergic reactions
- Guillain-Barré syndrome.

*Vaccine scares:* Diabetes mellitus.

## Pneumococcal Conjugate Vaccine (PCV 13)

Tridecavalent vaccine.

### Contents
- 13 antigens from serotypes 1, 3, 4, 5, 6A, 6B, 7F, 9V, 14, 18c, 19A, 19F, 23F conjugated to diphtheria carrier protein
- Aluminum
- Polysorbate
- Succinic acid, as acidity regulator
- Sodium chloride

### Diluents

*Ideal age at administration of pneumococcal conjugate vaccine (PCV 13):*
- Minimum age 6 weeks. Routine immunization is not recommended after 5 years of age.
- Minimum interval between two doses should be 4 weeks for those who get vaccinated before 12 months of age.
- Minimum interval between two doses should be 8 weeks for those who get vaccinated after 12 months of age.

### Dose and Schedule
- *Dose:* 0.5 mL
- *Schedule: See* Annexure
- *Route of administration:* Intramuscular
- *Site of administration:* Deltoid/thigh
- *Protective efficacy:* 95%
- Duration of protection: 2–3 years
- Catch-up vaccination:
  - 7–11 months two doses ≥4 weeks apart, one booster at 15–18 months
  - 12–23 months two doses ≥8 weeks apart
  - 24–59 months: one dose
  - >60 months: one dose only if in high-risk category
- *Storage:* + 2 to + 8°C
  - Keep away from light
  - To be stored at the top of the rack.

## Clinical Aspects

### General indications:
- All children below 2 years of age
- 2–65 years with chronic health conditions
- All adults 65 years of age and older.

### Conditions in which vaccine should be given:
- Alcoholism
- Asplenia
- Bone marrow transplant
- Cancers
- CSF leak
- Chemotherapy
- Drugs—steroids, immunosuppressants
- Diabetes
- Hematological—sickle cell anemia
- HIV/AIDS patients
- Heart disease
- Immunodeficiency
- High-risk groups who can develop complications:
  - Asplenia or hyposplenia
  - Brain problems—recurrent meningitis
  - Chronic liver, heart, kidney, lung diseases
  - Cochlear implants
  - Cerebrospinal leaks/fistula
  - Complement disorders
  - Coeliac disease
  - Cochlear implant
  - Diabetes mellitus
  - Hodgkin's disease
  - Hemoglobinopathy: Sickle cell anemia
  - Immunosuppression
  - Kidney disease—renal failure, nephrotic syndrome
  - Lung disorders
  - Liver disorders
  - Multiple myeloma
  - Nephrotic syndrome
  - Organ transplant recipients.

### Contraindications and cautions to pneumococcal conjugate vaccine:
- Age: Children under 6 weeks and more than 5 years of age

- Life-threatening reaction to a previous dose of vaccine
- Life-threatening allergy to any component of the vaccine
- Moderately or severely ill until they recover
- Lymphoreticular malignancies
- Patients on immunosuppressive therapy.

### Side effects of pneumococcal conjugate vaccine:

Mild side effects:
- Local: Local pain, induration, swelling, redness, and tenderness will be mild nature and will last for 1–2 days
- Systemic:
  - Adenopathy—lymphadenopathy
  - Appetite lost
  - Anaphylaxis
  - Behaviour—restlessness.
  - Breathing problems—wheezing
  - Crying—excessive
  - Diarrhea
  - Drowsiness
  - Emesis (Vomiting)
  - Fever
  - Fussy
  - Guillain-Barré syndrome
  - Irritability
  - Idiopathic thrombocytopenic purpura (Relapse)

The above symptoms are mild and self-limiting.

Rarely:
- Febrile convulsions
- Breath-holding spells.

Severe side effects:
- Severe allergic reactions
- Fever with fits
- Hives.

Rarely:
- Guillain-Barre syndrome
- Anaphylaxis
- Breathing problems
- Circulatory problems
- Relapse of ITP.

## QUESTIONS

**Q1. What is the advantage of pneumococcal conjugate vaccine (PCV 13) over polysaccharide vaccine?**
Polysaccharide vaccines will have low immunogenicity in children less than 2 years. Conjugate vaccines were developed to increase the immunogenicity below 2 years of age.

**Q2. What is PCV 7, PCV 9, etc.?**
- PCV 7 contains 7 serotypes
- PCV 9 and PCV 11 contain 9 and 11 serotypes, respectively.
- PCV 10 is available internationally and can be given from 6 weeks of age.

**Q3. Why polysaccharide vaccine cannot be used in children below 2 years of age when it is most required?**
Immune response is IgM type, short-lived, has low titers, does not induce IgA immunity, has low affinity, low avidity, and not have boosting effect in spite of repeated doses.
Hence this vaccine cannot be used in children below 2 years of age.

**Q4. What are the drawbacks of polysaccharide vaccines?**
- Affinity and avidity will be low
- Boosting effect not present in spite of repeated boosters
- Cannot be used in children below 2 years of age
- Duration of immunity: Short-lived immunity
- Polysaccharide vaccine being non T cell dependent will not induce a good immunity.
- Immune response is IgM type:
  - Low titers
  - Does not induce local IgA immunity
  - Pneumococci: Carrier state and Herd immunity—some studies have

shown nearly 50% reduction in the carriage with vaccine types but it is counter balanced by similar 50% increase in the nonvaccine types carriage leading to no net change in the prevalence of carriage rates.

|  | Unconjugated | Pneumococcal conjugated |
|---|---|---|
| Serotypes | • Polysaccharide<br>• 23 valent<br>• Contains 25 μg of polysaccharide of 23 serotypes in the vaccine<br>• Poorly immunogenic | • Polysaccharide linked to a protein carrier<br>• 13 valent<br>1, 3, 4, 5, 6A, 7F, 9V, 14, 18C, 19A, 9F, 23F |
| Herd immunity | • No herd effect<br>• No reduction in nasopharyngeal carriage<br>More than 2 doses should not be given in the life time | Herd effect present<br>Reduction in nasopharyngeal carriage resulting in decline in disease in unvaccinated contacts |
| Protective efficacy |  | • 95–99%<br>• Revaccination or further doses after primary series is not recommended |
| NIS schedule | Not included | Not included |
| IAP schedule | 3 doses ≥6 weeks apart one booster at 15–18 months | IAP schedule for PCV 3 doses at ≥ 6 weeks ≥ 4 weeks apart, booster at 15–18 months |

## Rotavirus Vaccine

Two types of vaccines are available—monovalent and pentavalent.

The following vaccines are available:
- *Rotarix:* Monovalent
  - Human monovalent vaccine
  - Contains one strain of G1P specificity
  - Prevents gastroenteritis caused by G1, non-G1 types G3, G4, and G9
- *Rotateq:* Live oral pentavalent

Human bovine reassortant pentavalent vaccine contains five reasserted rotavirus strains.
- *Rotavac* was used in India since 2014.
  - It is a live attenuated, monovalent vaccine.
  - Contains G9P human strain isolated from children in India.
  - Three doses 4 weeks apart beginning at 6 weeks and to be completed before 8 months of age.

### Technical Aspects

- Human monovalent live oral vaccine
- Human pentavalent live vaccine. Each 2 mL contains $2 \times 10^6$ infectious units of all the five reassortant strains.
- *Contents:*
  - Live attenuated virus monovalent
  - Human rotavirus strain 89-12 (G1-P8)
- *Diluents:* Sterile water
- *Ideal age at immunization*: First dose, 6–15 weeks
- *Dose and schedule of rotavirus vaccine*
  - Dose 5 drops
  - Minimum age 6 wks
  - Maximum age for first dose 14 wks 6 days
  - Maximum age for final dose 8 months
  - *Schedule of rotavirus vaccine:* See Annexure.
- *Route of administration of rotavirus vaccine*: Oral

- *Protective efficacy of rotavirus vaccine* is more than 80% (85–98%).
- *Storage*: + 2 to + 8°C
  - Keep away from light
  - To be stored at the top of the rack.

### Clinical Aspects

**Indications:**

- First dose minimum age 6 weeks
- First dose maximum age 14 weeks 6 days

**Contraindications of rotavirus vaccine:**

- Age less than 6 weeks and more than 8 months
- Acute gastroenteritis
- Breathing disorders: Wheezing
- Cancer or those on cancer treatment
- Drug—on long-term steroids
- Enteral malformations: Persons with uncorrected congenital malformation of gastrointestinal system that will predispose to intussusception
- Fructose intolerance, glucose galactose malabsorption, and sucrose isomaltase insufficiency
- Use with caution in gastrointestinal illness and growth retardation
- Hypersensitivity to any of the components or previous dose
- History of intussusception
- Immunodeficiency disorders: AIDS, severe combined immunodeficiency (gastroenteritis associated with vaccine was reported).

### Side Effects of Rotavirus Vaccine

**Mild side effects:**

- Irritability
- Mild diarrhea or vomiting
- Pyrexia
- Otitis media.

**Severe side effects or complications of rotavirus vaccine:**

- Allergy—rash
- Apnea—risk of apnea is present; monitoring for 48–72 hours is advised
- Abdominal pain or cramps
- Appetite—loss of appetite
- Anaphylaxis
- Breathing difficulty (chest tightness, feeling short of breath)
- Black out
- Burning micturition
- Bronchiolitis
- Bronchopneumonia
- Convulsions
- Crying
- Chest pain (stabbing in nature)
- Dizziness
- Diarrhea (severe)
- Ear pain (Otitis media)
- Emesis (Vomiting)
- Flatulence
- Fever
- Fatigue
- Gastroenteritis
- Gastric regurgitation of food
- Hematochezia
- Hand swelling
- Heart rate increased
- Irritability
- Intussusception within a week was reported even with the currently available vaccines. There is an increased risk of intussusception in children receiving rotavirus vaccine
- Kawasaki disease.

## QUESTIONS

**Q1. Why rotavirus vaccine is not recommended in children age above 8 months?**

It is because they are more likely to have complications. Also there is no much evidence about how it works in older children.

**Q2. What are the reasons for poor immunogenicity in developing countries like India?**

The efficacy of this vaccine is poor in developing countries like India. Oral vaccines have a poor record of immunogenicity and effectiveness in

India and other developing countries. This may be due to presence and transplacental transmission of antirotavirus antibody from the mother. Also this may be present in the breast milk.

**Q3. Can the rotavirus vaccine given along with oral polio vaccine?**

Concomitant use of oral polio vaccine may result in decreased efficacy of oral polio vaccine.

## Measles Vaccine

Live attenuated vaccine propagated on human diploid cell.

### Technical Aspects

*Contents:* Each dose 0.5 mL contains not less than 1,000 TCID of measles virus (Schwarz of Edmonston-Zagreb strain) grown in chick embryo cells on reconstitution with diluents.

**Ideal age at immunization:** At completed 9 months of age (270 days).

**Route of administration:** Subcutaneous (Do not inject intravenously).

**Site of administration of measles vaccine:** Right upper arm at the insertion of Deltoid.

**Precautions:** Should be reconstituted with diluent and should be administered within 4-6 hours as contamination with bacteria especially *Staphylococcus aureus* can occur. This may cause staphylococcal scalded syndrome or toxic shock syndrome.

**Dose and schedule of measles vaccine:**

Dose: 0.5 mL
Schedule of measles vaccine: *See* Annexure.
Measles: Maternal antibodies are in the child's circulation up to about 3-4 months which may neutralize the vaccine if given before 6 months. At the same time, a second dose of measles vaccine is advised to increase the efficacy. If the vaccine efficacy is good, then most of the children who had already infected or vaccinated will have antibodies which will neutralize the vaccine.

**Instructions to the mother after administration of measles vaccine:**

Mild fever with rash can occur 5-7 days after immunization.

**Protective efficacy of measles vaccine:**

Protective efficacy of measles vaccine is almost 95%.

**Storage:**
- Both heat and light sensitive
- Stored in the top rack
- Keep away from light
- *When vaccine is not in use:* + 2°C to + 8°C in the uppermost compartment of the refrigerator.
- During immunization + 2°C to + 8°C

**Q. What should be done for storage of vaccine in case of power failure?**

The measles vaccine should be kept in an ice box.

*Compatibility:* Vaccination of certain vaccines like measles before waning of maternal antibodies would result in failure of vaccine uptake.

Measles can be given with all vaccines.
It can be combined with mumps, Rubella, and vitamin A.

*Note:* Measles vaccine will be replaced by Measles-Rubella vaccine.

Use within 4-6 hours after reconstitution.

### Clinical Aspects

**Indications for Measles vaccine:**
- Recommended to all infants
- Age at administration: 9 months

**Contraindications and cautions for the use of Measles vaccine (Mnemonic A–I):**
- Acute illness
- Active tuberculosis or untreated tuberculosis (may flare up)

- ❖ Anaphylactic reactions to neomycin: History of severe allergic reactions to the constituents
- ❖ Blood or blood components transfusion (For 6 weeks following blood transfusion)
- ❖ Cancer: Leukemia, Hodgkin's disease
- ❖ Congenital immunodeficiency states
- ❖ Drugs: Cancers/malignancy treated with immunosuppressants or antimalignant drugs, antimetabolites, alkylating agents, corticosteroids
- ❖ Egg allergy (anaphylaxis)
- ❖ Febrile illness (Delay the dose until recovery)
- ❖ Gestational period (Should avoid pregnancy for 1 month after monovalent measles vaccine)
- ❖ Gammaglobulin administration (should be delayed for 6 weeks following immunoglobulin therapy)
- ❖ HIV/AIDS
- ❖ Immunodeficiency: Severely immunocompromised.

## Side Effects of Measles Vaccination

*Minor reactions:*
- ❖ Allergy—skin rash
- ❖ Burning sensation at the site of injection
- ❖ Blistering at the site of injection
- ❖ Catarrh
- ❖ Diarrhea
- ❖ Erythema
- ❖ Emesis
- ❖ Fever (over 103°F) with rash after 5–7 days

*Major reactions:*
- ❖ Anaphylaxis/allergic reactions (Urticaria)
- ❖ Angioneurotic edema
- ❖ Bruising
- ❖ Bronchial spasm
- ❖ Convulsions
- ❖ Double vision
- ❖ Encephalitis/encephalopathy
- ❖ Erythema multiforme
- ❖ Febrile convulsions in children with fever
- ❖ Gastrointestinal disorders
- ❖ Hematological—thrombocytopenia, purpura
- ❖ Stevens-Johnson syndrome
- ❖ Subacute sclerosing panencephalitis (SSPE).

## Serious Complications of Measles Vaccination

- ❖ Multiple sclerosis
- ❖ Exaggeration of tuberculosis
- ❖ Encephalitis
- ❖ Toxic shock syndrome due to contamination by *Staphylococcus aureus*
- ❖ Systemic lupus erythematosus
- ❖ Crohn's disease
- ❖ Pagets disease
- ❖ Shift of epidemiology—measles are occurring in older children with waning immunity for which some are proposing another dose at 12–15 years.

## QUESTIONS

**Q1. What are the causes of measles in an already immunized child?**

Causes of measles in an already immunized child are:
- ❑ Age at administration of vaccine: Immunization before 6 months of age. Maternal antibodies are in the child's circulation up to about 3–4 months which may neutralize the vaccine.
- ❑ Blood or blood components transfusion (which may neutralize the vaccine up to many weeks following blood transfusion depending upon the components transfused).
- ❑ Cold chain problems: Improper cold chain resulting in loss of potency.
- ❑ Drug administration: Simultaneous administration of immunoglobulin.
- ❑ Expired vaccines: Use of expired vaccine.
- ❑ Failure: Vaccine failure in 10–15% cases.
- ❑ Immunocompromised or congenitally immunodeficient individual.
- ❑ Impotent vaccine is used for immunization.
- ❑ Vaccine-induced measles.

**Q2. Will the measles vaccination affect the test for tuberculosis?**
If the test is done on the same day, the test will not be affected. But if it is not done on the same day, it should be postponed to at least 4 weeks because measles virus will inhibit the response to tuberculin.

**Q3. Why measles vaccine is contraindicated in children with severe egg allergy?**
It is because measles vaccine is produced in the chick embryo cell culture.

**Q4. Why measles vaccine is administered before 6 months of age?**
Measles infection may be seen from the age of 6-9 months and get lifelong immunity. But if you get vaccine by the age of 6 months, maternal antibodies present in the body will interfere with development of immunity.

**Q5. Can measles infection occur even after measles immunization?**
Yes, it can occur. Measles—there are 15% cases which are primary failure with the first dose of the vaccine.

**Q6. Why contamination is common in measles vaccine?**
The vaccine does not contain antibacterial preservatives and any bacteria contamination of the vaccine will multiply.

## Measles–Rubella Vaccine

Live attenuated vaccine induces both humoral and cell-mediated immunity.

### Technical Aspects

10 dose vials.

*Contents:* Measles—each dose contains 1,000 infective units of Edmonston-Zagreb strain.

*Rubella:* RA 27/3 strain propagated in human diploid strains.

*Form:* Lyophilized.

*Diluents:* Supplied with the vaccine each ampoule contains 5 mL for 10 dose vials.

*Ideal age at immunization:* At 9 months.

*Dose:* 0.5 mL.

*Schedule*: See Annexure.

*Route of administration:* Subcutaneous.

*Site of administration:* Right upper arm of the child.

*Precautions:*
- Should be protected from sunlight
- Discarded within 4 hours after reconstitution.

*Protective efficacy:* More than 85% when given at 9 months, more than 95% when given after 12 months for both measles and Rubella.
- Peak immune response will develop 6-8 weeks after vaccination
- Immunity will persist for 20 years.

*Storage:* + 2 to +8°C
- Keep away from light.

### Clinical Aspects

*Indications of the vaccine:* To all children aged 9 months to 15 years of age.

### Contraindications and cautions for MR vaccine:

- Allergic reactions to previous dose of measles or rubella or vaccine components
- Anaphylactic/anaphylactoid reaction to neomycin, gelatin other components in MR vaccine
- Blood or blood component transfused persons (vaccinate after 3–11 months)
- Convulsions
- Drugs: Long-term steroids, immunosuppressant drugs, antimalignant drugs, and alkylating agents
- Elevated body temperature (High fever >102°F)
- Full blown AIDS
- Gelatin allergy
- Gestational period (Pregnancy)
- Gammaglobulin administration
- Hospitalized children
- Heart disease (Decompensated)

- Immunocompromised
- Impairment of renal functions
- Ill patients—with serious disease, unconscious etc.

### Side Effects

*Local:* Mild pain and redness at the injection site.

*Systemic:*
- Allergic rash
- Anaphylaxis
- Arthralgia/Joint pain
- Aches: Muscle aches
- Fever (Low grade)
- Febrile seizure
- Thrombocytopenic purpura.

## QUESTIONS

**Q1. What is Measles–Rubella campaign?**
The aim is to vaccinate 100% of the children. Children aged 9 months to 15 years are provided with an additional dose of MR vaccine. The vaccine is given irrespective of previous vaccination or disease.

**Q2. Can the MR vaccine be administered to girl who is menstruating?**
Yes.

**Q3. Is HIV infection a contraindication to MR vaccine?**
No, HIV infection is not a contraindication. HIV infected children should be vaccinated early by 6 months of age. An additional dose should be given at the age of 9 months.

**Q4. Can MR vaccine be given to malnourished children?**
Yes.

### Measles, Mumps, Rubella Vaccine

- Live attenuated vaccine
- Measles, mumps, rubella (MMR) vaccine is available as human diploid cell vaccines.

### Technical Aspects

**Contents of MMR vaccine:** Each dose of 0.5 mL contains not less than 1,000 TCID of measles virus (Schwarz) grown in chick embryo cells on reconstitution with diluents.

- 1,000 TCID of live hyperattenuated measles virus
- 5,000 TCID of mumps virus of Jeryl-Lynn/Urabe strain
- 1,000 TCID of live attenuated rubella virus RA 27/3 strain.

**Nature:** Lyophilized form.

*Diluents—sterile water,* should be diluted in 0.5 mL of diluent.

Minimal age of immunization with MMR: 9 months.

**Ideal age at immunization:** Three doses

First dose: 9 months

Second dose: 15–18 months

Third dose: 5 years.

Dose: 0.5 mL.

Schedule: *See* Annexure.

**Route of administration of MMR vaccine:** Subcutaneous or intramuscular route.

**Site of administration of MMR vaccine:** Thigh/deltoid.

**Precautions:** This should not be given along with BCG vaccine.

**Instructions to be given to the mother after administration of MMR vaccine:** Mild fever with rash can occur 5–7 days after immunization.

**Seroconversion rate of MMR vaccine:** 80-95%.

**Protective efficacy:** is about 90–95%.

**Storage:**
- Freezer + 2° to + 8°C
- Keep away from light

- To be stored at the top of the rack
- Storage of MMR vaccine when vaccine is not in use: Stored at + 2°C to + 8°C.
- Storage of MMR vaccine during immunization: During immunization, the measles vaccine should be kept in an ice box.
- Storage of vaccine in case of power failure: The measles vaccine should be kept in an ice box.

## Clinical Aspects

**Indications of the vaccine:** Recommended to all infants at 15–18 months of age. Minimal age of administration—12 months of age.

**Contraindications and cautions for the use of MMR vaccine:**

- Anaphylaxis (Severe anaphylactic reactions to egg or neomycin, MMR vaccine)
- Blood abnormalities: Thrombocytopenia (should be carefully given in patients with thrombocytopenia purpura)
- History of thrombocytopenia following measles or MMR
- Cancer treatment with alkylating agents, antimetabolites, treatment with radiotherapy
- Drugs: Immunosuppressant drugs, steroids, alkylating agents, antimetabolites
- Severe allergic reactions
- Fever—acute febrile illness
- Gestational period: Pregnancy (MMR is contraindicated in pregnant women and pregnancy should be avoided for 28 days after vaccination)
- HIV infection
- Immunocompromised or immunodeficiency (severe)
- Illness: Moderate or severe
- Can be vaccinated 2 years after transplantation.

## Side Effects of MMR Vaccine

**Mild side effects:**

- Fever (mild) with rash after 5–7 days
- Sore throat
- Parotid swelling after 10 days
- Arthralgia
- Mild lymphadenitis after 7–10 days.

**Moderate side effects:**

- Allergy
- Bleeding/bruising
- Convulsions/seizures (febrile convulsions)
- Decreased platelet count (thrombocytopenia) resulting in bleeding
- Pain and stiffness of joints

**Serious adverse effects of MMR:**

- Aseptic meningitis
- Arthralgia
- Arthritis (Rubella)
- Allergic reactions (Serious)
- Anaphylaxis
- Ataxia
- Brain damage (Permanent)
- Bleeding
- Blood clotting disorder
- Coma
- Consciousness level lowered
- Colitis (Nonspecific colitis)
- Convulsions: Long-term seizures
- Cot death/Crib death/SIDS
- Deafness
- Degeneration—neuroregression
- Encephalopathy
- Encephalitis: Measles inclusion body encephalitis (MIBE)
- Fever
- Fits: Long-term seizures (6–11 days after MMR vaccination)
- Guillain-Barré syndrome
- Hypersensitivity reaction
- Hemolytic uremic syndrome
- Inflammatory bowel disease
- Idiopathic thrombocytopenic purpura (after 2 weeks of MMR vaccine)
- Joint pain
- Lymphadenopathy
- Myalgia
- Neuroregression
- Nodular lymphoid hyperplasia

- Ocular palsy
- Optic neuritis
- Otitis media
- Parotid swelling (transient parotitis)
- Peripheral neuropathy
- Polyneuritis
- Rhinitis
- Retrobulbar neuritis
- Sore throat
- Syncope
- Thrombocytopenic purpura
- Vaccine strain measles viral infection
- Autism: Initially the studies revealed that there is association between MMR vaccine and autism. But later it is said that there is no association between them.

**Adverse effects of mumps:**

- Aseptic meningitis
- Convulsions
- Encephalopathy
- Mild fever
- Guillain-Barré syndrome
- Hemolytic uremic syndrome
- Parotid swelling
- Mumps infection had occurred following mumps vaccination.

**Adverse effects of Rubella:**

- Arthralgia
- Fever
- Lymphadenopathy
- Peripheral neuropathy
- Sore throat
- Thrombocytopenia.

## QUESTIONS

**Q1. How long a female should not get pregnant after MMR vaccination?**
Female vaccinees should not become pregnant for at least 2 months after MMR vaccination.

**Q2. What is the protective level of Rubella antibody?**
Rubella antibody more than 10 IU/mL is protective. Test antibody levels for Rubella after 8 weeks following MMR vaccination.

## Hepatitis A Vaccine

Freeze dried live vaccine for subcutaneous use in children above 1 year of age. Vaccine induces neutralizing antibody and cell-mediated immune response. Vaccine is well-tolerated and highly immunogenic.

### Types of Hepatitis A Vaccine

Two types of vaccines are available:
1. Killed or inactivated vaccine: Formaldehyde-inactivated vaccines (Aluminum hydroxide adjuvanted and virosomal vaccine)
2. Live attenuated vaccines.

### Killed or inactivated vaccine:

Technical aspects:
- Contents: Inactivated vaccine killed formalin inactivated from 9R326, HM 175, aluminum hydroxide adjuvanted vaccine
  - Up to 18 years: 720 million ELISA units (MEU)
  - More than 18 years: 1,440 MEU
- Dose: Inactivated vaccine, 0.5 mL intramuscularly at Deltoid or thigh
- Schedule: *See* Annexure
- Minimal age at administration: 12 months of age
- Route of administration: Intramuscular
- Site of administration: Deltoid or thigh
- Protective efficacy: *Seroconversion rates*—range from 90-95% after two doses
- Immunogenicity lasts for 10 years
- Storage: + 2°C to + 8°C
  - Keep away from light
  - To be stored at the top of the rack.

Clinical aspects:

Indications: Can be given for children aged 1-15 years.

Hepatitis A is indicated for the following persons:
- Adolescents who are seronegative to HAV leaving home for residential schools
- Carriers of hepatitis B and hepatitis C
- Drugs: Children on hepatotoxic drugs
- Endemic area visitors: Travelers to countries with high endemicity for hepatitis A
- Gammaglobulin negative: HAV-IgG negative adolescents
- Hepatic disorders: Patients with chronic liver disease
- House hold contact of patients with hepatitis A infection within 10 days of onset of illness in index case
- Immunosuppressed individuals: congenital or acquired
- Laboratory personnel
- Transplant recipients

**Contraindications for hepatitis A vaccine**
- Allergic reactions: Any severe life-threatening allergic reaction to a previous dose, severe life-threatening allergic reaction to any vaccine component
- Moderately ill or severely ill should wait until recovery
- Contraindicated in severe immunodeficiency.

**Side Effects of hepatitis A vaccine**
Mild side effects:
- Headache
- Fever (Low grade)
- Appetite lost
- Soreness
- Tiredness.

Severe side effects:
- Fainting
- Serious life-threatening allergic reactions within minutes to hour after the vaccination.

**Live attenuated vaccines:**
Technical aspects:
- Contents: Live attenuated vaccine contains attenuated H2 strain of HAV

- Dose: Live attenuated vaccines—1 mL subcutaneously at Deltoid or thigh
- Schedule: *See* Annexure
- Minimal age at administration—One year
- Route of administration: Intramuscular
- Site of administration: Deltoid or thigh
- Protective efficacy—upto 95 to 100% after one dose

**Clinical aspects:**

**Indications:**
Hepatitis A is indicated for the following persons:
- HAV-IgG negative adolescents
- Patients with chronic liver disease
- House hold contact of patients with hepatitis A infection
- Can be given for children aged 1–15 years

**Contraindications for hepatitis A vaccine**
- Any severe life threatening allergic reaction to a previous dose
- Anyone with severe life threatening allergic reaction to any vaccine component
- Anyone with moderately ill or severely ill should wait until recovery
- Immunodeficiency

**Side effects of hepatitis A vaccine**
Mild side effects:
- Soreness
- Headache
- Loss of appetite
- Tiredness

Severe side effects:
Serous allergic reactions within minutes to hour after the vaccination

## Tetanus Toxoid (TT) Vaccine

Formalin treated exotoxin of tetanus bacilli.

### Technical Aspects
Killed vaccine.

**Contents:** Each 0.5 mL contains 4 Lf flocculation units of tetanus toxoid.

**Preservative:** Thimerosal
- Contains thimerosal, mercurial derivative (25 mg mercury/dose)
- Does not contain ammonium containing adjuvant.

**Nature:** Liquid, toxoid in isotonic sodium chloride.

**Ideal age at immunization:** After 7 years.

**Dose and schedule**
- Dose: 0.5 mL
- Schedule: *See* Annexure
- Six doses of tetanus containing vaccine starting in the age of 6 weeks of age
- First dose around 2 months of age
- Fifth dose by 4–6 years
- Interval between two doses should be 4 weeks
- Td and Tdap are recommended to older children above 7 years old instead DTwP, DTap/DT, and instead of TT in all ages
- *Boosters* once in 10 years.

**Route of administration:** Intramuscular.

**Site of administration:** Upper arm/deltoid/thigh.

**Preparation of the site of administration:**
- Clean with spirit
- Do not rub vigorously after injection.

**Precautions:**
- Should be used as boosters only after 7 years of age
- In bleeding disorders, use subcutaneous route
- Response will be poor when given with immunosuppressants or chemotherapy
- Should not be used for primary immunization
- Used only for booster
- Diphtheria containing toxoids and tetanus toxoid (Td) is preferred for tetanus alone

**Protective efficacy:**
*Duration of immunity*: Up to 6–8 years.

**Storage:**
- +2°C to +8°C
- Keep away from light
- Keep it in the middle or lower compartment of the fridge
- Do not freeze.

## Clinical Aspects of TT Vaccine
**Indications for tetanus toxoid:**
- Recommended to all children aged above 7 years for booster
- Two doses of TT to the pregnant mothers.

**Contraindications and cautions for tetanus toxoid:**
- Allergic or neurologic reactions to previous dose
- Allergy to latex
- Bleeding disorders, thrombocytopenic purpura
- Chemotherapy
- Drugs: Immunosuppressants, steroids
- Epidemics of polio: Avoid during outbreak of poliomyelitis
- Fever: Children with fever
- Guillain-Barré syndrome
- HIV/AIDS.

**Adverse effects of tetanus toxoid:**
- Erythema at the local site, pain, induration, fever, chills, enlargement of axillary lymph nodes, malaise, aches, and pains
- Hypotension
- Arthralgia
- Neurological disorders
- Tetanus toxoid adsorbed: Aluminum
- Allergy—hives, life-threatening allergic reaction
- Breathing difficulty
- Brachial neuritis (2–28 days following administration of tetanus containing vaccine)
- Fever
- Guillain-Barré syndrome within 6 weeks following previous dose of influenza vaccine
- Nausea

- Joint pain
- Light headedness.

## Side effects of repeated injections with tetanus toxoid:

Repeated TT injections will lead to:
- Amyloidosis
- Brachial neuritis
- Chills
- Decreased immunogenicity
- Hypersensitivity
- Hemolytic anemia
- Hemorrhagic disease of newborn (Increased risk)
- Joint pain
- Immunodeficiency.

# QUESTIONS

**Q1. What are the types of tetanus toxoid?**
Tetanus toxoid is of two types—fluid and adsorbed.

**Q2. What are the differences between fluid and adsorbed types of tetanus toxoid?**
Adsorbed types of tetanus toxoid will induce higher antibody titers and the duration of immunity will be prolonged.

**Q3. From what age tetanus toxoid can be given?**
TT can be given from 3 months of age.

**Q4. What type of injury is associated with increased risk of tetanus?**
This is indicated after any injury in an unimmunized child. Tetanus can occur after an injury. The risk is more in pinprick injuries like thorn prick. The tetanus spores will be present in the sand. When a thorn pricks the spores will be entering deep into the wound. There will be an anaerobic condition in pinprick injuries which will favor growth of tetanus spores and formation of tetanus toxin.

**Q5. Why TT should not be repeated within 5 years?**
It may provoke hypersensitivity reaction.

**Q6. What are the tetanus containing vaccines?**
DTap and DT are given to children below the age of 7 years.

Tdap and Td are given to those 7 years or older.

Small d and p indicate lower strength of diphtheria and pertussis.

## Diphtheria, Tetanus, Pertussis— Acellular Vaccine (DTaP Vaccine)

- Contains inactivated pertussis toxin.
- One or more additional pertussis antigen contains fimbrial antigen, pertussis toxin.

### Technical Aspects

**Contents:** The components of the pertussis bacilli are used for preparation of acellular vaccines.

DTaP vaccine contains—20-30 Lf of diphtheria toxoid and 5-25 Lf tetanus toxoid and 10 µg of detoxified acellular pertussis antigen.

**Nature:** Liquid vaccine.

**Ideal age at immunization:** 6 weeks.

**Dose and schedule:**
- Dose: 0.5 mL
- Schedule: *See* Annexure

**Catch-up vaccination:** *See* Annexure.

**Route of administration:** Intramuscular

**Site of administration:** Anterolateral aspect of thigh or deltoid

**Protective efficacy:**
- Diphtheria and tetanus: 95% after three doses
- Pertussis: 70-90%
- Efficacy of three doses: 82-96%
- Duration of immunity: Up to 6-8 years
- Storage: + 2°C to +8°C

Keep away from light.

## Clinical Aspects of DTaP Vaccine

### Indications:
To all infants.

### Contraindications for DTaP vaccine:
- Age: Should not be used in children aged 7 years or more due to reactogenicity
- Age below 6 weeks
- Allergic reactions to previous dose or life-threatening reactions to DTaP
- Brain or nervous system diseases within 7 days after a dose of DTaP should not get another dose
- Convulsions: Had a seizure after a dose of DTaP
- Cried nonstop for 3 hours or more after a dose of DTaP
- Degenerative or demyelinating disorders: Progressive neurological disease
- Encephalopathy after a dose of DTaP
- Fever 105°F after a dose of DTaP
- Fits after a dose of DTaP
- Moderately ill or severely ill until recovery.

### Side effects:
The incidence of adverse effects of DTaP will be only two thirds of those seen in DTwP. Hence, incidence are almost the same.

Adverse effects of DTaP:
- Mild side effects:
  - Local reaction: Redness, swelling, soreness, and tenderness
  - Sometimes swelling of entire arm in which the dose was given (will last for 1–7 days)
  - Fever, crying, irritability, and loss of appetite
  - Fussiness
  - Tiredness
  - Vomiting
- Moderate side effects:
  - Convulsions
  - Continuous nonstop crying for 3 hours or more
  - Fever: High fever 105°F or more.
- Severe problems:
  - Allergic reactions (Serious)
  - Brain damage (Permanent)
  - Consciousness: Lowered
  - Coma
  - Convulsions: Long-term seizures.

## QUESTIONS

**Q1. What is the problem faced due to immunization of all children below the age of 5 years?**

There is an increased adult susceptibility due to waning of acquired immunity in the absence of natural boosting or adult vaccination program.

With effective vaccination the epidemiology has shifted to the right with more adolescents and adults getting diphtheria and pertussis.

## Typhoid Vaccines

### Types of Typhoid Vaccine
- Phenol or acetone inactivated vaccines (TAB: Typhoid A and B)
- TA vaccine polysaccharide
- Vi polysaccharide vaccine
- Typhoid conjugate vaccine
- Ty21a oral vaccine.

Of these, Vi polysaccharide vaccine (T cell independent vaccine) for children aged more than 2 years and Typhoid conjugate vaccine (T cell dependant vaccine) for children aged more than 9 months of age are only available in the market.

### Age of Administration of Various Typhoid Vaccines
- Phenol or acetone inactivated vaccines (TAB—Typhoid A and B)
- TA vaccine polysaccharide
- Vi vaccine is not given before 2 years of age
- Ty21a vaccine oral after 6 years of age.

## Typhoid AKD Vaccine (Acetone Killed Vaccine)

**Technical aspects:**

**Contents:** Contains 1,000 million heat killed phenolized or acetone killed bacteria per mL.

**Dose:** 0.5 mL.

**Route of administration:** Subcutaneous.

**Site of administration:** Anterolateral aspect of thigh/deltoid.

**Dose and schedule for Typhoid AKD vaccine:**
- Dose and schedule: 0.5 mL for children more than 10 years and 0.25 mL for less age subcutaneously or intramuscularly.
- Boosters: Once in every 3 years.

The protective efficacy of Typhoid AKD vaccine: 70–80% lasting for 3–5 years

In endemic areas, booster dose of 0.1 mL subcutaneously will be required every 3 years.

Instructions to the mother after administration of vaccine: Child may develop fever and should be treated with antipyretics.

**Protective efficacy** is 51–73%.

**Clinical aspects:**

Indications for Typhoid AKD vaccine:
- Recommended to all children above 2 years
- Age at administration: Given after 2 years of age.

Contraindications for Typhoid AKD vaccine:
- Age below 2 years
- Allergy/Anaphylaxis: Any severe reaction to previous dose, severe allergy to any component of the vaccine
- Moderately or severely ill until their recovery.

**Side effects—Typhoid AKD vaccine:**

The side effects of AKD vaccine (acetone killed) are:
- Local: Pain, swelling, tenderness
- Systemic: Fever, malaise, headache, chills.

Relapse of chronic diseases like rheumatoid arthritis and compensated cardiac conditions.

## Typhoid Vi Polysaccharide Vaccine

**Technical aspects:**

Liquid form.

**Contents:** 0.5 mL.

**Dose:** 0.5 mL.

**Schedule:** Single dose, booster every 3 years.

**Ideal age at immunization:** At or after 2 years of age.

The dose should be repeated after 3–5 years.

**Route of administration:** Subcutaneously or intramuscularly.

**Site of administration:** Thigh/deltoid.

**Protective efficacy:** 70–80% lasting for 3–5 years.

**Storage:**
- + 2°C to +8°C; do not freeze
- Keep away from light
- To be stored at the middle or bottom of the rack.

**Clinical aspects:**

Indications of Typhoid Vi capsular polysaccharide vaccine:
- Recommended to all children 2–15 years of age
- Travelers
- Close contacts
- High-risk group

Contraindications and cautions of Typhoid Vi capsular polysaccharide vaccine:
- Age less than 2 years (Vi antigen is T-cell independent and will not produce immune response in children less than 2 years)

- Life-threatening reaction to a previous dose of vaccine
- Life-threatening allergy to any component of the vaccine
- Moderately or severely ill until they recover.

Side effects of Typhoid Vi capsular polysaccharide vaccine:

The side effects of Typhoid Vi capsular polysaccharide vaccine are:
- Local: Mild pain, swelling, induration
- Serious hypersensitivity, fever, headache.

Disadvantage of Typhoid Vi capsular polysaccharide vaccine:
- Cannot be given to children aged below 2 years
- Typhoid Vi capsular polysaccharide vaccine does not protect against paratyphoid A and B
- Duration of protection is short-lived.

## QUESTIONS

**Q1. Why typhoid Vi capsular polysaccharide vaccine should be given after 2 years of age?**
Should be given after 2 years of age because the antigen is T-cell Independent.

**Q2. Can an unimmunized child suffering from typhoid fever get immunized?**
An unimmunized child with enteric fever can be immunized 4 weeks after recovery.

### Typhoid Conjugated Vaccine (TCV)

**Technical aspects:**

Liquid vaccine.

**Contents:** Vi antigen conjugated with tetanus toxoid conjugate vaccine.

**Ideal age at immunization:** From 6 months of age.

**Route of administration:** Intramuscular.

**Site of administration:** Thigh/deltoid.

**Dose and schedule of conjugated Typhoid vaccine:** See schedule

**Protective efficacy of conjugated Typhoid vaccine:** More than 90% lasting for more than 10 years.

**Clinical aspects:**

Indications for conjugated Typhoid vaccine: All children aged 6 months to 2 years.

Contraindications of conjugated Typhoid vaccine:
- Diarrhea (persistent diarrhea)
- Emesis
- Fever
- Gestational period: Pregnant and lactating women
- Hypersensitivity to any constituents
- Infections: Severe infection

**Side effects:** Mild local pain, redness, induration, mild fever.

Advantages of conjugate vaccine:
- Long lasting protection
- Required less number of doses
- Can be provided to children less than 2 years of age
- GGAVI funding approved.

### Ty21a (Oral) Vaccine

Ty21a strain of *Salmonella typhi* that is a mutant strain which lacks the enzyme UDP galactose-4-epimerase. This enzyme is responsible for incorporation of galactose into cell wall polysaccharide. The galactose present in the intestine cannot be accumulated in the cell wall of the organism, as it cannot be converted into polysaccharide. Accumulation of intermediary products of galactose in the cell will cause disruption of cell membrane.

Continued faulty biosynthesis of cell wall polysaccharide will produce immune effect. Subsequent bacterial lysis will account for low virulence of this strain.

**Technical aspects:**
Oral capsules.

**Contents:** Ty21a strain of *Salmonella typhi*, a mutant strain.

**Dose and schedule of Ty21a (oral) vaccine:** *See* Annexure.

**Route of administration:** Oral.

**Precautions:** Should be taken with cool water 1 hour before food.

**Protective efficacy of Ty21a (oral) vaccine:** 70–80% lasting for 7 years.

**Storage:**
- + 2° to + 8°C
- Keep away from light
- To be stored at the top of the rack.

**Clinical aspects:**

Vaccine—indications of Ty21a (oral) vaccine: Recommended to all children above 6 years.

Contraindications and cautions for typhoid Ty21a (oral) vaccine:
- Age less than 6 years (as the child cannot swallow)
- Acute febrile illness
- Acute intestinal infection
- Congenital or acquired immunodeficiency
- Disease that affects the immune system: HIV/AIDS
- Drugs that affect the immune system, cancer therapy or treatment with radiation or drugs. Until at least 3 days after taking antibiotics or sulfa drugs
- Concurrent intake of the antimalarial mefloquine should not be taken along with the capsule.

**Side effects of typhoid Ty21a (oral) vaccine:**

The side effects of typhoid Ty21a (oral) vaccine are:
- Local: Diarrhea, vomiting, stomach pain (abdominal cramps)
- Systemic: Transitory exanthema, fever, headache.

Disadvantages of typhoid Ty21a (oral) vaccine:
- Cannot be used in children below 6 years of age
- Uptake of vaccine is slow and requires multiple doses
- GAVI, the vaccine alliance will not provide funding for Ty21a vaccine.

## QUESTIONS

**Q1. Why typhoral is not given to children aged less than 6 years?**
The capsule should be swallowed as a whole without biting or chewing. This is given only after the age of 6 years as the capsule has to be swallowed without biting. The dose should be repeated after 3–5 years. Three capsules; one on day 1, 3, and 5; should be taken in cool water 1 hour before food.

### Tdap Vaccine

**Technical aspects:**

Liquid vaccine.

**Contents:**
- Each 0.5 ml of Tdap contains
  - 5 Lf tetanus toxoid
  - 2 Lf diphtheria toxoid
  - 2.5–10 µg of the three pertussis antigens (acellular pertussis).
  - 2.5 µg of detoxified acellular Pertussis, 5 µg of FHA, 3 µg of PRN and 5 µg of combined FIM-2 and FIM-3.

**Ideal age at immunization:** Minimum 5 years if DTaP is not available; can be replaced with Tdap at 5 years booster; at 10 and 15 years of age the dose can be repeated followed by booster every 10 years.

**Dose and schedule:**
- Dose: 0.5 mL
- Schedule: *See* Annexure.

**Route of administration:** Intramuscular.

**Site of administration:** Thigh/deltoid.

**Protective efficacy:** 90%.

**Storage:**
- +2° to +8°C
- Keep away from light.

Tdap can be administered regardless the interval between the last dose of tetanus or diphtheria toxoid containing vaccines.

**Clinical aspects:**

Indications: All children and pregnant women.

**Contraindications:**
- Allergic reactions to DTwP/DtaP vaccines or its ingredients
- Coma or seizures within a week after receiving the vaccine.

**Side effects of Tdap vaccine:**
- Mild side effects:
  - Body ache
  - Chills
  - Diarrhea
  - Emesis
  - Fever (Mild)
  - Glands swollen
  - Gastrointestinal symptoms: nausea, stomach ache
  - Headache
  - Sore joints
  - Tiredness.
- Moderate side effects:
  - Emesis
  - Extensive swelling of the entire arm in which injection was given
  - Fever >102°F
  - GIT symptom: Nausea
  - Headache
  - Pain
  - redness.
- Severe side effects:
  - Allergy: Severe allergic reactions
  - Bleeding
  - Brachial neuritis
  - Fainting.

## Td Vaccine

Adsorbed vaccines.

*Technical Aspects*

Liquid vaccine.

**Contents:**
- Tetanus toxoid 5 Lf
- Diphtheria 2 Lf (Low dose)

**Ideal age at immunization:** Adolescents and adults after 7 years of age.

**Dose and schedule:** *See* Annexure
- Dose: 0.5 mL
- Schedule of td: Td/TdaP vaccine is used as replacement for DTwP/DTaP/DT for catch-up vaccination in children above 7 years of age.

WHO recommends Td/TdaP vaccine instead of TT in wound management prophylaxis against neonatal tetanus and maternal tetanus in pregnant women. Unpregnant women should be given a minimum of 2 doses of Td at 4–8 weeks interval and one dose in previously immunized women getting pregnant after 3 years of the previous dose.

**Booster:** Td should be repeated every 10 years.

**Route of administration:** Intramuscular.

**Site of administration:** Thigh or deltoid.

**Protective efficacy:** 100% for tetanus. More than 95% for diphtheria.

**Storage:**
- +2° to +8°C
- Keep away from light
- To be stored at the middle or bottom of the rack.

*Clinical Aspects*

**Indications:**
- This is used in children aged above 7 years instead of DTwP or DTaP.
- Can be used as replacement for TT at all ages above 7 years.

**Contraindications:**

- Allergy—severe allergic reaction to tetanus or diphtheria containing previous dose
- Age less than 7 years
- Guillain-Barré syndrome within 6 weeks after immunization with vaccine containing tetanus or diphtheria
- Those who received TT in the last 5 years.

**Side effects of Td vaccine:**

Mild side effects:
- Pain
- Redness
- Mild fever
- Headache
- Muscle soreness.

Moderate side effects:
Fever.

Severe side effects:
- Allergic reactions (Severe)
- Anaphylaxis
- Bleeding
- Breathing difficulties
- Convulsions
- Dizziness
- Edema—throat, tongue, lips
- Extensive swelling of the arm, bleeding in which injection was given
- Fainting
- Hives
- Swelling
- Severe pain.

**Immunization Schedule IAP**

Tdap and Td after 7 years of age; Td every 10 years.

## VACCINES USED ON SPECIAL OCCASIONS

### High-risk Group

High-risk group includes the following:
- Acquired immunodeficiency
- Asplenia
- Babies (newborn, infancy)
- Cancer: Malignancies
- Cancer therapy: Radiation therapy
- Congenital immunodeficiency group
- Chronic cardiac, pulmonary (like asthma treated with steroids for a long time), liver disease, hematologic, renal (like nephrotic syndrome)
- Cerebrospinal leak
- Cochlear implant
- Diabetes mellitus
- Drugs: Steroids—those on long-term corticosteroids
- Epidemics: During disease outbreaks
- Functional asplenia/hyposplenism
- Foreign visits: Travelers to foreign countries
- Geriatric age group
- Healthcare workers and laboratory personnel
- Immunocompromised: congenital or acquired
- International travelers.

### IAP Recommendations—Vaccines for High-risk Group

- Rabies vaccine
- Japanese encephalitis vaccine
- Meningococcal A+ vaccine
- Influenza vaccine
- Cholera vaccine
- Yellow fever vaccine
- Pneumococcal polysaccharide vaccine

### Influenza Vaccines

#### Technical Aspects

*Types of influenza vaccines:*

Two types of vaccines are available:
1. Influenza inactivated vaccine (whole virion vaccine, split virion vaccine and subunit vaccine)
2. Nasal spray flu vaccine is a live aerosol vaccine/inactivated aerosol vaccine,

## Influenza Inactivated Vaccine

### Technical aspects:

**Contents:** Contains three viral strains—two type A and one type B

**Nature:** Liquid

**Types:** Three types are present:
1. Whole virus
2. Split product
3. Sub unit surface antigen formulation

**Ideal age at immunization:** Age at administration of influenza vaccines—
- The vaccine is given for children aged 6 months to 59 months.
- This vaccine should not be given for children below 6 months of age.

**Route of administration:** Intramuscular.

**Site of administration:** anterolateral aspect of thigh
- *Preparation of the site of administration:*
  - Clean with spirit
  - Do not rub vigorously after injection.

**Protective efficacy:** Depends on the factors such as:
- Specific influenza strains
- Prior antigenic exposure
- Underlying disease condition of an individual.

**Duration of immunity:** 6 months to 1 year

**Storage:**
- + 2° to + 8°C
- Keep away from light
- Keep it in the middle or lower compartment of the fridge
- Do not freeze.

### Disadvantages:
- Antigenic shift occurs frequently
- Composition of vaccine is changed periodically in anticipation of the prevalent influenza strains
- Duration of immunity: Short 6 months to 1 year.

### Clinical aspects:

They should be given to the following who are at high-risk of serious complications, if get influenza infection.

It should be used in patients on long-term aspirin therapy. Immunosuppressants for patients with chronic pulmonary or cardiac diseases, diabetes mellitus, renal dysfunction, and hemoglobinopathies.

Indications for influenza vaccines (Mnemonic A-I):
- Age more than 6 months to 59 months
- Aspirin: Long-term therapy
- Bronchial asthma patients
- Chronic illness: Heart disease, cirrhosis, nephrotic syndrome, neurological disorders
- Chronic obstructive pulmonary disease
- Cystic fibrosis
- Chronic renal failure
- Care takers for infants
- Chronic metabolic diseases
- Diabetics
- Drug to suppress immune system
- Elder people
- 50 years or more of age
- Gestational period (Pregnant)
- Healthcare workers
- Household contacts
- HIV infection
- Hemoglobinopathies: Sickle cell anemia
- Immunosuppressed children and adults.

Contraindications and cautions for inactivated influenza vaccine:
- Allergy to egg protein
- Children under the age of 6 years
- Life-threatening allergies
- Severe egg allergy
- Severe reaction to previous dose of influenza vaccine
- Guillain-Barré syndrome within 6 weeks following previous dose of influenza vaccine
- Moderately or severely ill
- Oculorespiratory syndrome to previous dose

- Immune response in congenital or acquired immunodeficiency will be insufficient
- An inactivated flu vaccine called afluria should not be given to children below 8 years of age except in special circumstances. Fever and fever-related seizures were noted
- Those suffering from medical conditions that predispose them to influenza complications.

**Side effects of inactivated influenza vaccine:**

Mild side effects:
- Local side effects—pain, induration, redness, mild soreness.
- Systemic side effects:
  - rash, myalgia, sore, red or itchy eyes, shivering
  - Aches
  - Allergy: Life threatening allergic reactions/Anaphylaxis
  - Angioedema
  - Asthenia
  - Cough
  - Dermatological problems: Generalized skin reactions, urticaria, pruritis, nonspecific rash
  - Ecchymosis
  - Fatigue
  - Febrile convulsions
  - Fever
  - Guillain Barre syndrome (rare)
  - Headache
  - Hoarseness
  - Itching
  - Kidney problems: Vasculitis with transient renal involvement
  - Lymphadenopathy (Transient)
  - Neurological manifestations like Neuralgia, paresthesia, encephalomyelitis, neuritis
  - Oculo respiratory syndrome: Red eyes, cough, sore throat, hoarseness
  - Shock: Allergic reactions leading to shock
  - Thrombocytopenia.

## Live Attenuated Influenza Vaccines (LAIV)

**Technical aspects:**

**Contents:** Live attenuated reassortment of WHO recommended strains.

**Diluents:** Sterile water.

**Dose:** 0.1 mL each nostril one month apart, total 0.2 mL

**Schedule:** *See* annexure.

**Age:** 2–49 years.

**Route of administration:** Nasal spray.
Precautions to be taken before administering live attenuated influenza vaccine: This vaccine should not be administered for 48 hours after cessation of antiviral therapy.

**Protective efficacy:** For children more than 2 years laboratory confirmed influenza—82% and influenza like illness—33%

**Storage:** 2–8 degree celsius.

**Clinical aspects:**

Indications for live attenuated influenza vaccine:
- Used for healthy nonpregnant individuals aged 2 to 4 years of age
- Administered as nasal spray
- Age less than 5 years and more than 50 years
  - 5–50 years with high-risk disease (weakened immune system, long-term health problems such as heart disease, lung disease, asthma, kidney disease, diabetes or blood disorders)
- Household contacts
- Healthcare personel.
- Extreme obese persons.

Contraindications and cautions for live attenuated influenza vaccine:
- Age: Children below 6 months of age
- Allergic reactions (Severe): With previous dose of influenza or its components

- Anemia
- Asthma/reactive airway disease
- Blood disorders
- Chronic diseases
- Drugs: Patients on long-term aspirin therapy
- Diabetes
- Egg allergy (Severe)
- First trimester of pregnancy: Pregnant women
- Guillain-Barré syndrome (GBS) or history of Guillain-Barré syndrome (GBS) within 8 weeks after getting immunized with influenza vaccine
- Heart disease
- Immunodeficiency disorders
- Kidney
- Lung disease
- Liver disease
- Long-term health problems such as heart disease, lung disease, asthma, kidney disease, diabetes or blood disorders
- Muscle disorders
- Nerve disorders
- Patients who are moderately or severely ill should wait until they recover
- Should not be administered for first 48 hours of antiviral therapy
- Antiviral therapy should not be given for first two days after vaccination.

Side effects of live attenuated influenza vaccines:
- Mild side effects:
  - Abdominal pain/tenderness
  - Breathing problems—wheezing
  - Breast tenderness
  - Cough
  - Diarrhea
  - Emesis (vomiting)
  - Fever
  - Fatigue
  - Generalized weakness
  - Headache
  - Irritability
  - Muscle aches
  - Nasal congestion
  - Running nose
  - Sore throat
  - Tiredness
  - Wheezing
- Local reactions: Nasal discomfort, stuffy nose, running nose, nasal congestion, loss of smell, red eyes, lacrimation.
- Systemic reactions: Headache, chills, fatigue, sore throat, myalgia, arthralgia, irritability, loss of appetite
- Severe side effects:
  - Allergic reactions/Anaphylaxis (severe life-threatening)
  - Brain damage (Permanent)
  - Coma
  - Dry eyes
  - Eye problems like itching
  - Flu-like symptoms (running nose, sore throat, tiredness, cough, heavy head, etc.)
  - Guillain–Barré syndrome
  - Heavy head
  - Itching all over.

## Rubella Vaccine

Vaccine against German measles.

### Types of Rubella Immunization

- Active immunization
- Passive immunization.

### Technical Aspects

It is a human diploid cell culture vaccine.

Contains live attenuated rubella virus Wistar RA 27/3 strain 1,000 TCID per 0.5 mL

Age of rubella immunization:
- Active immunization should be given to girls before their marriage, from 1 year of age to puberty
- Passive immunization: Rubella gamma-globulin can be given to pregnant women exposed to rubella.

**Dose:** 0.5 mL.

**Schedule:** *See* Annexure.

**Site of administration:** anterolateral aspect of thigh.

**Route of administration:** Subcutaneous.

**Protective efficacy:** 95%.

**Duration of protection:** Lifelong protection.

**Storage:** 2–8°C.

## Clinical Aspects

### Indications of rubella (MMR) vaccination:
Recommended to all infants.

### Contraindications and cautions for rubella (MMR) vaccination:
- Anaphylaxis/anaphylactoid reactions to neomycin
- Blood transfusion antibody containing blood products with in past 11 months
- Cancers—leukemia, lymphoma
- Drugs—immunosuppressants
- Epilepsy (family or personal history of seizures)
- Fever >101°F
- Gestational period (Pregnancy)
- Gammaglobulin administration
- Hypogammaglobulinemia
- Immunocompromised/immunodeficiency
- Infections: Acute infectious diseases Active untreated tuberculosis HIV
- Pregnancy should be avoided up to 3 months after this vaccine.

### Side effects of rubella (MMR) vaccination

**Mild side effects:**
- Mild fever, rash, malaise, sore throat
- Transient arthralgia/arthritis—joint pain in adults
- Paresthetic pains
- Thrombocytopenia
- Peripheral neuropathy.

**Severe side effects:**
- Acute encephalitis
- *Staphylococcus aureus* 1 in 1,000,000 cases with MMR vaccine
- Meningitis

## QUESTIONS

**Q1. What are the precautions to be taken if the rubella vaccine is administered after puberty?**

After puberty, the vaccine should not be given to the pregnant women or they should avoid pregnancy for at least 8 weeks after the vaccination. The vaccine can be given after estimating hemagglutination inhibition antibody titer. This titer can be estimated in two samples at an interval of 3–6 weeks.

**Q2. Is termination of pregnancy indicated if you have accidentally given rubella vaccine during pregnancy?**

But the risk should be explained to the parents and they will have to decide about it.

## Pneumococcal Vaccines

- Unconjugated pneumococcal vaccine—23 valent polysaccharide
- Non-T-cell dependent and will not induce good immunity
- 7 valent vaccine—2 μg each of 4, 9, 14, 18C, 19F, 23F, and 4 μg each of 6B
- 9 valent vaccine—1, 5
- 11 valent vaccines
- Two different vaccines are available. Polysaccharide and conjugate vaccines are available.
- PPSV23 typically 23 valent
- Pneumococcal conjugated vaccine (PCV) typically 13 valent.

*Minimal age at administration of pneumococcal polysaccharide vaccine*: 6 weeks for conjugate vaccine and 2 years for polysaccharide vaccine.

### Pneumococcal Polysaccharide Vaccine (PPSV 23)

Polysaccharide vaccines will have low immunogenicity.

## Technical aspects:

**Contents:** PPSV 23 is a 23 valent vaccine containing serotypes 1, 2, 3, 4, 5, 6B, 7F, 8.9N.9V, 10A, 11A, 12 F, 14, 15 B, 17F, 18C, 19F, 19A, 20, 22F, 23F, 33F.

**Ideal age at immunization:**
Dose and schedule of pneumococcal polysaccharide vaccine (PPSV):
- Age: More than or equal to 2 years of age
- Dose: 0.5 mL
- Schedule: *See* Annexure
- Not more than two doses are required in the life time
- Repeated doses will result in immunologic hyporesponsiveness
- Boosters.

**Route of administration:** Subcutaneously/intramuscularly.

**Site of administration:** Thigh/deltoid.
*Preparation of the site of administration:*
- Clean with spirit
- Do not rub vigorously after injection.

**Protective efficacy:**
- Poorly immunogenic
- At best its efficacy is 70%
- Less than 2 years poor immunological memory.

**Storage:**
- + 2° to +8°C
- Keep away from light
- Keep it in the middle or lower compartment of the fridge
- Do not freeze.

## Clinical aspects:

Indications for pneumococcal polysaccharide vaccine:

PCV13 is recommended for children less than 5 years of age for the following children who are at risk for developing pneumococcal infection.

Pneumococcal vaccine is administered for children who are at high-risk to get infected with pneumococci. They are:
- Asplenia (functionally or anatomically asplenic)/before splenectomy (This vaccine should be given at least 2 weeks before splenectomy)
- Alcoholics
- Bone marrow transplant
- Cancers
- CSF rhinorrhea/CSF leak
- Chronic heart disease
- Chronic lung disease like asthma
- Children with chronic diseases (cardiac, pulmonary diseases)
- Diabetes mellitus
- Ear: Children with cochlear transplant
- Failure—kidney, cardiac
- Fracture—cribriform plate with CSF leak
- Geriatric age group (>65 years of age )
- Hemoglobinopathies: Sickle cell diseases, other sickle cell hemoglobinopathies, hemoglobin SS, hemoglobin S-C, hemoglobin S-β, thalassemia
- HIV infection
- Hematological—sickle cell anemia
- Immunodeficiency–B cell or T cell deficiency, phagocytic disorders, complement deficiency
- Immunocompromising conditions
- Kidney disease: Nephrotic syndrome, chronic renal failure
- Liver cirrhosis
- Long-term steroids children who received a solid organ transplant
- Leukemia
- Lung disorders
- Liver disorders
- Lymphoma: Hodgkin's
- Multiple myeloma
- Meningitis (Recurrent meningitis )
- Neoplasms
- Organ transplant patients
- Prosthesis—cochlear implant.

## Contraindications to pneumococcal polysaccharide vaccine (PPSV):

Age: Children under 2 years.

Allergy: Life-threatening reaction to a previous dose of vaccine or any components of the vaccine.

Bed ridden patients: Moderately or severely ill until they recover.

Cancers: Lymphoreticular malignancies.

Drugs: Patients on immunosuppressive therapy.

### Side effects of pneumococcal polysaccharide vaccine

**Mild side effects:**

Local—local pain, induration, swelling, redness, stiffness, tenderness will be mild nature and will last for 1–2 days

**Systemic:**
- Appetite: Loss of appetite
- Allergic reactions: Rash
- Breathing difficulties
- Chills
- Crying: Abnormal
- Drowsiness
- Dizziness
- Diarrhea
- Emesis (Vomiting)
- Fever
- Febrile or afebrile convulsions
- Fatigue
- Fainting
- Generalized weakness
- Guillain-Barré syndrome
- Headache
- Hemolytic anemia
- Irritability
- Joint pain
- Knee joint arthritis
- Lymphadenitis/lymphadenopathy
- Muscle ache
- Nausea
- Edema in the injected limbs
- Paresthesia
- Radiculoneuropathy
- Sleep disturbances (Decreased or increased sleep)
- Serum sickness
- Serositis
- Thrombocytopenia
- Urticaria.

Apnea is common when administered for preterm below 28 weeks of gestation. The vaccine recipient should be monitored for respiratory problems for at least 48–72 hours.

## QUESTIONS

Q1. What are the recent indications for pneumococcal polysaccharide vaccine?

For children under the age of 13 years, pneumococcal conjugate vaccine PCV 13 can be used as the response to PPSV 23 is poor.

*Unconjugated pneumococcal polysaccharide vaccine (PPSV 23)*: PPSV 23 is a T cell independent vaccine.

Q2. What are the disadvantages of pneumococcal polysaccharide vaccine PPSV 23?
- Poorly immunogenic in children aged less than 2 years
- Does not reduce nasopharyngeal carriage
- Does not produce Herd immunity
- Has low immune memory
- Protective efficacy only 70%
- Does not provide protection against non-bacteremic pneumonia/otitis media.
- PCV vaccine

### Meningococcal Vaccine

Endemic meningococcal infection is caused by Group B meningococci for which effective vaccine is not available. There are 13 clinically significant serogroups of which six serotypes A, B, C, Y, W135, and X are responsible for most of the diseases in humans.

### Types of Meningococcal Vaccine Licensed in India

1. Quadrivalent vaccine against four serotypes– A +C+Y+W135
2. Bivalent: Meningococcal A + C vaccine. It is a bivalent vaccine containing antigens of serotypes group A and C of *N. meningitides*
3. Monovalent group A.

## Unconjugated Polysaccharide Vaccine

Bi and quadrivalent vaccines. Conjugate vaccines are preferred due to T cell dependent immunity to produce memory B cells. Conjugate vaccines are preferred.

## Unconjugated Meningococcal Polysaccharide Vaccine (MPSV)

**Technical aspects:**

- Contents of unconjugated meningococcal polysaccharide vaccine:
- A, C, Y, and W135 effective in children above 2 years of age
- Each unit dose contains pure lyophilized polysaccharide of *Neisseria meningitidis* group A and C each 50 µg.
- There is no vaccine against serotype B.

Diluent: Distilled water

Ideal age at immunization: More than 2 years

Quadrivalent conjugate and polysaccharide vaccines are recommended for children above 2 years of age. Only under special circumstances like outbreaks/close household contacts, it can be given to children aged 3 months to 2 years.

### Dose and schedule of meningococcal vaccine:

Dose: 0.5 mL

Schedule: See Annexure

Route of administration of meningococcal vaccine: Subcutaneously or intramuscularly.

Site of administration of meningococcal vaccine: Deltoid or anterolateral aspect of thigh.

Protective efficacy: 85% protective antibodies will be formed in 10–14 days after vaccination.

### Instructions to the mother after administration of vaccine:

*Protective efficacy of meningococcal vaccine is 85–90%*

- Keep away from light
- To be stored at the top of the rack.

Storage:

- *When vaccine is not in use, + 2°C to + 8°C* in the upper most compartment of the refrigerator.
- *During immunization can be kept in ice and should be used within 2 hours.*
- *Storage of vaccine in case of power failure:* Keep in an ice box.

If the child is vaccinated before the age of 3–4 years, the vaccine should be repeated after 2–3 years.

## Quadrivalent Meningococcal Polysaccharide—Protein Conjugate Vaccine

Lyophilized vaccine.

**Diluent:** Distilled water.

**Advantages:**

The following three advantages are seen with conjugate vaccines for long-term protection:
1. Memory response
2. Herd immunity
3. Circulating antibody.

**Contents:** 4 µg each of A, C, Y, and W135 conjugated to 48 g of diphtheria toxoid .

**Dose:** 0.5 mL.

**Schedule:** First dose at 11–12 years

- Booster at 16–18 years
- Booster once in 5 years
- For those vaccinated at 2–6 years should be revaccinated after 3 years
- For those vaccinated after 7 years should be revaccinated after 5 years.

**Route of administration of meningococcal vaccine:** Deep intramuscularly.

**Site of administration of meningococcal vaccine:** Deltoid or thigh.

**Protective efficacy:** 85%. Protective antibodies will be formed in 10–14 days after vaccination.

**Instructions to the mother after administration of vaccine:**

*Protective efficacy of meningococcal vaccine is 80–85%.*

- Keep away from light
- To be stored at the top of the rack.

**Storage:**
- *When vaccine is not in use:* + 2°C to + 8°C in the uppermost compartment of the refrigerator.
- During immunization can be kept in ice and should be used within 2 hours.
- *Storage of vaccine in case of power failure:* Keep in an ice box.

If the child is vaccinated before the age of 3-4 years, the vaccine should be repeated after 2-3 years.

## Monovalent Serotype A Conjugate Vaccine

Lyophilized vaccine.

**Contents:** 10 µg of purified meningococcal A polysaccharide covalently bound to 10-33 µg tetanus toxoid.

**Adjuvant:** Alum.

**Preservative:** Thimerosal.

**Site of administration:** Intramuscular dose 0.5 mL

- Age: 1-29 years of age
- Monovalent conjugate group A vaccine can be used for children above 1 year of age.

**Schedule:** Single dose

- Need for booster dose not established
- Those vaccinated previously with polysaccharide vaccine can be revaccinated with conjugate vaccine.

## Clinical Aspects of Meningococcal Vaccines

**Indications:** High-risk group.

**Indications of meningococcal vaccine— currently not recommended for routine use:** It is indicated only for high-risk group during outbreaks.

- Anatomic asplenia
- Anemia—sickle cell anemia
- Before splenectomy (at least 2 weeks before)
- Complement deficiency—persistent complement or properdin deficiencies
- Close contacts as an adjunct to chemoprophylaxis
- Day care contacts
- Epidemics (As a part of outbreak control programs)
- Functional asplenia
- Group of people with high-risk: Health care workers, microbiologist exposed to meningococci
- Hyposplenia
- HIV cases
- Immunodeficiency—terminal complement component deficiency
- International travelers to endemic countries
- CDC recommendation: All 11-12 years old children are immunized with meningococcal conjugate vaccine. Booster dose is given at 16 years.

**Contraindications of meningococcal vaccine:**
- Allergic reaction to a previous dose of vaccine
- Life-threatening allergy to any component of the vaccine
- Moderately or severely ill until they recover
- Pregnancy
- It is not recommended for children below 3 months of age.

## Side Effects of Meningococcal Vaccine

**Mild side effects:**
- Mild fever
- Headache in older children
- pain at local site
- Redness
- Swelling
- Muscle or joint pain.

**Severe side effects:**
- Allergic reactions: Serious allergic reactions
- Brief fainting spells especially in adolescents

- ❖ Chills
- ❖ Diarrhea
- ❖ Edema
- ❖ Fever
- ❖ Guillain-Barré syndrome
- ❖ Hemolysis.

## QUESTIONS

**Q1. What are the steps for outbreak prevention and control of meningococcal infection?**
- ❑ Active case surveillance
- ❑ Beta lactam antibiotics in patients allergic to penicillin and cephalosporins
- ❑ B serogroup (recombinant) vaccines as B serotype is more common cause of meningitis
- ❑ Chemoprophylaxis of close contacts
- ❑ Drugs therapy for affected individuals: Antibiotics (Cephalosporins and penicillin)
- ❑ Empiric therapy
- ❑ Early diagnosis
- ❑ Fostering disease awareness within the community
- ❑ Government should take immediate action by forming a rapid response team
- ❑ High-risk group revaccination (household contacts, hospital staff)
- ❑ Isolation of patients for 72 hours.

**Q2. What are the healthcare workers included in rapid response team?**
- ❑ Medical professionals
- ❑ Microbiologist
- ❑ Epidemiologist.

**Q3. What are the functions of healthcare workers included in rapid response team?**
- ❑ Identify the cases
- ❑ Assist in management of critically ill patients.

**Q4. Can meningococcal vaccine given to pregnant women?**
Meningococcal vaccine can be given during pregnancy.

**Q5. What is the age at which Men ACWY-CRM and Men ACWY-D can be administered?**
- ❑ Men ACY W135-CRM—meningococcal serogroups A,C,W,Y vaccine: more than or equal to 2 months
- ❑ Men ACWY-D: More than or equal to 9 months.

**Q6. What is the chemoprophylaxis of meningococcal vaccine?**
Chemoprophylaxis to the contacts—antibiotics to prevent nasopharyngeal carriage of pathogenic microbes in the household members and contacts.

Ceftriaxone in a dose of 20 mg/kg in a single dose for 2 days, maximum dose of 600 mg.

**Q7. Why meningococcal vaccine is not given routinely to all children?**
Meningococcal vaccine is not given routinely to all children because the incidence of meningococcal disease is less.

**Q8. Can the quadrivalent meningococcal vaccine be given simultaneously along with PCV13?**
Interference with PCV13 was noted so at least 1 month interval should be present between them.

## Japanese B Encephalitis Vaccine

Types of Japanese B encephalitis vaccine:
- ❖ Live attenuated cell culture Japanese B encephalitis vaccine
- ❖ Inactivated cell culture Japanese B encephalitis vaccine
- ❖ Inactivated vero cell culture Japanese B encephalitis vaccine.

### *Live Attenuated, Cell Culture Japanese B Encephalitis Vaccine*

**Technical aspects:**

Liquid vaccine.

**Contents:**
- ❖ 5.4 log PFU of SA
- ❖ 14-14-2 strain of JE virus.

Ideal age at immunization:
- After 9 months
- Minimal age 8 months.

**Dose and schedule:**
- Dose: 0.5 mL
- Schedule:
  - First dose at 9 months along with measles vaccine
  - Second dose at 16–18 months.

**Route of administration:** Subcutaneous route.

**Site of administration:** Thigh/deltoid.

**Protective efficacy:** More than 90%.

**Storage:**
- + 2°C to +8°C
- Keep away from light
- To be stored at the top of the rack.

**Clinical aspects:**
- Indications of the vaccine:
  - People living in high-risk area
  - Travel to high-risk areas for more than 1 month
  - Stay in rural areas for more than 1 month
- Contraindications for administration of live JE vaccine
- Allergy to vaccine or any component of the vaccine
- Bacterial infection: Active untreated tuberculosis inpatient
- Convulsions/past history of convulsions
- Drugs: Immunosuppressants
- Ear infections: Otitis media, tympanitis
- Fever more than 38.5°C
- Gestational period: Pregnancy
- Gelatin hypersensitivity
- Hepatic, renal, and cardiac disease
- Hypersensitivity to gentamicin or kanamycin
- Household contacts of immunodeficiency patients
- Immunodeficiency: Congenital or acquired immunodeficiency
- Infections: Active untreated tuberculous infections.

The following are not contraindications for administration of Japanese B encephalitis vaccine:
- Minor illness like respiratory infection or diarrhea
- Family history of convulsions
- Corticosteroids use
- Stable neurological disorders like cerebral palsy
- Down syndrome.

There should be a gap of at least four weeks between administration of live JE vaccine and any other live vaccines.

**Side effects:**
- Local reactions: Redness, swelling, pain at the site of injection
- Systemic reactions:
  - Anaphylaxis
  - Fever
  - Headache.

## Inactivated Cell Culture Japanese B Encephalitis Vaccine

**Technical aspects:**

**Contents:** Lyophilized vaccine Nakayama NH strain.

**Diluents:** Sterile water.

**Minimal age at immunization:** 1 year.

**Dose and schedule:**
- Dose: Two doses of 0.25 mL for children aged more than or equal to 1 year to less than or equal to 3 years.
- Schedule: On days 0 and 28.

Route of administration: subcutaneous route.

Site of administration: Deltoid.

Protective efficacy: 80–90%.

Storage:
- + 2°C to +8°C
- Keep away from light
- To be stored at the top of the rack.

**Clinical aspects:**
- ❖ Indications of the vaccine:
  - People living in high-risk area
  - Travel to high-risk areas for more than 1 month
  - Stay in rural areas for more than 1 month
- ❖ Contraindications:
  - Serious hypersensitivity
  - Pregnancy
- ❖ Side effects:
  - Allergic reaction: Anaphylaxis
  - Neurological problems.

## Inactivated Vero Cell Culture Japanese B Encephalitis Vaccine

**Technical aspects:**

Ideal age at immunization: 1 year.

**Dose and schedule:**
- ❖ Dose: Two doses of 0.5 mL for children aged more than 1 year.
- ❖ Schedule: *See* Annexure

**Route of administration:** Intramuscular route.

**Site of administration:** Deltoid.

## Yellow Fever Vaccine

- ❖ Live attenuated vaccine
- ❖ Derived from 17 D strain of yellow fever virus
- ❖ Freeze dried preparation.

### Technical Aspects

**Contents:**
- ❖ Lyophilized
- ❖ Freeze dried.

**Diluents:** Sterile saline

**Ideal age at immunization:** After 9 months of age (Minimal age 9 months).

**Dose and schedule:**
- ❖ Dose: 0.5 mL
- ❖ Schedule: *See* Annexure.
- ❖ Booster: Every 10 years.

**Route of administration:** Subcutaneously or intramuscularly.

**Site of administration:** Deltoid—lateral aspect of upper arm/anterolateral aspect of thigh.

**Precautions:** This vaccine should be given at least 10 days before travel.

**Protective efficacy:** More than 90%

Immunogenicity will be attained from 10th day after vaccination and lasts for at least 10 years or lifelong.

**Storage:**
- ❖ + 2°C to +8°C
- ❖ Heat labile
- ❖ Keep away from light
- ❖ To be stored at the top of the rack
- ❖ Should be discarded within 1 hour after reconstitution.

### Clinical Aspects

**Indications of the vaccine:**
- ❖ To all travelers to yellow fever endemic zones like sub-Saharan Africa or few tropical South American countries.
- ❖ A certificate should be issued which will be valid from the 10th day after vaccination to 10 years or lifelong after vaccination.
- ❖ This vaccine is not for routine use in India.

**Contraindications and cautions (Mnemonic A–I):**
- ❖ Allergy to vaccine or vaccine components
- ❖ Age: Young infants below 6 months of age due to risk of vaccine associated neurotrophic or viscerotropic disease (better to delay ≥9 months of age)
- ❖ Breastfeeding/lactating women
- ❖ Cancers
- ❖ Drugs causing immunosuppression
- ❖ Egg allergy (Serious)
- ❖ Females who are pregnant
- ❖ Geriatric age: Elderly more than or equal to 65 years
- ❖ HIV infection (Symptomatic) CD4 less than 200/mm$^3$ or less than 15% of total in children less than 6 years

- Immunodeficiency: Primary immunodeficiency, immunocompromised, thymus disorders, HIV disease, congenital immunodeficiency, and symptomatic HIV patients.

### Precautions for Administration of Yellow Fever Vaccine

- Age: 6–8 months
- Age above 60 years
- CD4 count 200–499 mm$^3$ or 15–24% of total in children aged less than 6 years
- Pregnancy
- Lactating mothers.

### Adverse Effects

- Minor:
  - Pain
  - Swelling
  - Fever
  - Headache
  - Myalgia
- Serious systemic adverse effects:
  - Anaphylaxis
  - Hypersensitivity reactions
  - Bronchospasm
  - Rash
  - Urticaria
  - Neurologic disorders
  - Acute disseminated encephalomyelitis
  - Guillain-Barré syndrome (GBS)
  - Encephalitis
  - Meningoencephalitis.

### ADEM

- Viscerotropic disease
- Yellow fever vaccine associated viscerotropic disease (YEL-AVD)
- Yellow fever vaccine associated neurotropic disease (YEL-AND).

## QUESTIONS

**Q1. Why Yellow fever is contraindicated in infants less than 6 months?**
The incidence of neurologic and viscerotropic diseases is higher.

## Chicken Pox Vaccine (Varicella Vaccine)

The chicken pox vaccine (Varicella vaccine) is a live attenuated viral vaccine which induces both humoral and cell-mediated immunity.

### Technical Aspects

Lyophilized form.

**Contents:** Contains live attenuated virus derived from Oka-Merck strain of varicella zoster virus. The vaccine should contain minimum of 1,000 plaque forming units. It contains 10 PFU plaque forming units in 0.5 mL.

**Doses and schedule:** 5 mL

- *Schedule: See* Annexure
- *Catch-up vaccination: See* Annexure.

**Route of administration:** Subcutaneous (never intravenous).

**Age at administration:** The vaccine is recommended after the age of 1 year.

**Seroconversion rate:** 95–99% after single dose

- Post-exposure: 90% efficacy if given within 3 days following exposure.
- Protective antibodies are present even after 10 years of vaccination.

**Duration of immunity:** Immunity following vaccine will be for about 10–20 years.

**Storage:**

- Stored in refrigerator but should not be frozen. If frozen, should not be refrozen.
- Should be used within 30 minutes of its reconstitution.
- Should be protected from light.
- Diluents can be stored at room temperature.

**Compatibility:** This vaccine can be given with all other childhood vaccines. If not given simultaneously, then an interval of 4 weeks should be there between two live viral vaccines, except OPV.

## Clinical Aspects
**Indications:**
- IAP recommends for all children after 1 year of life
- After 12 years, the vaccine should be given for the following cases:
  - Age group: Susceptible adolescents
  - Adults confined to institutions and seronegative
  - Adults about to attend residential school and seronegative
  - Children attending day care centers
  - Chronic heart or lung disease
  - Drugs like steroids used for long term, chemotherapy, immunosuppressants, and long-term steroids as in nephrotic syndrome
  - Exposure to cases with varicella/chicken pox: Post-exposure immunization Family members/household contacts of immunosuppressed (for fear of transmission to them) should receive vaccine within 72 hours of exposure
  - HIV infection (asymptomatic) (when CD4 counts are >15%)
  - Leukemia (when in remission for one year or more).

**Contraindications and cautions for chickenpox vaccine:**
- Adverse reactions—who had life-threatening adverse reactions to previous dose of Hib
- Blood dyscrasias
- Blood or blood products transfusion (will interfere with the antibody formation)
- Congenital or acquired immunodeficiency
- Cancers affection bone marrow or lymphatic system like leukemia, lymphoma
- Drugs that affect the immune system, cancer therapy or treatment with radiation or drugs. Children on steroids, children with acute leukemia on chemotherapy (can be given after 11 months of completion of chemotheraphy, after 4 weeks of stopping steroids)
- Earlier varicella infection: Vaccination is not indicated in those who had already infected with chicken pox

Family history of congenital hereditary immunodeficiency in first degree relatives like parents or siblings
- Gestational period: Pregnancy—females should not get pregnant at least for 3 months after receiving the vaccine (during pregnancy can cause low birth weight and limb anomalies)
- Hypersensitivity to neomycin
- Humoral immunodeficiencies
- HIV (clinically manifested)/AIDS/Disease that affect the immune system
- Immunocompromised individuals—it should not be given along with other live vaccines
- Immunodeficiency: Severe T cell deficiency with absolute lymphocyte count less
- Ill patients: People who are moderately or severely ill at the time of vaccination
- Varicella vaccine need not be given for those who had already had infection earlier.

**Note:** Varicella zoster immunoglobulin can be administered to those persons to whom varicella vaccine is contraindicated and not already infected.

### Side Effects of Varicella Vaccine
- Local—pain, redness, swelling, at vaccination site, injection site papulovesicular eruption
- Systemic—mild fever, headache, pneumonitis, arthropathy, systemic varicella like rash

**Mild side effects:**
- Soreness
- Swelling
- Fever mild rash.

**Moderate side effects:**
Seizure (Jerking or staring).

**Severe side effects:**
- Pneumonia
- Severe brain reactions
- Low blood count.

## Complications of Chickenpox Vaccine
- Arthritis
- Breakthrough varicella
- CNS infections—meningitis
- Cerebellar ataxia
- Dehydration
- Encephalitis: Post-infectious encephalitis
- Failure: Vaccine failure especially following first dose/single dose
- Group A streptococcal infections
- Herpes zoster can occur both due to vaccine virus and wild virus. Since it is a live form attenuated virus and remains dormant in the dorsal root ganglia, herpes zoster can occur. This also can develop when the person immunized is immunocompromised. This also can occur when the patient develops malignancy.
- Infections: Secondary bacterial infections, Varicella pneumonia
- Vaccine strain varicella zoster infection with or without other organ involvement (pneumonia, encephalitis, meningitis, hepatitis are common in individuals with immunodeficiency)
- Reye's syndrome (If aspirin is taken during chickenpox. Avoid salicylates for 6 weeks following vaccination).

# QUESTIONS

**Q1. Why chickenpox vaccine was not used generally?**
Although the chicken-pox vaccine was developed in Japan in early 1970s, it was not in general use because of the following factors:
- Mild nature of chicken pox infection
- One infection provides long immunity
- Concern regarding incidence of Herpes zoster after vaccination.

Also WHO had not recommended for inclusion of chicken-pox vaccine in the immunization schedule in developing countries.

**Q2. Mention the high-risk group for chickenpox infection.**
- Newborns and infants
- Unvaccinated children and adults.

**Q3. Can MMR and varicella vaccine administered on the same day?**
Yes. If not administrated on the same day, they should be administered after 28 days.

**Q4. How will you prevent chickenpox in newborn when the mother is infected with chickenpox in the antenatal period?**
If the mother had infection 3 days before or 5 days after the delivery, the baby should receive varicella zoster immunoglobulin (VZIG). If the baby is not infected, the baby should be isolated from the infected mother for 21 days. Immunoglobulin should be given to the baby in a dose of 125 units/kg as soon as the baby is delivered. If the baby develops lesions the baby should be isolated until the scabs are formed.

**Q5. What is breakthrough varicella?**
Breakthrough varicella is defined as varicella developing more than 42 days after immunization and usually occurs 2–5 years following vaccination.

It may be mild with maculopapular rash with low or no fever and shorter duration of illness.

In some cases, it will be contagious and may be severe. Thus can result in outbreaks and has occasionally caused death.

The predisposing causes for breakthrough varicella are:
- Intake of steroids within 3 months of vaccination
- Increasing time since vaccination

- Young age at vaccination at 15 months or less
- Administration of varicella vaccine within 28 days of MMR vaccination
- Varicella vaccine virus can cause herpes zoster in the post-immunization period which will be more severe than the natural disease
- The rate of this was 2.6/100,000 vaccine doses distributed.

*Breakthrough infections:* More cases of breakthrough infections are reported today.

**Q6. Although varicella can be given from the age of 12 months, why it is advised at 15 months?**

Because the incidence of breakthrough varicella is low after 15 months.

## Anti-rabies Vaccine

Rabies can cause acute encephalomyelitis after dog bite. The incubation period is from months to years.

Prognosis: The disease is fatal.

*Types of anti-rabies vaccines:*
- Purified chick embryo vaccine (PCEV)
- Purified vero cell vaccine (PVCV)
- Human diploid cell vaccine (HDCV).

### Human Diploid Cell Vaccine
**Technical aspects:**

Lyophilized (Freeze dried).

Contents: Inactivated rabies virus grown on human diploid/chick embryo/vero cells:

Diluents: Sterile water provided with the vaccine.

Dose: 1 mL.

Schedule: *See* Annexure.

Pre-exposure—0, 7, and 28 days.

Post-exposure depends upon the class of bite 0, 3, 7, 14, and 30 days.

Route of administration: Intramuscular

(Intradermal route—small dose can be given intradermally at multiple sites)

Site of administration: Deltoid is the ideal site, anterolateral aspect of thigh for newborn, infants, and young children.

Gluteal region should be avoided as the response is poor due to excess fat at this site which will retard absorption of the antigen.

Precautions:
- Immunoglobulins should be administered in severe bite cases.
- Immunosuppressants should not be given during vaccination period.

Protective efficacy: 90–100%.

Storage:
- +2°C to +8°C
- Keep away from light
- To be stored at the top of the rack.

**Clinical aspects:**

Indications of the vaccine:
- Pre-exposure prophylaxis—for high-risk group
- Post-exposure prophylaxis—all cases of dog bite.

Contraindications:
- Pre-exposure prophylaxis: Severe reaction for previous dose
- Post-exposure prophylaxis: Severe reaction for previous dose
- Sensitivity to gelatin, neomycin, and chicken protein.

Side effects of tissue cell culture vaccine:
- Local—soreness
- Systemic reactions:
  - fever
  - Headache
  - Anaphylaxis
  - Malaise
  - Edema at the site of injection
  - Transient neuroparalytic illness of Guillain-Barré type.

## QUESTIONS

**Q1. What is the indication for Rabies immunoglobulin?**
Rabies immunoglobulin is indicated in all class III bites and should be infiltrated in and around the wound.

**Q2. What are the types of rabies prophylaxis?**
The types of rabies prophylaxis:
- **Pre-exposure prophylaxis**—three doses of cell culture vaccine 0, 7, and 21or 28 days will give 100% protection.
- **Post-exposure prophylaxis**—passive immunization with human rabies immunoglobulin 40u/kg body weight will give protection until antibody is produced by the rabies vaccine. Half of the dose should be given subcutaneously at the site of bite or scratch and the other half dose should be given intramuscularly.
   5 doses at day 0, 3, 7, 14, and 28 days (Essen schedule).
   4 doses with 1 mL of HDCV or PCECV at day 0, 3, 7, and 14 days along with immunoglobulin are as effective as 5 dose regimen.

**Q3. What is the schedule for already vaccinated dog bite cases?**
For already vaccinated with cell culture vaccine with adequate antibody titer 2 dose regimen will be enough.

**Q4. What is the schedule for dog bite cases who are immunocompromised?**
For immunocompromised, 5 dose regimen with antibodies should be given.

**Q5. What are the conditions in which the dog which has bitten the patient is considered as rabid dog?**
The conditions for considering the dog as a rabid dog are:
- Bite by stray dog
- Dog is not alive
- Dog is missing
- Dog is not traceable
- Unprovoked dog bite
- Dog had bitten many people
- Dog is aggressive (Rabid dog)
- Dog is calm (Dumb rabies)

**Q6. What are the conditions not considered as contraindications for the vaccine?**
- Infancy
- Pregnancy
- Old age
- Lactation period.

**Q7. What is the dose of immunoglobulin?**
40 IU/kg body weight up to 3,000 IU.

**Q8. What is the precaution to be taken while infiltration of immunoglobulins into the wound?**
- Avoid multiple injections into the wound
- The dose of immunoglobulin should not be in excess which may suppress antibody production by the body in response to the vaccine.

**Q9. Can the antirabies immunoglobulin be administered later?**
The immunoglobulins can be administered up to 7 days of administering the vaccine. After 7 days, the immunoglobulins may be produced by the body and external administration is not needed.

**Q10. What is the protective level of antirabies antibody?**
0.5 IU/mL.

**Q11. Can the vaccine be shifted from one brand to other?**
No shifting from one brand to other should be avoided.

## Human Papilloma Virus Vaccine

- Serotypes 16 and 18 are associated with invasive cervical cancer
- Serotypes 6 and 11 are associated with anogenital warts.

## Technical Aspects
- Liquid vaccine
- Recombinant DNA vaccines.

Two types of vaccines are available:
- Bivalent—16, 18
- Quadrivalent serotypes 6, 11, 16, 18 are effective in preventing genital warts, vaginal/vulvar intraepithelial neoplasia.

**Contents:** L1 protein, noninfective virus-like particle.

**Ideal age at immunization:** 11–12 years through 26 years of age.

### Dose and schedule:
- Dose: 0.5 mL
- Schedule—*See* Annexure.

**Route of administration:** Intramuscular.

**Site of administration:** Deltoid.

### Precautions:
- This vaccine should be administered before exposure to to HPV.
- As this vaccine can cause syncope, vaccine should be administered in sitting or lying down position.
- The vaccine recipients should be observed for 15 minutes after immunization.

*Catch-up vaccination:* Before initiation of sexual activity and can be given up to 45 years (26 years of age in USA).

*Protective efficacy:* More than 95%.

*Storage:*
- + 2°C to +8°C
- Keep away from light
- To be stored at the top of the rack.

*Compatibility:* Can be given with other vaccine like hepatitis B, Tdap.

## Clinical Aspects
**Indications of the vaccine:** To all females aged 10–12 to 26 years.

### Contraindications:
- Allergic reactions/Anaphylaxis to previous dose
- Pregnancy
- Severe illness
- Serious hypersensitivity

### Side effects:
- Pain
- Erythema
- Fainting
- Fever
- Headache
- Itching
- Swelling

### Severe side effects:
- Allergy/Anaphylaxis
- Blood clots
- Convulsions
- Demyelinating disorders
- Encephalomyelitis
- Fatigue syndrome (Chronic)
- Guillain-Barré syndrome.

## QUESTION
**Q1. Is HPV recommended in males?**
HPV 4 is recommended in males aged 11 years through 18 years for prevention of genital warts.

## Cholera
Cholera is caused by *Vibrio cholerae*. This spreads by fecal-oral route. Cholera will manifest as watery diarrhea.

### Cholera Vaccine
- Not recommended for routine use.
- Original vaccines contained live *vibrio cholerae* and were replaced due to the adverse reactions. This vaccine was a compulsory one for travelers in the past, but now very few countries insist on this.
- Minimal age of administration—1 year, two doses, 2 weeks apart for children above 1 year of age.

- Short-term protection.
- Oral vaccine is also available.

*The types of cholera vaccine:*
- Killed oral vaccine (V cholera $O_1$) with recombinant b subunit of cholera toxoid
- WC-rBS vaccine (Dukoral vaccine).

**Technical aspects:**
- Liquid vaccine
- Contents:
  - 6,000 million killed bacteria of Ogawa serotype of classical *Vibrio cholerae*
  - 6,000 million killed bacteria of Inaba serotype of classical *Vibrio cholerae*
  - 0.5% phenol is used as preservative.
- Dose:
  - 0.25 mL for less than 10 years
  - 0.5 mL for more than 10 years
- Schedule: 2 doses at 2 weeks interval
- Minimal age for immunization: 1 year
- Route of administration: Subcutaneous or intramuscular
- Site of administration: Deltoid or anterolateral aspect of thigh
- Instructions to the mother after administration of vaccine: If fever develops, it should be treated with antipyretics.

**Protective efficacy:**
- Parenteral killed vaccine:
  - 3 months efficacy of 45%
  - WC-rBS vaccine (Dukoral vaccine) 35–50%, does not exceed 50–60%
  - First 6 months 85% protection
  - By 2 years less than 50% protection
- Duration of immunity: Lasts for 3 months up to 2 years
- Storage: 2 to 8°C
  - When vaccine is not in use: Lowermost compartment of the fridge
  - During immunization keep at room temperature
- *Storage of vaccine in case of power failure:* Keep the vaccine in a cool and dark place.

**Clinical aspects:**

Advantages: When most of the population is immunized, it protects those who are not immunized, also known as Herd immunity.

Indications: Only during epidemics or for those who are residing or traveling to endemic or epidemic areas. Although it will not be useful in epidemics as the protective antibodies will be produced only after 2 weeks, the cholera vaccine can be given.

Contraindications:
- Age less than 2 years
- Acute illness
- Allergy—severe reaction to previous dose.

Side effects of cholera vaccine:
- Abscess formation
- Abdominal pain
- Allergy—rash
- Anaphylaxis (Rarely)
- Cramps
- Diarrhea
- Emesis
- Fever
- Flu-like symptoms
- GIT problems—nausea
- Headache
- Induration
- Joint pain
- Lymphadenopathy
- Malaise
- Numbness
- Pain (restriction of movement of limbs)

## QUESTIONS

**Q1. What are the disadvantages of cholera vaccination?**
- ☐ Duration of protection last for only 3 months
- ☐ Efficacy is less than 50%
- ☐ The vaccine is highly reactogenic
- ☐ Injectable vaccine does not produce any local immunity in the intestinal mucosa
- ☐ Antibodies will be produced only after 2 weeks.

## COMBINATION OF VACCINES

### Pentavalent Vaccine

This is a combined vaccine containing the following five components conjugated into one vaccine:
- Diphtheria, Pertussis, Tetanus (DPT) vaccine.
- Hib vaccine against *Haemophilus influenzae* type b.
- Hepatitis B vaccine.

### Technical Aspects

**Type of Vaccine—killed:**
- Liquid vaccine
- Multidose vial contains 10 doses
- Conjugated vaccine.

**Contents:**
- Diphtheria toxoid
- *Bordetella pertussis* (Whole cell)
- Tetanus toxoid
- Purified capsular Hib polysaccharide polyribosyl ribitol phosphate (PRP)
- Hepatitis B surface antigen-HBsAg (rDNA)

**Dose and schedule:**
- Dose: 0.5 mL
- Schedule: 6, 10, and 14 weeks.

**Route of administration:** Intramuscular.

**Site of administration:** Anterolateral aspect of thigh.

**Protective efficacy:** 85-95%.

**Storage:**
- + 2°C to +8°C
- Keep away from light
- To be stored at the top of the rack
- Ice lined refrigerator—in the basket
- Freeze sensitive vaccination.

### Clinical Aspects

**Indications of the vaccine:** To all children.

**Contraindications:**
- Severe allergic reactions to the vaccine or its components
- Children with moderate to severe illness
- Conditions in which the vaccine should be administered after admission into a hospital and observed for 24 hours following vaccination
- Preterm less than 36 weeks
- Hypotonic hyporesponsive episodes (HHE) reaction to previous dose of pentavalent vaccine
- Severe congenital anomalies requiring prolonged hospitalization during neonatal period
- Recent severe illness like pneumonia and neonatal sepsis requiring prolonged hospitalization.

**Side effects suspected to be caused by pentavalent vaccine:**
- Local: Pain, redness, and swelling at the injection site
- General: Fever, malaise, irritability
- Gastrointestinal: Diarrhea, vomiting
- Feeding disorders like loss of appetite
- Nervous system disorders—sleepiness
- Psychiatric disorders
- Severe side effects:
  - Anaphylaxis
  - Crying: Persistent inconsolable screaming for more than 3 hours
  - Encephalopathy
  - Fits/seizures
  - Hypotonic-hyporesponsive episodes.

**Complications:** Death was reported at few places.

## QUESTIONS

**Q1. Is booster dose of pentavalent vaccine required?**

The booster dose for pentavalent vaccine is not recommended but booster doses of DPT vaccine can be given at the age of 16-24 months and 5-6 years.

**Q2. How does pentavalent vaccine prevent the incidence and transmission of Hib?**
- By reducing the nasopharyngeal carriage of *H. influenzae* type b
- Herd immunity

**Q3. What is the age group in which Hib vaccine is recommended?**
Hib should be given for infants in the age group of 6 weeks to 1 year.

**Q4. What are the diseases caused by *H. influenzae* type b?**
- Pneumonia
- Meningitis
- Bacteremia
- Epiglottis
- Septic arthritis
- Osteomyelitis

**Q5. What are the precautions for preventing death following pentavalent vaccine?**
- Preterm less than 36 weeks of gestation
- Recent history of significant illness
- Severe congenital anomalies requiring prolonged hospitalization
- History of HHE to previous dose is not a contraindication
- The infants age 2 months receiving the first dose of pentavalent vaccine should get admitted in a suitable inpatient and kept under observation for 24 hours.

## Combination Vaccines

It contains two or more separate immunogens physically combined in a single preparation.

Example: DTP, MMR, Td, MMRV, TdaP
- DTwP + IPV
- DTwP + HepB
- DTwP + Hib + IPV + HepB
- DTaP + Hib
- DTaP + Hib + IPV
- Pentavalent (DTP + Hib + HBV, DTap + Hib + IPV)
- Hexavalent (DTwP + Hib + IPV + HBV, DTaP + Hib + IPV + HBV).

**Hep A + Hep B**
- 0, 1, and 6 months
- Rapid schedule for travelers—0, 7, and 21 days.

**DTaP + Hib**
Lyophilized form.

**Easy Four**
- It contains—diphtheria, tetanus, pertussis, *H. influenzae*
- Three doses at four weeks interval
- Dose 0.5 mL
- Booster at 15–18 months
- Route of administration: Intramuscular
- Site: Anterolateral aspect of thigh.

**Easy Five**
- It contains—diphtheria, tetanus, pertussis, hepatitis B, and *H. influenzae*
- Three doses at four weeks interval
- Dose 0.5 mL
- Booster at 15–18 months
- Route of administration: Intramuscular
- Site: Anterolateral aspect of thigh.

**Other Combination vaccines**
- DTwP + IPV
- DTwP + Hib + IPV
- DTaP + IPV
- DTaP + Hep B
- DTaP + IPV + Hep B
- DTaP + Hib + Hep B
- DTaP + IPV + Hib + Hep B

## QUESTIONS

**Q1. What are the combination vaccines?**
Combination vaccines are the vaccines that consist of two or more separate immunogens combined into a single product.

**Q2. What are the advantages of combination vaccines?**
- Scientific—synergism, shelf life-DTP
- Logistic—cost, easiness, visits, storage space-hexavalent

- Avoids multiple injections
- Reduced burden on cold storage and cold chain
- Reduced requirement of syringes and needles
- Easy record keeping.

**Q3. What are the disadvantages of combination vaccines in relation to Hib?**
- The immunological response to Hib is low as compared to when given separately
- Suboptimal immunogenicity
- Immune interference between various antigens
- Decreased stability of the combine vaccine.

**Q4. Name few combination vaccines?**
- MMR vaccine (Measles, Mumps, Rubella)
- HiB: Hepatitis B vaccine (*H. influenzae*, Hepatitis B vaccine)
- Hepatitis a: Hepatitis b vaccine
- Diphtheria; Tetanus; acellular pertussis; Hepatitis B; inactivated polio virus vaccine
- Pneumococcal conjugate vaccine.

*Technical Aspects*

This contains the following six components: (DTwP + HiB + IPV + HBV, DTaP+ HiB + IPV + HBV).

**Contents:** DTwP/DTaP + HiB + IPV + HBV

**Diluents:** Distilled water

**Ideal age at immunization:** At birth.

**Dose and schedule:** Same as Pentavalent

**Route of administration:** Intramuscular

**Site of administration:** Anterolateral aspect of thigh.

**Protective efficacy:** Same as pentavalent

**Storage:**
- +2°C to +8°C
- Keep away from light
- To be stored at the top of the rack.

**Indications of the vaccine:** To all children.

**Contraindications:** Same as pentavalent

**Side effects:** Same as pentavalent

**Complications:** Same as pentavalent

## Quadruple Vaccine

*Technical Aspects*

DTP-Hib vaccine.

**Type of vaccine—killed:**
- Liquid vaccine
- Multidose vial contains 10 doses
- Conjugated vaccine.

**Contents:**
- Diphtheria toxoid 25 Lf units
- *Bordetella pertussis* (Whole cell) 20× 10 (organisms per dose)
- Tetanus toxoid 10 Lf units
- Inactivated poliomyelitis virus
- *H. influenzae* type B

**Dose and schedule:**
- Dose: 0.5 mL
- Schedule: 6, 10, and 14 weeks.

**Route of administration:** Intramuscular.

**Site of administration:** Anterolateral aspect of thigh.

**Protective efficacy:** 85–95%.

**Storage:**
- +2°C to +8°C
- Keep away from light
- To be stored at the top of the rack

# Vaccines

- Ice lined refrigerator—in the basket
- Freeze sensitive vaccination.

## Clinical Aspects

**Indications of the vaccine:** To all children.

**Contraindications of quadruple vaccine:** Same as pentavalent.

**Side effects of quadruple vaccine:** Same as pentavalent.

## DURATION OF PROTECTION OFFERED BY VACCINES

Duration of protection offered by vaccines will vary with each vaccine. The duration of protection after all doses is given in the following table:

| Vaccine | Estimated duration of protection after all doses |
|---|---|
| Diphtheria | Around 10 years |
| Pertussis | 4–6 years |
| Tetanus | 13–14 years |
| Poliomyelitis | 18 years |
| H. influenzae | >9 years |
| Measles | Lifelong |
| Mumps | >10 years |
| Rubella | >15 to 20 years |
| Pneumococcal vaccine | >4–5 years |
| Human papilloma virus vaccine | >5–8 years |
| Varicella | >14 years following two doses |
| Hepatitis B | >20 years |

No vaccine is 100 % protective.

## CONTRADICTIONS PRECAUTIONS FOR IMMUNIZATION

- *Nursing care* should be available.
- *Dates and schedule* for immunization should be verified.
- *Route of administrations* should be followed strictly as it varies for different drugs. There are incidences where vaccines supposed to be given parenterally were provided through oral route.
- *Site of administration* should be verified for each vaccines:
  - BCG should be given in the left arm
  - Measles should be given in the right arm
  - DPT should be given in the anterolateral aspect of the thigh.
- *Contraindications* for each vaccines should be kept in mind.
- *Complications and adverse effects* following vaccination should be known by the person who is administering the vaccines.
- *Observation:* The child should be observed at least 15 minutes after administration of the vaccine.

  The parents or caretakers should be advised to observe for the adverse events following vaccination.
- Recording: The details regarding the administration of vaccines should be recorded in the immunization chart.

  The date of next visit should be informed to the parents or caretakers.
- *National immunization days:* Medical professionals, nurses, parents should be aware of dates of the National immunization days for immunizations programs like pulse polio and MR vaccines. Also they should be aware of the places of administration of vaccines.
- *Cold chain system* should be maintained.
- *Aseptic precautions:* Strict aseptic precautions should be maintained.

The fluid in which the site of administration of vaccine should be cleaned should be known.
- *Diluents:* The diluents also vary with each vaccine.
- *Maintenance of records:*
  - The registers, stocks with date of expiry
  - Organization of immunization camps

- Updating the information about the immunization, changing trends, etc.
- Reporting about adverse events following immunization.
❖ Multidose vials should be discarded after 1 hour after opening the vial if there is no preservative.
❖ If the vaccine contains preservative, the vials should be discarded after 3 hours.

## VACCINATION FAILURE

*Vaccination failure* breakthrough diseases can occur after immunization against that organism against which vaccine was administered.

*Causes of vaccination failure are:*
❖ Persistence of maternal antibody
❖ Waning immunity
❖ Simultaneous use of antibodies.

*Primary vaccination failure:* Administration of recommended doses does not result in immune response sufficient to protect disease.
This is seen in poliomyelitis.

*Secondary vaccine failure*: Administration of recommended doses will result in immune response sufficient to protect disease. But infection occurs. This is seen in pertussis, typhoid, and BCG.

Vaccine failure is very rare after measles, diphtheria, and tetanus immunizations.

### Poor Efficacy of a Vaccine

Poor efficacy is due to:
❖ High population densities
❖ Malnutrition
❖ Poor sanitation
❖ Poor vaccine efficacy due to improper maintenance of cold chain
❖ Monovalent and bivalent polio vaccines are more effective as the competition between different polio viruses is eliminated

❖ Presence of maternal antibodies will interfere with good immune response.

## VACCINE STORAGE

Vaccines should be stored carefully to avoid loss of potency.

### Cold Chain

Cold chain is the system of storage, transport, and distribution of vaccines in a potent state at a recommended temperature from the point of manufacture to the point of use. The cold temperature should be maintained from the site of manufacture to the site of delivery to maintain the potency of vaccines which are heat labile. The vaccine with live attenuated organisms like poliomyelitis, measles, and BCG can be killed on exposure to higher temperature than recommended. Hence, they will lose their potency. It is important to maintain a cold chain because once the vaccine potency is lost it cannot be restored.

Guidelines are set for the manufacturers, transporters and stockists, practitioners and others who are involved in the immunization practices.

### Equipment Used for Maintenance of Cold Chain

The cold chain equipment consists of the following two aspects:

*I-Set chain:*
❖ Walk in cold rooms (WIC) or walk in freezers
❖ Deep freezers
❖ Ice lined refrigerators (ILRs)
❖ Refrigerators.

*II-Mobile chain:*
❖ Isothermic boxes
❖ Vaccine carriers
❖ Cold boxes
❖ Day carriers
❖ Ice packs

# Vaccines

| Type | Equipment | Temperature | Uses/Duration of storage |
|---|---|---|---|
| Set chain | Walk in cold rooms or walk in freezers | −20°C | Regional level storage for 4–5 districts up to 3 months |
| | Deep freezers: 140–300 L capacity | −15°C to −25°C | At district and PHC levels used for preparation of ice packs |
| | Ice lined refrigerators (ILRs) Refrigerators | 2°C to 8°C | At district and PHC levels |
| Mobile chain | Isothermic boxes/Cold boxes | 2°C to 8°C (fully frozen ice packs placed at the sides and bottom) | Collection and transport of large amount of vaccines for outreach places/centers, subcenters, villages |
| | Vaccine carriers | Four ice packs are used | Carry small quantities of vaccines of about 16–20 vials for out reach stations |
| | Day carriers | Two fully frozen ice packs | Only for few hours |
| | Ice packs | | Used for cold boxes and vaccine carriers |

- DPT, DT, and TT should not be kept in direct contact
- Diluents should be stored at 2°C to 8°C.

| Level of storage | Method |
|---|---|
| National level | Cold room (0–8°C) Freezer room (−15°C to −25°C) Ice lined freezers (ILRs) |
| Regional level | Ice lined refrigerators (ILRs) |
| District level | Medium capacity freezer Medium capacity refrigerator |
| PHC level | Small ILR Small top opening freezer |

## Set chain:

- *Walk in cold rooms or walk in freezers.* (Serves as a distribution point):
  - Storage of vaccines at manufacturer, state, and regional levels
  - Temperature: Freezers will be −15°C to −25°C
- *Walk in freezers:*
  - Size 16.5 feet
  - 32 cubic meters
  - Temperature −20°C
  - Bulk storage for vaccines like OPV, measles vaccines. Serves as a distribution point.
- *Deep freezer:* Temperature −15°C to −25°C
- *Ice lined refrigerators:* Refrigerators specially designed for storage of vaccines.

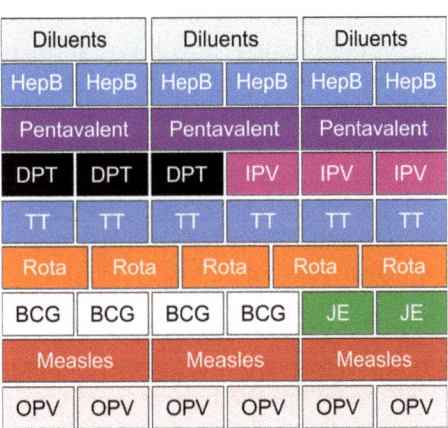

**Fig. 7.1:** Vaccine storage color code.

## Storage of vaccines inside the ILR (Fig. 7.1)
## Color code for ILR (Fig. 7.2)

- *Refrigerators:* It should have the following features—
  - Auto door closure
  - Auto defrost
  - Bins with adjustable heights
  - Built in holders
  - CFC free
  - Double door refrigerator, one door for each compartment
  - Enough space should be present for storage
  - Free of leakages of water and coolants

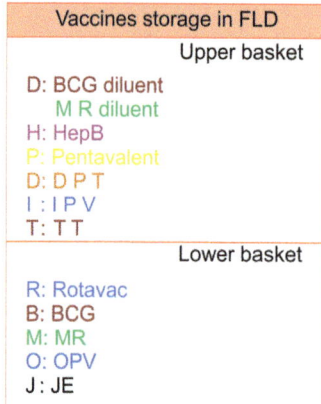

**Fig. 7.2:** Vaccine storage.

- Fluctuations in voltage can be prevented using a voltage stabilizer should be present
- Freeze watch indicators
- Full extension transparent drawers so that contents inside it are visible, so that the contents can be seen without opening
- Quiet without making much noise.

## Cautions for use of refrigerator:

- Temperature should be maintained at −4°C to 0°C in the freezer compartment and 2°C–8°C in the main compartment.
- Should not be used for any other purpose.
- Should be kept away from sunlight and heat.
- Should have ice packs in the freezer compartment and water bottles in the door which will maintain the temperature for some time in case of power failure.
- Vaccines should not be stored in the baffle tray or door shelves.
- Defrosting should be done periodically.
- Household refrigerators and flasks are not recommended.
- Other items should not be stored in the cold systems.
- The door of the cold system should not be frequently opened.
- The doors should be closed air tight.

*Storage of vaccines inside a refrigerator:*

| Compartment | Vaccines stored |
|---|---|
| Freezer compartment | OPV |
| Top shelf | BCG, Measles, MMR |
| Middle shelf | DTwP, DTaP, DT, TT, Tdap, typhoid (T-series vaccines) Combination vaccines, HPV, hepatitis A, Hib IPV Influenza PCV Rotavirus |
| Lower shelf | Hepatitis B, varicella |
| Crisper compartment | Diluents |
| Baffle tray | Should be kept empty |
| Doors | No vaccines should be stored |

- Ice packs should be kept in the freezer which will be helpful in maintaining temperature for some time of about 3 to 4 hours during power failure.
- Temperature should be recorded at least twice a day.
- The refrigerator used to storage of vaccines should not be used for any other purpose like storage of food, beverages, pathology specimens, and other medications.
- The refrigerator should be kept at least 10 cm away from the floor and the walls to allow free air circulation.
- The refrigerator should not be overloaded.

## Refrigerator (Fig. 7.3)

### Mobile chain:

*Isothermic boxes or cold boxes are* well-insulated, solid tight sealed boxes with frozen ice packs at the bottom, sides, and top. This is available in 5L and 20 L capacities.

Uses:
- Used for collection and transport of large amount of vaccines at 2°C to 8°C for outreach places.
- Emergency storage during periods of electricity (power) failure.
- Storage of vaccine during maintenance of refrigerator.

# Vaccines

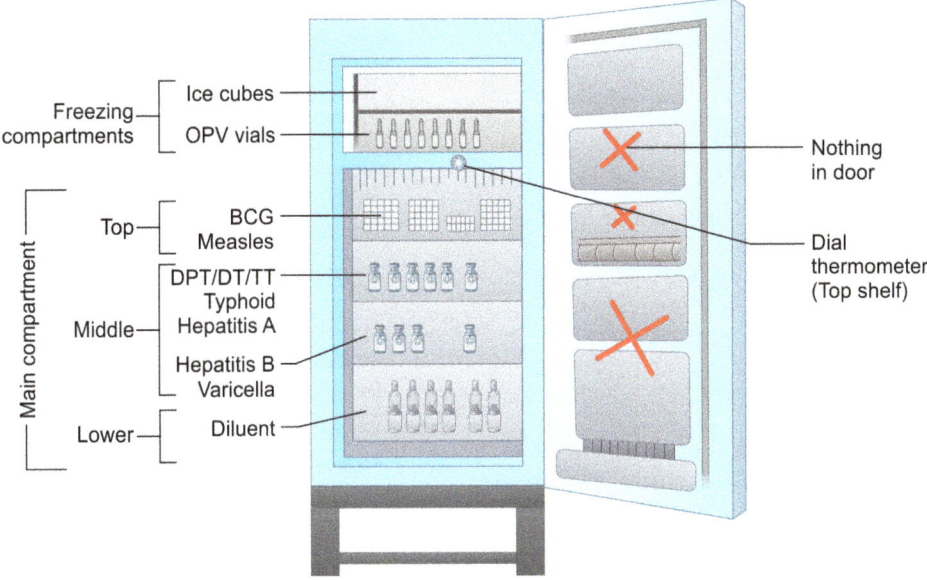

**Fig. 7.3:** Refrigerator showing vaccines stored correctly in clinic setup.

Advantages: The vaccine can be maintained at recommended temperature for 5 days.

❖ *Vaccine carriers:* Are small versions of cold boxes that can carry small quantities of vaccines of about 16-20 vials. These have frozen ice packs lining the sides. The conditioned ice packs instead of frozen ice packs will prevent cold injury.

Uses: Used to carry small quantities of vaccines for distribution of outreach places within the same day.

## QUESTIONS

**Q1. Mention the heat-sensitive vaccines.**
Many vaccines will be degraded following exposure to heat. Repeated exposure to heat will have cumulative effect. The potency lost by exposure to heat cannot be reverted back by replacing the vaccine in recommended temperatures.

The following vaccines and their combinations are sensitive to heat:
❑ Live attenuated influenza vaccine
❑ BCG
❑ OPV
❑ Measles
❑ MMR (few brands)
❑ MMRV (few brands)
❑ Varicella (few brands)
❑ Rotavirus
❑ Yellow fever.

**Q2. Mention the freeze-sensitive vaccines.**
Freeze-sensitive vaccines should not be sued if they are exposed to temperature less than 0°C. All aluminum adjuvanted vaccines are freeze-sensitive.

The following vaccines and their combinations etc. should not be freezed:
❑ Hepatitis A containing vaccines
❑ Hepatitis B containing vaccines
❑ Meningococcal C conjugate vaccine
❑ DTP containing vaccines
❑ TT vaccine
❑ DT vaccine
❑ Td vaccine
❑ Hib vaccine
❑ HPV vaccine

- Influenza vaccine
- Japanese B encephalitis vaccine
- Pneumococcal vaccine PCV 7
- Rabies vaccine
- All reconstituted vaccines
- Vaccine diluents.

The following vaccines can be frozen:
- Oral polio
- Lyophilized measles
- MMR
- BCG
- Varicella
- MMRV.

**Q3. Mention the light-sensitive vaccines.**
The following vaccines and their combinations are susceptible to light and should not be exposed to light:
- BCG
- Measles vaccine
- DTaP containing vaccines
- Oral polio vaccine
- Reconstituted MMR vaccine
- Monovalent Rubella vaccine
- Rotavirus
- Human papilloma virus
- Varicella zoster vaccine.

The Advisory Committee on Immunization Practices (ACIP) had issued recommendations for storage and handling of vaccines. Also Centers for Disease Control and Prevention (CDC) had issued certain guidelines.

**Q4. What are the time limits for using vaccines after reconstitution?**

| Vaccine | Time limits for using vaccines after reconstitution |
| --- | --- |
| BCG | 4–6 hours |
| DTaP/Hib combination | 30 minutes |
| Measles | 4–6 hours |
| MMR | 4–6 hours |
| MMRV | 30 minutes |

*Contd...*

*Contd...*

| Vaccine | Time limits for using vaccines after reconstitution |
| --- | --- |
| Meningococcal vaccine polysaccharide single dose vial | 30 minutes |
| Varicella | 30 minutes |
| Yellow fever | One hour |

**Q5. What are the vaccines that can be stored in the freezer compartment?**
BCG, OPV, measles, MMR.

**Q6. What are the vaccines that can be stored in the top shelf?**
OPV, Measles, MMR, Varicella.

**Q7. What are the vaccines that can be stored in the middle shelf?**
Hepatitis B, DTwP, DTaP, DT, TT, Tdap, combination vaccines, IPV, HPV, Typhoid, Hepatitis A, Hib, PCV, Influenza, Rotavirus.

**Q8. What are the vaccines that can be stored in lower shelf?**
Diluents.

**Q9. What are the vaccines that can be stored in the door?**
No vaccines should be kept in the door.

**Q10. What are the vaccines that can be stored in the baffle tray?**
Baffle tray should be kept empty.

**Q11. What are the vaccines that can be frozen?**
- BCG
- Measles
- Polio
- Yellow fever

**Q12. What are the vaccines that cannot be frozen?**
- DPT
- TT
- Typhoid.

**Q13. What are the vaccines that should be stored in the top shelf?**
OPV and measles.

**Q14. What are the vaccine that should be stored in the middle shelf?**
BCG, DPT, TT, Diluents.

**Q15. What are the vaccines that should be stored in the shelf?**
No vaccine should be stored in the lower shelf.

**Q16. How many times will you record the temperature in the fridge used for storage of vaccines?**
Temperature should be recorded at least twice a day.

**Q17. What are the vaccines that are considered for removal from cold chain?**
DTwP, DTap, TT, DT, Td, hepatitis B to eliminate the risk of freezing.

**Q18. What is VAERS?**
Vaccine associated adverse event reporting system.
The VAE child be reported to IAP immunization website www.iapcoi.com.

**Q19. What is the advantage of temperature buffered probe?**
This will be useful than measuring the vaccine temperature rather than the ambient air temperatures.

**Q20. What is the disadvantage of using Cyclic defrost refrigerator?**
In cyclic defrost refrigerator is associated with wide temperature control. The temperature often goes above the ideal recommended due to heating cycles.

**Q21. What are the steps in conditioning of ice packs?**
The frozen ice packs are kept outside until there is sweating of ice packs. After this the ice packs should be shaken and sound of water should be heard.

## Monitoring of Cold Chain

Vaccine vial monitor

Potency test

Change in color.

## Temperature Monitoring

Temperature recording should be continuous, calibrated, and certified. Temperature should be monitored continuously.

*Vaccine monitoring tools:* The following tools are used to monitor the temperature—
- Thermometers can be used to record the temperatures:
  - Dial thermometers
  - Stem thermometers
  - Electronic thermometers
- Indicators:
  - Vaccine vial monitor
  - Freeze watch indicators: Freeze tag

### Vaccine Vial Monitor (Fig. 7.4)

*Vaccine vial monitor (VVM)* is label containing heat-sensitive material placed on a vaccine vial to register heat exposure due to combined effects of time and temperature causing the inner square to darken gradually and irreversibly.

The vaccine vial monitor is a circle with a small square inside it. It is printed on the product label or to the cap of the vaccine vial or at its side. The VVM was first introduced in the polio vaccine vials and now used for other heat and light sensitive vaccines also. A vaccine monitor (VVM) placed on a vaccine vial which will register cumulative heat to which the vial is exposed. VVM

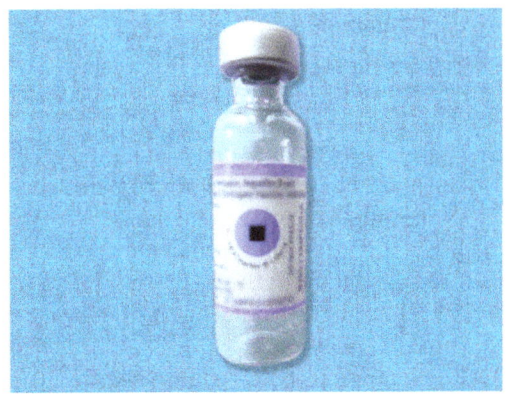

**Fig. 7.4:** Vaccine vial monitor.

contains heat-sensitive material which will change color on exposure to temperature over a period of time. The combined factors of time and temperature cause the monitor to change color, which will be gradual and irreversible.

The heat sensitive component in the VVM will register a gradual color change with exposure to heat. The inner square will be lighter in color than outer surrounding circle. When the level and/or duration of heat do not damage the vaccine, the inner square remain lighter than the outer circle. The discard point is at a point when the inner square is the same color as the surrounding circle. This is an unacceptable level of exposure to heat which will have damaged the vaccine.

There is a direct relationship between the rate of color change and temperature:
- Lower the temperature, slower will be the color change.
- Higher the temperature, faster will be the color change.

Stages of changes in VVM

| Stage | Color change |
|---|---|
| I | Inner square lighter than outer circle |
| II | Inner square still lighter than outer circle |
| III | Color of inner square matches the outer circle |
| IV | Color of inner square darker the outer circle |

*The interpretation of the rules for reading the vaccine vial monitor:*

The point to focus on is the color of the inner square relative to the color of the surrounding circle:
- Rule 1: If the inner square is lighter than the outer circle and the expiry date is not passed, the vaccine can be used.
- Rule 2: If the inner square is the same color or darker than the outer circle and the expiry date is not passed, the vaccine must not be used.

The change in color will be applied the particular vial to which the VVM is attached. It does not indicate the potency for other vaccines stored in the same container.

## Advantages of VVM

- The VVM indicates the total accumulated heat exposure for which the vaccine in the vial has been subjected to.
- Easy to use: A simple glance at the VVM will be enough to show the vaccine can be used or not.
- VVMs can be used on vaccine vials, droppers or ampoules.
- Useful in outreach programs.
- Low cost.
- Avoid vaccine wastage.
- Prevent children from receiving ineffective or low potency vaccines.

## Disadvantages of VVM

- Vaccine vial monitor does not measure the vaccine potency.
- The vaccine vial monitor does not directly measure vaccine potency but it does give information about the main factor which affects potency; heat exposure over a period of time.
- Vaccine vial monitor does not register information about other factors contributing to the vaccine degradation, such as sunlight and age (time).
- Vaccine vial monitor does not provide information about cold injury to the vaccines.

*Heat stability:* The vaccine vial monitor reflects the heat stability of the vaccine to which it is attached and does not, therefore, change color immediately with a brief exposure to moderate heat.

Vaccines have a level of heat stability which enables them to withstand temperatures outside the cold chain, above 8°C, for a limited amount of time. The rate at which the vaccine vial monitor changes color reflects the rate at which the quality of the vaccine changes with heat exposure.

# QUESTIONS

**Q1. At room temperature, what will be the time taken for the vaccine vial monitor to change form the "start point" to the "discard point"?**

This depends on the room temperature which will vary according to the season, place, and time of the day.

The table showing the times recorded for a vaccine vial monitor attached to a vial of OPV.

| Constant temperature, day and night | Time for VVM to reach "discard point" |
|---|---|
| Room temperature at 20°C | 20 days |
| Room temperature at 25°C | 8 days |
| Refrigerator at 4°C | 500 days |

**Q2. Will the color change of the VVM get reversed if vaccine is returned to a refrigerator after being outside the cold chain for a long time?**

The color change of VVM is irreversible.

**Q3. Will the VVM register any change if the vaccine freezes?**

The VVM is not affected by freezing temperature and does not give any information with regard to freezing.

## Ice Lined Refrigerator (ILR) and Freezer (Fig. 7.5)

- Fix the equipment to a voltage stabilizer
- Keep the equipment locked
- Don't store any other drug, food or drinking water
- Do not open frequently, open only when necessary
- Do not keep more than one month requirement
- Do not keep drugs with expired dates.

## Excipients Used in a Vaccine

- Aluminum salts and gels are used as adjuvants

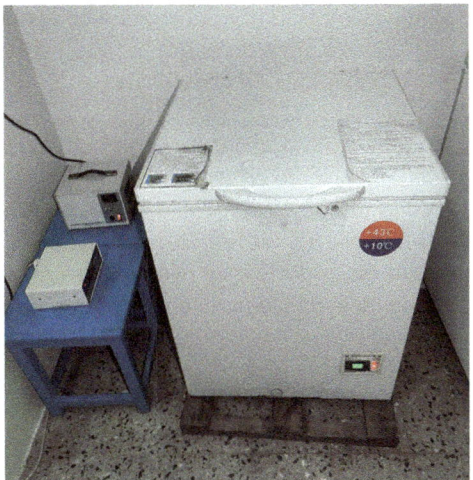

**Fig. 7.5:** Ice lined refrigerator and freezer.

- Antibiotics
- Egg protein is present in influenza and yellow fever vaccines
- Formaldehyde
- Monosodium glutamate and 2-phenoxy-ethanol are used as stabilizers
- Thimerosal is a mercury-containing preservative used in vials that will prevent contamination and growth of potentially harmful bacteria.

*Preservatives used in a vaccine are*: Thimerosal, phenoxyethanol, and formaldehyde.

The foreign substances injected into the human body can cause many adverse effects.

## ADVERSE EVENTS FOLLOWING VACCINATION

### Introduction

An adverse event following vaccination (AEFI) is defined as an untoward event or medical incident that occurs after an immunization caused by the vaccine product or vaccination process and causes concern and is believed to be caused by immunization.

Adverse events following immunization can be minor local reactions to serious allergic reaction.

Serious adverse event is defined as which is fatal or life-threatening or results persistent or significant disability, incapacity or results in or prolongs hospitalization or the patient leads to congenital defects or birth defects. The adverse events that are not resulting in death or hospitalization or but may jeopardize the patient also will be considered as serious. In many countries a significant number of babies less than one year suffer serious life-threatening illness and medical events like sudden infant death syndrome. Also many congenital events will become evident in the first year of life. It will be difficult to determine if the event is directly related to a vaccination. Hence a detailed study has to be done regarding this.

Most of the vaccines are having one or other side effects. Everyone should have a thorough knowledge about the side effects for each vaccine.

## Classification of Side Effects

### Predictable or Idiosyncratic

Local reactions—pain, swelling, redness at the injection site

- *Predictable generalized side effects*: Fever, rash
- *Unpredictable generalized side effects:* Anaphylaxis, idiopathic
  10% of children will fail to develop immunity to live measles vaccine.
- *Unpredictable idiosyncratic side effects:*
  - Anaphylaxis
  - Idiopathic thrombocytopenic purpura
  - Hypotonic hyporesponsive episodes (HHEs)

### Classification of Adverse Reactions

*Adverse vaccine reactions (vaccine-induced reactions)*: VAPP following polio vaccine, anaphylaxis.

- *Vaccine potentiated reactions—Trigger reaction:* Febrile convulsions following vaccination in a predisposed child.
- *Side effects due to program errors*—are said to be the most common cause of serious adverse events and death following measles vaccination due to toxic shock syndrome. Resulting from improper reconstitution or storage of measles vaccine.
- *Injection reactions: Injection-related side effects* are syncope due to pain of vaccination, injection site abscess, sciatic nerve damage, transmission of blood borne pathogens like HIV, HBV/HVC.
- *Coincidental:* An adverse event that occurs after immunization but is not caused by vaccine.
- *Unknown*: The cause of an adverse event cannot be determined.

## Classification of Adverse Reactions based On Casual Association

- Definitely
- Probably
- Possibly
- Unlikely

## Classification Cases at the End of Assessment for Causal Association to Immunization

1. *Cases with adequate information:*
   A. Consistent with causal association to immunization
      A1. Vaccine product related
      A2. Vaccine quality defect related
      A3. Immunization error related
      A4. Immunization anxiety related
   B. Indeterminate
      B1. Consistent temporal relationship but insufficient definite evidence for vaccine causing the event
      B2. Reviewing factors result in conflicting trends of consistency and inconsistency with causal association to immunization
   C. Inconsistent with causal association to immunization (Coincidental)
      Conditions caused by exposure to any other things other than vaccine.
2. *Cases without adequate association:*
   The events are classified as unclassifiable as they require additional information to determine the causality.

## Classification of Adverse Effects According to Severity

- ❖ Minor: Pain, fever
- ❖ Severe: Anaphylaxis, dissemination of infection.

### Minor adverse vaccine reactions:

These are casually related to vaccine:

Local: Pain, erythema, induration. These will increase with repeated doses.

Systemic: Fever which will not lost for more than 48 hours. These will decrease with increasing age or repeated doses.

### Severe adverse reactions:

Allergic—severe allergy or anaphylaxis or anaphylaxis like reactions (generalized urticaria or hives, wheezing, swelling of mouth and throat, difficulty in breathing, hypotension, shock. The allergic reaction may be due to the vaccine antigen, residual animal protein like egg, stabilizers like gelatin, preservatives like thimerosal.

Any one with a history of serious allergy to any of the vaccine constituents should not receive the vaccine. Occurrence of anaphylaxis to any vaccine cannot be predicted. So any one getting vaccinated should be observed for 15 minutes after vaccination.

## Program Errors Leading to Adverse Events

| Program errors | Adverse events |
|---|---|
| • Nonsterile needle use/reuse of needle<br>• Improperly sterilized syringe or needle<br>• Contaminated vaccine or diluents<br>• Reuse of reconstituted vaccine | Infection. Local suppuration at injection site, abscess, cellulitis |

The most common program error is nonsterile injection predisposing to iatrogenic infection.

*Incorrect preparation of vaccines*

- Incorrect preparation of vaccines
- Incorrect dilution
- Substitution for vaccines or diluents
- Local reaction or abscess
- Effect of drug—muscle relaxant, insulin

Incorrect diluents used can result in adverse effects.

*Injection at wrong site*

| Injection at wrong site | Gluteal region—sciatic nerve damage |
|---|---|
| BCG given subcutaneously (instead of intradermal) | Local reaction or injection site abscess |
| Toxoid vaccines given too superficially | Sciatic nerve damage Hepatitis B and rabies will be ineffective |

Infection can occur at the injection site

| Vaccine stored or transported incorrectly | Increased local reaction from frozen vaccine |

## Adverse Reactions due to Contraindications Ignored

Can result in severe adverse reactions.

*Death following vaccination*—deaths due to AEFI can be considered.

- ❖ Certain/very likely if it occurs immediately after vaccination and if no other disease or drug is found as the reason.
- ❖ Probable if it happens within a reasonable time after vaccination.

## Vaccination Scares

Public scare occurs for various vaccines. The diseases are believed to be caused by the vaccines administered. Vaccine scares will result in a portion of people forgoing vaccination. The following are some of the vaccines and the scares:

| Vaccines | Adverse effects |
|---|---|
| Pertussis (Whole cell) | Encephalopathy, epilepsy, learning disorders |
| DPT | Sudden death (cot death/sudden infant death syndrome) |
| Influenza vaccine | Diabetes mellitus |

*Contd...*

Contd...

| Vaccines | Adverse effects |
|---|---|
| Hib | Autism spectrum disorders, Diabetes mellitus |
| Hepatitis B | Multiple sclerosis, lupus, diabetes |
| MMR | Autism spectrum disorders, inflammatory bowel disease, chronic arthropathy |
| Rubella | Congenital anomalies |
| Thimerosal containing vaccines | Neurodevelopmental disorders, autism spectrum disorders, muscular fibrosclerosis |
| Aluminium containing vaccines | Autism spectrum disorders, asthma, muscular fibrosclerosis |
| Various vaccines | Autoimmune disorders<br>Inflammatory bowel disease<br>Chronic fatigue syndrome<br>Deaths -Cot death<br>Leukemia<br>Learning disorders<br>Immune deficiency |

All vaccines should be administered where personnel and equipment for recognition and treatment of anaphylaxis are available.

## QUESTIONS

**Q1. What are the vaccines associated with life-threatening allergic reactions?**
The following six vaccines are associated with severe life-threatening allergic reactions like anaphylaxis in yeast sensitive persons:
1. MMR vaccine
2. Varicella vaccine
3. Influenza vaccine
4. Tetanus containing vaccines
5. Meningococcal vaccine
6. HPV vaccine

Syncope can occur with any vaccine.

**Q2. What are the predisposing factors for adverse reactions to vaccines?**
- Faulty administration
- Faulty storage
- Inherent properties of vaccines.

**Q3. What are the types of adverse reactions to vaccines?**
Local or generalized.

**Q4. What are the diseases associated with vaccines?**
The following diseases are also known to be caused by various vaccines:
- Asthma
- Autoimmune diseases
- Chronic fatigue syndrome
- Learning disorders
- Increase in criminal activities
- Diabetes mellitus
- Immunodeficiency.

Many other diseases like dyslexia, autism, cancers are on the rise even though it is said that the standard of living and healthcare has increased. It is important to find if the newly seen disorders are due to vaccines also.

**Q5. What are the recommended criteria for events that should be reviewed by the medical health officer?**
- All events managed as anaphylaxis
- All neurological events including febrile or afebrile convulsions
- Allergic events
- All events that required medical attention
- All serious events resulting in residual disability, hospitalization, congenital malformation or death.
- Events which the medical officer considers to confer precautions, contraindications or reason to postpone future immunization.

## Antibodies: A Double Edged Weapon

Antibodies are formed when a foreign antigen (substance or organism) enters the body. The immune system will recognize them as foreign substance and form antibodies which will destroy them. These antibodies will cause damage to the foreign substance or microorganism. Sometimes the antibodies will be formed against one's own body cells causing damage to the body cells or organs. There will be mutation in our body cells which may result in malignancy. But the immune system will recognize those cells as foreign and form antibodies against them and destroy them. When the immune system becomes weak in old age or due to AIDS, the cancer cells will not get destroyed and will grow resulting in malignancy.

Vaccines will induce antibody production. These antibodies can have nonspecific actions. So it is important to watch for any complications after vaccinations. Antibodies have both beneficial effect and deleterious effect on our body. They will be beneficial when they act against pathogens or cancer cells. At the same time if it acts against one's own body cells it can modify or destroy the cells.

All antibodies can have nonspecific actions which result in damage to other body cells. For example, in Rheumatic fever, antibodies formed against *Streptococcus* will cause damage to the human tissues including cardiac, nervous, joint tissues, skin, etc. Similarly, the antibodies formed in response to the vaccines will have nonspecific actions thereby causing damage to other body tissues. So it is important to observe for those nonspecific actions and report them to appropriate authorities. Any unacceptable adverse reactions should be recognized and reported so that steps can be taken to prevent those complications in other children getting vaccinated with that particular vaccine. Any adverse event following vaccination with a particular vaccine should be considered as caused by that vaccine unless proved otherwise. A high index of suspicion is necessary. Also the adverse event need not occur immediately after vaccination, but can occur even after many hours, days, weeks, months or years after vaccination. For example, subacute sclerosing pan-encephalitis can occur about 7-10 years after measles vaccination.

*Rheumatic fever:* The disease is due to the antibodies formed against the streptococcal organisms. The antibodies formed against various components of *Streptococcus* will destroy the bacteria. At the same time those will also destroy the body cells like heart (Endocardium, myocardium, and pericardium), brain (Caudate nucleus) which resembles the various components of the *Streptococcus*. This will cause rheumatic valvular heart diseases like mitral valve stenosis, mitral valve regurgitation, etc., rheumatic chorea, rheumatic arthritis, subcutaneous nodules, erythema marginatum, etc. This indicates that antibodies produced *Streptococcus* have nonspecific actions and can destroy various human body cells causing permanent damage.

*Dengue:* When we consider Dengue fever, the whole problem is due to the antibodies formed against the Dengue virus. The antibodies will act on the blood vessels and increase the permeability. This will result in extravasation of fluid from intravascular compartment to extravascular compartment thereby predisposing to hypovolemic shock.

Thus all antibodies have one or other nonspecific actions which can be beneficial or harmful to the humans. When this destroys important parts like brain, heart, etc., permanent sequelae will occur and the child will have lifelong problems.

As the complications can occur even after months to years after administration of drugs or vaccines, children should be carefully monitored for any complications. These complications should be reported to appropriate authorities, so that if the same adverse effect is observed at many places, they can be analyzed and studied further.

Imagine a vaccine or drug is administered to a child or adult which is followed by a severe adverse reaction. There is an argument that the same drug or vaccine from the same vial or ampoule is given for other children, but they had not developed those adverse events or complications. So it should be considered that the adverse effects are not due to that drug or vaccine. Penicillin is given to many children from the same vial, but only few children develop adverse effects like anaphylaxis or even death. That does not mean that the anaphylaxis is not due to penicillin. Each and every human body will react differently to same stimulus. Also few people are allergic to sea foods like prawns. Even death has occurred after consuming sea foods. If a person develops allergy/anaphylaxis after eating sea foods like prawns, you cannot argue that the same sea food or prawn was eaten by others, but they did not develop allergy and so the allergy cannot be due to sea foods like prawn. Remember each human reacts in a different way for same drugs or vaccines. As a medical practitioner should always expect any adverse effect following any drug or vaccine. Keep the equipment and emergency drugs ready to manage emergencies whenever you administer any medicines or injections. Even drugs like cefotaxime had caused serious adverse effects including death. Also discuss about both positive and negative aspects of each and every drug or vaccine. The parents and caretakers also should be aware of both the positive and negative aspects of each and every drug or vaccine administered to them or their children.

The adverse effects following immunization are discussed in this book so that those who are involved in vaccination should observe for these adverse events and inform to the concerned authorities. This list is not an end, many other adverse events can occur and should be observed carefully. The parents also should observe for complications adverse events following immunization and inform them to the concerned authorities.

*Autoimmune disorders:* Antibodies will develop against one's own body cells and will damage them.

*Dengue:* Antibody will cause damage to the vessel wall and increase the permeability and fluid leak. This results in decreased effective blood volume and decreased tissue perfusion.

*Sympathetic ophthalmia:* Injury to one eye will expose the lens to the blood. There will be formation of antibodies to the lens which will cause damage to the other eye also.
- Antibodies are proteins.
- Increased protein load.

## Reporting of Adverse Events Following Vaccination

All adverse events following immunization should be reported to appropriate authorities. If there is any doubt if the event is to be reported or not be proactive and report the event.

*Vaccine adverse event reporting system:* Adverse events following immunization should be reported to monitor the vaccine safety. Reporting the adverse events will be useful for the following:
- Assess the potential casual association
- Biological plausibility where the events may be explained by the associated with natural history, biological mechanisms of the disease, and laboratory investigations.
- Causality assessment for serious AEFI, clusters of AEFI, events occurring above the expected rate or of unusual quality and other significant events of unexplained cause occurring 30 days after vaccination or events causing significant concern to the parents, care takers or community.
- Clusters of adverse events, the cause for each case should be identified separately.
- Detailed epidemiological studies to compare the events among the vaccines to the unvaccinated.
- Establish trends
- Generate hypothesis.

## When to report the adverse events following immunization:

| Classification | Adverse events |
|---|---|
| Minor | Local redness<br>Induration<br>Tenderness<br>Painful limbs<br>Crying<br>Agitated<br>Drowsy<br>Irritable<br>Loss of appetite<br>Swelling<br>Fever<br>Arthralgia<br>Myalgia |
| Moderate | High fever as high as 40°C<br>Pronounced drowsiness<br>Prolonged drying<br>Irritability |
| Major | Guillain-Barré syndrome |

Major reactions should be reported within one day of occurrence.

Moderate reactions should be reported immediately upon the knowledge of adverse reaction.

Minor reactions need not be reported unless the number of minor reactions is increasing.

## Any adverse event following immunization should be immediately reported:

| Time of occurrence following immunization | Adverse events |
|---|---|
| Within 24 hours | Anaphylaxis<br>Anaphylactoid reaction<br>Persistent inconsolable crying or screaming for more than 3 hours<br>Hypotonic hyporesponsive episodes (HHE) |
| Within 5 days | Toxic shock syndrome (TSS)<br>Sepsis<br>Injection site abscess<br>Severe local reaction |
| Within 15 days | Seizures<br>Febrile seizures (Measles, MMR 6–12 days, DTP 0–2 days)<br>Encephalopathy (Measles, MMR 6–12 days, DTP 0–2 days) |

*Contd...*

*Contd...*

| Time of occurrence following immunization | Adverse events |
|---|---|
| Within 3 months | Acute flaccid paralysis (OPV recipient 4–30 days, contact 4–75 days)<br>Brachial neuritis (2–28 days following administration of tetanus containing vaccine) |
| Within 1 year | Thrombocytopenia (15–35 days following measles vaccine)<br>Lymphadenitis<br>Disseminated BCG infection<br>Osteitis<br>Osteomyelitis |
| After 12 months | |
| No time limit | Death<br>Hospitalization<br>Unusual events thought by health workers related to immunization |

Events following immunization should be reported which include all SAR, irrespective of the casual association, non-serious adverse events unexpected in nature, severity, frequency or outcome, vaccine failures, and all usage in pregnancy.

- Minor AEFI should be reported to ANM or village health nurses who will report them to the medical officer primary health center/CHC.
- Private practitioners should report to the medical officer primary health centre/CHC or DIO.
- The AEFI can be directly reported to the DIO.
- DIO will report to the state.
- The report should contain:
  - Description of the event
  - Timing of the event in relation to the immunization
  - Vaccines given
  - Identifying details of the patients

Vaccine adverse event reporting system (VAERS) is available in many countries to pick up previously unrecognized adverse effects and generate further data.

*Events that should not be reported:*
- Local injection site reactions lasting for less than 4 days
- Non-specific systemic reaction like headache, myalgia unless that occur more frequently or more severely than expected
- Events clearly attributed to other causes for which another cause is present
- Fever that is not accompanied by any other symptoms
- Vasovagal syncope without injury.

*Events that should be reported are:*
- Serious life-threatening events
- Events requiring urgent medical attention
- Unusual or unexpected events that are not noted previously like oculorespiratory syndrome following influenza vaccination or events that had been identified before but occurring more frequently
- Cluster of events following vaccination that occurs in a geographic area.

## QUESTION

**Who should report the AEFI ?**
Healthcare professionals including physicians, nurses, and pharmacists can inform about any adverse events following immunization. Vaccine recipients or their parents or care takers may report the AEFI to the physicians or directly to public health authorities.

## Reporting of Side Effects
- All side effects should be reported to appropriate authorities.
- In some countries there are free applications available for both iOS and Android devised for reporting the adverse effects.
- Yellow card schemes are available to report the side effects on line.

## NATIONAL VACCINE INJURY COMPENSATION PROGRAM

This program was started in 1980s in US. This was started as there was a rise in cases filed against the vaccine companies. National Vaccine Injury Compensation Program (VICP) was created to provide a Federal Fault System for compensating vaccine related injury or death. The persons who had experienced an injury or died due to administration of vaccines covered under this program can seek compensation. Vaccine injury compensation are given in USA for those individuals who are proved to be harmed by vaccine administration. Every year the number of cases getting this compensation is on the rise.

National Childhood Vaccine Injury Act of 1986 came into effect from October 1, 1988. This is an alternative to civil litigation. All vaccines can cause side effects.

The National Vaccine Injury Compensation Program will provide compensation to those who are affected by VCIP-covered vaccine.

## Criteria
- The vaccine should be recommended by CDC for administration to children or pregnant women.
- The injuries covered are listed in the vaccine injury table.
- The first symptom of these injuries should have occurred within the specified time period.
- It should be presumed that the vaccine caused the injury unless proved otherwise.
- If the above criteria are not met, it should be proved with enough evidence with expert witness, medical records, or medical opinion.
- The effects lasted for more than 6 months, or resulted in inpatient hospitalization or surgical intervention or resulted in death.

## Procedure

Any one irrespective of age who believes that he is affected by administration of vaccine can file a petition. The claims must be first adjudicated through this program before civil litigation can be pursued. A table with the list of vaccines covered by the programme is available. This also includes the list of injuries, disabilities, illness, and conditions including death for which compensation can be awarded. The time during which the first symptom or substantial aggravation of an injury must appear after vaccination to be eligible.

The claimants can also claim for the adverse events not listed in the table, if the causation by the vaccines are proved.

## Time Frames

The petition should be filed within specified time depending upon the type of injury:
- Injury within 3 years
- Death within 2 years or death within 4 years of the first symptom or manifestation of onset or of the significant aggravation of the injury from which the death resulted
- In few conditions the time limit may be relaxed by the court.

All vaccines and diluents are stored at 2–8°C except varicella containing vaccines.

## Vaccine Controversy

*A vaccine controversy* is a dispute over the morality, ethics, effectiveness, and poor safety of vaccinations. There is an argument that the immunity provided by vaccines are short-lived and needed boosters, whereas natural infection results in long immunity.

A vaccinated child should be followed for a minimum of 30–60 minutes following immunization. Also an emergency kit and a basic knowledge about management of anaphylaxis should be available. But unfortunately this is ignored. Measles vaccine related deaths were reported in many places. Few were said to be due to toxic shock syndrome and few were due to anaphylaxis both of them could have be prevented.

## Conditions in Which Immunization Should be Delayed

- Delay measles/MMR vaccination for 6 weeks if the child has received immunoglobulin therapy.
- Live vaccine can be delayed during severe febrile illness.
- If the child had taken antibiotics effective against *Salmonella typhi* within past 1 week.

Many wonder why one should receive a vaccination against a disease that do not see to exist at all. Many myths and misinformation about a vaccine are abound to confuse parents who are trying to make sound decision about their children's healthcare.

The negative aspects of the vaccines are not discussed with the parents; one has to consider both the positive and negative aspects of a vaccine before it is administered to the recipients.

*If the benefits outweigh the risks you can give the vaccine and if the risk outweigh the benefits it is better to avoid the vaccine.*

## Vaccine Adverse Event Reporting System

VAERS table:

| Event | Interval from vaccination |
|---|---|
| Anaphylaxis/anaphylactic shock | 7 days |
| Brachial neuritis | 28 days |
| Vasovagal syncope | 7 days |
| Guillain-Barré syndrome | 36 days (6 weeks) |
| Intussusception | 21 days |
| Shoulder in injury related to vaccine administration | 7 days |
| Acute sequelae | Not applicable |
| Death | Not applicable |

General information regarding VAERS is available at: https:vaers.hhs.gov/index.html
Information for healthcare providers are available at the following site: https:vaers.hhs.gov/resources /infoproviders.html

# CHAPTER 8

# Supplement on Vaccines—2019

## CHAPTER OUTLINE

- Immunization Schedule of Vaccines
- High-risk Group
- Immunization Schedules
- Catch-up Vaccination
- Vaccine Schedule for an Unimmunized Child

## INTRODUCTION

The schedule for each vaccine should be known so that the doses are not missed or extra doses are not given. The schedule for the vaccines are discussed in this chapter.

## IMMUNIZATION SCHEDULE OF VACCINES

### General Vaccines Dose and Schedule

#### Bacillus Calmette-Guérin (BCG) Vaccine—Live Attenuated Vaccine

- ❖ *Dose:* 0.05 mL for children below 4 weeks of life.
  - 0.1 mL after 4 weeks of life.
  - Preterm and low birth weight (LBW): In clinically stable babies.
- ❖ *Route of administration:* Intradermal.
- ❖ *Site of administration:* Left upper arm at the insertion of deltoid.
- ❖ *Schedule:*
  - *National schedule:* Single dose at birth.
  - *Indian Academy of Pediatrics (IAP) schedule:* Single dose at birth.
  - *Catch-up vaccination*
- ❖ *National Program:* No upper age specified (as early as possible).
- ❖ *Indian Academy of Pediatrics schedule:* Up to 5 years.

### Oral Polio Vaccine—Live Attenuated Vaccine

- ❖ *Dose:* 2 drops
- ❖ *Route of administration:* Oral
- ❖ Schedule
  - **UIP 2019:**
    - ♦ *Zero dose:* At birth
    - ♦ *Primary doses:*
      1st dose: 6 weeks
      2nd dose: 10 weeks
      3rd dose: 14 weeks
      4th dose: 15–18 months
      5th dose: 4–5 years.
    - ♦ Pulse polio immunization (irrespective of the immunization status).
    - ♦ On all NIDs for children less than 5 years of age 2 doses per year.
    - ♦ On all SNIDs.

**Catch-up vaccination:** Up to 5 years of age
- *Indian Academy of Pediatrics 2012 schedule:* Sequential oral poliovirus vaccine/inactivated polio vaccine (OPV/IPV) schedule
  - 0 dose: At birth—OPV
  - 1st dose: 6 weeks—IPV
  - 2nd dose: 10 weeks—IPV
  - 3rd dose: 14 weeks—IPV
  - 4th dose: 9 months—OPV
  - 5th dose: 15-18 months—IPV
  - 6th dose: 4-5 years—OPV
- Pulse polio immunization (irrespective of the immunization status).
- On all NIDs for children less than 5 years of age 2 doses per year.
- On all SNIDs.
- *Catch-up vaccination:* Up to 5 years of age.

## Hepatitis B Vaccine—Recombinant Subunit Vaccine

- *Dose:*
  - 0.5 mL (10 µg) in children less than 18 years.
  - 1 mL (20 µg) in adults more than 18 years.
  - 40 µg for high-risk groups (hemodialysis, etc.).
- *Route of administration:* Intramuscular.
- *Site of administration:* Anterolateral aspect of mid-thigh (younger than 6-7 years or deltoid (> 7 years).
- *Schedule:*
  - UIP 2019: At birth, 6, 10, 14 weeks.
  - Indian Academy of Pediatrics 2019: At birth, 6 weeks, 6 months or birth +6, 10, 14 weeks or birth, 6 and 14 weeks or 0, 1, and 6 months:
    - Preterm: Less than 2 kg—at birth (not counted), 1 dose at month, then along with DPT+Hib.
      Hbs Ag positive mother: Hepatitis B immune globulin (HBIG) with vaccine at birth.
    - Post-exposure prophylaxis—check for antibody titer, 0.5 mL at 0, 1, and 6 months along with immunoglobulin.
- *Catch-up vaccination for previously not immunized:* 0-18 years
- *Children who are not previously vaccinated must receive 3 dose series:* Complete 3 dose series with second dose more than or equal to 4 weeks and third dose more than or equal to 8 weeks from the previous dose at any age. 0, 1 and 6 schedule is used for catch-up vaccination.

## DTwP Vaccine—Diphtheria, Tetanus Toxoid with Whole-cell Pertussis Vaccine

- *Dose:* 0.5 mL
- *Route of administration:* Intramuscularly
- *Site of administration:* Anterolateral aspect of the thigh.
- *Schedule:*
  - UIP 2019: Primary—three doses at 6 weeks, 10 weeks, and 14 weeks.
    - Booster at 15-18 months and 5 years given as pentavalent with *Haemophilus influenzae* type b (Hib) and hepatitis B virus (HBV).
  - Indian Academy of Pediatrics: Primary—three doses at 6 weeks, 10 weeks and 14 weeks.
    - Booster either DTwP or diphtheria, tetanus, and acellular pertussis (DTaP) at 15-18 months and 4-5 years followed by tetanus, diphtheria, pertussis vaccine for adult/diphtheria toxoids (TdaP/Td) at 10-12 years and 15 years, Td/TdaP every 10 years.
  - *Catch-up vaccination:* Catch up less than or equal to 5 years—0, 1, and 6 months.
    - Catch-up more than 5 years TdaP, Td and at 0, 1, and 6 months.
    - Second booster, the fifth dose is not required if the last dose was given after the age of 4 years.

## Enhanced Injectable Polio Vaccine—Killed Vaccine

- *Dose:* 0.5 mL
- *Route of administration:* Intramuscular or intradermal: Fractional IPV is given in a dose of 0.1 mL, intradermal in national program.
- *Site of administration:* Anterolateral aspect of thigh for IM route, right arm for intradermal route.
- *Schedule for IPV for children:*
  - UIP 2019: 2 dose at 6 and 14 weeks.
  - Indian Academy of Pediatrics schedule: 6, 10, 14 weeks, booster at 15–18 months.
  - Participants of national program should be offered with 1 dose 0.5 mL intramuscular IPV in first year with booster at 15–18 months.
- *Catch-up vaccination for IPV:* Up to 5 years of age gives 3 doses at 0, 2 and 6 months two doses at 2 months apart booster after 6 months after the previous dose.
  - If the 3rd dose is given at the age of more than or equal to 4 years of age, the fourth dose is not need.

## Haemophilus Influenza Type b Vaccine Killed Conjugated Vaccine

- *Dose:* 0.5 mL in children.
- *Route of administration:* Intramuscular.
- *Site of administration:* Anterolateral aspect of thigh
- *Schedule:*
  - UIP 2019: Primary series 6, 10, 14 weeks with booster at 12 months through 18 months.
  - Indian Academy of Pediatrics schedule: 6, 10, 14 weeks and booster dose at 15–18 months.
- *Minimal age of administration:* 6 weeks.
- *Maximal age of administration:* The third dose should be administered at the age of 12 months through 15 months and at least 8 weeks after the second dose.
- *Catch-up vaccination:* It is recommended only up to 5 years of age.
  - 7–11 months—2 primary doses more than or equal to 4 weeks apart and one booster at 16–18 months.
  - 12–14 months—one primary dose and one booster at 15–18 months.
  - 15–59 months—one single dose.
  - 5 years—not recommended.

## Pneumococcal Conjugate Vaccine (PCV-13, PCV-10)—Killed Conjugated Vaccine

- *Dose:* 0.5 mL
- *Route of administration:* Intramuscular.
- *Site of administration:* Anterolateral aspect of thigh or deltoid.
- *Schedule:*
  - UIP 2019: Pilot project in 6 states (PCV 13). 6, 10, 14 weeks and booster at 15–18 months.
  - Indian Academy of Pediatrics schedule 2016: PCV 13 or PCV 10—4 dose schedule at 6, 10, 14 weeks and a booster dose at 15–18 months. For children age 6–18 years with underlying medical conditions like sickle cell disease, HIV infection, immunocompromised, cochlear implant, CSF leak, give one dose of PCV13 followed by pneumococcal polysaccharide vaccine (PPSV 23) by 8 weeks later. PCV is recommended in adults and older peoples also in high-risk groups as mentioned above.
- *Catch-up vaccination:*
  - 7–11 months 2 doses more than or equal to 4 weeks apart, 1 booster at 15–18 months.
  - 12–23 months—2 doses more than or equal to 8 weeks apart.
  - 24–59 month—one dose should be administered for all healthy children

aged 24-59 months who are not completely vaccinated for their age more than 60 months one dose if high-risk category.
- For PCV 10 it is recommended that a minimum of 2 doses at 8 weeks apart has to be given at any age.

## Rotavirus Vaccine—Oral Live Attenuated Vaccine

- *Dose:*
  - RV1 (Rotarix)—1 mL lyophilized (liquid reconstituted 1.5 mL).
  - RV5 (RotaTeq)—2 mL prefilled liquid.
  - ORV 116E (monovalent oral rotavirus vaccine 116E)—used in national program—liquid both single dose and multidose vials (single dose: 0.5 mL, multidose 5-10 mL doses).
- *Route of administration:* Oral.
- *Schedule:*
  - UIP 2019: 6, 10, and 14 weeks.
  - *Indian Academy of Pediatrics*: RV 1—two doses/RV 5—three doses or ORV116E—3 doses:
    - First dose—at 6-14 weeks.
    - Second dose—at least more than or equal to 4 weeks later so that the second dose is completed before 32 weeks.
- Minimal age—6 weeks of age second dose at 6-8 weeks interval before 32 weeks of life.
- Maximal age for first dose is before 15 weeks.
- Maximal age for final dose—8 months
- Vaccination series should not be initiated at the age of 15 weeks 0 days or older.
- The final dose should be completed before 12 months of age.
- 2 dose series with Rotarix or 3 dose series with RotaTeq. If any dose in the series is not known default to 3 dose series.

## Measles Vaccine—Live Attenuated Vaccine (Measles Alone not in use in India. Instead using Measles with Rubella or Mumps Measles and Rubella Vaccine)

- *Dose:* 0.5 mL.
- *Route of administration:* Subcutaneous.
- *Site of administration:* Right upper arm at the site of insertion of deltoid.
- *Schedule of measles vaccine:*
  - UIP 2019: 9 months
    - First dose: After 9 months
    - Second dose: 16-24 months.
    - But during outbreaks first dose can be given at more than or equal to 6 months. But again 2nd dose at 12-15 months to be given.
- *Catch-up vaccination:* It can be given up to 5 years if not given by 9-12 months.
- *Indian Academy of Pediatrics 2012:*
  - First dose—at 9 months.
  - Second dose as measles, mumps and rubella (MMR)—at 15 months.
  - Third dose as MMR—at 5 years (4-6 years) (optional).
- *Catch-up vaccination:* Up to 18 years—2 doses of MMR 3 months apart.

## Hepatitis A

### Hepatitis A: Formalin inactivated vaccine

- Efficacy is more with killed vaccine.
- *Dose:* 0.5 mL —720 U or junior below 18 years and 1 mL—1440 U for more than 18 years.
- *Route of administration:* Intramuscular.
- *Site of administration:* Deltoid or thigh.
- *Schedule:*
  - UIP 2019: Not included.
  - *Indian Academy of Pediatrics schedule:* Two doses beyond one year of age 6 months apart.
- *Catch-up vaccination:* One dose followed by booster after 6 months.

## Hepatitis A
### Hepatitis A: Live attenuated vaccine
- *Dose:* 0.5 mL
- *Route of administration:* Subcutaneously or intramuscular
- *Site of administration:* Deltoid or thigh
- *Schedule:*
  - UIP 2019 : Not included.
  - Indian Academy of Pediatrics schedule: Risk group 2 doses 6 months apart, one dose in healthy single dose after 1year. Boosters are not necessary.
  - Minimal age for immunization: 12 months.
- *Catch-up vaccination:* Single dose at any age—boosters are not necessary.

### Aluminum hydroxide adjuvant vaccine:
Aluminum hydroxide is the most commonly used chemical as an Adjuvant in Vaccines. Adjuvants will enhance the immune response. The disadvantage of the aluminum hydroxide is that the vaccines cannot be frozen. Also adjuvants can cause adverse effects.

### Virosomal vaccine (Not Available Now)
- It does not contain aluminum hydroxide so pain will be less.
- Booster—after 6 months.
- Dose—5 mL equivalent to 24 IU.

## Tetanus Toxoid (Td)
- *Dose:* 0.5 mL
- *Route of administration:* Intramuscular
- *Site of administration:* Upper arm or deltoid or thigh.
- *Schedule:*
  - UIP 2019
  - Indian Academy of Pediatrics schedule: Two doses of Td at 10 years, 16 years.
  - Boosters once in every 10 years.
- *Catch-up vaccination:*
  - For unimmunized school aged children primary Td immunization with 2 doses of Td 4 weeks apart.
  - In the antenatal period for unimmunized mothers, two doses at one month interval with the last dose at least 2 weeks before delivery.
  - In already immunized mother one dose will be enough.
  - After completion of full course of 7 doses, additional dose is not needed during pregnancy for next 10 years. After 10 years a single Td will be enough to boost the immunity for next 10 years.
- *Recent advances:* Diphtheria toxoid vaccine is given instead of Td.

## DTaP Vaccine—Diphtheria, Tetanus Toxoid with Acellular Pertussis Vaccine
- 2 component, 3 component, 5 component are available in the market.
- *Dose:* 0.5 mL
- *Route of administration:* Intramuscular.
- *Site of administration:* Anterolateral aspect of thigh or deltoid.
- *Schedule:*
- UIP 2019: Not included.
  - Indian Academy of Pediatrics schedule: Three doses at 6 weeks, 10 and 14 weeks (Only for high-risk groups like allergies, serious adverse events following immunization (AEFIs), progressive neurological conditions and international travelers going to some countries where DTaP alone is given—primary vaccine with DTaP is indicated).
  - Boosters—at 18 months and 5 years.
- **Catch-up vaccination:** Catch-up less than or equal to 7 years—0, 1 and 6 months. Catch-up more than 7 years Tdap at 0 month, Td at 1 month and 6 months.

## Typhoid Vaccines—Three Types
- Typhoid Vi polysaccharide vaccine
- Typhoid conjugate vaccine
- Typhoral vaccine (Ty21a oral vaccine)

### Typhoid Vi polysaccharide vaccine
- *Dose:* 0.5 mL
- *Route of administration:* Intramuscularly.

- *Site of administration:* Thigh or deltoid.
- *Schedule:*
  - UIP 2019: Not included.
  - Indian Academy of Pediatrics schedule: Single dose after 2 years of age. T-cell independent vaccine hence short lasting immunity. Booster every 3 years.
- *Catch-up vaccination:* Single dose booster every 3 years.

### Typhoid conjugate vaccine

- *Dose:* 0.5 mL can be used from 6 months of age.
- *Dose:* 9 months onwards—No booster recommended now.
- *Route of administration:* Intramuscular.
- *Site of administration:* Thigh or deltoid.
- *Schedule:*
  - UIP 2019: Not included.
  - Indian Academy of Pediatrics schedule: Being T-cell dependent immunity this can be given in children below 2 years of age.

### Typhoral vaccine (Ty21a oral vaccine)

- This vaccine is not available.
- *Dose:* 3 to 4 capsules on alternate days.
- *Route of administration:* Oral.
- *Schedule:*
  - UIP 2019: Not included.
  - Indian Academy of Pediatrics schedule: One capsule on alternate days for 3 days a total of three capsules. This is given only after the age of 6 years as the capsule has to be swallowed without biting. The dose should be repeated after 5 years. Three capsules one on day 1, 3 and 5 should be taken in cool water 1 hour before food.

### Tetanus, Diphtheria, Pertussis Vaccine for Adult (TDAP) Vaccine

- *Dose:* 0.5 mL
- *Route of administration:* Intramuscular.
- *Site of administration:* Thigh or deltoid.
- *Schedule:*
  - UIP 2019: Not included
  - Indian Academy of Pediatrics schedule: Minimum 5 years if DTaP is not available can be replaced with TdaP at 5 years booster at 10 years and 15 years of age the dose can be repeated followed by booster every 10 years.

### Diphtheria Toxoids (Td) Vaccine

- Contains usual dose of tetanus and only 2 units of diphtheria toxoid.
- *Dose:* 0.5 mL
- *Ideal age at immunization:* Adolescents and adults after 7 years of age.
- *Route of administration:* Intramuscular.
- *Site of administration:* Thigh or deltoid.
- *Schedule:*
  - UIP 2019 : Not included.
  - IAP schedule
  - Diphtheria toxoids vaccine or tetanus, diphtheria, pertussis vaccine for adult (Td/TdaP) is used as replacement for DTwP or DTaP or DT for catch-up vaccination in children above 7 years of age.
  - World Health Organization recommends Td or TdaP vaccine instead of tt in wound management prophylaxis against neonatal tetanus and maternal tetanus in pregnant woman. All pregnant women who are not immunized should be given a minimum of 2 doses of Td at 4-8 weeks interval and one dose in previously immunized women getting pregnant after 3 years of the previous dose.
  - Two doses at 10 years and 16 years.
- *Booster:* Td should be repeated every 10 years.

Quadrivalent (DTwP + HBV or DTap + Hib), pentavalent vaccines (DTwP + Hib + HBV or DTap + Hib + HBV or DTap + Hib + eIPV), hexavalent (DTwP + Hib + HBV + eIPV or DTap + Hib + HBV + eIPV), are available in the market.

- *Dose:* 0.5 mL
- *Route of administration:* Intramuscular.
- *Site of administration:* Anterolateral aspect of left mid-thigh.

Diphtheria tetanus (DT) vaccine previously used at 5 years in UIP now not in use.

## HIGH-RISK GROUP

High-risk group include the following:
- Acquired immunodeficiency
- Asplenia
- Babies (newborn, infancy)
- Cancer: Malignancies
- Cancer therapy: Radiation therapy
- Congenital immunodeficiency group
- Chronic cardiac, pulmonary (like asthma treated with steroids for a long time), liver disease, hematologic, renal (like nephrotic syndrome).
- Cerebrospinal leak
- Cochlear implant
- Diabetes mellitus
- Drugs-steroids: Those on long-term corticosteroids.
- Epidemics: During disease outbreaks.
- Functional asplenia or hyposplenism
- Foreign visits: Travelers to foreign countries
- Geriatric age group
- Healthcare workers and laboratory personnel
- Immunocompromised: Congenital or acquired
- International travelers.

## Indian Academy of Pediatrics Recommendations: Vaccines for High-risk Group

- Rabies vaccine
- Japanese encephalitis vaccine
- Meningococcal A+ vaccine
- influenza vaccine
- Cholera vaccine
- Yellow fever vaccine
- Pneumococcal polysaccharide vaccine

## IMMUNIZATION SCHEDULES

Various immunization schedules are followed. These schedules are changed from time to time.

## Expanded Program on Immunization

The Government of India started the Expanded Program on Immunization (EPI) in January 1978 to reduce the incidence of common infectious diseases such as diphtheria, tetanus, pertussis, polio, tuberculosis and typhoid fever. The target populations were children one year of age and pregnant women.

## Universal Immunization Program

In 1985, Universal Immunization Program (UIP) was introduced in India. The target populations were the children under 1 year of age. The vaccines recommended were BCG, DPT, OPV and measles.

### UIP 2019

Difference between UIP 2019 and Indian Academy of Pediatrics schedule is given in Table 8.1.

## CATCH-UP VACCINATION

The aim of catch-up vaccination is to complete the recommended vaccination schedule in a shortest and most effective time frame so that optimal protection against diseases are provided. The scheduled interval between the doses may be short or longer than the standard interval. Also as the age of the child is advanced the number of doses change as they become less vulnerable to the infections. A catch-up schedule should be recommended for missed or overdue vaccinations Table 8.2.

## VACCINE SCHEDULE FOR AN UNIMMUNIZED CHILD

An unimmunized child should be immunized as per the schedule given in the Table 8.3.

**Table 8.1:** Immunizations schedules.

| Age | UIP schedule 2019 | IAP schedule 2019 |
|---|---|---|
| 0 (At Birth) | BCG, OPV 0, HBV 1 | BCG, OPV 0, HBV 1 |
| 6 Weeks | DTwP 1 + HBV 2+ Hib 1 + Rotavirus 1 + IPV 1* + OPV 1 | DTwP1/DTaP1 + HBV2 + Hib1 + Rotavirus 1 + IPV1** + PCV1 |
| 10 Weeks | DTwP2 + HBV3 + Hib2 + Rotavirus 2 + OPV 2 | DTwP2/DTaP2 + HBV3 + Hib2 + Rotavirus 2 + IPV2 + PCV2 |
| 14 Weeks | DTwP3 + HBV4 + Hib3 + Rotavirus 3 + IPV2 + OPV3 | DTwP3/DTaP3 + HBV4 + Hib3 + Rotavirus 3 + IPV3 + PCV3 |
| 6 Months | — | TCV + Flu (Yearly) |
| 9 Months | MR1 + JE1 | MMR1 + OPV2+ MCV1 |
| 12 Months | — | Hep A1 + JE1 + MCV2 |
| 13 Months | — | JE2 |
| 15 Months | — | MMR 2 + Varicella 1 + PCV- B1 |
| 16–18 Months | DTwP- B1 + OPV -B1 + MR2 + JE2 | DTaP-B1 + OPV- B1 + IPV- B1 + Hep A2 + Hib- B1 |
| 2–3 Years | — | MCV 3 |
| 4–6 Years | DTwP- B2+ OPV -B2 | DTaP-B2 + OPV- B2 + Varicella -B + MMR3 |
| 10 Years (9–11 Years) | Td | Tdap, PCV, HPV1 and 2 |
| 16 Years | Td | Td/Tdap, HPV1, 2, 3 |
| Pregnancy | Td 2 doses | Tdap |

UIP schedule: Universal Immunization Programme Schedule; IAP schedule: Indian Academy of Pediatrics Schedule; DTwP: Diphtheria, tetanus, whole cell pertussis vaccine; DTaP: Diphtheria, tetanus, acellular pertussis vaccine; DT: Diphtheria, tetanus vaccine; HBV: Hepatitis B vaccine; Hep A: Hepatitis A vaccine; Hib: H. influenza vaccine; HPV: Human papilloma virus vaccine; Rot: Rotavirus vaccine; IPV: Injectable polio vaccine; JE: Japanese encephalitis vaccine; MCV: Menigococcal vaccine; MMR: Measles, mumps, rubella vaccine; MR: Measles, rubella vaccine; PCV: Pneumococcal conjugate vaccine; TCV: Typhoid conjugate vaccine; B: Booster; Pentavalent vaccine: DTwP1 + HBV2 + Hib1

*National schedule IPV is administered in a dose of 0.1 mL intradermally
**IAP schedule 0.5 mL, intramuscularly.

**Table 8.2:** Catch-up vaccination.

| Vaccine | Catch-up vaccination | Age |
|---|---|---|
| BCG | Up to 5 years | |
| Hepatitis B | 0, 1 and 6 months | |
| Measles | Beyond 12 months give MMR | |
| MMR | 2 doses at 4 months interval | |
| Varicella | • 2 doses for all aged 7 through 18 years with no evidence of immunity<br>• If one dose is administered give second dose. | 12 months through 12 years —at minimum interval of 3 months<br>>13 years at minimum interval of 4 weeks |
| Hepatitis A | 2 doses 6 months apart. | |
| Typhoid | Catch-up given up to18 years | |
| HPV | Females 13–45 year routine schedule for catch-up | |
| Td | 2 doses 4 weeks apart | |

- Arthus type hypersensitivity reactions can occur in persons who had received multiple boosters previously. This is characterized by severe local reactions starting about 2-8 hours after the injection.
- For unimmunized pregnant women 2 doses of Td 4 week apart. The last dose should be given at least 2 weeks before delivery.

**Table 8.3:** Vaccine schedule for an unimmunized child.

| Age | Age < 5 years | Age > 5 years |
|---|---|---|
| First visit | BCG, OPV, DPT, HB | Td, HB |
| Second visit (1 month later) | OPV, DPT, HB | Td, HB |
| Third visit (1 month later) | OPV, DPT, MMR/measles, typhoid | MMR, typhoid |
| 1 year later | OPV, DPT, HB | HB |
| Every 3 years | Typhoid booster | Typhoid booster |

No other vaccine should be administered along with measles/MMR vaccine.

# Annexure

## IMMUNIZATIONS SCHEDULES.

| Age | UIP schedule 2019 | IAP schedule 2019 |
|---|---|---|
| 0 (At Birth) | BCG, OPV 0, HBV 1 | BCG, OPV 0, HBV 1 |
| 6 Weeks | DTwP 1 + HBV 2+ Hib 1 + Rotavirus 1 + IPV 1* + OPV 1 | DTwP1/DTaP1 + HBV2 + Hib1 + Rotavirus 1 + IPV1** + PCV1 |
| 10 Weeks | DTwP2 + HBV3 + Hib2 + Rotavirus 2 + OPV 2 | DTwP2/DTaP2 + HBV3 + Hib2 + Rotavirus 2 + IPV2 + PCV2 |
| 14 Weeks | DTwP3 + HBV4 + Hib3 + Rotavirus 3 + IPV2 + OPV3 | DTwP3/DTaP3 + HBV4 + Hib3 + Rotavirus 3 + IPV3 + PCV3 |
| 6 Months | — | TCV + Flu (Yearly) |
| 9 Months | MR1 + JE1 | MMR1 + OPV2+ MCV1 |
| 12 Months | — | Hep A1 + JE1 + MCV2 |
| 13 Months | — | JE2 |
| 15 Months | — | MMR 2 + Varicella 1 + PCV- B1 |
| 16–18 Months | DTwP- B1 + OPV -B1 + MR2 + JE2 | DTaP-B1 + OPV- B1 + IPV- B1 + Hep A2 + Hib- B1 |
| 2–3 Years | — | MCV 3 |
| 4–6 Years | DTwP- B2+ OPV -B2 | DTaP-B2 + OPV- B2 + Varicella -B + MMR3 |
| 10 Years (9–11 Years) | Td | Tdap, PCV, HPV1 and 2 |
| 16 Years | Td | Td/Tdap, HPV1, 2, 3 |
| Pregnancy | Td 2 doses | Tdap |

UIP schedule: Universal Immunization Programme Schedule; IAP schedule: Indian Academy of Pediatrics Schedule; DTwP: Diphtheria, tetanus, whole cell pertussis vaccine; DTaP: Diphtheria, tetanus, acellular pertussis vaccine; DT: Diphtheria, tetanus vaccine; HBV: Hepatitis B vaccine; Hep A: Hepatitis A vaccine; Hib: H. influenza vaccine; HPV: Human papilloma virus vaccine; Rot: Rotavirus vaccine; IPV: Injectable polio vaccine; OPV: Oral polio vaccine; JE: Japanese encephalitis vaccine; MCV: Menigococcal vaccine; MMR: Measles, mumps, rubella vaccine; MR: Measles, rubella vaccine; PCV: Pneumococcal conjugate vaccine; TCV: Typhoid conjugate vaccine; B: Booster; Pentavalent vaccine: DTwP1 + HBV2 + Hib1

*National schedule IPV is administered in a dose of 0.1 mL intradermally
**IAP schedule 0.5 mL, intramuscularly.

# RECOMMENDATIONS FOR CATCH-UP IMMUNIZATION UP TO 18 YEARS OF AGE

**Catch-up vaccination**

| Vaccine | Catch-up schedule |
|---|---|
| BCG | • NIS–Catch-up schedule up to 1 year if missed<br>• IAP–Catch-up schedule up to 5 years if missed |
| DTwP or DTaP | • Catch-up ≤ 7 years–DtaP or DTwP at 0, 1 and 6 months<br>• Catch-up ≥ 7 years–Tdap at 0, 1 and 6 months<br>• Catch-up ≥ 7 years–Tdap at 0 months and Td at 1 and 6 months |
| OPV | • NIS–up to 5 years if missed<br>• IAP–up to 5 years if missed |
| IPV | Up to 5 years–3 doses at 0, 2 and 6 months |
| Measles | • <12 months administer measles<br>• ≥12 months administer MMR vaccine, beyond 12 months MMR 2 doses at 4 months interval<br>• Measles catch-up <1 year MR vaccine |
| MMR | Two doses ≥ 4 weeks apart, one dose if already received one dose of MMR |
| Hib | • 6–12 months–2 doses ≥ 4 weeks apart with one booster at 15–18 months<br>• 12–15 months–one dose and one booster at 15–18 months<br>• 14–16 months–one dose<br>• >5 years not recommended |
| Hepatitis B | Complete 3 dose series dose 1 and 2 are ≥ 4 weeks apart and 2 and 3 are ≥ 8 weeks apart (0, 1 and 6 months) |
| Varicella | Complete two dose series with minimum interval of 3 months in between (≥ 4 weeks if ≥ 12 years old)<br>• 2 doses for all aged 7 through 18 years with no evidence of immunity<br>• If one dose is administered give second dose. 12 months through 12 years —at minimum interval of 3 months >13 years at minimum interval of 4 weeks |
| Rotavirus | • Maximum age for first dose 14 weeks 6 days<br>• Maximum age for last dose 8 months 0 days |
| Typhoid | One dose beyond 2 years of age. Catch-up given up to 18 years |
| PCV | • 7–11 months two doses ≥4 weeks apart, one booster at 15–18 months<br>• 12–23 months two doses ≥8 weeks apart<br>• 24–59 months–one dose<br>• >60 months–one dose only if in high-risk category |
| Hepatitis A | 2 doses 6 months apart. Complete two doses at an interval of ≥ 6 months<br>If ≥ 10 years old screen for HAV antibody first and if negative administer |
| HPV | Females before initiation of sexual activity. 13–45 years routine schedule for catch-up |
| Japanese B encephalitis | One dose in susceptible children up to 15 years of age during outbreak |
| TT | 2 doses 4 weeks apart for unimmunized pregnant women 2 doses of TT 4 week apart. The last dose should be given at least 2 weeks before delivery |

# Index

Page numbers followed by *f* refer to figure and *t* refer to table.

## A

Abdomen 186, 188, 232
   lateral radiograph of 123
   X-ray 122, 123*f*, 186, 187, 191, 233, 252
   plain 192
Abdominal tuberculosis, types of 192
Abscess 172
   site of 161
   types of 161
Acellular pertussis vaccine 558
Acellular vaccine 509
Acetazolamide 411
Acetone killed vaccine 511
Acetylcholine 326
Achalasia cardia 245, 245*f*
Achondroplasia 215
   radiological findings 215
Acidosis 312
Acquired megacolon 268
Acrodermatitis enteropathica 40
Actinomyces 279
Acycloguanosine 308
Acyclovir 308
Adenosine monophosphate 423
Adrenaline 329
Adverse vaccine reactions, minor 547
Afluria 517
Aganglionic megacolon, congenital 266
Agathi keerai 23, 23*f*
Air
   beyond stomach single bubble sign, absence of 246*f*
   bronchogram 154*f*
   filled viscus 263*f*
   leak syndrome 164, 227
Airways 86, 113
   indications for 114
   measurement of 114

Albendazole 319
Albers-Schönberg disease 212, 213
   radiological findings 212
Albumin 476
Alpha blockers 339
Alpha methyldopa 346
Aluminum hydroxide adjuvant vaccine 558
Alveolar edema 177*f*
Alveoli causing pneumomediastinum, rupture of 138
Amikacin 295
Aminoglycosides 293, 294
Aminophylline 349, 350
Amla 28, 28*f*
Amlodipine 345
Ammonia 425
Amoxycillin 284, 285
Amphotericin B 312
Ampicillin 285
   derivatives of 286
Anemia 40
Angel wing sign 137
Angiotensin-converting enzyme inhibitor 348
Animal foods 34
Anorectal anomalies 123*f*, 125*f*, 269, 270
Antecubital fossa, veins in 57
Anthelmintics 319
Antibodies 548
Anticholinergics 357
Anticholinesterase poisoning, features of 328
Anticoagulants 421
Antiepileptics, newer 369, 382
Antioxidant activity 451
Anti-rabies vaccine 530
Antituberculous drugs 303
Antral nipple sign 246
Antropometry 48
   tapes 50

Aorta
   coarctation of 136*f*, 149, 150*f*
   shape of 130
   size of 130
Apnea 86
Apple 28, 28*f*
Artemether 315
Artesunate 316
Ascariasis 190
Ascending colon loop, fixed 252*f*
Aspiration 154*f*
Asthma 174
   devices 108
Atria, localization of 128
Atrial septal defect 143, 143*f*
Atrophic rickets 205
Atropine 324, 326, 327
   administration of 48
Attenuated vaccine, oral live 557
Autoimmune disorders 550
Azithromycin 298
Azotemia 312

## B

Bacterial infections 164
*Bacteroides fragilis* 285
Bag 91
   contraindications of 100
   resuscitator 99
   uses 99
Bajra 15, 16, 16*f*
   nutritive values 16
Baker's yeast 491
Banana 28, 28*f*
Barbiturate 369, 457
   poisoning
      acute 370
      chronic 371
Bare area sign 167
Barium
   contrast 192

enema 192, 250f, 265, 265f
   signs 263
   study 261f
   swallow 245
Barley 14
   nutritive values 14
Barrel chest 176
Barton's disease 210
Battered baby syndrome 202, 203, 210
Batwing appearance 176, 177f
BCG
   complex 488
   natural history of 486
   side effects of 487
   test 488
   vaccination 485, 487, 554
      complications of 487
Beak sign 246
Beau's lines 44
Beclomethasone 356
Bed's syndrome 41
Beet root 25f
Bell's staging, modified 255
Belladonna 326
   poisoning 326
Bengal gram 18f
Benzathine penicillin 288, 291
Benzodiazepines 358
Benzyl penicillin 288-290
Beriberi 40
Beta carotene 449
Beta-blockers 341
Beta-lactam antibiotics 284
Betamethasone 389
Beverages 34
   types of 34
Bilateral consolidation 153f
Bilateral hilar
   adenopathy sarcoidosis 134f
   node enlargement 134
   over lay sign 236
Biopsy gun 72, 72f
   advantages 72
   complications 73
   disadvantages 73
   indications 72
   uses 72
Biopsy needles 67
Bird beak sign 263
Birth injuries 234
Bitot's spots 40, 452
Bivalent polio vaccine 490
Bleeding problems 40

Blood
   collection, sites for 57
   culture bottle 117, 117f
   pressure 55
      apparatus 55, 55f
      measure 55
      normal 56
   products 465, 482
   transfusion set 92, 92f
   vessels 180
Bone 127, 212
   age 201, 202
      delayed 194f
   dead 218
   density 204f
   long 206
   metaphysis of rapidly growing 204
Bone marrow 70
   aspiration 70
      contraindications for 71
      needle, indications for 70
      procedure for 70
   biopsy needle 70
      parts of 70
   trephine biopsy 71
      complications of 71
      procedure of 71
Bony cage 127
Boot shaped heart 141, 144, 145f
Bowel atresia, small 248
Bowel cleaning 426
Bowel gas 238
   pattern 187, 233
   analysis of 187
Bowel obstruction, large 189
Bowel related signs 257
Bowel sign, bowel in 259
Bowing legs, causes of 205
Bradycardia 86
Breathing unit bag, artificial manual 99, 99f
Brittle bone disease 210, 211
Brock's syndrome 155, 158
Bronchial asthma 165, 350
Bronchial obstruction, causes of 156
Bronchiectasis 156, 158
   left lower lobe 156f
   sicca 158
Bronchiolitis 163, 165
   complications of 164
   management of 164
Bronchodilators 349

Budesonide 356
Bulb sucker 107, 107f
   advantages 107
   disadvantage 107
   precautions 107
   uses 107
Bulging fissure sign 155
Bull's eye 259
Burlow's test 220
Burning feet syndrome 41
Butterfly needles 62

## C

Cabbage 22, 22f
Caffeine citrate 412
Calcium 384
   channel blockers 343
   gluconate 413, 414
   indications for 413
Calmpose 358
Captopril 348
Carbamazepine 368, 369, 379
   therapeutic level of 380
Carbohydrate 1
   effects of 1
   metabolism 384
Cardiac
   asthma 350
   glycosides 401
   shadow 128
   silhouette 139, 176
   toxicity 404
Cardiogenic pulmonary edema 179
Cardiomediastinum, contours of 129
Cardiomegaly 147, 147f, 177f, 222
   criteria for 147
Cardiomyopathy 41
Cardiorespiratory arrest 64
Cardiovascular system 138, 222, 234
Carotene, absorption of 451
Carpal bones 201, 207f
Catch-up immunization 564
Catch-up vaccination 485, 555, 556, 558, 560, 561t, 564
Catecholamines 329, 339
Catheters 87
   suction 87
Caudate nucleus 549
Cauliflower 24f
Cecal volvulus 262
Cefotaxime 291-293

# Index

Ceftriaxone 291, 293
Cell culture Japanese B
    encephalitis vaccine 524
Central venous
    catheter 89, 89f
        complications of 90
        types of 89
    line 90
        advantages of 90
        indications for 89
        veins for 89
Cephalexin 291
Cephalosporins 291
    generation
        first 291
        fourth 291
        second 291
        third 291
Cereals 11
    milling of 13
    soaking of 12
Cervical rib 219
    significance of 219
    X-ray of 219f
Cervicothoracic sign 134
Cetirizine 323
Chamber enlargement 130
Champagne flute sign 253
Chana 20
    dal 20f
Cheilosis 41
Chelating agents 407
Chest 156, 216
    barium study 263f
    X-ray 125, 147, 186, 222, 236
        normal 128f, 132, 139f
Chickenpox
    infection 529
    vaccine 527-529
Chloramphenicol 376
Chloroquine 317
    overdose 318
    resistant malaria 318
Chlorpheniramine maleate 322
Cholera 532
    vaccine 532, 533
Chromosomal disorders 194
Cimetidine 376
Ciprofloxacin 283
Clarithromycin 298
Clavulanic acid 285
Claw sign 259
Clinical thermometer 53

*Clostridium difficile* 284, 293, 298, 308
Clotrimazole cream 313
Coconut 26, 26f
Coiled-spring sign 259
Coin test 170
Collapse 172
    causes of 174
    lung margins 168f
Colloids 465, 475
Colon cut off sign 191, 259
Colon, cone-shaped 266
Colonic aganglionosis 265
Condiments 33
    benefits of 33
Congestive cardiac failure 41, 237
Consolidation 153
Constipation, habitual 276, 277f
Continuous diaphragm sign 256
Contrast enema 232
Cooking cereals, method of 12
Cornea, vascularization of 47
Corneal ulcer 41
Corneal xerosis 41
Corner fractures 202
Cortical hypercalcinosis 196
Corticosteroid 355, 356, 373
    treatment with 385
Costophrenic sulcus, posterior 167
Co-trimoxazole 281
Cranial walls 219
Crescent sign 259
Cromolyn sodium 357
Crystalloids 464, 467
Cupola sign, X-ray of 258f
Cushing's syndrome 388
Cyanocobalamin 453
Cyanosis, without 181
Cyclopam 415
Cystic fibrosis 232

# D

Dale's vasomotor reversal 332
Dance sign 259
Dead in bed syndrome 41
Decubitus film 258f
Deelee oral mucus trap 97f
Deferiprone 407
Delee oral mucus trap 97
Dementia 41
Dengue 549, 550

Depression 41
Dermatitis 41
Desferrioxamine 407, 408
Developmental dysplasia of hip 219, 220, 220f, 221
    types of 221
Dexamethasone 388
Dextran 477
Dextrocardia 128f, 141
    causes 142
    embryology 141
    mirror image 142
    types 142
    X-ray of 142f
Dextroposition, X-ray of 142f
Dextrose 468, 469
Diaminopyrimidines 281
Diamond sign 246
Diaphragm 131, 188, 243
    development of 243
    eventration of 243, 244f
Diaphragmatic hernia 244
    congenital 243
Diaphysis 204
Diarrhea 41
Diazepam 358, 360, 361, 363
    infusion 361
Diclofenac sodium 416
Dicumarol 376
Dicyclomine 417
Digital X-rays 125
Digitalis toxicity 404, 405
Digoxin 401, 403, 406, 457, 497
    contraindications for 403
    intravenous dose of 402
    oral dose of 402
    side effects of 404
Diphtheria, tetanus
    acellular pertussis vaccine 561
    pertussis 509
    toxoid 555, 558
    vaccine 559, 561
    whole cell pertussis vaccine 561
Diphtheria, toxoids vaccine 559
Dislocation, true 220
Distal microcolon 271f
Distended stomach 262f, 263f
Diuretics 396, 457
    classification of 396
Dobutamine 337, 339
Dock's sign 136, 137
Doge's cap sign 253, 256

Dome, sign of 256
Dome, X-ray of sign of 257f
Dopamine 334, 338, 339
   adverse reactions of 336
   toxicity 336
Double bubble sign 190, 248, 249f
Double diaphragm sign 168
Double track sign 246
Double wall sign 257
Doughnut sign 259
Down syndrome 194, 195, 195f
Doxycycline 302
Drugs 278-448
   antiasthmatics 349
   antibacterials 279
   antibiotics 279
   anticonvulsants 368
   antiepileptic 368
   antifungals 312
   antihistaminics 322
   antihypertensives 339
   antiprotozoal 315
   antivirals 308
   cholinergic 324
   corticosteroids 384
   glucocorticoids 384
   H2-receptor blockers 408
   hormones 390
   inotropic 329
   miscellaneous 306
   opioids 363
   sedatives hypnotics 358
   sympathomimetic 329
Drumstick leaves 22, 23f
Dry fruits 27
Dry powder inhalers 110
   advantages 111
   disadvantages 111
   precautions 111
Duck neck sign 266
Duodenal atresia 248, 249f
Dyssebacea 42

# E

Ebstein's anomaly 151
   X-ray 151f
Edema 42
Egg 35
   composition of 35
   minerals 35
EGG, part of 36
Electrolyte 35, 384
Elephant ear appearance 195f
Ellis curve 166

Emphysema 169, 175
   compensatory 175, 176f, 185
   types of 175
Empyema 160
   necessitans 160
   thoracis 159, 159f, 160
Enalapril 348
Endocrine system 192, 233
Endotracheal intubation 84
   complications of 85
   contraindications for 85
Endotracheal tube 83, 84
   malposition of 86
   obstruction of 86
   sizes of 83
   types of 83
   universal adaptor 83f, 87
Enterocolitis 266f
Eosinophilic pneumonia 152
Epicardial fat pad sign 236, 237
Epidermoid tumor 64
Epilepsy, therapy of 360
Epinephrine 329, 331
   dose of 330
Epiphyseal dysgenesis 193f
Epiphysis 203, 233
   absence of 193f
   absent 234f
   appearance of 201
Erlenmeyer flask deformity 212
Erythromycin 296
Esophageal
   anomalies 239
   atresia 237
   pouch 238
Esophagus 86
Ethambutol 305
Ethosuximide 381
Ewart's sign 237
Extraluminal gas, abnormal 187

# F

Face mask 98, 98f
Falciparum ligament sign 257
   X-ray of 253f
Fat 5, 31
   intake, effects of 5
   metabolism 384
   pad 236
Feeding tube
   abnormal placement of infant 76
   infant 74, 75
Feeds, excess intake of 40

Femur
   causes of fracture of 234
   fracture of 234f
   shaft of 234
   lower end of 234f
Ferrous sulfate 418
Fetal fluid, retained 223
Fetal hydantoin syndrome 378
Fetus, lung maturation in 227
Fever 55
   continuous 54
   intermittent 54
   Pel-Ebstein 55
   quartan 55
   remittent 54
   saddle back 55
   step ladder 55
   tertian 55
   types of 54
   undulant 55
Fibrosis 184
Figure of 8 141
   appearance 149f
Fish 38
Flow-inflating bags 100, 101
Fluconazole 313
Fluid
   resuscitation 469
   type of 237
Flunarizine 345
Fluoroquinolones 283
Fluoroscopy 238
Foley's catheter 87, 87f
   complications 88
   contraindications 88
   disadvantages 88
   indications 88
   method 88
   parts 87
   sizes 87
   uses 88
Foley's tube, problems with 88
Folic acid 378
Follicular hyperkeratosis 42
Food containing niacin 45
Food items, nutritive values of 11
Football sign 253, 257
   X-ray of 253f
Foreign body
   aspiration 185
      radiological findings 185
   obstruction 175, 176f
Formalin inactivated vaccine 557
Free gas, X-ray of 253f
Fresh frozen plasma 482

# Index

Fruits 26
 juices 34
 nutritive value of 27
Furazolidone 299
Furosemide 396
 mechanism of action of 396
 side effects 397

## G

Gabapentin 382
Galeazzi's sign 220
Gas relief sign 257
Gasless abdomen 238
 causes of 190
Gastric outlet obstruction,
 congenital 245
Gastric volvulus 262, 262f, 263, 263f
Gastroesophageal reflux 154f, 189, 189f
Gastrointestinal problems 64
Gastrointestinal system 231, 245
Gastrointestinal tract, parts of 233
Gelatin 481
Genitourinary system 196, 271
Gentamycin 293, 295
Glossitis 42
Glycopeptides 300
Goiter 42
Golden S-sign 173
Gopalan's feet 42
Gram, black 18, 18f
Grapes 29, 29f
Great vessels, transpositions of 148
Green gram 18, 18f
Grierson-Gopalan syndrome 41
Ground-glass appearance 225
Groundnut 26, 27f
Growth plate 205
Growth retardation 43
Guava 29, 29f
Guedel airway 113
Guedel oropharyngeal airway 114f
Guillain-Barré syndrome 63, 489, 518
Gums, lacerations of 86
Guttoral pigmentation 43

## H

Haemaccel 479
*Haemophilus influenzae* 496, 535
 type B vaccine 496, 556

Hair loss 43
Hair-on-end appearance 198f
Haloperidol 420
Headache 64
Healing rickets 205
Heart
 abnormal silhouette of 140
 mitralization of 146
 normal 138, 139, 139f
 shape of 129
 size of 130
Hematology 198
Hemithorax 167
Hemolysis 43
Hemolytic anemia 40
Heparin 421, 422
 antagonist 423
 sodium 421
Hepatitis
 A 557, 558
  vaccine 506
 B 492
  infection, chronic 310
 B vaccine 490, 555
Hepatosplenomegaly 214
Herd immunity 533
Herpenden caliper 52, 52f
Hetastarch 480
Hilar node enlargement 134
Hilar region 132
Hilar shadow-silhouette sign, right 186f
Hilum convergence sign 134
Hirschsprung's disease 232, 265, 265f, 266, 266f, 267
 grading of 266
 radiological signs of 265
Honey 33
Hoover's sign 160, 163
Hormones 390
Horse gram 19, 19f, 20
Human diploid cell vaccine 530
Human papilloma virus vaccine 531, 563
Hyaline membrane disease 152, 225, 225f, 226, 227
Hydrating fluids 466
Hydrocortisone 355, 387
 indications for 387
Hydronephrosis 197, 275, 275f
 acquired causes 198
 causes of 197
 complications of 198
 congenital causes 197

Hydropneumothorax 171, 171f
 causes of 171
 X-ray findings 171
Hydroureteronephrosis
 bilateral 197f, 276f
 right 197f, 276f
Hyperkalemia 442
Hyperlucency 162
Hyperphosphatemia 210
Hypertonic saline 474
Hypertransfusion 200
Hypertrophic pyloric stenosis 245, 247
Hyperventilation, bilateral 174
Hypervitaminosis A
 acute 450
 chronic 450
 features of 450
Hypocalcemia 415
 causes of 215
Hypokalemia 442, 467
Hypomagnesemia 427, 428
Hyponatremia 467
Hypophosphatasia 211
Hypothalamo-hypophyseal-adrenal axis 387
Hypothyroidism 192, 193f, 194, 233, 234, 394, 395
 newborn with 192
 radiological feature 233
Hypotransfusion 200
Hypoxia 86

## I

Iatrogenic complications 171
ICD, complications of 82
Ice lined refrigerator and freezer 545f
Idiopathic hypertrophic pyloric stenosis 245
Ileal atresia 250
Ileus, mechanical 233
Iliac spine
 advantages of posterior superior 70
 anterior superior 195f
Immunization
 and vaccines 483
 contradictions precautions for 537
 passive 492
 schedule 560, 561t, 563
Indian Academy of Pediatrics schedule 561

Indian Council of
   Medical Research
   recommendations 39
Indian gooseberry 28
Indomethacin 423
Indomethacin, contraindications
   for 424
Infant feeding tubes, uses of 76
Infantometer 49, 49f
   advantages 50
   technical aspects 49
   uses 49
Infection 64, 86
Influenza
   inactivated vaccine 516
   vaccine 515, 563
Infusion
   pump 115, 115f
   sets 92
      parts of 92
   type of 115
Inhaler 108, 109f
   advantages 109
   problems with 109
   types 109
Instruments 48
   and procedures 48-118
Insulin 390
   syringe 73, 73f
Intellectual disability 43
Intercostal drainage
   bag 91
   indications for 80
   tube 79
   tube insertion 168f
      empyema left side after
         160f
Interface sign 167
Interferon 309
Interlobar
   effusion 135
   hydrothorax 135
Intestinal atresia 250, 250f
Intestinal gangrene 191
Intestinal malrotation 264
Intestinal obstruction 125f, 188,
   188f, 189, 250f, 251
   multiple fluid levels 251f
Intestinal perforation 191, 256
   radiological findings 256
   sign of 191
Intestine
   lower part of 191
   tuberculosis of 192
Intracranial pressure 219

Intracranial tension 219
   increased 123, 218
Intraluminal gas, abnormal 187
Intramural gas 255
Intramuscular diazepam 360
Intramuscular injection
   method of 56
   site of 56
Intraosseous transfusion 71
Intraspinal epidermoid tumor 64
Intravenous cannula, risks of 58
Intravenous colloids fluids 465
Intravenous crystalloids fluids 464
Intravenous extension tube 82,
   82f
Intravenous fluid 464-82
   infusion set 92, 92f
   types of 464
Intravenous infusion 57
Intravenous needle insertion,
   complications of 58
Intubation, stylet for 84, 84f
Intussusception 259, 259f, 260
   radiological signs of 259
Inverted V sign 257
   X-ray of 258f
Invertogram 188, 269f
Ipratropium bromide 357
Ipsilateral atelectasis 175
Iron
   chelation therapy 200
   chelators 201
   deficiency anemia 40, 419
   sources of 40
Isolyte P 471
Isoniazid 303
Isonicotinylhydrazide 376
Ivermectin 320

**J**

Jackson Rees circuit 96
   advantages 96
   disadvantages 97
   indications 97
   parts 96
Jaggery 32, 32f
Jamshidi bone marrow needle 71f
Japanese encephalitis vaccine
   561, 563
Jarisch-Herxheimer reaction 288
Jaundice 43
   causes of 248
Jejunal atresia 249, 250f
Joint space 205

Jowar (sorghum) 15, 16, 16f
   nutritive values 16
Jug handle appearance 143f
Jugular venous pulse 235

**K**

Kadalai paruppu 20
Kambu 16, 16f
   nutritive values 16
Kartagener's syndrome 157
Keratomalacia 43
Kerley B lines 177f, 178, 178f
Kerley lines 177, 180
Keshan disease 43
Ketoconazole 314
Kidney biopsy
   contraindications for 69
   procedure for 69
Killed vaccine 484, 556
   advantages of 484
   conjugated 556
   disadvantages of 484
*Klebsiella* pneumonia 153
Knee 212
   joint, X-ray of 204f
Koilonychia 43
Korasakoff
   psychosis 43
   syndrome 43
Kwashiorkor 43

**L**

Lactulose 425
   mechanism of action of 425
Lamotrigine 382, 383
Laryngoscope 105f
   size of 105
   sterilization of 106
   uses of 105
   with detachable blades 105
Leather bottle appearance 147f
Left colon syndrome 232
Legumes 16
Lemon 29, 29f
Lethargy 43
Leukotriene receptor antagonist
   358
Levetiracetam 383
Limbs 216
Linezolid 306
Lingular consolidation, left 154f
Liquid paraffin 427
Live and killed vaccines 484

Live attenuated
 influenza vaccines 517
 vaccine 483, 554, 557, 558
Live vaccines 483
 advantages of 484
 contraindications of 484
 disadvantages of 484
Liver 37
 edge sign, absent 259
 failure 426
Liver biopsy 67
 complications of 68
 contraindications of 68
 indications for 67
 needles 67
 procedure of 67
Lobar emphysema, congenital 240, 240f, 241
Lobar overinflation, congenital 175, 240
Lobar pneumonia
 causes of 155
 stages of 155
Loculated effusions 166
Loeffler's pneumonia 152
Lorazepam 361, 362, 363
Lower lobe collapse
 left 173
 right 173
Lumbar puncture 64
 complications of 64
 contraindications for 64
 indications for 63
 needle 62, 62f
 procedure 62
Lung 241
 abscess 160, 161, 161f, 173t
 agenesis of 229, 229f
 disease, chronic 230, 231, 231f
 fibrosis of 183
 maturation of 228
 metastasis 183, 184f
 shadow 130

# M

Macleod syndrome 157
Macrocephaly, causes of 214
Macrolides 296
Magnesium sulfate 427
Maize 14
 nutritive values 14
Malecot catheter 88
 parts 88
Malnutrition 44

Malrotation, X-ray of 264f
Mango 30, 30f
Mannitol 398
Marasmic kwashiorkor 44
Marasmus 44
Marble bone disease 213
Marfan's syndrome 170
Mask ventilation 100
Massive cardiomegaly 147f
Mast cell stabilizers 357
Measles vaccination
 complications of 502
 side effects of 502
Measles vaccine 501, 557
Measles, mumps, rubella vaccine 561, 563
 side effects of 505
Measles-rubella
 campaign 504
 vaccine 503, 557, 561, 563
Meat 37
 and meat products 37
Mebendazole 321
Meconium 229, 232
 aspiration syndrome 228, 228f
Meconium ileus 191, 231, 232, 233f, 271
 radiological findings 231
Mediastinal widening 133, 134f
Mediastinum 131
Medullary hypercalcinosis 196
Megacolon, congenital 265, 268
Megaloblastic anemia 40, 455
 causes of 455
Meissner plexus 265
Menigococcal vaccine 521, 523, 561, 563
Meningococcal polysaccharide vaccine, unconjugated 522
Meniscus sign 259
Menkes disease 202
Meropenem 306
Mesenteroaxial gastric volvulus 261f
Mesenteroaxial volvulus 262f
Mesocardia 142
Metabolic side effects 459
 serum 459
 urine 459
Metastatic calcification 196
Metered dose inhaler 110
 advantages 110
 disadvantages 110
 parts 110
 priming 110

Methyldopa, side effects of 347
Methylxanthine 412
Metoclopramide 429
Metoprolol 430
Metronidazole 318
Microcolon 250f
Microcytic hypochromic anemia 200
Micturating cystourethrogram 273
 normal 271, 271f, 272
Midazolam 361
Middle lobe
 collapse, right 173
 consolidation, right 154f
 syndrome 155, 157
Midgut volvulus 262, 263
Miliary mottling 182, 182f
 radiological findings 182
Miliary tuberculosis 183f
Milk 34
 and dairy products 34
 nutritive value of 34
 product 34, 35
Miller's triad 229
Millets 11, 14
 types of 14
Minerals 8, 35, 39
Mitral stenosis 146, 146f
Mitralization 146f
Money bag appearance 141
 pericardial effusion 236f
Monoclonal antibody 164
Monovalent serotype A conjugate vaccine 523
Morphine 363, 366
 sulfate 363
 withdrawal syndrome 366
Motion artifacts 132
Mounier-Kuhn syndrome 157
Mouse tail 246
Mucopolysaccharidosis 206, 206f, 207f, 208
Multiple fluid levels 188f
Mumps measles 504, 547
Muscle 384
Musculoskeletal system 201
*Mycobacterium tuberculosis* 82, 161
*Mycoplasma pneumonia* 151

# N

Nail changes 44
Naloxone 367, 368

Nasal cannula 93, 93f
　advantages 93
　disadvantages 93
Nasal intubation 84
Nasal oxygen catheter 93
　advantages 94
　disadvantages 94
Nasogastric feeding tubes 74
Nasogastric tube 74, 75f
　complications of 75
　length of 75
　size of 75
　types 74
　uses 75
Nasopharyngeal airway 115
Nasopharyngeal oxygen catheter 94
　advantages 94
　disadvantages 94
National Vaccine Injury Compensation Program 552
Natural glucocorticoids 387
Nebulizers 112
　advantages 112
　contraindications 112
　disadvantages 112
　indications 112
　parts 112
　types 112
Neck 219
Necrotizing enterocolitis 252, 252f
　pneumatosis cystoides intestinalis 252
Needles 56
　intramuscular 56
　intravenous 57
Neostigmine 327
Nephrocalcinosis 196
Nephrotoxicity 312
Net protein utilization 4
Neural tube defects 44
Neurotoxicity 304
Nevirapine 310
　prophylaxis 311
Nifedipine 343
Night blindness 44
Nitrofuran derivatives 299
Nitroglycerin 431
Nocardia 279
Nonaccidental trauma 202
Noncardiogenic pulmonary edema 179
Non-rebreather mask 95

Noradrenaline
　dosage of 333
　side effects of 333
Norepinephrine 332
Norfloxacin 284
Nutrition 1–47
Nutritional deficiency disorders 40
Nutritional disorders 40
Nutritional rickets 457
Nuts 26
　and oil seeds 25, 26f
Nyctalopia 44

## O

Obstructive emphysema 175, 176f, 185
　radiological findings 185
Obstructive lung disease 175
Oil 31
　seeds nutritive value 26
Oligemic lung fields, features of 121
Oncogenic rickets 205
Ondansetron 432
Ophthalmoplegia 44
Oral airway, technique of insertion of 114
Oral chloroquine, adverse effects of 317
Oral intubation 84
Oral iron
　side effects of 418
　treatment with 418
Oral polio vaccine 554, 561, 563
Oral poliomyelitis immunization, complications of 489
Oral rehydration 433
　solution 432, 433
Oral vaccine 512
Orange 30, 30f
Oreo cookie sign 236
Orogastric tube, tracheoesophageal fistula coiling of 238f
Oro-oculo-genital syndrome 44
Oropharyngeal airway 113
Ortolani's test 220
Osmotic diuresis 398
Osteoclasts, functions of 214
Osteogenesis imperfecta 210, 211
　treatment of 212
Osteomyelitis 217, 217f
　acute 218

　chronic 218
　complications of 218
　radiological changes in 217
　types 217
Osteopetrosis 212-215
　complications of 214
　femur and tibia 213f
　pathogenesis of 214
　types of 213
Osteoporosis 44
Overfeeding 40
Overnutrition 40
Oxygen
　delivery systems 93
　tube 87, 87f
Oxygen hood 94
　advantages 94
　disadvantages 94
　precautions 94
Oxygen mask 95, 95f
　advantages 95
　disadvantages 95
　precautions 95
Oxygen reservoir
　bag 96
　　advantages 96
　　non-rebreathing mask with 96f
Oxygen tent 94
　advantages 95
　disadvantages 95

## P

Paladai 116, 116f
Paracetamol 439
Paralytic ileus 191, 233, 251, 261
Paralytic poliomyelitis, vaccine associated 489
Parapneumonic effusion 160
Parrot, pseudoparalysis of 209
Peak flow meter 113, 113f
　advantages 113
　disadvantages 113
　types 113
Pearl millet 15
Pediatric breathing circuit 96
Pediatric surgery 234
Pelkan's spur 209
Pellagra 45
Pelvis 122, 195f, 216, 219
Penicillin 286
　adverse effects of 287
　G 288, 289
　intrathecally 288

intravenously 288
modified 289
shortcomings of 288
treatment 288
types of 288
V 289
Pentavalent vaccine 534
Pericardial effusion 236, 237
causes of 237
signs in large 236
Peripheral neuropathy 45
Peripheral vein
infusion 58
transfusion, veins for 58
Peritoneal ligament related signs 257
Peritoneum, free gas in 257*f*
Peritonitis 261
Pernicious anemia 40
types of 455
Petechiae 45
Petit mal epilepsy 374
Phantom tumor 135
Pheniramine maleate 323
Phenobarbitone 369, 371-373, 378
mechanism of action of 371
Phenoxybenzamine 340
Phenoxymethylpenicillin 289
Phentolamine 340
Phenytoin 336, 369, 373, 374, 376, 378
in diabetics 378
toxicity 377
Pheochromocytoma 347
Phrynoderma 45
causes of 45
Pig tail deformity 266
Piptaz 307
Plantain 28
*Plasmodium falciparum* 318
Platelets concentrate 482
Plethoric lung fields, features of 122
Pleural effusion 160, 165
massive right 166*f*
Pleural tap
complications of 80
indications for 79
Pneumatocele 162, 172, 172*f*, 173*t*
causes 172
Pneumatosis cystoides intestinalis 254*f*
Pneumatosis intestinalis, X-ray of 253*f*

Pneumococcal conjugate vaccine 497, 498, 556, 561, 563
side effects of 498
Pneumococcal polysaccharide vaccine 519, 521
Pneumococcal vaccines 519
Pneumomediastinum 137, 235, 137*f*
causes of 137
signs in 137
Pneumonia 151, 221
types of 152, 152*t*
Pneumopericardium 234, 235, 235*f*, 253, 256
Pneumoperitoneum
air under diaphragm 256*f*
football sign 258*f*
signs of 256
X-ray of 253*f*, 257*f*
Pneumothorax 80, 86, 167, 168*f*, 169, 170
bilateral sided 168*f*
left-sided 168*f*
small 168
X-ray findings 167
Polio 495
switch over 490
Polio vaccine 556
inactivated 495
injectable 563
oral live attenuated 488
vaccination, side effects of inactivated 495
Poliomyelitis vaccine 488
Polysaccharide vaccine 498
unconjugated 522
Pork 37
Portal vein 253*f*, 256*f*
Postexposure prophylaxis 492, 531
Potassium
administration 442
chloride 441, 442
phenoxymethylpenicillin 289
sparing diuretics 400
Pouch-perineal distance 270
Poultry 38
chicken 38
Prader orchidometer 116
Pralidoxime 438
Prazosin 339
Prednisolone 389
Pressurized metered dose inhalers 110
Procaine penicillin 288, 290
Promethazine 443

Prophylaxis 460
pre-exposure 531
Propranolol 341, 342
adverse effects of 342
toxicity 343
Protein 2
conjugate vaccine 522
effects of 2
efficiency ratio 4
metabolism 384
Proton-pump inhibitors 408
Provitamin A 451
Pseudobronchiectasis 157
Pseudokidney sign 259
Pseudopneumoperitoneum 258
Pulmonary adenomatoid malformation, congenital 241, 241*f*
Pulmonary agenesis 229
Pulmonary artery 130
Pulmonary edema 176, 177*f*, 179
cardiogenic 180
noncardiogenic 180
treatment of 180
Pulmonary fibrosis 184
Pulmonary function tests 226
Pulmonary interstitial emphysema 231*f*
Pulmonary oligemia 145*f*, 182, 182*f*
unilateral 145
Pulmonary plethora 147*f*, 180
causes of 181
Pulmonary sequestration 243
Pulmonary surfactant 446
Pulmonary vascular markings 129
Pulmonary vasculature 182
normal 181
Pulmonary venous congestion 180
Pulses 16
nutritive values 17
Pumps, types of 115
Pyknodysostosis 215
Pyloric stenosis string sign 247*f*
Pylorus caterpillar sign, cephalic orientation of 246
Pyrazinamide 304

# Q

Quadriplegia 45
Quadrivalent meningococcal polysaccharide 522
Quinolones 283

# R

Rabies
  immunoglobulin 531
  prophylaxis 531
Rachitic rosary 203f
Radiological signs 257
Radiology (X-rays) 119–277
  basics 119
Radiolucent stones 196
Ragi 15, 15f
  nutritive value of 15, 16
Ramstedt's pyloromyotomy 248
Ranitidine 410
Reactions, injection 546
Recombinant subunit vaccine 555
Record vital signs, instruments to 53
Rectal gas absent 250f
Rectal thermometer 53
Red blood cells 482
Red gram 19, 19f
Red man syndrome 301
Renal biopsy 68
  complications of 69
  indications for 69
  precautions for 69
  procedure 72
  types of 68
Renal calculus 196
Renal stones 196
Respiratory distress syndrome 226
Respiratory syncytial virus 164
Respiratory system 151, 223, 237
  differential diagnosis 159
  infections 151
Resuscitation, newborn 97
Retinol
  sources of 451
  transported 451
Retrosternal rib notching 137
Rheumatic fever 549
Rib
  beading of 203f
  notching 136
    causes of inferior 136
    inferior 136, 136f, 150f
    single 136
    superior 136
    unilateral 136
  osteopetrosis of 213f
Ribavirin aerosol 164

Rice 11
  grain, parts of 11
Rickets 45, 203, 204f
  bones in 203
  tumor 205
  types of 205, 457
  white line of 205
Rifampicin 304, 376
Right pleural effusion, moderate 166f
Rigler's sign 253, 257
Ringer lactate 472
Roesler sign 136
Rotahaler 109
  advantages 110
  indications 109
  method 109
  parts of 109
  precautions 110
  procedure 109
Rotavirus vaccine 499, 557, 563
  side effects of 500
Rubella vaccine 504, 518, 557
  side effects of 519
Ryle's tube 76, 76f
  indications for 76

# S

Saber en boot 141
Saddle bag sign 258f
Sail sign 132, 133f
Salah and Klima needle 70f
Salbutamol 350
Saline, normal 473
*Salmonella typhi* 512
Sandwich sign 259
Saw-tooth appearance 266
Scalp vein set 61, 61f
  disadvantages of 62
  over straight needle, advantages of 61
  parts of 61
Scrotal dermatitis 42
Scurvy 46, 208, 209f
  line 209
  signs in 209
Sea foods 38
Seborrheic dermatitis 41
Self-inflating bags 101
Sepsis
  early neonatal 222
  neonatal 222
Septicemia 222, 222f

Serum magnesium level 428
Shaken infant syndrome 202
Shakirs tape 51, 51f
Shoulder sign 246, 247
Sigmoid volvulus 262
Signet-Ring sign 209
Silence classification 211
Silhouette sign 134, 138, 138f, 173, 186
Silicone 88
Silver sign 257
Single bubble sign 245f
Situs 142
Situs inversus 142f
  heart 128f
  totalis 142
Skeleton 203
Skinfold
  caliper 52
  thickness
    normal 53
    significance of 53
    sites in 52
Skull 198f, 218
  changes in rickets 205
Snowman appearance 141
Sodium
  absorption 433
  bicarbonate 415, 444
  cromoglycate 357
  valproate 368, 378
Soft drinks 34
Soft tissue 127
  swelling 218
Soyabeans 19, 19f
Spacer 111, 111f
  advantages 112
  cleaning 111
  method 111
  precautions 111
Sphygmomanometer, parts of manual 55
Spices 33
  benefits of 33
Spinal cord, subacute combined degeneration of 46
Spine 194, 206
  X-ray of 207f
Spinnaker sail sign 137
Spironolactone 400, 401
Splenectomy 201
Spontaneous pneumoperitoneum 259
Spring sign 259
Stadiometer 50, 50f

*Staphylococcus aureus* 285, 502
Steeple sign 121
Steroids 355, 384
Streptococcal pneumonia, group B 151
*Streptococcus* 549
Streptomycin 295, 296
String sign 190, 245, 246
Subpulmonic effusion 166, 184, 185*f*
Sugar 32, 32*f*
   salt solution 434
Sulfamethoxazole 281, 282
Sulfonamides 279
   action of 279
   effects of 279
Sunburst appearance 223*f*
Supertransfusion 200
Surfactant
   dose of 226
   types of 446
Swyer-James syndrome 157
Sympathetic ophthalmia 550
Sympathomimetic amines 326
Synthetic glucocorticoids 387
   advantages of 387
Syringes 73
   parts of 73
   tip of 56
   uses 73

## T

Tar syndrome 276*f*
Target sign 247, 259
Tegretol 379
Temperature 53
   assessment 53
   range 53
   thermometers 53
Temporal lobe epilepsy 374
Tender coconut 38
Teratogenic effects 368
Terbutaline 354
Testicles, orchidometer measuring volume of 116*f*
Tetanus
   diphtheria, pertussis vaccine 513, 514, 559
   toxoid 558
   vaccine 507, 508
Tetracycline 301
Tetralogy of Fallot 144, 145*f*
Thalassemia 198, 198*f*, 199

splenectomy in 200
Theophylline 352
Thermometer 53*f*
   types of 53
Thiamine, food rich in 40
Thoracoabdominal sign 134
Thoracocentesis 79
Thoracoscopic surgery, video-assisted 161
Three-way
   connector 117*f*
   stopcock 117*f*
Thrombocytopenia absent radius syndrome 275, 276
Thymus 132
   normal 133*f*
Thyroxin 393, 395
Tolerance 373
Tongue 46, 86
   depressor 115, 115*f*
Total anomalous pulmonary venous
   connection 148
   drainage 148
   return 148, 149*f*
Toxicity 288, 306, 325, 328
   acute 450
   chronic 450
   long-term 312
Toxoids 484
Trace elements 39
Trachea, perforation of 86
Tracheoesophageal fistula 237, 238, 238*f*, 239
   congenital 239
Tram track sign 246
Tramadol 447, 448
Transdermal administration 431
Transient tachypnea 223, 223*f*, 224
Triangle sign 257
Triangular sign 256*f*
Trimethoprim 281, 282
Triple bubble sign 250*f*
Tropical eosinophilia 183
Trucut needle 67, 67*f*
Tube 74
   catheters 132
   confirm position of 85
   features of 83
   feeds, indications for 75
Tuberculin syringe 74
   uses 74
Tuberculosis, abdominal 192

Tyndall effect 423
Typhoid
   vaccine 510, 558
      conjugate 512, 559, 561, 563
      polysaccharide 511, 558
Typhoral vaccine 559

## U

Ulcer 47
   conjunctival 41
Ultrasonogram, sign in 255
Umbilical cord clamp 107, 108*f*
Umbilical ligament sign, lateral 257
Universal Immunization Program 485, 560
   schedule 561
Upper lobe 172
   collapse, right 173
   consolidation, right 154*f*
   herniation 240*f*
Upper quadrant sings, right 258
Ureterocele 274
Urethral valve, posterior 272, 273, 273*f*
Urinary bag 91
   complications 91
   indications 91
   precautions 91
   types 91
Urine collection bag, infant 91*f*

## V

Vaccination
   adverse events following 545
   failure 538
   scares 547
Vaccine 483-553
   adverse event reporting system 551, 553
   carriers 541
   combination of 534, 535
   controversy 553
   dose and schedule 554
   for high-risk group 515, 560
   freeze-sensitive 541
   heat-sensitive 541
   immunization schedule of 554
   inactivated 484
   incorrect preparation of 547
   light-sensitive 542

poor efficacy of 538
quadruple 536
scares 496
storage 538, 540*f*
   cold chain 538
   color code 539*f*
   refrigerator 540
   temperature monitoring 543
subunit 484
supplement on 2019 554-62
types of 488
vial monitor 543, 543*f*
Valproate 369
Valproic acid 378
Vancomycin 300, 301
Vanishing lung tumor 135
Vanishing tumor 180
Varicella vaccine 527, 528
Vegetables 20, 23
Venflon 59, 59*f*
  advantages of 60
  color code 60*f*
  sizes of 60
Ventricular hypertrophy, right 145*f*
Verapamil 344
Vero cell culture, inactivated 526
Vertebra 206*f*, 216
Vertebral bone 64
Vesicoureteral reflux 274
  bilateral 275*f*
Virosomal vaccine 558
Vitamin 30, 31, 35, 39, 449-463
  A 39, 449, 450*t*
    daily requirement of 449
    deficiency 450, 452
    forms of 451
    functions of 451
    precursors of 451
    prophylaxis program 450
    sources of 451
    stored 451

B 39
B12 453
  daily requirement of 453
  forms of 454
  functions of 453
  sources of 454
B12 deficiency 453
  causes of 454
  secondary 454
C 39
  containing foods 46
  deficiency 210
  sources of 209
D 39, 455
  daily requirement of 457
  deficiency of 456
  functions of 455
  sources of 457
  treatment of rickets with 205
E 39, 458
  clinical features of 458
  deficiency 458
  excess 459
K 39, 459
  complications of 460
  daily requirement of 459
  deficiency 461
  dependent 460
  functions of 459
  sources of 460
Volume infusion sets 93*f*
  measured 93
Volvulus 261

## W

Warfarin 376
Water 384
  bottle sign 236
Weakness 47
Weech's formula 49
Weighing machine 48, 48*f*
  precautions 49

significance 49
types of 48
Wernicke encephalopathy 47
Wernicke Korsakoff syndrome 47
Wet lung 223
  syndrome 223
Wheat 13
  nutritive values 13
Whirlpool sign 263
White metaphyseal line of Frankel 209
Whole-cell pertussis vaccine 555
Williams-Campbell syndrome 157
Wimberger's ring sign 209
Wrist 122, 203
  ossification centers in 201
  widening of 204*f*, 205
  X-ray of 204*f*

## X

Xerophthalmia 47
Xerosis 47
  conjunctival 41

## Y

Yellow fever vaccine 526, 527
Yellow nail syndrome 157
Young syndrome 157

## Z

Zidovudine 311
Zinc 8
  functions of 8
  uses of 8
Zinc deficiency
  causes of 8
  side effects 9
Zinc rich foods 8
  animal sources 8
  plant sources 8

EU GSPR Authorised Reprsentative
Logos Europe, 9 rue Nicolas Poussin
1700, La Rochelle, France
Phone: +33 (0) 6 67 93 73 78
E-mail: contact@logoseurope.eu

www.ingramcontent.com/pod-product-compliance
Ingram Content Group UK Ltd.
Pitfield, Milton Keynes, MK11 3LW, UK
UKHW050430150426
5217IPUK00019B/1318